MEDICAL RADIOLOGY

Diagnostic Imaging and Radiation Oncology

Springer
Berlin
Heidelberg
New York
Barcelona
Budapest
Hong Kong
London
Milan
Paris
Santa Clara
Singapore
Tokyo

J. F. Debatin · G. Adam (Eds.)

Interventional Magnetic Resonance Imaging

With Contributions by

G. Adam · C.J.G. Bakker · R. Bernays · T.L. Boaz · C. Boesch · R. Botnar · A. Bücker
J.F. Debatin · M. Drobnitzky · C.L. Dumoulin · J. Felblinger · C. Frahm · H.-B. Gehl
A. Glowinski · S. Göhde · R.W. Günther · M.A. Hall-Craggs · A.F. Heuck · K. Hynynen
F.A. Jolesz · G.M. Kacl · Th. Kahn · J. Kettenbach · R. Kikinis · S. Kollias · C. K. Kuhl
M. E. Ladd · G. Lenz · J.S. Lewin · M.G. Mack · G.U. Müller-Lisse · J.M. Neuerburg
R. Newman · E.A. Penner · H. H. Quick · B. J. Romanowski · J.F. Schenk
H.-J. Schwarzmaier · H.F.M. Smits · R. Speetzen · U. Spetzger · P. Steiner · J. Tacke
F. Ulrich · J.J. Van Vaals · T.J. Vogl · G.K. von Schulthess · D. Vorwerk · S. Wildermuth
G.G. Zimmermann

Series Editor's Foreword by

A.L. Baert

Forewords by

R. W. Günther and G.K. von Schulthess

With 193 Figures in 342 Separate Illustrations, 58 in Color

Springer

PD Dr. Jörg F. Debatin
Leitender Arzt, Institut für Diagnostische Radiologie
MR Zentrum
UniversitätsSpital Zürich
Rämistraße 100
CH-8091 Zürich
Switzerland

PD Dr. Gerhard Adam
Klinik für Radiologische Diagnostik
Klinikum der RWTH Aachen
Pauwelsstraße 30
D-52057 Aachen
Germany

MEDICAL RADIOLOGY · Diagnostic Imaging and Radiation Oncology

Continuation of
Handbuch der medizinischen Radiologie
Encyclopedia of Medical Radiology

ISSN 0942-5373

ISBN-13: 978-3-642-64329-3 e-ISBN-13: 978-3-642-60272-6
DOI: 10.1007/978-3-642-60272-6

Library of Congress Cataloging-in-Publication Data. Interventional magnetic resonance imaging/ J.F. Debatin, G. Adam (eds.). p. cm. -- (Medical radiology) Includes index. ISBN 3-540-62587-9 (alk. paper) 1. Interventional magnetic resonance imaging. I. Debatin, J.F. (Jörg F.), 1961- . II. Adam, Gerhard. III. Series. RD33.56.I58 1997 617'.05--dc21 97-21329 CIP

Softcover reprint of the hardcover 1st edition 1998

Cover design: de'blick, Berlin
Typesetting: Verlagsservice Teichmann, Mauer

SPIN: 10565743 21/3135 – 5 4 3 2 1 0 – Printed on acid-free paper

Foreword

One of the most amazing and spectacular developments in modern radiology has been the rapid growth and expansion of so-called interventional radiology, which can also be described as minimally invasive therapy guided by radiological imaging. Many applications of this method are now widely in use in different organs, particularly in the vascular system.

Everybody is well aware of the shortcomings and drawbacks of the radiological modalities currently used for guiding minimally invasive procedures. Ultrasound, although it has the advantage of being absolutely harmless to the patient and the operator, cannot be used for many procedures because it does not provide the precise anatomical information needed for a safe performance of these procedures. Röntgen rays provide superb anatomical insight to guide delicate manipulations inside the human body, but as operations tend to become longer and more complicated, the radiation dose for patients, as well as for operators, is becoming an increasing source of concern.

It is therefore logical that we should explore the possibilities for interventional radiological procedures provided by the latest imaging modality - magnetic resonance imaging - taking advantage of the specific physical properties of this method and the absence of ionizing radiation. It soon became evident that this new approach represents a tremendous challenge involving the development of new hardware and software, new catheters and other material that can be used in a magnetic environment, etc.

During the past few years, all over the world groups of enthusiastic investigators have started to explore unknown avenues in order to develop interventional procedures with the help of magnetic resonance imaging. A wealth of information is now emerging from different sources, and although the field is still subject to rapid change some distinct facts and strategies can already be discerned.

Two dynamic young European radiologists actively involved in interventional magnetic resonance research have now taken on the difficult task of editing a book on interventional magnetic resonance imaging. Dr. Debatin and Dr. Adam should be complimented not only on bringing together a superb group of highly qualified and internationally renowned interventional magnetic resonance investigators, but also for their outstanding performance in producing this book in such a short period of time. Less than a year only has elapsed between the first discussions on the concept of this volume and its publication; even taking into account the modern technical possibilities for book printing and production, this is a remarkable achievement.

Leuven

Albert L. Baert

Foreword

Evolution and progress in science often culminate in knowledge which may lead to new approaches in diagnosis and therapy. MR has reached that stage and is positioning itself at the cutting edge of the developments in the field of interventional radiology. Since the introduction of X-rays into clinical use over a century ago, MR has, more than any other modality, demonstrated the potential to completely change the field of medical imaging, displaying so many interesting facets that are beyond the capacity of radiography. One of the most exciting new aspects is the use of MR for percutaneous and minimally invasive interventions, where it can be employed for guidance, monitoring, and follow-up.

As with other rapidly developing imaging technologies, interventional MR has advocates who look upon it as the ultimate tool, the hypothesis being that any kind of intervention currently performed using X-ray techniques or ultrasound could, in the future, be carried under MR guidance. The most obvious advantage that MR has over X-ray techniques is that the procedures are performed without any radiation exposure. It is even expected that an ever-widening range of therapeutic possibilities may be opened up by MR as practitioners become aware of and comfortable with the application of functional imaging, thermosensitivity and other features.

Many obstacles have to be overcome on the way to the full realization of interventional MR, which presents a great challenge. Several scientific groups in the world are contributing to this goal of creating a clinical "tool for the future", a future which in some senses has already begun. The editors, who work at two European universities –in Aachen, Germany and Zürich, Switzerland – where the topic is dealt with intensively, have attempted to bring together in this book experts from Europe and the US who can demonstrate the state-of-the-art in this emerging field. We have no doubt that interventional MR is poised for a period of rapid growth during which it may well substantially and indelibly alter the perspectives of interventional radiology.

Aachen

Rolf W. Günther

Foreword

The terms interventional MRI, intraprocedural MRI and intraoperative MRI all identify a methodology where MR imaging is used to guide therapeutic rather than diagnostic procedures. When the first MR scanners were introduced in the mid-1980s nobody thought of using these systems for guidance of interventional procedures, for two main reasons: patients were not accessible inside a typical MR magnet, and MRI was so slow in image generation that guidance of real time processes was out of the question. Some pioneers started to use MRI for biopsy guidance in the late 1980s, mainly because of the excellent soft tissue contrast of the method, but the clinical success of these MR-guided biopsies was certainly not impressive enough to warrant widespread use, and the interest in interventional MRI remained minimal.

At the University of Zurich we became interested in interventional MRI in 1991, when it was decided to install a system capable of echoplanar imaging due to the simple reasoning that with the advent of real-time MRI an essential prerequisite to guide interventions was met, while we were confident that the manufacturers would eventually solve the challenge of providing more accessible MR systems. We therefore embarked on a program of producing instruments such as catheters and guidewires which can be visualized under MR guidance. When the undersigned started to show his early results during some lectures on ultrafast MRI, initially a large fraction of the audience thought that he was out of his mind, mainly because many of the potential applications could be dealt with using conventional X-ray guided techniques. However, over the past several years, the doubters have receded and the number of enthusiasts of interventional MRI has increased substantially. What are the reasons why interventional MRI may become very important ? First and foremost, MRI has excellent tissue contrast and 3D imaging capabilities without using ionizing radiation. Hence, information needed to guide an intervention may be much more substantial than that obtainable by an X-ray based technique, thus potentially allowing for many new applications. Also, the absence of ionizing radiation is an important advantage for the patient, but even more so for the interventionalist. Second, MR can be visualized actively, i.e. the computer system "knows" where, for example, the tip of a tool is positioned. Hence, interventional MRI may well become an important environment for robot surgery or "virtual reality" surgery. Finally, MRI provides not only morphological information, but also functional information on blood flow, tissue perfusion and the like. This is a potentially important advantage, for example, when performing vascular interventions under MR control.

As a result of the work of many research groups and the new strong interest of the manufacturers in the field, the future of interventional MRI in 1997 certainly looks bright and may yet turn out to be the most exciting new clinical development in MRI in the 1990s. All the potential advantages of using MRI as a tool to guide interventions enumerated above can now be considered to be within technical reach. The manufacturers have indeed met the challenge of producing MR systems in which the patient is more accessible, and a range of prototypes and products is now available. On the systems available, experience has increased to the point that one can be confident that some applications await further developments. As an example, the ideal magnet system for vascular interventions awaits construction. Hence, in some applications we cannot expect to perform clinical routine interventional MRI before the turn of the century. The editors of this text have done an excellent job in summarizing the avenues currently taken in interventional MRI and describing both techniques with immediate impact and developments whose introduction into a clinical environment will probably still take a few years.

Zürich GUSTAV K. VON SCHULTHESS

Preface

Driven by a continuous stream of technological advances, radiology has undergone tremendous change in recent decades. While all aspects of radiology have been affected by this process, the greatest strides have, in the past few years, been made in magnetic resonance imaging and interventional radiology. Progress in these areas has been facilitated by a general trend in medicine towards reduced invasiveness.

MRI has several attractive characteristics, including high contrast and spatial resolution, multiplanar imaging capabilities, inherent sensitivity to flow and, last but not least, unique sensitivity for temperature changes. These combine to permit improved detection and characterization of mass lesions throughout the body, frequently obviating the need for further investigations. Vast progress has also been made in the area of vascular imaging. Based on ultrafast, three-dimensional data acquisition strategies, entire vascular territories can be imaged noninvasively with a diagnostic quality comparable to – or in some cases superior to – that of conventional catheter angiography.

Although the original appeal of MR was founded in its noninvasiveness nature, it soon became evident that it could also be used to plan, guide and monitor minimally invasive procedures. To date, dedicated X-ray imaging techniques such as digital subtraction angiography and computed tomography are used for that purpose. Countless procedures, most of them replacing a surgical alternative, have been developed and introduced into clinical practice over the past several years. For instance, CT-guided percutaneous biopsy and drainage have almost completely replaced open surgery in various anatomic regions like the mediastinum, the lung, the upper abdomen, the retroperitoneum and the axial and peripheral skeletal system. Interventional uroradiology, percutaneous interventions of the biliary system, endovascular embolization techniques, percutaneous transluminal angioplasty and the development of endoluminal vascular prostheses (stents) are only some of the important milestones of the last two decades. Nowadays, the interventional radiologist must also become familiar with sophisticated and more aggressive procedures such as transjugular portosystemic shunts and the percutaneous placement of aortic endoprostheses.

The integration of MR and interventional radiology has culminated in the field of interventional MR. With the advent of open MR imagers and high-end, ultrafast MRI technologies, the vision of MR-based guidance, control and monitoring of minimally invasive interventions has evolved from a hypothetical concept to a practical possibility.

This book strives to provide a comprehensive overview of these developing and fascinating techniques. The opening chapters familiarize the reader with the basic principles underlying currently available hardware and software configurations, the current status of MR-compatible instruments, and the safety aspects of interventional MR. Following sections present the details of percutaneous MR-guided interventions, the principles of MR-guided interstitial therapy and preliminary clinical experience with these techniques. Finally, the book tries to take a look into the future, discussing the potential role of MRI in the operating theatre and as a guidance tool for intravascular procedures. The authors have striven to maintain a critical perspective in their analysis of the current status of clinical applications of interventional MR. Their attempt to provide a reasonable comparison with state-of-the-art interventional radiology should help the reader to realize that interventional MR is still in its infancy and that its clinical practicality and value still need to be determined.

We have enlisted experts from around the world to report upon first-hand experience in their respective areas. In recognition of the rapid technical progress characterizing this field, we have placed great emphasis on a quick turnaround to permit timely publication of this book. We would like to express our thanks to the authors for their expeditious work and for helping us both to adhere to a stringent publication deadline and maintain high quality. We are indebted to Antoinette Schumacher, Zurich, for administration and editorial support. Thanks also to Dr. David Hunter, Minneapolis, who spent many hours editing manuscripts during his stay in Aachen. Finally, we would like to acknowledge the contribution of Ursula Davis and the staff of Springer-Verlag and K. Teichmann production company.

Zürich — Jörg F. Debatin
Aachen — Gerhard Adam

Contents

MR Imager Configurations

1 Interventional MRI with an Open Low-Field System

G. LENZ and M. DROBNITZKY

CONTENTS

1.1 Introduction

The past decade has seen a dramatic change in the healthcare environment: a shift from fees for scan services to a managed care industry. As a consequence, the number of minimally invasive, interventional procedures on an outpatient basis is steadily increasing. While the interest in tissue-conserving methods with the associated low number of complications was dominant in the past, the focus today is on improving the cost-effectiveness of medical services by shorter hospitalization and faster recuperation.

Many of these interventional procedures require image-assisted methods to control the instruments or monitor the therapy. Conventional X-ray fluoroscopy, computed tomography, and ultrasound have been used for interventional diagnostic and therapeutic procedures. With the advent of open magnet technology and progress in fast imaging techniques, magnetic resonance (MR)-guided interventional procedures are being developed (JOLESZ and KIKINIS 1995; LUFKIN 1995; SCHENK et al. 1995). Besides radiation-free imaging, MRI offers unique advantages such as excellent soft tissue contrast, the ability to acquire images in any arbitrary slice orientation and, most importantly, the ability to image tissue response to thermal treatment (DEPOORTER et al. 1995; LEBIHAN et al. 1989; MATSUMOTO et al. 1994; SINHA et al. 1995).

A serious paradox is the fact that indications for MR-guided procedures at the moment exist only in areas where ultrasound or X-ray fluoroscopy are insufficient. On the other hand, investment in expensive technology cannot be justified unless a baseline number of procedures is performed. With the current lack of reimbursement for MR-guided procedures, dedicated interventional MRI systems will be limited to a few research centers being able to perform only a small number of patient studies. The ideal solution seems to be an open MR scanner that combines diagnostic and interventional imaging at the same time, hence minimizing the financial risk. This approach allows the study of the potential of interventional MRI on a worldwide basis, even if some compromises are made.

1.2 Technical Prerequisites for Interventional MRI with an Open Low-Field System

The most important prerequisite for interventional MRI is a magnet system that allows access to the patient during the procedure (LENZ and DEWEY 1995). The C-shaped magnet of the Magnetom Open unit (Siemens, Erlangen) has a vertically oriented field of 0.2 T between horizontal poles (Fig. 1.1). This design allows lateral patient access of roughly 280° circumferentially for interventional and intraoperative procedures (Fig. 1.2). In particular, claustrophobic or obese patients appreciate the patient-friendly design, but advantages exist also for pediatric imaging or imaging of emergency patients requiring ventilation. Since the system was designed as an all-purpose imager, the maximum field of view (FOV) of more than 36 cm is sufficient for all body interventions. The use of a resistive instead of a permanent magnet enables the magnet to be switched off in less than 1 s in case of an emergency or when not in use. The small magnetic fringe field at 0.2 T results in

G. LENZ, PhD, Siemens AG, Medical Engineering, MR Applications, P.O. Box 3260, D-91050 Erlangen, Germany
M. DROBNITZKY, PhD, Siemens AG, Medical Engineering, MR Applications, P.O. Box 3260, D-91050 Erlangen, Germany

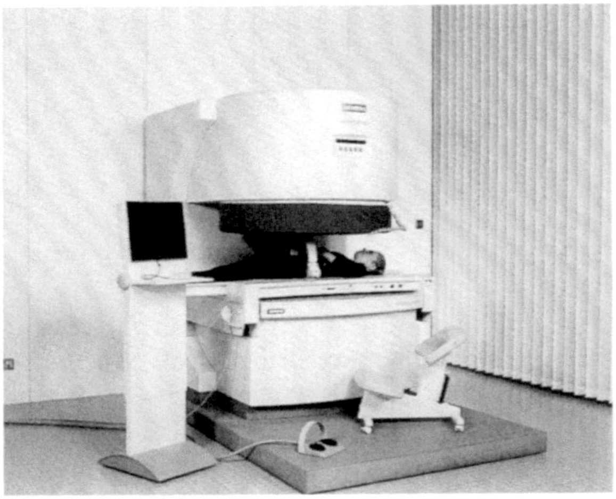

Fig. 1.1. A Magnetom Open unit with the in-room MR console (*left*) and components of the MR-guided procedure package, such as inbore light, foot switch, open body coil, sterile drape, and ergonomic knee chair

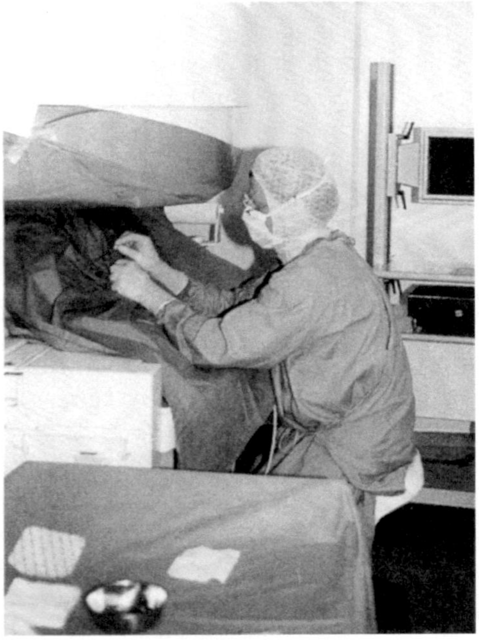

Fig. 1.2. Demonstration of patient access during an MR-guided procedure with an in-room MR console in the background

space requirements of less than 320 square feet (30 m^2) and enables convenient siting in existing radiological suites or operating rooms. More important, however, is the fact that MR-guided procedures require physician and patient to be exposed to a magnetic field for extended periods of time. Based on the American Conference of Governmental Industrial Hygienists (ACGIH) standards, this low-field system allows for up to 7 h exposure per day. That means that one person can do multiple procedures in a day, if necessary. This provides a safe environment for both the patient and the hospital staff.

Because of the vertical magnetic field alignment, very effective annular coils developed for interventional purposes can be used as receiver coils. These flexible coils are simply placed around the patient's body and covered with a sterile drape. The physician has an interventional field on either side of the coil in which all sterility requirements can be fulfilled without the receiver coil being an obstruction. From an economic point of view it is important that these coils can be reused. With a slightly tilted orientation of the annular coil relative to the long axis of the patient's body, the region of interest can be positioned in the center of the coil, providing the best signal-to-noise ratio (SNR) and the shortest possible access from the side at the same time.

MRI can be used during interventional procedures, first, to control the actual position of instruments with sequences providing a good contrast-to-noise ratio and showing small susceptibility artifacts, and second to guide instruments with real-time measurement protocols. Prerequisite for fast imaging is a powerful gradient system with a high duty cycle. The Magnetom Open features a flat, actively shielded gradient system with 15 mT/m and an ultra-short rise time of 900 μs for 15 mT/m. Due to water cooling, a maximum duty cycle of 100% becomes possible. The fastest MRI technique is in general echo planar imaging (EPI). Unfortunately, EPI is very sensitive to any local field distortion caused by interventional instruments and has so far not been successfully used for interventional MRI. At low field strength, steady-state gradient-echo sequences provide maximum SNR per unit time. Combined with rectangular FOV for improved resolution, image frame rates of less than 1 s are possible, sufficient for real-time guidance of instruments.

Passive interventional tools by themselves are not directly visible in MR, but are depicted by the local susceptibility artifact they create in the MR image. The size of the artifact and augumented width of the instrument depends among sequence parameters also on the field strength and the material (Luedecke et al. 1985; Shellock et al. 1993). At low field strength, the typical materials used today for instruments, such as stainless steel or titanium alloys, create an acceptably small artifact, while at higher field strength the artificial augmentation of the tool size increases, thus decreasing the positional accuracy (Lewin et al. 1996).

To comply with the high safety requirements of interventional procedures and to provide immediate image feedback, a local monitor is used as in X-ray fluoroscopy. It is placed close to the magnet bore. Because of the magnetic stray field, only liquid crystal display (LCD) technology is recommended. With the mobile and adjustable in-room MR console, a large LCD screen shielded from radiofrequencies (RF) can be operated inside the RF room without disturbing image acquisition. The resolution is sufficient to display up to four images simultaneously in addition to the menu bar and all control and operating windows. Using a shielded mouse the in-room MR console allows operation of the MR scanner next to the patient.

Besides the in-room MR console, fluoroscopic sequences, and accessible receiver coils, a few other components complete a commercially available MR-guided procedures package. A customized drape covers the upper pole shoe of the magnet to guarantee sterility. A specially adapted knee chair for the physician ensures an ergonomic sitting position during an interventional procedure. A fiber-optic lamp with a goose-neck extension provides a cold light source for the interventional working area. The autodisplay software ensures that all images that have already been measured and reconstructed are displayed immediately on the local monitor during the ongoing measurement. Thus, a continuous acquisition mode similar to fluoroscopy can be implemented in the Magnetom Open. It is operated by a footswitch similar to X-ray fluoroscopy. The physician performing the interventional procedure can concentrate on the patient and still operate the system interactively.

A problem encountered when performing interventional procedures under MR guidance is the proper localization of the needle insertion point. The most straightforward approach is simply to use the physician's finger interactively to match the location of the current image plane with the patient's body. Likewise, a small tube filled with contrast agent can be used. Alternatively, an MR-visible grid positioned on the patient during the acquisition of the localizer images is available for procedure planning. A more sophisticated solution is the integration of a three-dimensional (3D) tracking system to interactively control the scan plane (Silverman et al. 1995). Although active optical systems always require a free line of sight, these systems are currently most accurate and versatile. With a digitizer probe, procedure planning is made easy and the optimal insertion point and slice angulation can be determined quickly. Since the interventional instrument does not always follow a straight line, it is in practice often necessary to interactively change the position or orientation of the imaging plane to ensure that the instrument is always visible. This can be accomplished with an MR-compatible version of the optical tracking system POLARIS (Northern Digital, Waterloo Ont., Canada) where the digitizer probe serves as instrument holder. The actual position information of the instrument holder is communicated to the measurement control system of the Magnetom Open and used for the next measurement (Fig. 1.3). Since optical markers are also attached to the cover of the MR scanner at a fixed known distance from the isocenter of the magnet, the camera system can be easily repositioned between interventional procedures without the need for time-consuming calibration procedures to match the coordinate system of the imager and the tracking system. When an additional marker is placed directly on the patient or on the patient table, the optical tracking system can be used even when the patient table is pulled out of the magnet.

As interventional MRI is a fairly new field, various fundamental questions must be clarified initially, such as:

1. Which interventional procedures today controlled by other imaging methods can be replaced by MR-guided interventions, making use of the specific advantages of MRI? Apart from radiation-free imaging and the better soft-tissue contrast, the possibility of arbitrary slice orientation and 3D imaging as well as the availability of safe contrast must be considered advantageous.
2. Which interventional procedures will be made safer owing to MR guidance?
3. Which new interventional procedures can be developed using minimally invasive techniques with the potential to ultimately improve healthcare outcome?

Currently, several centers and Siemens clinical collaboration partners are performing multiple studies to demonstrate the benefits of interventional MRI, if possible accompanied by a cost advantage. Among the potential applications of interventional MRI are:

1. Diagnostic biopsy of lymph nodes and metastases in the head/neck area, the liver, and the lower pelvis (Duckwiler et al. 1989; Frahm et al. 1996; Silverman et al. 1995)
2. Drainage of cysts, abscesses, and hematomas (Gehl et al. 1996)

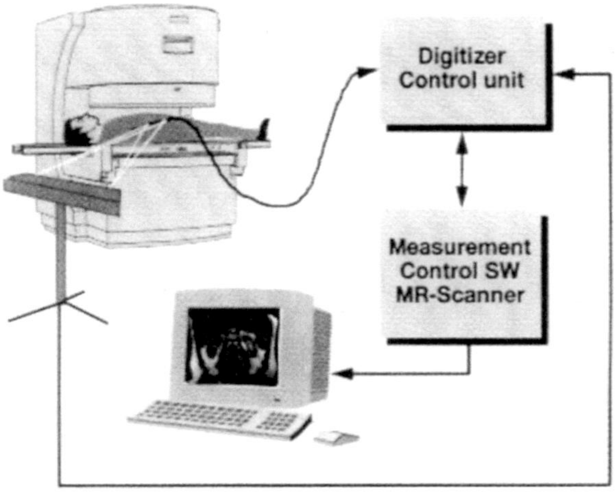

Fig. 1.3. The principle of the MR-compatible optical tracking system, Polaris, integrated into the Magnetom Open-unit

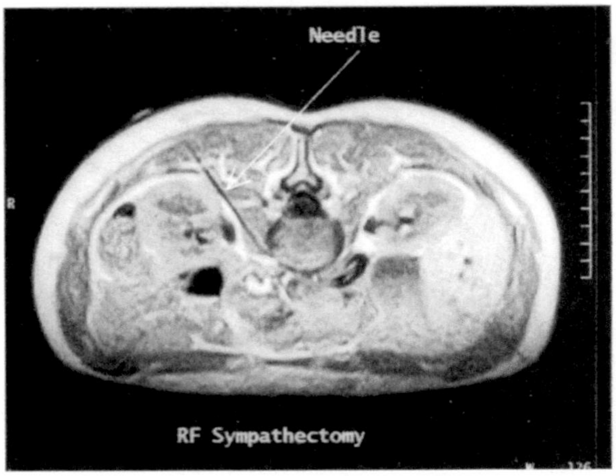

Fig. 1.4. MR-guided radiofrequency (RF) ablation of the sympathetic ganglia in the lumbar spine of a 33-year-old woman with hyperhidrosis of the lower extremities. The patient was placed in prone position and the RF probe was advanced via the posterolateral approach, with the tip at the anterolateral margins of the vertebral bodies. (Courtesy of Dr. R. Lufkin, University of California, Los Angeles)

3. Degenerative treatment of diseases with pain syndrome and nerve root treatment (Groenemeyer et al. 1995) and MR-guided sympathectomies (Fig. 1.4)
4. Interstitial laser therapy (Kahn et al. 1994; Pushek et al. 1995; Vogl et al. 1995)
5. Local tumor therapy with RF ablation (Anzai et al. 1995; Farahani et al. 1995)
6. MR-guided focused ultrasound (Cline et al. 1995, Hynynen et al. 1996)
7. MR-guided cryosurgery (Pease et al. 1995)
8. Local drug therapy and chemoablation (Bartolozzi et al. 1994; Sironi et al. 1994)
9. Vascular interventions (Wildermuth et al. 1997)

1.3 Technical Prerequisites for Intraoperative MRI with an Open Low-Field System

Apart from the development of minimally invasive approaches to therapy, MRI has particularly attracted interest in the field of neurosurgery (Huang et al. 1995; Jolesz and Shtern 1992). One reason for this is the outstanding demarcation of pathological structures in the region of the brain and the spinal cord offered by routine preoperative MRI diagnosis. Furthermore, particularly in the field of neurosurgery, complex surgical planning and intraoperative neuronavigation techniques based on 3D imaging data are already being applied today. Use of the same MR scanner for surgical planning, intraoperative therapy, monitoring, and postoperative control, and in exceptional cases for preoperative diagnosis as well, ensures a higher degree of imaging system utilization.

The main goal of using navigation systems in neurosurgery is to improve both the microsurgical precision and to minimize the amount of residual tumor tissue. The boundaries of certain invasive tumors often cannot be clearly demarcated even by microsurgery. In neuronavigation, certain position points in the operating area are therefore projected into the preoperative MR data, thus allowing the surgeon to determine the position of lesions located deeper within the operating area. The main disadvantage of all systems of this type, regardless of whether they are of mechanical, optical, acoustic, or electromagnetic design, lies in the fact that they are all based solely on preoperative image data. A discharge of cerebrospinal fluid after the cranial cap and dura have been opened and the use of brain spatulas during tumor resection will alter the cerebral morphology (see also Chap. E.6). With intraoperative MRI, these alterations of brain structures can be detected. As a result, an increase in the spatial accuracy of neuronavigation can be expected, which in turn should yield a reduction in morbidity and further improvement of surgical precision.

In two neurosurgical departments (University of Heidelberg, Germany and University of Erlangen, Germany) the Magnetom Open is installed inside the operating room. Procedures are performed under the guidance of an institutional review board (Fig. 1.5). Anesthesia and life-support systems were

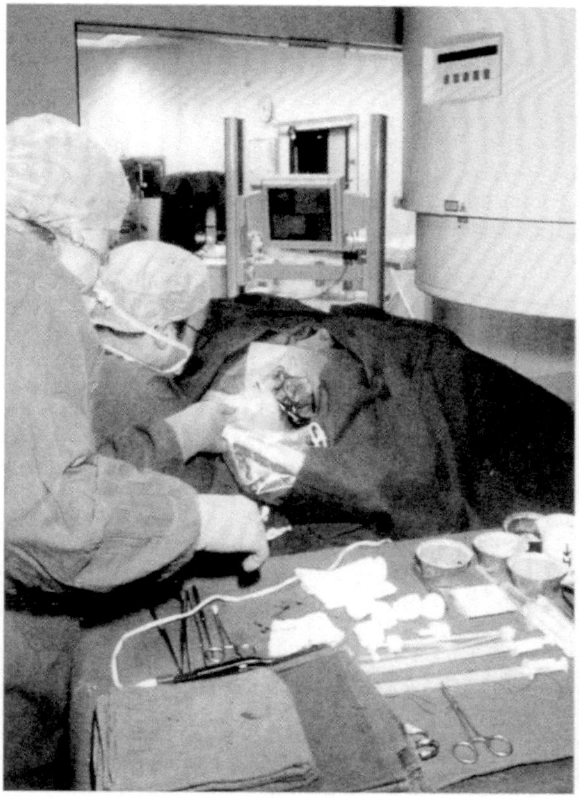

Fig. 1.5. Intraoperative installation of the Magnetom Open at the University of Heidelberg showing the adjacent operating room in the background. The actual neurosurgical procedure is performed at the patient table of the MR scanner. Intraoperative control images can be acquired during the procedure whenever necessary

carefully chosen for MR-compatibility and lack of interference with the RF system of the MR scanner. As a prerequisite for intraoperative MRI, an MR-compatible head holder is attached to the patient table. The head holder made of ceramic material with plastic screws and ceramic tips (Brandis, Weinheim, Germany, in conjunction with the German Cancer Research Institute, Heidelberg) provides a completely metal-free support that avoids any additional susceptibility artifacts. A specially designed receive head coil attached to the head holder allows unobstructed patient access. Its upper part can be easily removed and sterilized for use after craniotomy. With this setup, neurosurgical procedures can be performed under MR guidance inside the scanner, such as free-hand brain biopsies (Fig. 1.6), drainage of cysts and abscesses or catheter placement for brachytherapy.

Working with an MR-compatible surgical microscope at the far end of the table position range allows certain procedures to be performed next to the

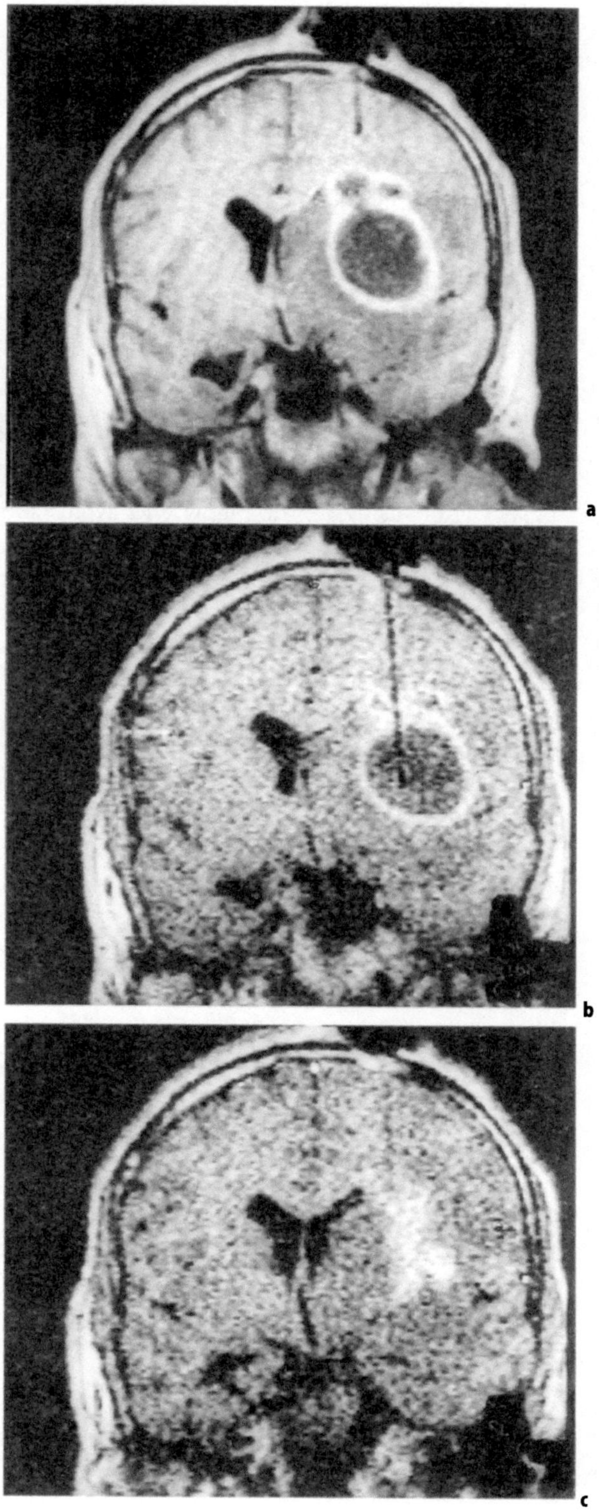

Fig. 1.6. Drainage of a brain abscess: **a** shows the contrast medium-enhanced intraoperative control image after the burr hole was set; **b** demonstrates the needle in the center of the abscess, acquired with a fast sequence protocol. The drainage of the abscess was performed under MRI control, and **c** shows the empty abscess cavity after aspiration of 20-ml of pus. (Courtesy of Dr. Tronnier, Department of Neurosurgery, University of Heidelberg)

magnet. Transsphenoidal pituitary surgery, for example, can benefit from an immediate MRI control image after surgery to guarantee no tumor is left. If necessary, surgery can be continued until completion. As MR-compatible endoscopes become commercially available, the range of intraoperative procedures is likely to grow.

In addition to the above two scenarios (Fig. 1.6), a patient transport system provides a third application. Sophisticated surgical microscopes with a built-in neuronavigation system provide stereotactic guidance to the surgeon. Since these systems are not MR compatible, the patient is moved after craniotomy to the MR scanner in the operating room (OR). A specially designed transport system ensures shock-free transportation using an air pillow and avoids the need for patient repositioning during surgery (Brandis, Weinheim, Germany, in conjunction with the German Cancer Research Institute, Heidelberg). The updated, intraoperative 3D-data set ensures the highest possible precision for the remaining stage of the surgery. The time-consuming preparation of the tumor is best done in the usual environment of the OR. If required, intraoperative control images can be repeated prior to tumor resection. The acquisition of contrast-enhanced MRI control image after tumor resection reduces the risk of residual tumor (Tronnier et al. 1997).

1.4 Conclusion

Open low-field scanners provide a viable means for interventional and intraoperative research and development. While interventional procedures such as MR-guided biopsies are already done routinely in several institutions, new approaches to therapeutic treatment such as interstitial laser therapy or local tumor therapy using RF ablation have to be the goal. These MR-guided procedures will require continuous clinical research over the next years. Initial clinical results, however, reveal the great potential of this development. The technology and instrumentation exist today to move interventional MRI beyond the feasibility stage. Clinical validation, outcome analysis, and prospective randomized clinical studies are now needed. It can be expected that dedicated MR scanners will be developed to support those procedures in an optimal fashion. Most likely no single design will satisfy all needs, but dedicated scanners for different types of procedures will probably be available in the not too distant future.

References

Anzai Y, Lufkin RB, DeSalles A, et al (1995) Preliminary experience with MR-guided thermal ablation of brain tumors. AJNR Am J Neuroradiol 16:39-48

Bartolozzi C, Lencioni R, Caramella D, et al (1994) Hepatocellular carcinoma: CT and MR features after transcatheter arterial embolization and percutaneous ethanol injection. Radiology 191:123-128

Cline HE, Hynynen K, Watkins RD, et al (1995) Focused US system for MR imaging-guided tumor ablation. Radiology 194:731-737

De Poorter J, De Wagter C, De Deene Y, et al (1995) Noninvasive MRI thermometry with the proton resonance frequency (PRF) method: in vivo results in human muscle. Magn Reson Med 33:74-81

Duckwiler G, Lufkin RB, Teresi L, et al (1989) Head and neck lesions: MR-guided aspiration biopsy. Radiology 170:519-522

Farahani K, Mischel PS, Black KL, et al (1995) Hyperacute thermal lesions: MR imaging evaluation of development in the brain. Radiology 196:517-520

Frahm C, Gehl HB, Weiss HD, et al (1996) Technik der MRT-gesteuerten Stanzbiopsie im Abdomen an einem offenen Niederfeldgerät: Durchführbarkeit und erste klinische Ergebnisse. Rofo Fortschr Geb Roentgenstr Neuen Bildgeb Verfahr 164:64-73

Gehl HB, Frahm C, Schimmelpenning H, et al (1996) Technik der MRT-gesteuerten abdominellen Drainage an einem offenen Niederfeldmagneten. Rofo Fortschr Geb Roentgenstr Neuen Bildgeb Verfahr 165:70-73

Groenemeyer DHW, Seibel RMM, Melzer A, et al (1995) Image-guided access techniques. Endosc Surg 3:69-75

Huang AY, Lufkin RB, Anzai Y, et al (1995) Interventional MRI for neurosurgery. Perspect Neurol Surg 6:44-59

Hynynen K, Freund WR, Cline HE, et al (1996) Clinical, non-invasive, MR imaging-monitored ultrasound surgery method. Radiographics 16:185

Jolesz FA, Shtern F (1992) The operating room of the future. Invest Radiol 27:326-328

Jolesz FA, Kikinis R (1995) Intraoperative imaging revolutionizes therapy. Diagn Imaging 9:62-68

Kahn T, Bettag M, Ulrich F, et al (1994) MRI-guided laser-induced interstitial thermotherapy of cerebral neoplasms. J Comput Assist Tomogr 18:519-532

LeBihan D, Delannoy J, Levin RL (1989) Temperature mapping with MR imaging of molecular diffusion: application to hyperthermia. Radiology 171:853-857

Lenz GW, Dewey C (1995) An open MRI system used for interventional procedures: current research and initial clinical results. In: Lemke HU, Inamura K, Jaffe CC, Vannier MW (eds) Computer Assisted Radiology 1995, Springer Verlag, Berlin Heidelberg, New York, pp 1180-1187

Lewin JS, Duerk JL, Jain VR, et al (1996) Needle localization in MR-guided biopsy and aspiration: effects of field strength, sequence design, and magnetic field orientation. AJR Am J Roentgenol 166:1337-1345

Luedecke KM, Roeschmann P, Tischler R (1985) Susceptibility artifacts in NMR Imaging. Magn Am J Roentgenol Reson Imaging 3:329-343

Lufkin RB (1995) Interventional MR imaging. Radiology 197:16-18

Matsumoto R, Mulkern RV, Hushek SG, et al (1994) Tissue temperature monitoring for thermal interventional therapy: comparison of T1-weighted MR-sequences. J Magn Reson Imaging 4:67-70

Pease GR, Wong STS, Roos MS, et al (1995) MR image-guided control of cryosurgery. J Magn Reson Imaging 5:753-760
Pushek T, Farahani K, Saxton RE, et al (1995) Dynamic MRI-guided interstitial laser therapy: a new technique for minimally invasive surgery. Laryngoscope 105:1245-1252
Schenck JF, Jolesz FA, Roemer PB, et al (1995) Superconducting open-configuration MR imaging system for image-guided therapy. Radiology 195:805-814
Shellock FG, Morisoli S, Kanal E (1993) MR procedures and biomedical implants, materials, and devices. Radiology 189:587-599
Silverman SG, Collick BD, Figueira MR, et al (1995) Interactive MR-guided biopsy in an open-configuration MR imaging system. Radiology 197:175-181
Sinha S, Sinha U, Mather R, et al (1995) Temperature measurements using phase-shift imaging on an open 0.2T interventional MR scanner. Radiology 197(P):423
Sironi S, De Cobelli F, Livraghi T, et al (1994) Small hepatocellular carcinoma treated with percutaneous ethanol injection: unenhanced and gadolinium-enhanced MR imaging follow-up. Radiology 192:407-412
Tronnier VM, Wirtz R, Knauth M, et al (1997) Intraoperative Diagnostic and Interventional Magnetic Resonance Imaging in Neurosurgery. Neurosurgery 40:
Vogl TJ, Mack MG, Müller P, et al (1995) Recurrent Nasopharyngeal tumors: preliminary clinical results with interventional MR imaging-controlled laser-induced thermotherapy. Radiology 196:725-733
Wildermuth S, Debatin JF, Leung DA, et al (1997) MR imaging-guided intravascular procedure: initial demonstration in a pig model. Radiology 202:578-583

2 Interventional MR with a Mid-Field Open System

E.A. Penner

CONTENTS

2.1 Introduction

Back in 1988, a group of more than 40 researchers and engineers started developing a truly innovative MR imaging system at General Electric's (GE) corporate research and development center in Schenectady, N.Y. The unit, called Signa SP, consists of a dedicated open magnet system with a cryogen-free, superconducting, 0.5-T magnet with imaging capabilities similar to a standard diagnostic scanner. In addition, the unique vertical opening of the Signa SP magnet allows the physician direct access to the patient during the procedure. Even during scanning patient access is not restricted, thus permitting true intraoperative MR imaging (iMRI).

With this system design, existing MR imaging capabilities are merged with existing therapy techniques. The combination of these technologies has the potential to deliver significant benefits to patients, while reducing costs at the same time. Current research is focussed on traditionally high-cost procedures requiring long hospital stays where the benefits of conversion to a minimally invasive procedure under MR guidance may decrease patient morbidity and mortality, and provide significant savings to the health care system as well.

E.A. Penner, PhD, GE Medical Systems Germany, Praunheimer Landstr. 50, D-60488 Frankfurt am Main, Germany

Prior to the installation of the first prototype in January 1994 at the Brigham & Women's Hospital (Boston, Mass.) several technical hurdles had to be overcome (Jolesz and Blumenfeld 1994; Schenck et al. 1995). Key developments required include:

- High-temperature superconducting magnet coils
- "Hidden" gradients, not obstructing the imaging volume
- Flexible transmit/receive coils
- New pulse sequences for fluoroscopic and temperature sensitive imaging on a 0.5-T imager
- Development and integration of guidance and tracking systems
- Integration of therapy devices, such as lasers, cryoprobes and electrocoagulation devices

In addition to the technical developments, new clinical applications have to be developed and evaluated to prove the clinical and economic advantages to the health care system. For this purpose, GE Medical Systems is collaborating with about a dozen leading medical institutions from around the world in a common research program entitled Clinical Investigators Program (CIP). The first CIP installation took place in September 1995 at the University Hospital of Zurich, Switzerland (Fig. 2.1). As of mid-1997, 11 systems will have been installed and will be fully operational.

2.2 Clinical Requirements

In this section the requirements for an ideal iMRI system are outlined from a clinician's point of view.

2.2.1 Rationale

It has been demonstrated that replacing open surgical procedures with minimally invasive therapy

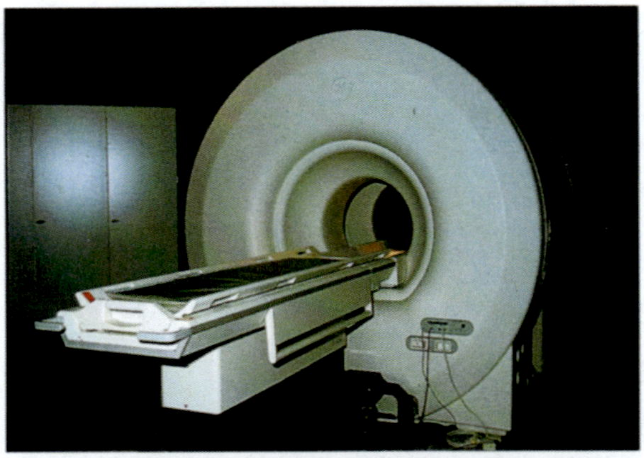

a

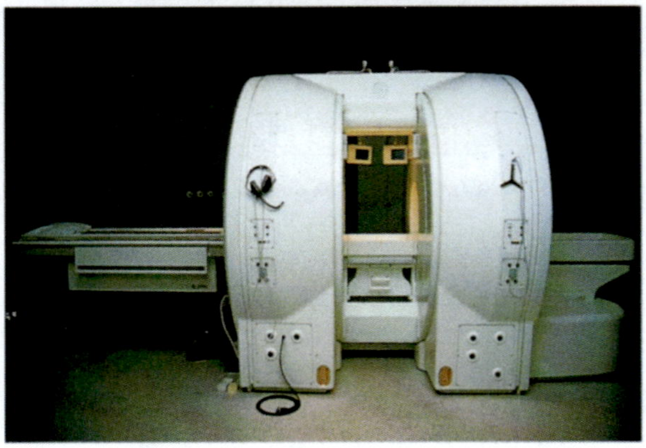

b

Fig. 2.1. Signa SP (University Hospital Zurich): **a** Front view, **b** side view

(MIT) can reduce morbidity and mortality, as well as the length of stay in the hospital, while patient outcomes are improved at the same time. Examples include laparoscopic cholecystectomy, arthroscopic knee procedures, and angioplasty procedures. Sometimes MIT procedures even enable conversion from inpatient to outpatient procedures, thereby dramatically reducing costs.

The key to maximal safety and effectiveness of most MIT procedures is pre-, peri-, and post-procedural imaging, providing data about the target region as well as surrounding structures. Expanded visualization is the key to increasing feasibility and cost effectiveness of minimally invasive procedures (Moriarty et al. 1996; Silverman 1996).

There are three major tasks an intraoperative imaging modality has to accomplish:

1. Planning
2. Guidance
3. Monitoring

Planning enables the physician to establish the optimal approach on-line, before the actual procedure starts or even during a procedure, if modifications turn out to be necessary.

Guidance provides a global view and depicts the tip of the instrument relative to the surrounding anatomy. Furthermore, an integrated guidance system should be able to calculate the projected path the instrument will take, if the instrument is advanced as planned. Hence, the guidance system will provide answers for the two most important questions during the positioning of an instrument: "Where am I?" and "Where am I going?" Monitoring is crucial when the actual therapy is being performed.

Monitoring permits assessment of the success of the therapy, limited to the intended target area and not beyond.

2.2.2 Why MRI?

MRI has several unique imaging features, which predispose it as an intraoperative imaging modality:

- Lack of ionizing radiation
- No blocking interfaces such as air or bone
- Excellent soft tissue discrimination
- High resolution imaging with high geometrical accuracy
- Multiplanar imaging capabilities
- Ability to acquire volumetric data in three-dimensional (3D) space
- Ability to measure multiple physical or functional parameters including spin density, relaxation times, diffusion, perfusion, flow, temperature, chemical shift, and others.

A comparison of MRI with other imaging modalities like X-ray, CT, and ultrasound shows that MRI is the only modality which combines real-time imaging capabilities of intuitively selected slices with temperature mapping (Table 2.1). Also, while providing excellent tissue discrimination, MRI does not expose the patient or the physician to unnecessary radiation.

2.2.3 Potential Applications

The most promising applications are:
- Replacement of high-cost, open surgery procedures by lower cost, less invasive, MR-guided interventions
- Procedures where the microscopic or endoscopic surface view is not sufficient

Table 2.1. Comparison of intraoperative imaging modalities

	X-ray	CT	Ultrasound	MR
Real-time capabilities	•	–	•	•
Intuitive selection of oblique slices	•	–	•	•
Three-dimensional imaging capabilities	–	•	–	•
Temperature-sensitive imaging	–	–	–	•
Not blocked by air or bone	•	•	–	•
No ionizing radiation	–	–	•	•

•, yes; –, no

Table 2.2. Examples of novel diagnostic procedures

Kinematic joint imaging (shoulder, spine, knee)
Dynamic weight-bearing knee study
Loaded spine
Dynamic cervical motion study, upright position
Esophagography
Female incontinence
Defecography

- Procedures where preplanning is unreliable owing intraoperative motion
- Thermal monitoring
- Novel diagnostic procedures

Examples of novel diagnostic procedures are given in Table 2.2 and of therapeutic procedures in Table 2.3; some of these procedures are described later in this book.

2.2.4 Design Requirements

From the applications outlined in Sects. 2.2.1 to 2.2.3 one may derive a list of design requirements for an iMRI scanner from the clinician's point of view:

- Unobstructed access to the patient
- Sufficient room for instruments above and around the patient
- Capability to install intraoperative tracking and guidance system(s)

Table 2.3. Examples of MR-guided procedures

Frameless stereotactic brain biopsy
Brachytherapy placement in brain
Interstitial laser therapy for tumor ablation in brain
Fenestration of cysts in brain ventricles under combined MR and endoscopic guidance
Frameless stereotactic craniotomy
Skull base surgery
Endoscopic sinus surgery
Cervical microdiskectomy
Laser disc decompression
Breast biopsy
Open breast surgery
Abdominal biopsies and drainages
Cancer staging
Angioplasty
Transjugular intrahepatic portosystemic shunt
Percutaneous tumor ablation in liver by means of laser, radiofrequency, microwave, or cryotherapy
Reduction of congenital hip displacements in newborns
Thermal surgery of the prostate, breast, liver, and kidney

- Capability to operate in fluoroscopy mode, i.e., short measurement times and excellent image quality
- MR-compatible instruments and equipment
- Installation in an operating room

2.3 System Design

Besides the clinical requirements discussed in the previous section there are some physical limitations which have to be taken into account as well. The resulting design of GE's Signa SP is described in this section.

2.3.1 Design Approaches

One of the most important parts of an iMRI system is the actual magnet, including the main coils to generate the static magnetic field, the gradient coils to provide spatial resolution, and the radiofrequency (RF) coil for transmission and reception of the MR signal. Currently available "open" magnet design approaches may be grouped into three categories:

1. A high-field, closed, short and wide bore magnet with limited patient access but excellent image quality owing to the high field strength.
2. A medium-field, vertical gap magnet providing the physician with access to the patient during scanning.
3. A low-field, horizontal gap magnet.

The systems belonging to category three might be further subdivided into:

- One-post, C-shaped magnets providing patient access from the front only (see Chapter 1)
- Two-post magnets providing patient access from the four corners
- Four-post magnets, resembling a temple, providing patient access from three sides

All of the horizontal gap magnets have potential for some interventional applications, but patient access is limited owing to the two large diameter magnet pole pieces. A common disadvantage of the horizontal gap systems is the very limited amount of space above the patient – horizontal openings typically extend only 40–45 cm including the space occupied by the patient.

Trade-offs between one-, two-, and four-post magnets are openness, weight, homogeneity, fringe field, and mechanical stability. In general, one-post magnets offer the greater, though still very limited, patient access than two- and four-post magnets. On the other hand, the four-post magnets are the lightest and most homogeneous magnets with the smallest fringe field and the highest mechanical stability. The two-post magnets are intermediate in every respect (Kaufman et al. 1996).

GE's Signa SP with its unique 58 cm vertical gap belongs into the second group. It offers the greatest patient access, combined with the highest static magnetic field of all open magnets available today.

2.3.2 Magnet Technology

When comparing other superconducting magnets with the Signa SP magnet, the most prominent difference is the absence of cryogens (Table 2.4). This is achieved by using a novel type of high-temperature superconductor, niobium-tin (Nb_3Sn), which can be operated at more than twice the temperature of conventional superconducting material (niobium-titanium, NbTi,): The new Nb_3Sn superconductor is operated at temperatures of around 10 K, instead of 4.2 K for the conventional NbTi. Therefore, it is no longer required to have a bath of liquid helium for cooling. Instead, cooling can be achieved by enclosing the main coils in a vacuum vessel and using conduction cooling to maintain the low temperatures. Major advantages of conduction cooling compared with cooling by means of liquid helium are: (1) no cryostat is required as the coils are enclosed in a vacuum vessel instead and (2) no space-occupying insulation around the outside of the vacuum vessel is required.

Because the vacuum vessel does not need to be designed like a cryostat's pressure vessel, which has to be able to take high pressure in case of a quench, it can be made much lighter. This permits a split magnet configuration with a wide vertical gap of as much as 58 cm and a bore diameter of 60 cm. The traditional single, cylindrical solenoid-type coil is replaced by a Helmholtz pair of coils installed in two separate doughnut-shaped half magnets.

Table 2.4. Comparison of conventional superconducting magnets with the Signa SP magnet

	Conventional superconducting magnet	Signa SP magnet
Type of construction	Cylinder	Two donuts
Main coil	Single solenoid	Split, Helmholtz pair
Gradient coils	Cylinder inside main coil	Split, "hidden" in donuts
Superconductor	Niobium-titanium (NbTi)	Niobium-tin (Nb_3Sn)
Cooling	Liquid helium	Conduction cooling
Insulation	Insulated cryostat	Vacuum vessel
Temperature (main coil)	4.2 K	≈10 K

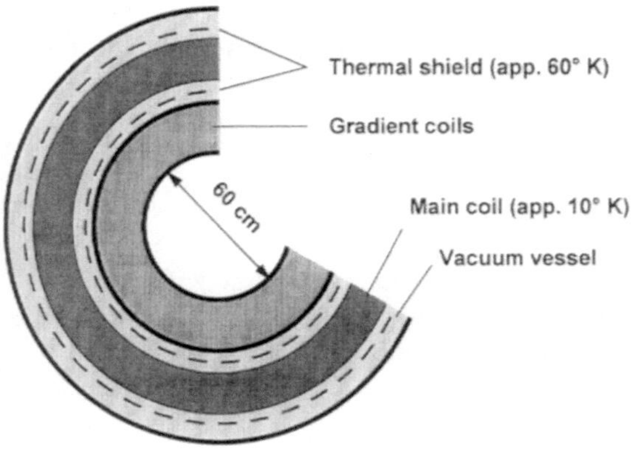

Fig. 2.2. Cross section of a "donut", showing how the main coil (generating the static magnetic field) is enclosed in the vacuum vessel

Figure 2.2 shows a cross-sectional cut through one of the "donuts". Since there is no need for insulation, the outside surface of the vacuum vessel containing the main coil is synonymous with the outside surface of the magnet at room temperature. A thermal shield is installed inside the vacuum vessel to reduce radiation heating. Next to the inner surface of the vacuum vessel are mounted the gradient coils, with an inner, non-obstructed opening 60 cm in diameter. The main coils are cooled by Gifford-McMahon cycle cryocoolers, which reduce the temperature of special structural components. The coils are cooled via thermal conduction through these structural components. The inner construction of the coils had to assure avoidance of unnecessary transmission of heat into the magnet coils. Key parts are the mounting points of the main coils and the electrical leads, which are needed during "ramp-up" and "ramp-down" of the magnet. For these leads, a special material had to be engineered, offering excellent electrical conductivity, while thermally representing an isolator at the same time. Use of a high-temperature superconducting material such as DYBCO (dysprosium-beryllium-copper-oxide), with a critical temperature exceeding 100 K, constituted an elegant solution to this problem.

Another major challenge was the production of coils using Nb_3Sn superconducting wire. Because Nb_3Sn is a brittle ceramic possessing the A15 crystallographic structure it cannot be formed into a superconducting wire in the same manner as the conventionally used NbTi alloy. NbTi magnets are wound from a composite wire in which strands of NbTi alloy filament wire are encased in a copper matrix which is subsequently drawn into a round wire. In contrast, the Signa SP magnets are wound from a very thin, flat Nb_3Sn tape wrapped in copper foil. The production of this tape is one of the key proprietary technologies developed by GE, enabling production of the Signa SP. The basic idea is to take advantage of the increased critical current density J_C, which is 40 times higher for Nb_3Sn than for NbTi (Table 2.5). Therefore, the active, superconducting area of Nb_3Sn wire can be made much smaller, thus allowing for the use of a very thin, flat structure instead of a round wire. The superconducting tape consists of a core of niobium tape, which is coated with tin and reacted to Nb_3Sn at the boundaries only. It is finally bonded to a copper foil and wound to coils afterwards.

The design and production of the gradient coils (Fig. 2.2) was another technical challenge that needed to be overcome. In conventional solenoid-type magnets it is relatively easy to control gradients in the imaging volume. In a split magnet configuration

Table 2.5. Properties of conventional niobium-titanium (NbTi) and high-temperature niobium-tin (Nb3Sn) superconducting wire

	NbTi	Nb_3Sn
Critical temperature T_C versus flux density B		
B = 0 T	≈ 9 K	≈ 18 K
B = 8 T	≈ 5 K	≈ 12 K
Critical flux density B_C	≈ 11.5 T	≈ 22 T
Critical current density J_C (B = 8 T)	≈ 500 A/cm^2	≈ 20 000 A/cm^2
Miscellaneous	Metallic alloy	Brittle ceramics
	Drawing of composite Cu-NbTi wires possible	Production of wires NOT possible

it is easy to maintain a stable and fairly linear gradient along the z axis pointing through the openings of the donuts. However, for the x and y axes it is much more difficult to attain gradients and keep the field linear. Linearity of the gradients, however, is crucial if the spatial information from the MR images is to be used for intraoperative guidance: any non-linearity might reduce spatial accuracy, giving rise to misregistrations which result in localization errors. The gradient design problems were overcome with the development of new concepts in magnetic field gradient control. The underlying idea in this case is the projection of the gradient fields into an open space (Superconductivity 1994). The current design employs water-cooled, high-performance gradients delivering 12 mT/m. Owing to the epoxy filling they are low in noise.

For best spatial accuracy a method was developed to correct for gradient non-linearity by software in 2D or 3D space. The method is based on a model of the gradient system, including its imperfections, and removes non-linearity by inverse operations. As with other magnets, the introduction of low-magnetic matter, or even the patient himself, may still create a substantial distortion of the magnetic fields adversely affecting spatial accuracy. According to the specifications, the spatial errors are less than 3 mm inside the whole imaging volume. As listed in Chap. 10, the actual errors are much lower.

The final, but not least significant hurdle to overcome was the design of flexible RF coils for transmission and reception of the MR signal. Figure 2.3 shows an example of such a coil. The coils are available in different sizes and shapes, including the butterfly design shown in Fig. 2.3, a single loop coil, or a circular coil. All of them are fully flexible and have openings to allow the physician access to the patient to perform the intervention. Sterile coil covers are available to maintain a sterile field.

2.3.3 Integration in the Operating Room Environment

Special attention has been paid to fulfilling requirements for installing the Signa SP unit in an operating room (OR). Basically, all instruments and equipment required in today's OR will be needed for intraoperative MRI. Consequently, the designers of the Signa SP integrated as much OR support as possible. This includes (see Fig. 2.4):

- Surgical table top
- Sterile coil covers and magnet drapes
- Flexible axial or transverse table entry
- Two display monitors inside the gap to display MR images, guidance information, endoscopic views, or other video sources
- Lighting of the operating field
- Video cameras to monitor and document the procedure
- Intercom for communication with the scanner technologist, the anesthesiologist, and the patient
- Ports for anesthesia gases, vacuum, and air
- Dedicated display and communication circuits for the anesthesiologist
- Ports for electrocautery, laser, and other therapy units
- Integrated tracking and guidance systems
- Interactive scan plane control

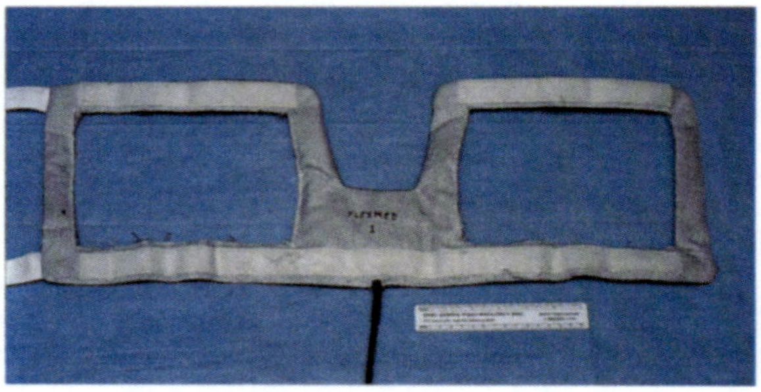

Fig. 2.3. Flexible transmit/receive coil with sterile covers and interventional openings

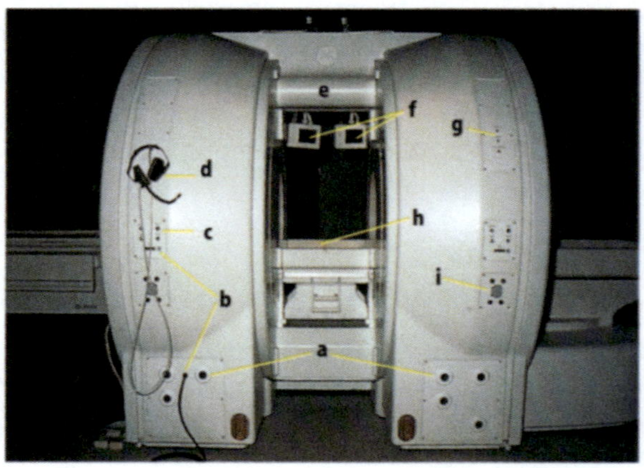

Fig. 2.4. Integrated operating room support: Ports for anesthesia gases, vacuum, and air (*a*); ports for patient monitoring (*b*); display and communication circuits for the anesthesiologist (*c*); intercom for the physician (*d*); upper magnet bridge containing a video camera to monitor and document the procedure, sensors for the integrated guidance system, and lighting for the operating field (*e*); liquid crystal display monitors (*f*); ports for the integrated guidance and tracking systems (*g*); surgical table top (*h*); ports for electrocautery, laser, and other therapy devices (*i*)

Table 2.6. Properties of Flashpoint tracking and MR tracking

	Flashpoint tracking	MR tracking
Information provided	Current location	Current location
	Projected trajectory	
Maximum tracking rate	10 positions per second	20 positions per second
Spatial error	±3 mm in a 30-cm sphere	±2 mm in a 20-cm field of view
Effect on imaging rate	None	Interleaving of imaging and tracking required
Miscellaneous	Suitable for rigid devices only	Suitable for rigid and flexible devices
	Requires specific handpieces to hold device	Requires integration of tracking coil(s) in each device
	Tracks up to four handpieces	Tracks up to four coils

Most important are the integrated tracking and guidance systems called Flashpoint tracking (Image Guided Technologies, Boulder, Colo.; SILVERMAN et al. 1995; SILVERMAN 1996; STEINER et al. 1996; MORIARTY et al. 1996) and MR tracking (DUMOULIN et al. 1993). These systems provide an intuitive, interactive means for the physician to control the scan plane in addition to localizing the tip of an instrument anywhere within the imaging volume (Table 2.6).

The Flashpoint tracking system is based on the detection of infrared light-emitting diodes (LEDs) mounted on top of an instrument holder. This system is ideal to determine the position and orientation of rigid instruments. It may be used very similar to an ultrasound probe to select the desired scan plane. Hence, it provides an intuitive means for rapid selection of oblique or double-oblique sections with respect to the instrument. For a more detailed description of the Flashpoint system please refer to Chap. 10.

MR tracking is based on the detection of a localized MR signal using one or more tiny reception coils mounted at the tip of the instrument. Particularly for flexible devices, MR tracking provides an excellent way to locate the tip or other parts of the instrument. The position of the coil might be used to define the location of the next acquired slice. Chapter 8 provides a more complete description of the features available when using MR tracking.

Both tracking systems are capable of indicating the actual position of the tracked instrument on an MR image. Because the tracking data can be acquired at a rate of up to 20 positions per second any movement of the instrument will be displayed in real time. The physician standing in the gap of the magnet may look at MR images acquired in the plane containing the instrument he is using. For convenience, both the MR image and a cursor indicating the actual position of the tip of the instrument in the image is displayed on the in-bore liquid crystal display (LCD) monitors in direct view of the physician.

2.4 Summary

As documented in this chapter, a lot of clinical considerations and technical know-how have been incorporated into the design of the Signa SP. The Signa SP is the world's first system specifically designed for intraoperative MRI (Table 2.7). Right

Table 2.7. Key features of the Signa SP

- Cryogen-free superconducting magnet with vertical gap
  - Field strength: 0.5 T
  - Homogeneity: better than ±7.5 ppm in a 30 cm sphere
  - High-temperature superconductor: Nb_3Sn
  - Operating temperature: ≈ 10 K
  - Gradients: "Hidden" in donuts, 12 mT/m
  - Bore diameter: 60 cm
  - Gap size: 58 cm wide, more than 130 cm in height
  - Weight: 8 t
- Flexible transmit/receive coils, allowing patient access through openings
- Dedicated image sequences providing real-time imaging
- Integrated tracking and guidance systems
  - Flashpoint tracking
  - MR tracking
  - Two LCD monitors inside the magnet gap
- Integrated operating room support
  - Surgical table top
  - Lighting
  - Ports for anesthesia gases, patient monitoring, intercom
  - Ports for ancillary equipment
- Flexible patient positioning
  - Mobile table with front and side docking
  - Chair for vertical patient positioning

now, we are still just at the beginning of iMRI development. The Signa SP, and iMRI in general, will eventually have the potential to revolutionize the surgical OR, and may lead to a redefinition of medical practice as we know it today.

References

Anonymous (1994) General Electric preparing to announce extraordinary new MRI system. Superconductivity News 6:1–12

Dumoulin CL, Souza SP, Darrow RD (1993) Real-time position monitoring of invasive devices using magnetic resonance. Magn Reson Med 29:411–415

Jolesz FA, Blumenfeld SM (1994) Interventional use of magnetic resonance imaging. Magn Reson Q 10:85–96

Kaufman L, Carlson J, Li A, Crooks L, Zha L, Arakawa M, Breneman B, Hsu YH, Matsutai K (1996) Open magnet for MRI. Adm Radiol 6:28–35

Moriarty TM, Kikinis R, Jolesz FA, Black PM, Alexander E (1996) Magnetic resonance imaging therapy – intraoperative MR imaging. Neurosurg Clin North Am 7:323–331

Schenck JF, Jolesz FA, Roemer PB, Cline HE, Lorensen WE, Kikinis R, Silverman SG, Hardy CJ, Barber WD, Trifon Laskaris E, Dorri B, Newman RW (1995) Superconducting open configuration MRI system for image-guided therapy. Radiology 195:805–814

Silverman SG (1996) Percutaneous abdominal biopsy: recent advances and future directions. Semin Interv Radiol 13:3–15

Silverman SG, Collick BD, Figueira MR, Khorasani R, Adams DF, Newman RW, Topulos GP, Jolesz FA (1995) Interactive MR-guided biopsy in an open-configuration MR imaging system. Radiology 197:175–181

Steiner P, Schoenenberger AW, Penner EA, Erhart P, Debatin JF, von Schulthess GK, Kacl GM (1996) Interaktive, stereotaktische Interventionen im supraleitenden, offenen 0,5-Tesla-MR-Tomographen. Fortschr Roentgenstr.

3 Interventional MR with a Hybrid High-Field System

J. J. van Vaals

CONTENTS

3.1 Introduction

Magnetic resonance (MR) imaging provides high soft tissue contrast and easy visualization of vessels at the same time. In addition, image contrast can be manipulated, depending on the sequence used. Its oblique, multiplanar, three-dimensional imaging capabilities greatly enhance accuracy and aid visualization of complex anatomy. MR can provide functional information as well and can be used for perfusion studies and qualitative and quantitative flow studies. Subsecond imaging is possible, although with low resolution.

These abilities have facilitated the growth of MR as a diagnostic imaging modality. These same advantages make it attractive for interventional applications as well. The wealth of information obtainable with MR is the driving force behind using MR as a tool to improve the clinical outcome of classic interventional procedures and possibly initiate new ones (Lufkin 1995). Consequently, it is obvious that an interventional MR scanner should not compromise unnecessarily on MR functionality.

Therefore, a 1.5-T state-of-the-art MR system with a short bore and open aperture was developed to investigate the potential value of MR for interventional procedures. Additionally, an angiography system is placed in-line with the MR scanner such that the patient can be moved on a floating table between the two systems (Fig. 3.1). This hybrid research platform facilitates evaluation of procedures combining MR imaging and X-ray fluoroscopy.

3.2 Clinical, Safety, and Economic Considerations

The clinical drive to pursue MR guidance of interventional procedures is to demonstrate clear clinical advantages over other methods. The extended anatomical and functional information available with MR may aid in directing or shortening the interventional procedure, thus improving clinical outcome or preventing a follow-up procedure. Opportunities, restrictions, requirements, and consequences for different clinical applications are discussed in Sect. 3.4 of this chapter.

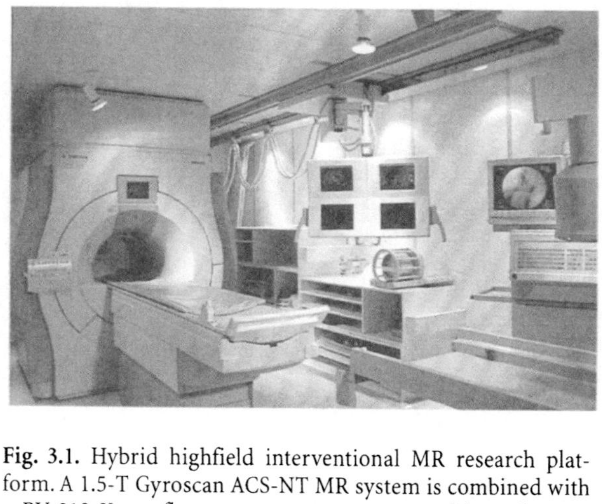

Fig. 3.1. Hybrid highfield interventional MR research platform. A 1.5-T Gyroscan ACS-NT MR system is combined with a BV-212 X-ray fluoroscopy system connected by a floating table (Philips Medical Systems, Best, The Netherlands). In-room viewing of both MR and X-ray images is possible on a set of four ceiling-suspended LCD screens

J. J. van Vaals, PhD, Philips Medical Systems, Clinical Science MR, P.O. Box 10 000, 5680 DA Best, The Netherlands

One of MRI's primary advantages is that it does not use conising radiation. Although this is not an issue in many X-ray procedures, there is growing concern with respect to situations where X-ray exposure may be excessive (Bieze 1993; Wagner et al. 1994). This is especially the case for exposure of the patient subject to increasingly complex and lengthy procedures, and in general for the occupational dose accumulated by the interventionist. Potential safety effects in the interventional MR environment, such as patient and occupational limits of static field, dB/dt, RF, and acoustic noise exposure are discussed in the chapter on safety issues (Chap. 11).

Cost has always been a stumbling block when MR has been compared to other imaging modalities. Even if MR can offer superior images, it will not be accepted if another modality can produce equally relevant clinical information at a lower cost. One area where interventional MR may prove its worth is in enhancing the efficacy of many minimally invasive procedures (Bieze 1994). By doing so, these procedures could replace more invasive surgery. By eliminating the need for general anesthesia and a hospital stay, MR could decrease the cost of therapy. One possible example may be monitoring of ablation therapy, if it can be validated that such a percutaneous procedure is efficacious and can reduce the need for more invasive surgical procedures. Another example is a selected class of otherwise more complicated biopsies, such as certain brain biopsies. If stroke patients can be diagnosed and treated successfully, the reduction in direct and subacute costs can be huge (Matchar and Duncan 1994). Cost effectiveness can be further augmented by using a standard MR system equipped with optional functionality for the interventional procedures, so that the same scanner can also be used for the routine diagnostic workload.

3.3 Hybrid High-Field System

In order to judge the value of MR for interventional procedures, an approach was chosen where the full range of MR functionality could be evaluated. Therefore, a high-field system is mandatory. This makes it possible to use without any limitations the most advanced MR features, such as fast, high-quality diffusion and perfusion imaging, functional MR, MR angiography and quantitative flow information, and real-time interactive imaging, and in general to achieve the highest image quality in terms of signal-to-noise ratio, resolution, and scan time.

The MR system is combined with a fluoroscopic angiography system to create a research platform which can be used to study the feasibility and requirements for MR guidance of procedures that cannot yet be performed completely without X-ray fluoroscopy or procedures. X-ray equipment can thus be used initially to validate the results obtained with MR guidance or is valuable as a fallback option.

Additionally, in order to evaluate the potential of focused ultrasound therapy, an MR-compatible focused ultrasound probe fully integrated into the tabletop has been developed.

3.3.1 General Description and Siting

A 1.5-T Gyroscan ACS-NT MR system is positioned in-line with a BV-212 X-ray C-arm system (both Philips Medical Systems, Best, The Netherlands) in an MR room of, typically, 5.5 by 9.5 m. Both systems are basically fully functional standard MR and X-ray systems. The combination of two X-ray-based imaging systems such as an angiography system with CT has been demonstrated before (Damascelli et al. 1992; Capasso et al. 1996). However, this is the first time that angiography has been combined with MR in the same room, thereby widely expanding imaging possibilities. Previously, such a combination was not possible due to the sensitivity of the X-ray image intensifier for even small magnetic fields. With the hybrid system, X-ray image quality is not comprised thanks to the very small fringe field of the 1.5-T MR system used.

Patient transport is possible with a floating tabletop over the complete length of the combined setup, allowing fast and smooth transport between the two modalities within seconds. When the table is at the MR or X-ray position, there is ample space between the two systems for personnel to move around freely. The patient can be repositioned in the MR system with 1-mm accuracy, even when the floating table has been moved back and forth between the MR and X-ray system. Table position is indicated on LCD displays at both ends of the magnet. When the table is not being moved, its position can be fixed by an air-pressurized brake. At the BV-212 location, the X-ray-compatible MR tabletop is mounted automatically on an AD-5 angiography table (Philips Medical Systems), allowing normal operation as in a standard angiography room. When moving the tabletop to the

MR system, the BV-212 is automatically switched off to prevent image artifacts due to possible RF interference from the electronics of the X-ray system. When the patient is moved back to the C-arm, the BV-212 again powers up automatically and is ready for imaging within seconds. At this position, because of the small fringe field, alternative imaging equipment can also be operated, such as ultrasound.

At one location, in order to facilitate minimally neurosurgical invasive procedures, the floor is lowered by about 30 cm at the back of the magnet. This makes it possible for the surgeon to work comfortably when a patient is positioned on the table. The table can be pulled out by 40 cm at the back of the magnet, so that a surgical team can approach the patient's head from all sides. Alternatively, since the distance from the end of the bore to the edge of the imaging volume at the isocenter of the magnet is less than 70 cm, and because of the flared opening of the magnet bore, which effectively further reduces this distance substantially, the brain can be easily approached from the back of the magnet even during imaging.

In case of clinical complications requiring emergency treatment, the floating table can be moved within seconds from the MR system to the AD-5 table pedestal at the BV position. At this position, the magnetic fringe field of the MR system is small enough (less than 5 G) to allow the use of non-MR-compatible instrumentation such as cardiac defibrillation equipment or any surgical instruments. Optionally, the AD-5 table is mounted on a swivel, so that the table can be rotated in order to allow even better access to the brain if needed. Alternatively, the patient table can be lowered onto an MR-compatible trolley and the patient transported out of the room completely.

In order to allow procedures normally performed in a room classified as an angiography or operating room, further modifications were required. Air supply and the electrical installation arrangements for protective earth grounding and potential equalization of the RF enclosure were adapted to comply with the general or critical care area requirements. All in-room equipment with exposed metal parts is connected to an equipotential point inside the room. No electrical ground loops are possible inside the examination room. Since both MR and X-ray are used in this room, the examination room is not only a Faraday cage but also has additional X-ray shielding in the walls, floor, ceiling, windows, and doors.

Extra filter-box and wave-guide feedthroughs in the RF enclosure of the room were installed to support passage of (laser) fibers and additional interconnections into the MR room. Several outlets were installed in the room to provide medical gases. MR-compatible anesthesia (Ohmeda) monitoring (In Vivo) and contrast injector (MedRad) equipment is used. For safety, all equipment in the room that is not fully MR-compatible is fixed or secured to the wall or floor or is limited in other ways to prevent unexpected movements due to the magnetic forces close to the magnet.

The ceiling is provided with reinforced connection points to allow installation, without corrupting the RF enclosure, of a surgical floodlight and a rail system supporting ceiling-suspended LCDs for in-room viewing of images when standing next to the MR system. Communication between the personnel inside and outside the room is possible via an intercom system. The entrance to the MR room is optionally equipped with two doors to provide a lock corridor, so that personnel can move in and out of the room without disrupting the Faraday enclosure and scanning can continue without interruption or introduction of artifacts from RF interferences. Apart from an area for the operator console and a room for technical equipment such as gradient amplifiers, additional rooms are available for patient and animal preparation and for handling of sterile devices.

Most procedures are performed with standard flexible surface coils, or the body coil. For neuro-interventions, a dedicated interventional head coil was developed. This coil consists of two circular coils on flexible arms mounted on the tabletop. All coils are wrapped in sterile drapes whenever needed. An example of an MR-compatible surgical head frame developed by Elekta (Stockholm, Sweden) and combined with interventional head coil elements is shown in Fig. 3.2.

3.3.2 The MR System

The Philips Gyroscan ACS-NT 1.5-T system is basically a standard system with commercially available state-of-the-art sequences such as EPI and GRASE. The results obtained with the interventional hybrid high-field MR system presented here are all still achieved using gradients with a slew rate of 50 mT/m per second, a rise time of 0.3 ms, and a maximum strength of 15 mT/m. Interventional systems will be equipped with a gradient system featuring a maximal strength of 23 mT/m and a rise time of 0.2 ms. The full strength and short rise time can be

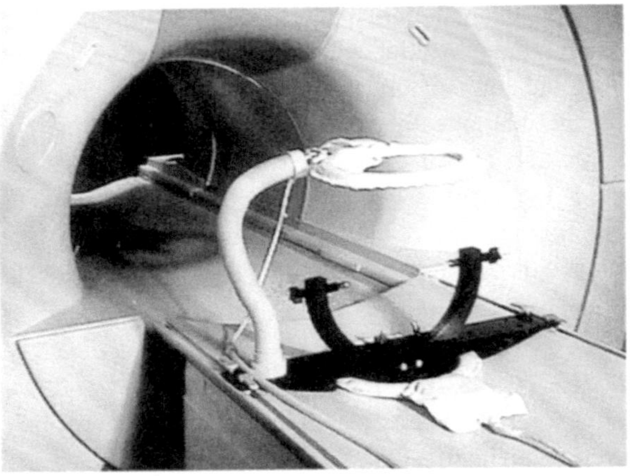

Fig. 3.2. MR-compatible surgical carbon-fiber head frame developed by Composite Manufacturing (San Clemente, Calif., USA) in collaboration with Elekta (Stockholm, Sweden) combined with interventional MR head coil elements. In this setup, one of the circular RF coil elements is placed under the frame, while the other one is mounted on a flexible arm and is freely positionable

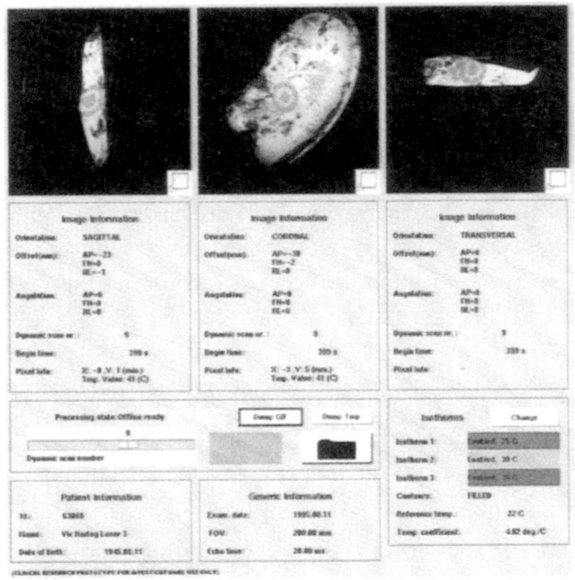

Fig. 3.3. Temperature mapping tool. Isotemperature contours are displayed over a reference image of an excised liver sample treated by laser ablation. The "background" image can be freely selected from any previous scan with the same geometrical location. Several parameters such as the reference temperature and the values of the temperatures for which the contours are calculated can be set. The temperature contours are updated on the fly during the procedure. In the present implementation, up to three slice orientations can be simultaneously monitored. Additionally, at any given moment the temperature at a point in the image indicated by the cursor is displayed

applied to any scan technique, including TSE, EPI and GRASE (see Chap. 12). There are no limitations with regard to duty cycle, (double-oblique) slice orientation, or nonstandard k-space sampling routes such as radial or spiral. Since the total length of the MR system is only 180 cm, with a bore diameter of 60 cm at the center, extending to 100 cm at the flared openings, accessibility of the patient is adequate for most procedures.

Several investigational techniques are under evaluation, such as the real-time LoLo (local look) or zoom-imaging sequence (van Vaals et al. 1994; Feinberg et al. 1985), advanced diffusion and perfusion imaging, interactive and radial scanning, catheter imaging methods, and a temperature mapping tool.

With the temperature mapping tool, isotemperature contours calculated from the 0.01 ppm per degree Celsius frequency shift of the water resonance frequency observed with gradient echo scans (Hindman 1966; Ishihara et al. 1992) are visualized "on the fly" as overlays on an anatomical reference image (Fig. 3.3). Typically, depending on the gradient echo scan used, temperature contours are updated at a rate of 2–20 s per image.

Interactive real-time imaging is implemented allowing on-the-fly manipulation of geometrical and contrast parameters. This can be done in noncontinuous or continuous mode. In noncontinuous mode, single images are acquired following a proceed command issued by the clinician, or after changing interactive parameters. Alternatively, in continuous mode, images are acquired consecutively without interruption, and modified parameters are immediately effective for the next image. In both situations the images are reconstructed and displayed immediately following acquisition. Latency is in the order of 0.1–0.5 s. Parameters can be adjusted using the keyboard, or the mouse at the operator's console, or using a remote control from within the MR room while standing next to the patient (Fig. 3.4). Images are displayed on the console as well as on a set of four MR-compatible LCD screens positioned next to the MR system. The screens are attached to a flexible arm and can be moved freely along a ceiling-mounted rail system. This makes in-room viewing during interventional procedures possible at any location, i.e., at the front as well as at the back of the magnet. During selection of interactively adjustable parameters, appropriate menus appear on the image screen to guide selection (Fig. 3.5).

At present, interactive scanning is usually performed with a fast gradient echo method (scan time per image typically 1–3 s), a zoom-imaging scan

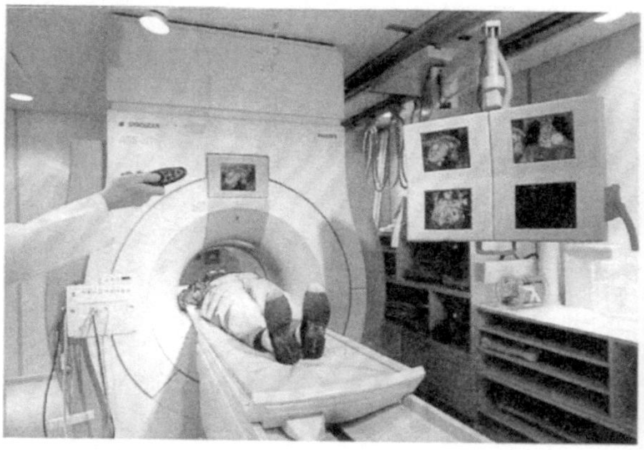

Fig. 3.4. Interactive MR imaging with on-the-fly image display on a set of four ceiling-suspended LCD screens. In the MR room, the interactive scans can be started, suspended, and stopped, and scan parameters can be adjusted on the fly during the scan using a remote control. The LCD screens can be freely positioned at both ends of the MR system

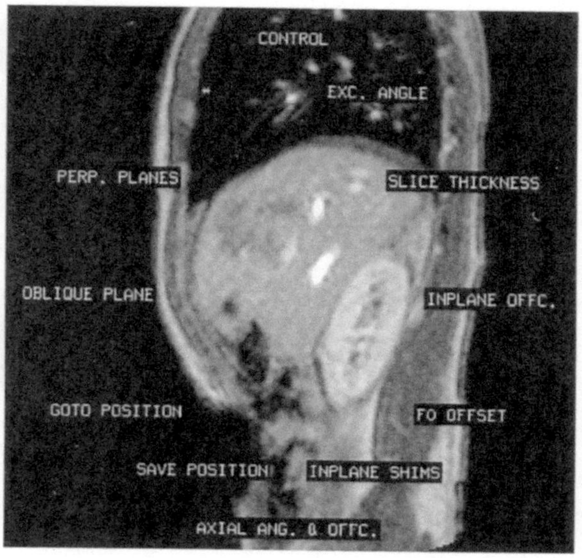

Fig. 3.5. Example of menu displayed on-screen for selection of interactive parameters. Upon selection of a particular mode, appropriate choices become available

(typically 50–500 ms per image), or the radial scan technique (Rasche et al. 1995). With radial scanning, 23 images per second are reconstructed and displayed with a 256 × 256 matrix using partially updated k-space according to the principle presented by Riederer (Riederer et al. 1988). Although the actual scan time to refresh all k-profiles is in the order of 1 s, the fast update rate mimics truly real-time imaging at fluoroscopy rate. Radial scanning can be adapted for simultaneous imaging and catheter tracking, using a catheter equipped with an RF microcoil (Rasche et al. 1997). The position of the catheter is determined and displayed in real-time as a moving point in the image. The catheter position is also fed back to the scanner to automatically adjust the slice position and follow the catheter tip on the fly.

3.3.3
The X-Ray Angiography System

The Philips BV-212 mobile X-ray C-arm has a 31-cm image intensifier and can be used for fluoroscopy, digital subtraction angiography, road mapping, and in maximal opacification mode.

To prevent any image distortions in the residual field of about 3–4 G at the working position of the BV-212, additional mu-metal screening has been applied. This allows operation of the image intensifier within the normal homogeneity specifications.

Since the total aluminum equivalent of the MR tabletop and the conventional angiography table at the BV-212 position on which it is positioned just exceeds the standard, operation of the BV-212 with the table positioned between the patient and the image intensifier is not permitted. As this setup is hardly ever needed, the consequences of this limitation for the functionality of the system are minimal.

3.3.4
The Focused Ultrasound Device

In order to investigate the feasibility of MR-guided focused ultrasound ablation, a fully MR-compatible focused ultrasound device has been developed and integrated into the MR tabletop (Fig. 3.6). The flat top of the construction stays well below the edges of the curved tabletop. The ultrasound probe is a 12-ring phased-array piezo-composite transducer with a diameter of 8.6 cm, operating 1.5 MHz with 50 W electrical power per channel. The distance between the probe and the focal point can be adjusted electronically over a range of 5–12 cm. In the plane parallel to the probe, the focal point can be moved hydraulically over a circular area of 10 cm, controlled by optical position indicators.

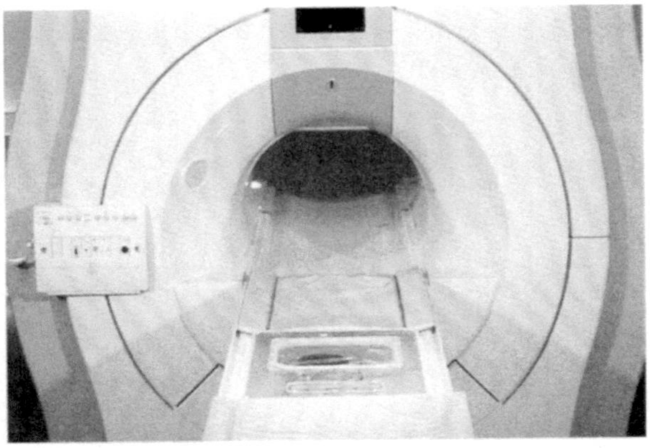

Fig. 3.6. The MR-compatible focused ultrasound device incorporated into the tabletop

3.4 Clinical Applications

3.4.1 Minimally Invasive Surgery

The most promising area of surgical intervention where MR may play a relevant role is in minimally invasive neurosurgical procedures (Jolesz 1996). MR guidance of most other surgical procedures is either not feasible with the present interventional MR systems, or there is no clinical or economical benefit expected from additional imaging during surgery (with an expensive modality complicating the working environment). Surgery where a complete surgical team needs full access to the patient during actual imaging would require a virtually "invisible" MR system. However, for neurosurgical procedures such as brain biopsies or targeted local drug delivery, limited access to the patient may be sufficient. On-line additional information from MR images, such as the actual location and boundaries of lesions, vessels, and functional areas, especially when brain deformation occurs during the procedure (e.g. due to CSF leakage), can be very helpful for the surgeon. Also the ability to perform intraoperative MR imaging and check during the surgical procedure, e.g. during a craniotomy or laminectomy, for residual tumor tissue is very useful.

With the high-field MR scanner, such information is readily available, including the possibility of obtaining functional information. To facilitate neurosurgical procedures, in the interventional MR suite at the University of Minnesota the floor has been lowered about 30 cm at the back of the magnet to create the so-called "surgical pit", allowing the surgeon to operate in a comfortable position. Additional spotlights are provided, and for image viewing the ceiling-suspended LCDs can be maneuvered to this location. Apart from the standard head coil, the interventional head coil is usually used. This coil consists of two freely positionable, flexible circular surface coil elements wrapped in sterile drapes mounted on flexible arms. Each coil element can be set up as an individual receiver coil or the two coils can be configured to act as a synergy or phased-array combination. When standing in the surgical pit, the surgeon can easily reach the magnet bore to approach the patient's head positioned in the isocentric imaging volume during imaging and simultaneously view the real-time images next to any other previously acquired images on the LCD screens. Alternatively, for unhibited access, the floating patient table can be moved up to 40 cm out of the magnet, as can be seen for the neurosurgical procedure depicted in Fig. 3.7. At this position, special nonmagnetic surgical instruments are required (Shellock and Shellock 1996). In case of an emergency or complication, the patient can be moved within seconds on the floating tabletop from the MR to the AD-5 pedestal, where the magnetic fringe field allows the use of any type of equipment, including non-MR-compatible devices. Additionally, at this position the table can be swivelled to allow even more access. An example of an MR-guided brain biopsy is shown in Fig. 3.8. Brain biopsies and craniotomies are now performed routinely on the high-field interventional MR system.

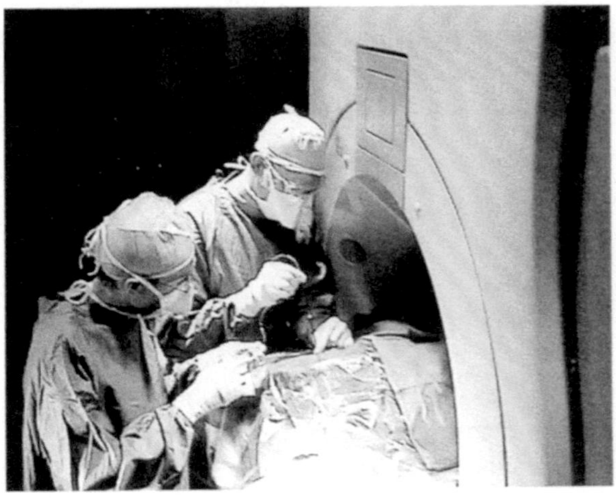

Fig. 3.7. An MR-guided brain biopsy using the MR-compatible head frame depicted in Fig. 3.2. This photo shows the surgical pit at the distal end of the magnet. The circular surface coil is centered on the burr hole and the biopsy needle is inserted into the brain. (Courtesy of C.L. Truwit and W. Hall, University of Minnesota)

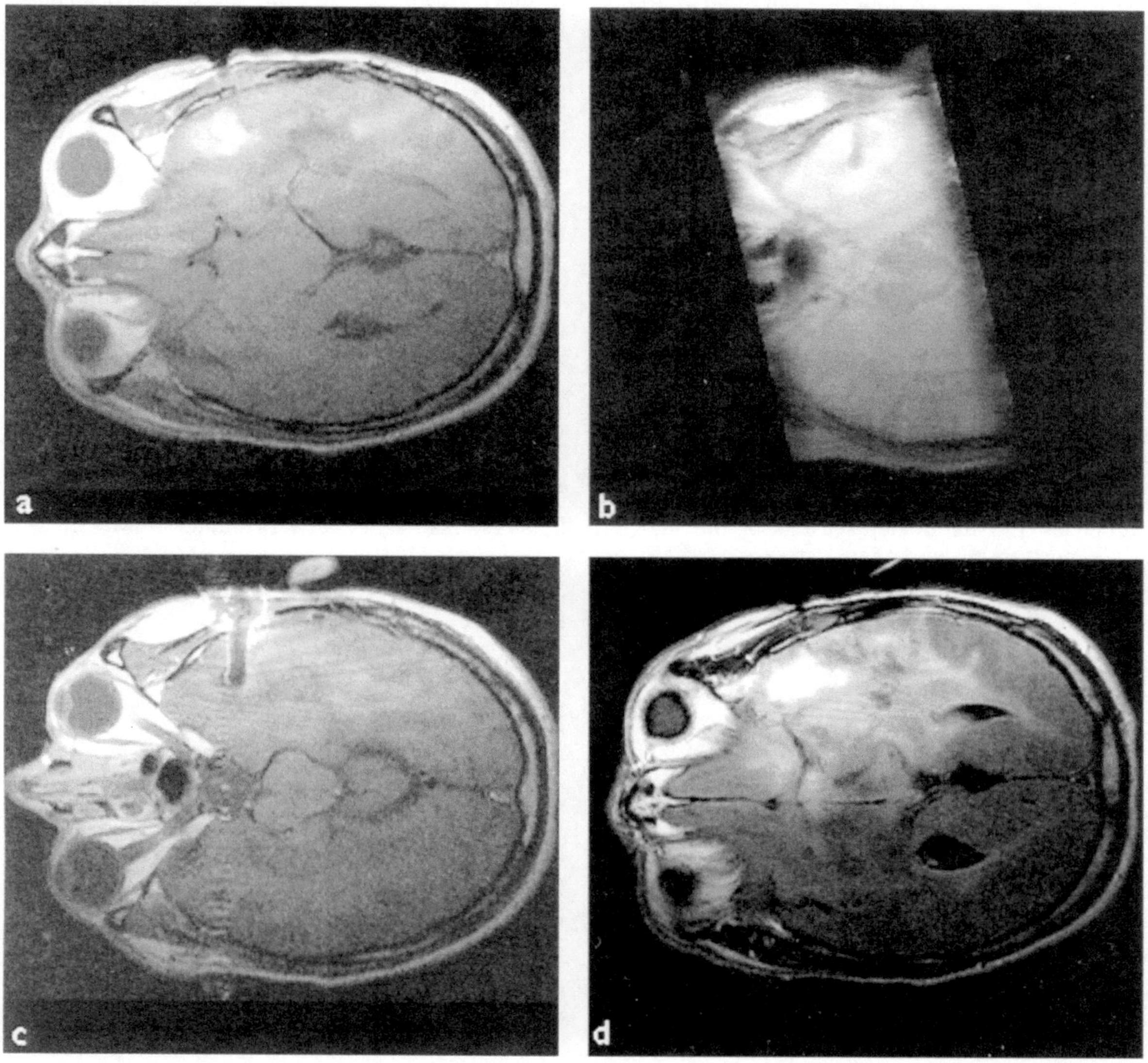

Fig. 3.8a-d. Several images of an MR-guided brain biopsy. A patient with a known oligodendroglioma was admitted to distinguish the enhancing portion of the temporal lobe lesion between recurrent tumor and radiation necrosis. The complete procedure was performed in the interventional MR system. **a** Image taken after a burr hole was created and immediately prior to biopsy. The location of the burr hole was first confirmed with a skin marker in a Gd-enhanced image. **b** Interactive MR scanning was performed during biopsy needle placement with the LoLo or zoom-imaging technique scanned at a refresh rate of 1/s to obtain T2 weighting. A flexible circular receiver coil centered on the burr hole was used during the interventional procedure. The prototype titanium biopsy needle was developed by Elekta (Stockholm, Sweden). **c** Since the enhancing part of the lesion was to be biopsied, a 1-min T1-weighted scan with the biopsy needle in place was also performed to confirm positioning. **d** Immediately after the interventional procedure, the patient was scanned with conventional MR techniques to determine whether significant hemorrhage had occurred as a result of the procedure. This turboflair image demonstrated a small hematoma at the biopsy site. (Courtesy of C.L. Truwit and W. Hall, University of Minnesota)

3.4.2 Image-Guided Biopsies

The majority of biopsies, aspirations, localizer-wire or electrode placements, and similar procedures can be performed perfectly well using ultrasound or other means of guidance. However, if the targeted tissue is difficult to distinguish from surrounding tissue using ultrasound or CT, or if passage is complicated, MR is an attractive option due to its excellent soft tissue contrast, vessel depiction, and stereotactic capabilities.

MR-guided biopsies can be applied to the brain, head and neck, breast, abdomen, pelvis, and bones (Mueller et al. 1986; Lufkin et al. 1987, 1988; Duckwiler et al. 1989; Hathout et al. 1992;

Silverman et al. 1995; Leung et al. 1995; Adam et al. 1997). Several cases are described in other chapters. For example, breast biopsies, biopsies of the abdomen and pelvis, bone biopsies and brain biopsies in a high-field MR system are currently considered clinical routine. For bone biopsies, a special MR-compatible bone drill has been developed, as described in Chapter 15. For these procedures, the patient is moved back and forth between the MR and fluoroscopic X-ray systems to guide and confirm needle placement (Fig. 3.9).

The susceptibility properties of interventional devices such as biopsy needles determine their appearance in the images. This is closely tied to the strength of the main magnetic field, the orientation relative to the main field, and the phase-encoding direction of the imaging technique, as well as to the properties and parameter settings of the imaging sequence (Lüdeke et al. 1985; Lewin et al. 1996; Ladd et al. 1996), as described in Chap. 12. Examples of biopsy needle visualization in the 1.5-T MR system using the LoLo or zoom-imaging technique are given in Chap. 12.

3.4.3 Endoscopy

MR may be used to guide flexible endoscopes, for example in the paranasal sinuses, where navigation solely by the optical endoscopic image can be very difficult (Langsaeter et al. 1997). MR guidance of such an endoscope can be achieved by technical means similar to those under development for catheter visualization. For local inspection by high-resolution MR imaging of tissue in or just beyond the wall of an endoscopically approached lumen, a small RF coil can be incorporated into the endoscope (Martin et al. 1992, 1996; Ocali and Atalar 1997). An important application may be the evaluation of plaque constitution in occluded vessels to determine the optimal treatment method.

Virtual endoscopy may become an alternative or adjunct to some fiberoptic endoscopic procedures (Rubin et al. 1996). It uses a high-quality MR or CT three-dimensional scan and advanced computers to construct a surface- or volume-rendered model of, for example, the bronchi, vessels, sinuses, or colon. The radiologist can fly through this virtual model and inspect the lumen. This may be advantageous, for example, in assessing the exact position and size of the nidus of an aneurysm or the status of a dissection (Fig. 3.10). Similarly, inspection of body cavities or organs – e.g. the heart – not accessible with an endoscope is possible, as is the use of virtual arthrography for joints. Apart from the educational benefits, this may be an easy way to rapidly inspect a large three-dimensional data set, and has clinical advantages providing a better impression of pathology.

3.4.4 Ablation Therapy

Ablation techniques are used to destroy tissue by heat (laser, RF, microwave, focused ultrasound), cold (cryogens), or chemicals (ethanol). Currently, there is no established gold standard to adequately observe and monitor ablation therapy. However, qualitative and quantitative assessment of ablation during the procedure is essential in most situations. As a consequence of, for example, tissue perfusion, heat distribution in living tissue is very dependent on individual factors. Tissue structure can greatly affect the distribution of alcohol ablation. Although ultrasound is occasionally used to monitor ablation procedures, it suffers from the requirement of an

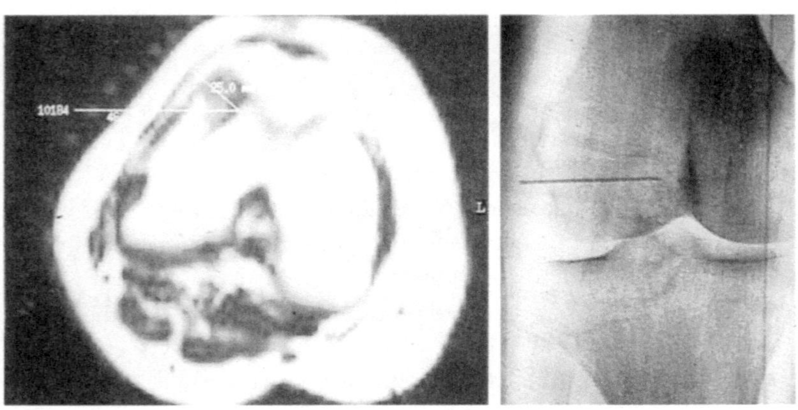

Fig. 3.9a, b. Bone biopsy. **a** The MR image is used to establish the entrance point for the biopsy. **b** The X-ray image is used to guide and confirm the needle placement in the lesion. The patient is moved between the two modalities with the floating table connecting the two systems. (Courtesy of J. Neuerburg, University of Aachen)

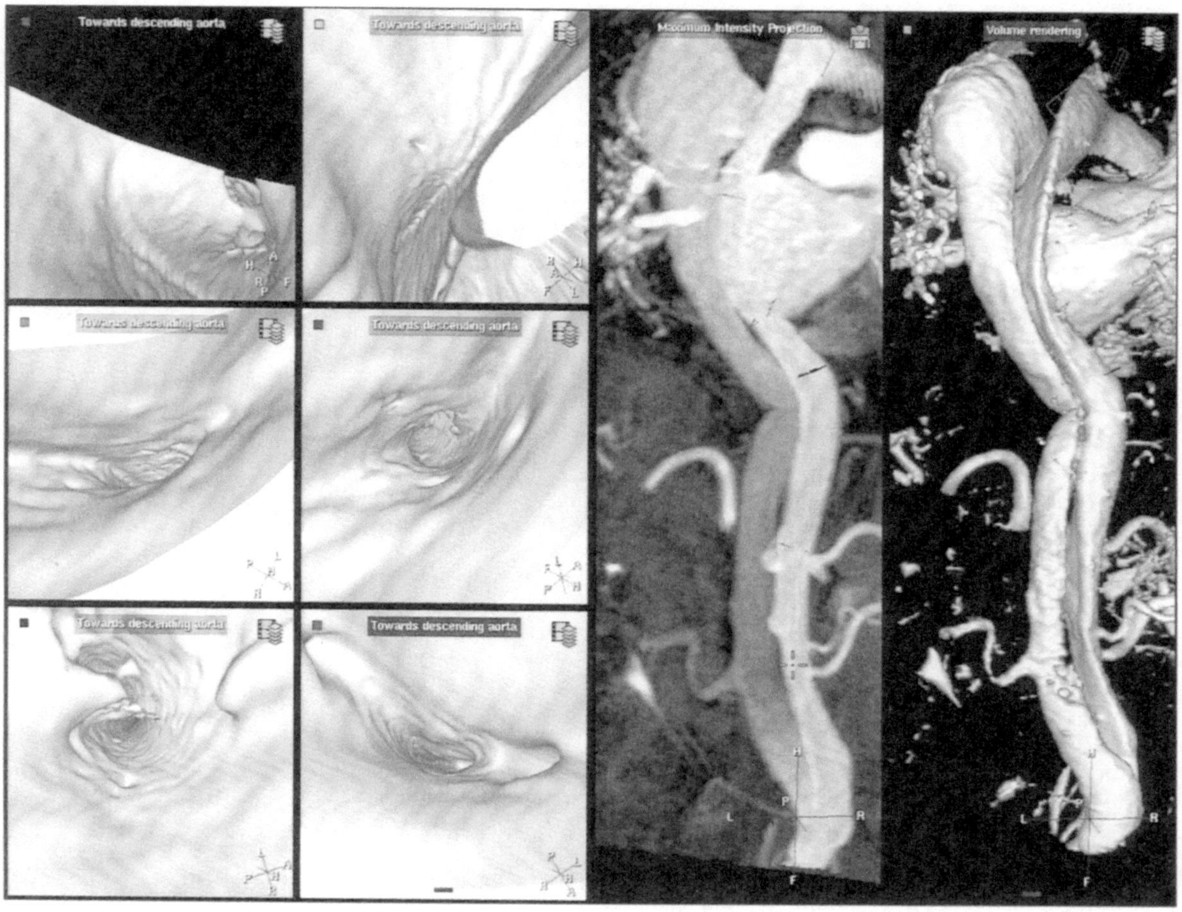

Fig. 3.10. Virtual endoscopy. The original images were acquired by contrast-enhanced MR angiography and processed on an EasyVision workstation with the EndoView package (Philips Medical Systems, Best, The Netherlands). The lumen of an abdominal aorta with dissection is shown at different locations. The viewpoints are indicated in the maximum intensity projection and the volume-rendered representations of the aorta. (Courtesy of H. Ahlström, University of Uppsala)

acoustic window. Furthermore, in cryogen ablation, ultrasound cannot look beyond the iceball, nor is heat deposition reliably and quantitatively observable with ultrasound. MR may play a very important role in monitoring any of the ablation techniques. Since these procedures do not require an open MR system, they may be applied in any MR system capable of imaging the ablation effect.

In cryoablation, any MR imaging technique will nicely show the growing iceball as a black hole, due to the lack of observable signal from the frozen, solid tissue (Rubinsky et al. 1993; Pease et al. 1995). In alcohol ablation, the distribution of the injected fluid may be followed with MR using a technique providing appropriate contrast, if necessary enhanced by mixing the ethanol with a small amount of contrast material. For laser, RF, microwave, or focused-ultrasound ablation, MR is a versatile tool to measure temperature changes during the procedure (Tanaka et al. 1981; Parker et al. 1983; Jolesz et al. 1988). This can be achieved by observing diffusion or T1-time contrast changes or by measuring proton chemical shift (Fig. 3.11).

Diffusion is very sensitive to temperature variations, with a change in the diffusion constant of 2.4% per degree Celsius but is rather insensitive in terms of signal-to-noise (LeBihan et al. 1989; Delannoy et al. 1991; Souza 1992). Since the diffusion technique detects extremely small molecular displacements, it is difficult to obtain reliable results in moving tissue.

Contrast changes are dominantly, although not exclusively, determined by the change in T1 relaxation. Unfortunately, this change is quite tissue-dependent and can vary between 0.2% and 1.2% per degree Celsius (Stollberger et al. 1992). Although this

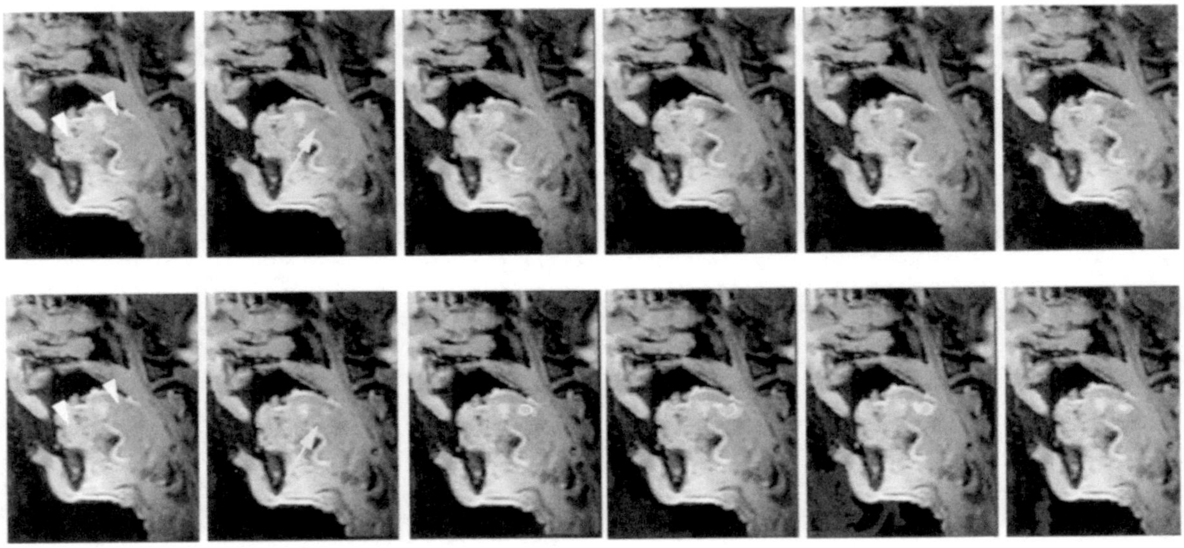

Fig. 3.11. MR-monitored laser ablation of a recurrent tongue tumor. The patient was fully anesthetized to reduce motion artifacts. The *upper row* shows a selection of the acquired T1-weighted images where the heated area appears *dark*. The lower row shows the corresponding temperature-mapping images. The laser fiber is indicated by the *arrowheads*, the ablation region by the *long arrow*. Laser ablation is started after the first image and stopped after the fourth image shown. (Courtesy of G. Adam, University of Aachen)

method is rather simple and straightforward to use with fast T1-weighted scans, caution is required when interpreting the results (Young et al. 1994). Changes in contrast are difficult to interpret quantitatively by eye. They are tissue-dependent, may be obscured by partial volume averaging induced by motion, and appear to be inaccurate at lower temperatures. However, the simplicity of use of the method where the change in contrast is used to monitor the temperature changes make it attractive for situations where an accurate assessment of the temperature and the ablation boundaries is not critical (Vogl et al. 1995).

The proton chemical shift method seems to be the potentially most accurate method (Hindman 1966; Ishihara et al. 1992, 1995; Stollberger et al. 1993; Young et al. 1994; Vitkin et al. 1997). The Larmor frequency of the spins changes by approximately -0.01 ppm/°C. This change is very small but can be measured quite accurately using gradient echo sequences. Phase images are subtracted from a baseline image and temperature contours are displayed on-line over an anatomical reference image so that therapy can be monitored. However, this method also has its limitations. Primarily, since it is based on subtraction, the method is sensitive to bulk tissue motion. Since fat has a different molecular structure than water, the temperature coefficient for fat is very small and temperature changes cannot be measured in fat. Accuracy is also affected by a slight change in the local susceptibility of the tissue at higher temperatures (de Poorter 1995; Young et al. 1996; Stollberger et al. 1997), and vessels may render additional flow-induced artifacts in the temperature maps. Nevertheless, in stationary tissue in vivo an accuracy of about 2–4 °C may be possible. The problems associated with this method in areas such as the liver where the tissue moves significantly may be overcome by employing new techniques such as echo-shifted sequences to reduce the scan time (Moonen et al. 1992; de Zwart et al. 1996). Prospective navigator-based slice-following is another technique, recently applied successfully in coronary imaging (Ehman and Felmlee 1989; Oshinski et al. 1996; McConnell et al. 1997). For critical applications where motion is absent or can be eliminated or corrected, the chemical shift method appears to be the most promising and accurate approach, providing objective and quantitative temperature maps.

Contrary to high-temperature ablation, monitoring of hyperthermia procedures requires much higher accuracy of at least 1°C, and preferably 0.1°C, since tissue heating should not exceed about 42°C. Evidently, the accuracy achievable in vivo with MR is still insufficient for these applications. Also, MR measures only the temperature change and not the absolute temperature, unless a spectroscopic approach is used (Kuroda et al. 1996). Temperature-sensitive agents may provide an alternative solution (Frenzel et al. 1996).

Focused ultrasound is different from the other techniques in that it is totally noninvasive (JOLESZ and JAKAB 1991; Cline et al. 1992; HYNYNEN et al. 1993; HILL and ter HAAR 1995). A major limitation of this procedure is obviously the requirement that the lesion targeted with focused ultrasound be accessible through a cone-shaped acoustic path. Furthermore, there should be no intermediate tissue layers with greatly varying ultrasound properties in order to maintain the focusing properties of the ultrasound beam. Another technical complication is the small focal volume, typically an ellipsoid of 1–2 by 8–10 mm, where ablation is achieved per focused ultrasound shot. In order to cover a complete lesion of 1–4 cm in diameter, many focused ultrasound shots are needed, each well targeted so that no parts of the lesion are missed. This is a daunting task, especially when aiming at lesions in moving tissue such as metastases in the liver. In order to avoid intermediate tissue heating, continuous ultrasound energy deposition for ablation cannot be performed, resulting in an extended procedure time. The noninvasive nature of this procedure makes it worth while to consider means to overcome those limitations. MR is mandatory to direct, possibly in real-time, the focal spot, to monitor and prevent excessive intermediate tissue heating, and to assess the result of the ablation in the target area. An example is given in Fig. 3.12 where focused ultrasound ablation is monitored by MR using the temperature mapping method.

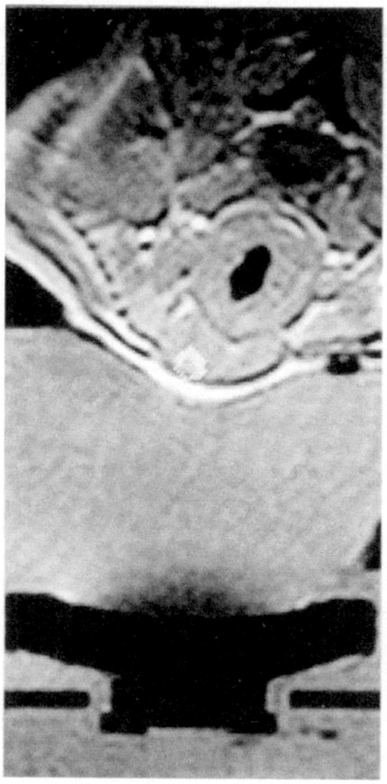

Fig. 3.12. Focused ultrasound therapy of the thyroid of a pig. The temperature increase during treatment is indicated by the colored contours. (Courtesy of A. Bücker, University of Aachen)

Recently, focused ultrasound has also been proposed for local induction of expression of the gene coding for the heat-inducible hsp70 promoter, opening up the possibility of local gene therapy under MR control (MOONEN et al. 1997).

3.4.5 Endovascular Procedures

Many endovascular interventions are performed perfectly well under X-ray guidance, without substantial radiation dose to the patient and with great ease of use and accuracy. However, there are complex procedures where the cumulative radiation dose to the patient is a risk factor (WAGNER et al. 1994). In addition, there is increased concern with respect to the occupational dose received by the interventionalist (BIEZE 1993). Therefore, dose elimination is considered relevant for some procedures. For example, some neurointerventional procedures, such as treatment of an arteriovenous malformation or aneurysm under fluoroscopy, require high radiation doses, making this an area where interventional MR can offer clear safety advantages.

Clinically, MR can contribute by showing both the vascular tree and the soft tissues in any orientation. This makes it possible to evaluate vascularization relative to a tumor and to the surrounding tissue, to monitor tissue or lesion displacement during the intervention, and to visualize the thrombosed part of an aneurysm and the surrounding lumen. MR can show the vasculature distal to a stenosis or occlusion, demonstrate reperfusion after an occlusion has been treated, and measure flow quantitatively. It may be used to monitor the effect of embolization agents or lysis and to observe the incidence of cytotoxic or vasogenic edema during the procedure.

Possible applications are highly accurate stent placement, more easily navigated angioplasty of renal arteries and other vessels, shorter procedure times for AVM and aneurysm treatment, or facilitated navigation in TIPS procedures employing the three-dimensional capabilities of MR. The most challenging and potential beneficial application is the diagnosis and treatment of ischemic stroke

(Camarate et al. 1994). With MR, stroke can be diagnosed and quantified (Bahn et al. 1996). The ultimate goal is to diagnose and contiguously treat acute stroke patients in the MR system while monitoring the effect of catheter-directed intra-arterial selective thrombolysis at the location of the occlusion (Higashida et al. 1995; Barnwell 1977). MR monitoring of vessel patency and brain tissue perfusion should indicate when treatment is sufficiently effective, while detecting any side effects as early as possible. This should increase the feasibility and safety of the procedure and would greatly expedite stroke treatment, where time is a critical factor.

A high-field system is considered imperative for clinical application of MR-guided endovascular interventions, since the ultimate in resolution, speed, and signal-to-noise ratio is desired for these procedures. This is important for obtaining anatomical and functional information not available with alternative modalities, such as diffusion parameters, tissue perfusion, flow, and the relation between vessels and lesions.

It is clear that excellent MR angiography is needed to guide endovascular interventions as well. Major improvements are already demonstrated ubiquitously using contrast-enhanced subtraction techniques (Prince et al. 1993, 1997; Kouwenhoven 1997). Furthermore, experimental blood pool contrast agents (developed, among others, by Nycomed, Schering/Berlex, Guerbet, Biomedical Frontiers, and Epix) are under investigation, and clinical trials using this approach are underway.

Catheter and guidewire manipulation can be performed with the fluoroscopy unit of the hybrid interventional MR system. Subsequently, the patient can be moved into the MR scanner on the floating tabletop without any danger of dislocation of the catheter tip, allowing early clinical investigations of the actual benefits of monitoring the interventional procedure with MR. However, the final goal is to also visualize catheter and guidewire manipulation with MR. Different techniques based on passive, active, or field-inhomogeneity effects are under development. Especially in the case of catheters, where conducting wires and small RF coils are employed, safety hazards need to be analyzed carefully before the techniques can be applied in humans. All three principles are evaluated in the hybrid interventional MR system and have been described in detail elsewhere (Köchli et al. 1994; Bakker et al. 1996, 1997; Ackerman et al. 1986; Dumoulin et al. 1993; Rasche et al. 1997; Glowinski et al. 1996, 1997). They are also discussed in this book (Chaps. 4, 5, 7–9).

Since all methods of catheter visualization have their specific advantages and disadvantages, the method of choice will most likely depend on the application, and it may even be expedient to combine different methods.

3.5 Conclusions

The clinical utility of interventional MR remains largely unexplored. However, it has already shown potential to greatly benefit both patient and physician.

The combination of MR with X-ray fluoroscopy as a research platform to investigate the requirements for interventional MR procedures is valuable in the initial phase of projects where X-ray guidance can facilitate parts of the procedure, and it is important as a check and a fallback scenario in the early phase of clinical studies. Employing a high-field MR system has the major advantage that there are no upfront compromises on MR functionality.

Both technically and clinically, interventional MR is still in its infancy. Outcome, efficacy, and economic viability still have to be proven for many potential interventional MR procedures. However, the apparent clinical, technical, and commercial benefits motivate the continued development of interventional MR.

References

Ackerman JL, Offut MC, Buxton RB, Brady TJ (1986) Rapid 3D tracking of small RF coils. In: Book of abstracts, 5th Annual Meeting of Society of Magnetic Resonance in Medicine, 19–22 Aug 1986, Montreal. Society of Magnetic Resonance in Medicine, Berkeley, p 1131

Adam G, Neuerburg J, Bücker A, et al (1997) Interventional MR: first clinical experience on a 1.5 T MR system combined with C-arm fluoroscopy. Invest Radiol 32:191-197

Bahn MM, Oser AB, Cross DT (1996) CT and MRI of stroke. J Magn Reson Imag 6:833–845

Bakker CJG, Hoogeveen RM, Weber J, van Vaals JJ, Viergever MA, Mali WPTM (1996) Visualization of dedicated catheters using fast scanning techniques with potential for MR-guided vascular interventions. Magn Reson Med 36:816–820

Bakker CJG, Hoogeveen RM, Hurtak WF, van Vaals JJ, Viergever MA, Mali WPTM (1997) MR-guided endovascular interventions: susceptibility-based catheter and near-real-time imaging technique. Radiology 202:273–276

Barnwell SL (1997) Thrombolytic therapy for acute stroke: indications, technique, and results. In: Proceedings, SCVIR

22nd Annual Scientific Meeting, Washington DC, 8–13 March, J Vasc Intervent Radiol 8 [Suppl]:28–32
Bieze J (1993) Radiation exposure risks haunt interventionalists. Diagn Imag 8:68–79
Bieze J (1994) Image guidance lowers costs, risks of surgery. Diagn Imag 4:53–61
Camarate PJ, Heros RC, Latchaw RE (1994) "Brain attack": the rationale for treating stroke as a medical emergency. Neurosurgery 34:144–158
Capasso P, Trotteur G, Flandroy P, Dondelinger RF (1996) A combined CT and angiography suite with a pivoting table. Radiology 199:561-563
Cline HE, Schenck JF, Hynynen K, Watkins RD, Souza SP, Jolesz FA (1992) MR-guided focused ultrasound surgery. J Comput Assist Tomogr 16:956–965
Damascelli B, Marchiano A, Spreafico C, et al (1992) CT and fluoroscopy: toward a dual unit. J Intervent Radiol 7:91-96
Delannoy J, Chen C, Turner R, et al (1991) Noninvasive temperature imaging using diffusion MRI. Magn Reson Med 19:333–339
de Poorter J (1995) Noninvasive MRI thermometry with the proton resonance frequency method: study of susceptibility effects. Magn Reson Med 34:359–367
de Zwart J, van Gelderen P, Kelly DJ, Moonen CTW (1996) Fast magnetic-resonance temperature imaging. J Magn Reson 112:86–90
Duckwiler G, Lufkin RB, Teresi L, et al (1989) Head and neck lesions: MR-guided aspiration biopsy. Radiology 170:519–522
Dumoulin CL, Souza SP, Darrow RD (1993) Real-time position monitoring of invasive devices using magnetic resonance. Magn Reson Med 29:411–415
Ehman RL, Felmlee JP (1989) Adaptive technique for high-definition MR imaging of moving structures. Radiology 173:255–263
Feinberg DA, Hoenninger LE, Kaufman CL, Watts JC, Arakawa M (1985) Inner volume MR imaging: technical concepts and their application. Radiology 156:743–747
Frenzel T, Roth K, Koßler S, Radüchel B, Bauer H, Platzek J, Weinmann H-J (1996) Noninvasive temperature measurement in vivo using a temperature-sensitive lanthanide complex and ^{1}H magnetic resonance spectroscopy. Magn Reson Med 35:364–369
Glowinski A, Adam G, Bücker A, Neuerburg J, van Vaals JJ, Günther RW (1996) Catheter visualization for interventional MR by actively controlled locally induced field inhomogeneities. In: Proceedings of 4th Meeting of International Society of Magnetic Resonance in Medicine, 27 April–3 May 1996, New York. Society of Magnetic Resonance in Medicine, Berkeley, p 51
Glowinski A, Adam G, Bücker A, Neuerburg J, van Vaals JJ, Günther RW (1997) Catheter visualization using locally induced, actively controlled field inhomogeneities. Magn Reson Med 38 (in press)
Hathout G, Lufkin R, Jabour B, Andrews J, Castro D (1992) MR-guided aspiration cytology in the head and neck at high field strength. J Magn Reson Imaging 2:93–94
Higashida RT, Tsai FY, Halbach VV, Barnwell SL, Dowd CF, Hieshima GB (1995) Interventional neurovascular techniques in the treatment of stroke: state-of-the-art therapy. J Intern Med 237:105–115
Hill CR, ter Haar GR (1995) High intensity focused ultrasound – potential for cancer treatment. Br J Radiol 68:1296-1301
Hindman JC (1996) Proton resonance shift of water in the gas and liquid states. J Chem Phys 44:4582–4592
Hynynen K, Darkazanli A, Unger E, Schenck JF (1993) MRI-guided noninvasive ultrasound surgery. Med Phys 20:107–115
Ishihara Y, Calderon A, Watanabe H, et al (1992) A precise and fast temperature mapping method using water proton chemical shift. In: Proceedings of 11th Meeting of Society of Magnetic Resonance in Medicine, 8–14 Aug, 1992, Berlin. Society of Magnetic Resonance in Medicine, Berkeley, p 4803
Ishihara y, Calderon A, Watanabe H, Okamoto K, Suzuki Y, Kuroda K, Suzuki Y (1995) A precise and fast temperature mapping using water proton chemical shift. Magn Reson Med 34:814–823
Jolesz FA (1996) Image-guided procedures and the operating room of the future. Radiology 201(P):23
Jolesz FA, Jakab PD (1991) Acoustic pressure wave generation within an MR imaging system: potential medical applications. J Magn Reson Imaging 1:609-613
Jolesz FA, Bleier AR, Jakab PD, Ruenzel PW, Huttl K, Jako GJ (1988) MR imaging of laser-tissue interactions. Radiology 168:249–253
Köchli VD, McKinnon GC, Hofmann E, von Schulthess GK (1994) Vascular interventions guided by ultrafast MR imaging: evaluation of different materials. Magn Reson Med 31:309–314
Kouwenhoven M (1997) Contrast-enhanced MR angiography, methods, limitations and possibilities. Acta Radiol Suppl (Stockh) 412:57-67
Kuroda K, Suzuki Y, Ishihara Y, Okamoto K, Suzuki Y (1996) Temperature mapping using water proton chemical shift obtained with 3D-MRSI: feasibility in vivo. Magn Reson Med 35:20–29
Ladd ME, Erhart P, Debatin JF, Romanowski BJ, Boesiger P, McKinnon GC (1996) Biopsy needle susceptibility artifacts. Magn Reson Med 36:646–651
Langsaeter L, Hill DLG, Keevil SF, Summers PE, Zhao J (1997) Tracking of an MR-compatible microendoscope for interventional MRI of the paranasal sinuses. In: Proceedings of 5th Meeting of International Society of Magnetic Resonance in Medicine, 14–18 April, 1997, Vancouver. Society of Magnetic Resonance in Medicine, Berkeley, p 1929
LeBihan D, Delannoy J, Levin RL (1989) Temperature mapping with MR imaging of molecular diffusion: application of hyperthermia. Radiology 171:853–857
Leung DA, Debatin JF, Wildermuth S, et al (1995) Real-time biplanar needle tracking for interventional MR imaging procedures. Radiology 197:485–488
Lewin JS, Duerk JL, Jain VR, Petersilge CA, Chao CP, Haaga JR (1996) Needle localization in MR-guided biopsy and aspiration: effects of field strength, sequence design, and magnetic field orientation. Am J Roentgenol 166:1337–1345
Lüdeke KM, Röschmann P, Tischler R (1985) Susceptibility artifacts in NMR imaging. Magn Reson Imaging 3:329-343
Lufkin RB (1995) Interventional MR imaging. Radiology 197:16–18
Lufkin R, Teresi L, Hanafee W (1987) New needle for MR-guided aspiration cytology of the head and neck. Am J Roentgenol 149:380–382
Lufkin R, Teresi L, Chiu L, Hanafee W (1988) A technique for MR-guided needle placement. Am J Roentgenol 151:193–196
Martin AJ, Plewes DB, Henkelman RM (1992) MR imaging of blood vessels with an intravascular coil. J Magn Reson Imaging 2:421–429
Martin AJ, McLoughlin RF, Barberi EA, Rutt BK (1996) An expandable intravenous RF coil for imaging the artery wall. In: Proceedings of 4th Meeting of International Society of Magnetic Resonance in Medicine, 27 April–3

May, 1996, New York. Society of Magnetic Resonance in Medicine, Berkeley, p 402
Matchar DB, Duncan PW (1994) Cost of stroke. In: Grotta JC (ed) Stroke: clinical updates, vol 5(3). National Stroke Association, Englewood, Colo, pp 9–12
McConnell MV, Khasgiwala VC, Savord BJ, Chen MH, Chuang ML, Edelman RR, Manning WJ (1997) Prospective adaptive navigator correction for breath-hold MR coronary angiography. Magn Reson Med 37:148–152
Moonen CTW, Liu G, van Gelderen P, Sobering G (1992) A fast gradient-recalled MRI technique with increased sensitivity to dynamic susceptibility effects. Magn Reson Med 26:184–189
Moonen CTW, Madio D, Olsen A, DesPres D, van Gelderen P, Fawcett T, Holbrook N (1997) On the feasibility of MRI guided focused ultrasound for local induction of gene expression. In: Proceedings of 5th Meeting of International Society of Magnetic Resonance in Medicine, 14–18 April 1997, Vancouver. Society of Magnetic Resonance in Medicine, Berkeley, p 526
Mueller PR, Stark DD, Simeone JF, et al (1986) MR-guided aspiration biopsy: needle design and clinical trials. Radiology 161:605–609
Ocali O, Atalar E (1997) Intravascular magnetic resonance imaging using a loopless catheter antenna. Magn Reson Med 37:112-118
Oshinski JN, Hofland L, Mukundan S Jr, Dixon WT, Parks WJ, Pettigrew RI (1996) Two-dimensional coronary MR angiography without breath holding. Radiology 201:737–743
Parker DL, Smith V, Sheldon P, Crooks LE, Fussel L (1983) Temperature distribution measurements in two-dimensional NMR imaging. Med Phys 10:321-325
Pease GR, Wong STS, Roos MS, Rubinsky B (1995) MR image-guided control of cryosurgery. J Magn Reson Med 5:753–760
Prince MR, Yucel EK, Kaufman JA, Harrison D, Geller SC (1993) Dynamic gadolinium-enhanced three-dimensional abdominal MR arteriography. J Magn Reson Imaging 3:877-881
Prince MR, Grist TM, Debatin JF (1997) 3D contrast MR angiography. Springer, Berlin Heidelberg New York
Rasche V, de Boer RW, Holz D, Proksa R (1995) Continuous radial data acquisition for dynamic MRI. Magn Reson Med 34:754–761
Rasche V, Holz D, Köhler J, Proksa R, Röschmann P (1997) Catheter tracking using continuous radial MRI. Magn Reson Med 37:963-968
Riederer SJ, Tasciyan T, Farzaneh F, et al (1988) MR fluoroscopy: technical feasibility. Magn Reson Imaging 8:1–15
Rubin GD, Beaulieu CF, Argiro V, et al (1996) Perspective volume rendering of CT and MR images: applications for endoscopic imaging. Radiology 199:321–330
Rubinsky B, Gilbert JC, Onik GM, Roos MS, Wong STS, Brennan KM (1993) Monitoring cryosurgery in the brain and in the prostate with proton NMR. Cryobiology 30:191-199
Shellock FG, Shellock VJ (1996) Ceramic surgical instruments: ex vivo evaluation of compatibility with MR imaging at 1.5 T. J Magn Reson Imaging 6:954–956
Silverman SG, Collick BD, Figueira MR, et al (1995) Interactive MR-guided biopsy in an open-configuration MR imaging system. Radiology 197:175–181
Souza SP (1992) Uncertainties in temperature mapping via diffusion imaging. In: Proceedings of 11th Meeting of Society of Magnetic Resonance in Medicine, 8–14 August, 1992, Berlin. Society of Magnetic Resonance in Medicine, Berkeley, p 1214
Stollberger R, Ebner F, Fan M, Ascher PW (1992) Temperaturmapping mittels MR-imaging am Beispiel der Laserkoagulation von Gehirngewebe. Biomed Tech (Berlin) 57:209–211
Stollberger R, Fan M, Ebner F, Ascher PW, Kleinert R (1993) Monitoring of temperature changes in heterogeneous tissues for the monitoring of hyperthermia. In: Proceedings of 12th Meeting of Society of Magnetic Resonance in Medicine, 14–20 August, 1993, New York. Society of Magnetic Resonance in Medicine, Berkeley, p 156
Stollberger R, Huber D, Renhard W, Glanzer H (1997) Influence of the temperature dependent susceptibility on monitoring of interstitial tissue coagulation using the proton resonance frequency method. In: Proceedings of 5th Meeting of International Society of Magnetic Resonance in Medicine, 14–18 April, 1997, Vancouver. Society of Magnetic Resonance in Medicine, Berkeley, p 1963
Tanaka H, Eno K, Kato H, Ishida T (1981) Possible application of noninvasive thermometry for hyperthermia using NMR. Nippon Acta Radiol 41:897–899
van Vaals JJ, van Yperen GH, Hoogenboom TLM, Duijvestijn MJ (1994) Local Look (LoLo): zoom-fluoroscopy of a moving target. In: Proceedings of 1st Meeting of Society of Magnetic Resonance, 5–9 March 1994, Dallas. J Magn Reson Imaging 4(P):38
Vitkin IA, Moriarty JA, Peters RD, et al (1997) Magnetic resonance imaging of temperature changes during interstitial microwave heating: a phantom study. Med Phys 24:269–277
Vogl TJ, Müller PK, Hammerstingl R, et al (1995) Malignant liver tumors treated with MR imaging-guided laser-induced thermotherapy: technique and prospective results. Radiology 196:257-265
Wagner LK, Eifel PJ, Geise RA (1994) Potential biological effects following high X-ray dose interventional procedures. J Vasc Interv Radiol 5:71-84
Young IR, Hand JW, Oatridge A, Prior MV (1994) Modeling and observation of temperature changes in vivo using MRI. Magn Reson Med 32:358-369
Young IR, Hajnal JV, Roberts IG, Ling JX, Hill-Cottingham RJ, Oatridge A, Wilson JA (1996) An evaluation of the effects of susceptibility changes on the water chemical shift method of temperature measurements in human peripheral muscle. Magn Reson Med 36:366-374

Instrument Visualization in the MR Environment

4 Principles of Passive Visualization

M.E. Ladd

CONTENTS

4.1 Introduction

Prerequisite to the safe execution of an interventional procedure is the ability to accurately visualize any instruments in relation to the MR image. These interventions might involve a percutaneous route, such as a biopsy, or endovascular or endoluminal access. In contrast to X-ray, visualization of interventional instruments in MR has proven to be difficult. Excellent contrast between the instrument and surrounding tissue can be obtained in X-ray through the use of high-atomic number metals such as gold or tungsten. These materials provide large attenuation of incident X-rays, rendering the instrument visible with high resolution.

Ideally, techniques used to render instruments visible in MR would be characterized by high spatial and temporal resolution, and provide a high-contrast signal, making it easy to pick out the instrument in the MR image.

M.E. Ladd, MSEE, MRI Center, Department of Medical Radiology, University Hospital Zurich, Rämistraße 100, CH-8091 Zurich, Switzerland

4.2 What Is 'Passive' Visualization?

Passive visualization of instruments is any technique which makes an instrument visible as part of the normal imaging process. The instrument under consideration is seen in the image, without requiring any additional hardware or post-processing. Passive visualization is used in X-ray fluoroscopy, where the high attenuation of interventional instruments renders them easily visible on a normal image.

In MR, techniques for making an instrument passively visible can be grouped into three categories. The first group relies on displacement of water by the instrument itself to create a signal void. The second group, the most commonly used, exploits the artifact created by magnetic susceptibility differences between various materials and human tissue. The third strives to create positive contrast by using contrast agents to enhance the signal from the device.

4.3 Signal Voids

The MR signal is generated by hydrogen protons in the human body, most of which are bound in water molecules. Conventional MR imagers are only sensitive to fluids. Molecules in the solid state have transverse magnetization coherence times too short to be detected (Callaghan 1991). This explains MR's excellent soft-tissue contrast, but poor presentation of the bony cortex.

An interventional device composed of solid materials will displace a certain amount of tissue, blood, or other signal source as it is inserted through the body. The contrast between the signal void of the device and the signal of the surrounding tissue will allow the device to be seen in the MR image. Visibility of the device is determined solely by the image resolution. Low in-plane resolution or thick sections will reduce the contrast due to partial voluming of the instrument and the local surroundings.

If the materials of the device have magnetic susceptibilities which are different from human tissue, an additional artifact will be created around the instrument, as described in Sect. 4.4.

Unfortunately, MR is known for its rather poor temporal resolution. The MR image must be rapidly updated as the instrument is inserted, preferably at least once per second. High imaging speeds are traditionally obtained by sacrificing in-plane image resolution, which leads to even poorer contrast. Also, a thick image section is often desirable, since if the plane of the device is unknown, which is the case for flexible instruments such as catheters and vascular guidewires, a thick section ensures that the device falls within the imaging plane. Otherwise, multiple contiguous images must be acquired, leading to an increase in total image acquisition time (for short-TR pulse sequences).

Thus, instrument visualization based on signal voids will work well only with large diameter instruments. Thin devices are poorly visualized, reflecting limited in-plane and through-plane image resolution. Fig. 4.1 displays a 5-F catheter, showing the much poorer visualization due to partial voluming.

Signal voids also fail in procedures such as laparoscopy or lung biopsies, where the interventional device is passed through air-filled cavities of the body. No signal-producing tissue is available around the device to provide the necessary contrast.

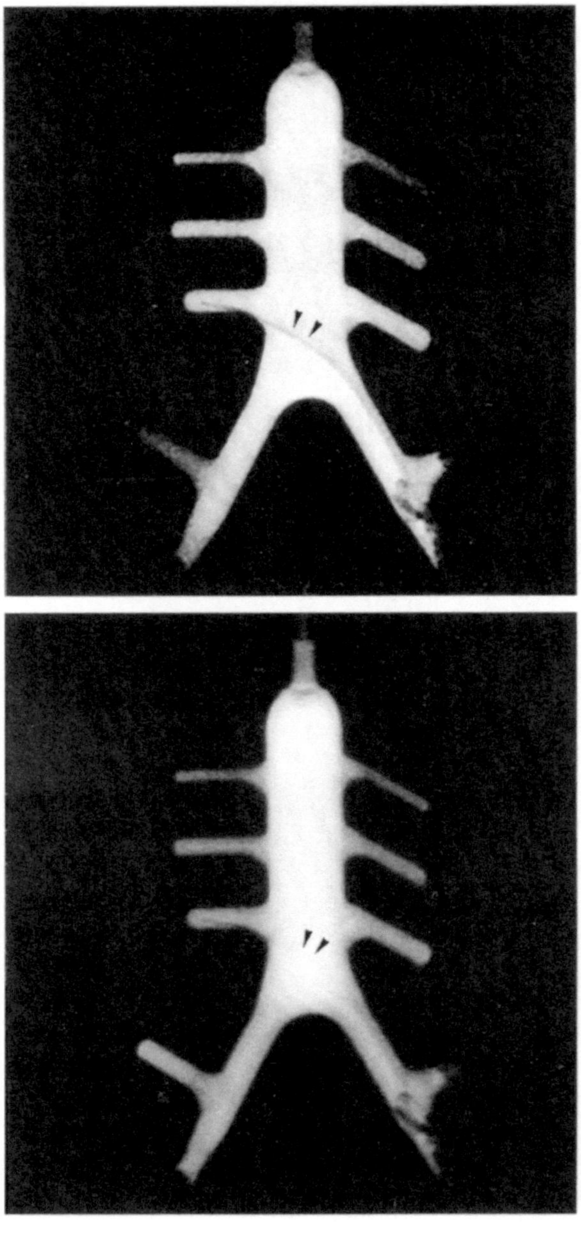

a

b

Fig. 4.1a, b. Signal-void based imaging. A 5-F catheter (*arrows*) imaged using a spoiled gradient-echo sequence with a TR400/TE 5.7 ms, NEX 2, FOV 20 cm, matrix 256 × 256, section thickness 7 mm and b matrix 256 × 128, section thickness 20 mm. The catheter is more difficult to detect with decreasing resolution owing to partial voluming. Note, in addition, that the imaging times (208 and 106 s, respectively) are unrealistic for interactive interventional guidance

4.4 Susceptibility Artifacts

Some of the most common artifacts encountered in MRI are based on magnetic susceptibility differences. Differences in magnetic susceptibility cause local inhomogeneities in the static magnetic field, B_0. These inhomogeneities in turn lead to geometric distortion and intra-voxel dephasing. The human body is filled with areas of non-uniform magnetic susceptibility, the most obvious of which can be found at tissue/air boundaries in the paranasal sinuses, the lungs, or the bowel.

4.4.1 Magnetic Properties of Materials

In a magnetic field intensity H, the magnetic flux density B is given by (Marshall and Skitek 1987)

$$B = \mu H \tag{4.1}$$

where μ is a constant of the medium called permeability. B can be also expressed as

$$B = \mu_r \mu_0 H \tag{4.2}$$

where μ_0 is the permeability of free space and μ_r is the relative permeability. For free space, $\mu_r = 1$.

Most materials can be classified into three types based upon their relative magnetic permeabilities and magnetic properties (MARSHALL and SKITEK 1987). The first group of materials, referred to as "diamagnetic", is characterized by $\mu_r < 1$. These materials are weakly repulsed when placed in a magnetic field. This effect is derived from orbital changes of the electrons.

The second group are "paramagnetic" and have $\mu_r > 1$. These materials have a net magnetic dipole moment at the atomic or molecular level. The dipoles tend to align with an external magnetic field, overwhelming the opposing effect of the electron orbits. These materials are thus attracted to magnets, albeit weakly.

The final group, referred to as "ferromagnetic", are characterized by $\mu_r >> 1$. These materials not only have a net magnetic dipole moment like the paramagnetics, but it is energetically favorable for the microscopic dipoles to align with their neighbors. When placed in a strong magnetic field, magnetic domains are formed, where the constituent dipoles are aligned in a common direction. Domains that are aligned with the field grow preferably to other domains. The result is that these materials can themselves exhibit a remnant magnetization when removed from the field.

The last group, the ferromagnetics, are usually excluded from consideration for use in interventional instruments because of their strong attraction to the magnet of the imager. Not only is a strong translational force created, but an associated torque attempts to align the device with the field.

For purposes of visualizing interventional instrumentation, therefore, only the paramagnetics and diamagnetics will be considered further. The relative permeabilities of both of these groups are very close to 1. So close, in fact, it proves useful to introduce another parameter, called the 'magnetic susceptibility' χ, given by

$$\chi \equiv \mu_r - 1 \tag{4.3}$$

The magnetic susceptibility of water (and, roughly, human tissue) is -9.05×10^{-6} (SCHENCK 1996), revealing it as a diamagnetic substance. The magnetic susceptibilities of a sampling of other materials is given in Table 4.1. For a much more thorough discussion of the magnetic properties of materials and the impact on MRI, see SCHENCK (1996).

Table 4.1 Volume magnetic susceptibility of several materials (SCHENK 1996)

Material	Susceptibility $\times 10^6$
Gold	−34
Silver	−24
Carbon (diamond)	−21.8
Aluminum oxide (Al_2O_3)	−18.1
Lead	−15.8
Pyrex glass (Corning 7740)	−13.88
Copper	−9.63
Water (human tissue)	−9.05
Silicon nitride (Si3N4)	−9.0
Zirconium oxide (ZrO2)	−8.3
Deoxygenated red blood cell	−6.52
Liver (heavy iron overload)	~0.0
Air	0.36
Magnesium	11.7
Aluminum	20.7
Tungsten	77.2
Titanium	182
Platinum	279

4.4.2 Magnetic Susceptibility and MR – Theory

Consider a uniform medium with magnetic susceptibility χ_{medium} immersed in a static magnetic field B_0. When an object with different susceptibility χ_{object} is inserted into the medium, the magnetic field is distorted. The exact distortion is dependent on the shape of the object, but can be calculated analytically for simple geometries such as cylinders and spheres (BAKKER et al. 1993, 1994; LÜDEKE et al. 1985), or numerically for more complicated shapes.

The local change in the magnetic field causes geometrical image distortion (BAKKER et al. 1993, 1994; LÜDEKE et al. 1985). Consider first the slice selection. If the desired slice is z, then the actual slice selected, $z'(x,y)$, will be

$$z'(x,y) = z + \Delta B_z(x,y,z')/G_{slice} \tag{4.4}$$

where $\Delta B_z(x,y,z')$ is the induced change in the z component of the main magnetic field over the xy plane and G_{slice} is the gradient amplitude in the slice-select direction. The distortion in the selected slice can be mapped over the entire slice if $\Delta B_z(x,y,z')$ is known. It is clear that the distortion can be minimized by using a large slice-select gradient amplitude, G_{slice}.

The local magnetic field changes also cause geometrical distortion in the plane of the image, but only along the direction of the frequency-encoding gradient. Similar to the slice-select distortion, a pixel at position x will be imaged onto another pixel location given by

$$x' = x + \Delta B_z(x,y,z)/G_{frequency}, \quad (4.5)$$

where $G_{frequency}$ is the amplitude of the frequency-encoding gradient. There is no distortion in the phase-encoding direction.

In addition to geometric distortion, a spatially dependent phase offset is introduced, given by (Bakker et al. 1993, 1994)

$$\Delta\Phi(x,y,z) = \gamma \, TE \, \Delta B_z(x,y,z), \quad (4.6)$$

where γ is the gyromagnetic ratio and TE is the echo time. This offset is compensated for by the 180° refocusing pulses in spin-echo sequences. In gradient-echo sequences, however, this effect is not compensated, and the phase offset introduces intra-voxel dephasing, essentially reducing the T2* time.

4.4.3 Magnetic Susceptibility and MR – Practice

To effectively utilize the susceptibility artifact, it is useful to understand how the size and appearance of the artifact changes under different conditions.

4.4.3.1 Magnetic Susceptibility (χ)

As the difference between the susceptibility of the object and the susceptibility of the surrounding medium is increased, the severity of the artifact increases (Lüdeke et al. 1985). The change in the magnetic field, $\Delta B_z(x,y,z)$, is linearly proportional to $\chi_{medium} - \chi_{object}$.

4.4.3.2 Size of Object

The larger the instrument itself, the smaller the relative distortion caused outside the object. That is to say, the diameter of the artifact as measured in terms of the physical diameter of the object will decrease as the physical diameter of object is increased (Lüdeke et al. 1985; Schenck 1996).

4.4.3.3 Orientation to B_0

In order to calculate $\Delta B_z(x,y,z)$, the orientation of the object to B_0 must be known if the object is asymmetrical, since $\Delta B_z(x,y,z)$ will be a function of orientation (Bakker et al. 1993, 1994; Lüdeke et al. 1985). A cylinder positioned parallel to the main magnetic field induces a magnetic field change limited to the interior of the cylinder. Exterior spins remain unaffected. If the cylinder is positioned perpendicular to the magnetic field, however, the disturbance in the magnetic field extends outside the cylinder to include voxels with signal-producing spins. This implies no artifact with the cylinder parallel to B_0 and the most severe artifact perpendicular to B_0 (Fig. 4.2). For orientations in between the two extremes, the distortion can also be calculated (Ladd et al. 1996).

4.4.3.4 Main Magnetic Field (B_0)

A stronger static magnetic field produces a more severe artifact (Farahani et al. 1990; Frahm et al. 1996a).

4.4.3.5 Spin Echo Versus Gradient Echo

The 180° refocusing pulses of spin-echo sequences make them less sensitive to any kind of disturbance in local magnetic field homogeneity, including susceptibility-induced differences. The refocusing pulses compensate for the phase offset and resultant intra-voxel dephasing. As a consequence, geometric distortion is the dominant effect, and can lead to signal intensity distortion around the object.

For purposes of illustration, a biopsy needle is imaged in a gel phantom (Fig. 4.3). A spin-echo image through the cylinder is shown in Fig. 4.3a. The cylinder itself is dark because it is not a source of MR signal. However, pixels from the interior of the cylinder are stretched out and distorted along the frequency-encoding direction, so that the size of the cylinder is exaggerated. Outside the cylinder, multiple object pixels can be imaged onto the same pixel, leading to local areas of high signal intensity border-

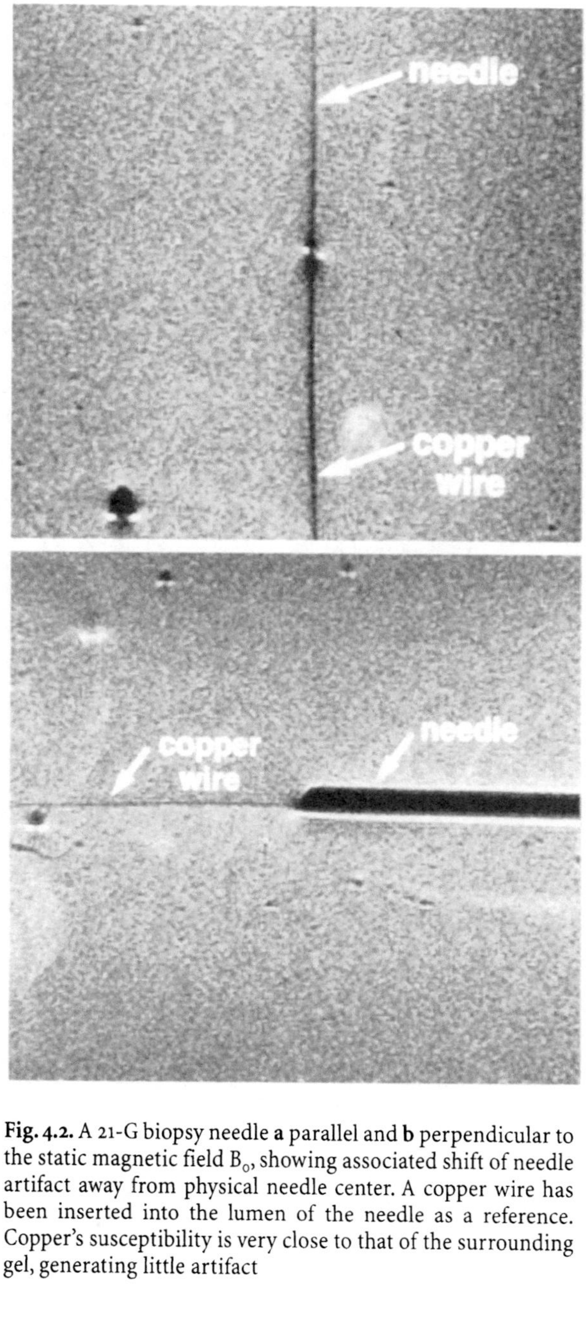

a

b

Fig. 4.2. A 21-G biopsy needle **a** parallel and **b** perpendicular to the static magnetic field B_0, showing associated shift of needle artifact away from physical needle center. A copper wire has been inserted into the lumen of the needle as a reference. Copper's susceptibility is very close to that of the surrounding gel, generating little artifact

ing the cylinder where more than one object pixel overlap.

Gradient-echo sequences, on the other hand, are dominated by intra-voxel dephasing. Especially for long echo times, this causes large regions of signal drop-out. For comparison, the same cylinder is imaged with a gradient-echo sequence in Fig. 4.3b, c. Here, the cylinder size is exaggerated by the signal-poor area around it.

Both geometrical distortion and intra-voxel dephasing lead to intensity distortions. For a spin-echo sequence, where geometrical distortion is the dominant effect, areas of higher intensity are the

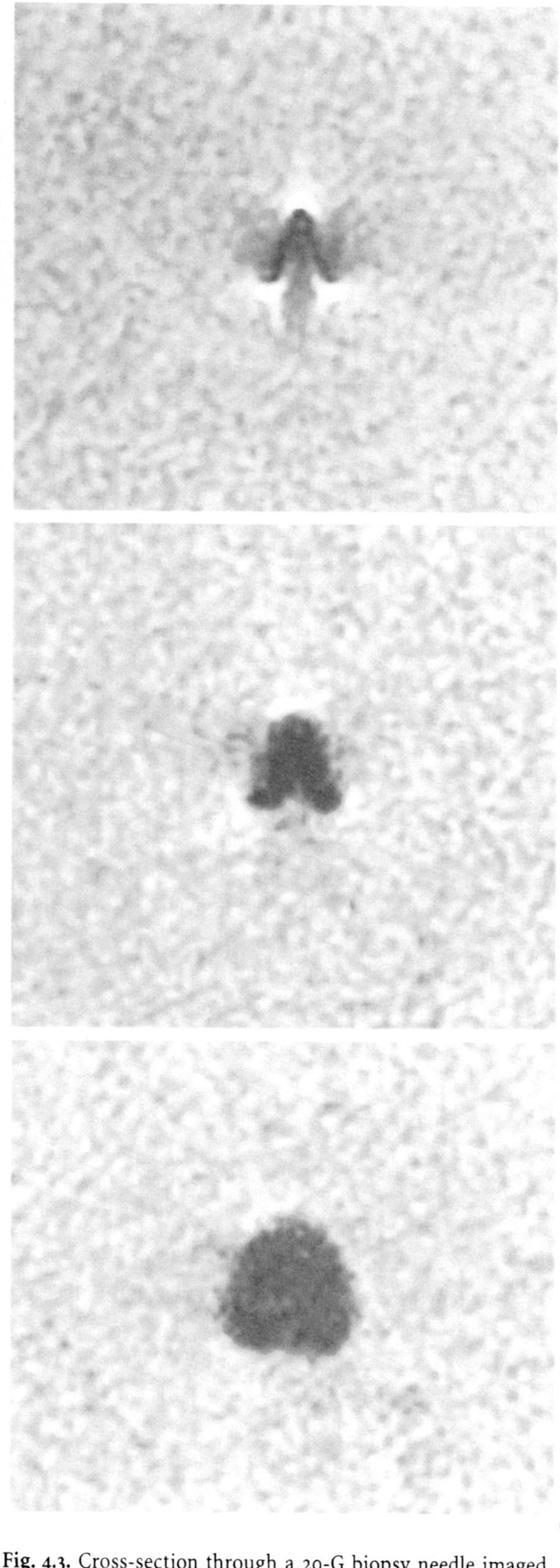

a

b

c

Fig. 4.3. Cross-section through a 20-G biopsy needle imaged with **a** a fast spin-echo sequence (TR 3000/TE 32) and **b** a spoiled gradient-echo sequence (TR 400/TE 6.4, flip angle 60°). **c** The same spoiled gradient-echo sequence with a longer echo time (TE 20). The frequency-encoding direction is vertical in all cases result. For a gradient-echo sequence, especially with a long TE, the intra-voxel dephasing dominates, resulting in a dark region around the object. Since variants of gradient-echo sequences are generally preferred for real-time guidance and monitoring of interventional procedures owing to their shorter imaging times, both geometrical distortion and intra-voxel dephasing must be kept in mind when dealing with materials of different magnetic susceptibility.

4.4.3.6
Echo Time (TE)

As the echo time is increased, the time for intra-voxel dephasing to take place is also increased, resulting in more signal drop-out for gradient echo sequences (Bakker et al. 1993, 1994; Fig. 4.3b, c). Spin-echo artifacts, on the other hand, remain fairly independent of TE, since intra-voxel dephasing does not play a dominant role.

4.4.3.7
Frequency-Encoding Direction

The geometric distortion effect follows along the frequency-encoding direction. For a cylinder with its axis perpendicular to B_0, the appearance and severity of the artifact can be dramatically altered by frequency-encoding either along or perpendicular to the axis of the cylinder (Frahm et al. 1996a; Ladd et al. 1996; Fig. 4.4).

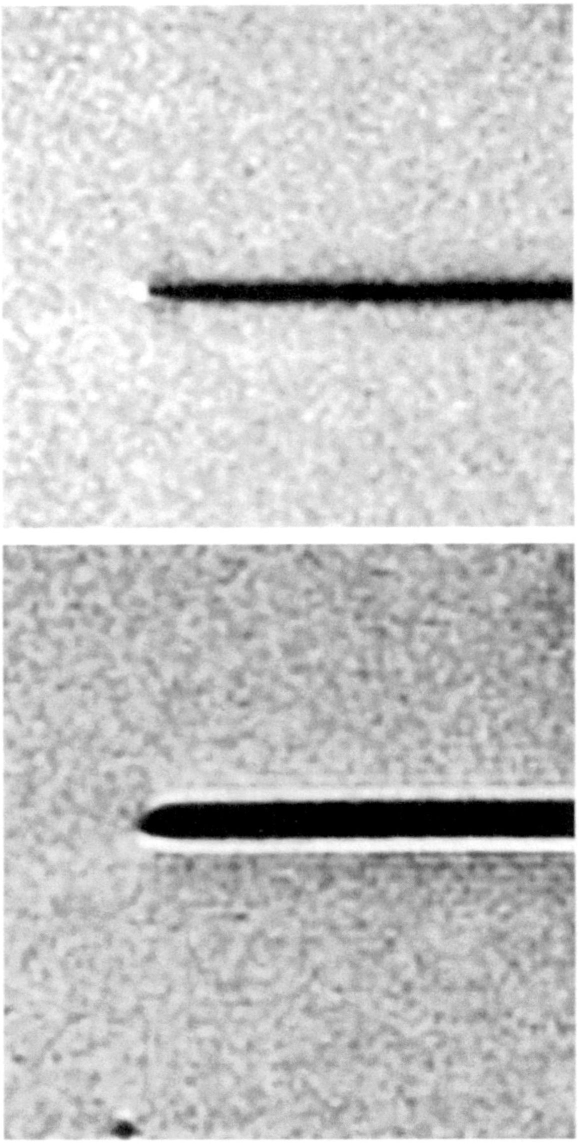

a

b

Fig. 4.4. A 20-G biopsy needle perpendicular to B_0, with frequency-encoding direction **a** parallel and **b** perpendicular to the needle

4.4.3.8
Gradient Amplitude

Slice-select and in-plane geometric distortion can be diminished by increasing gradient strength. For geometric distortion, where

$$x' = x + \Delta B_z(x,y,z)/G_{frequency}, \tag{4.7}$$

the imaged location, x', will approach x as $G_{frequency}$ is increased.

4.4.3.9
Receiver Bandwidth and Field of View

Susceptibility artifacts can also be affected by changes in receiver bandwidth or field of view. As the receiver bandwidth is increased, for example, artifact severity is reduced. The dependencies can best be understood in terms of gradient amplitude, which is given by

$$G_{frequency} = BW / (\gamma\, FOV), \tag{4.8}$$

where BW is the receiver bandwidth, γ is the gyromagnetic ratio, and FOV is the field of view. When the receiver bandwidth is increased, the underlying frequency-encoding gradient amplitude is also increased, leading to the artifact reduction.

4.4.4
Interventional Use

Exploitation of the susceptibility artifact has been the most common method used to make percutaneous devices visible in MR images to date. As a first step in the development of interventional MR, most efforts have concentrated on developing strategies for MR-guided biopsies (FRAHM et al. 1996b; LEWIN et al. 1996; LUFKIN et al. 1987; MUELLER et al. 1986; OREL et al. 1994; SILVERMAN et al. 1995; VAN SONNENBERG et al. 1988). A second area where the susceptibility artifact has been applied is for vascular interventions. Both catheters and guidewires can be visualized with the artifact (BAKKER et al. 1996; KÖCHLI et al. 1994; LENZ et al. 1996; RUBIN et al. 1990).

Unfortunately, the large number of dependencies on orientation and pulse sequence parameters make the consistent portrayal of devices difficult. Additionally, although a large artifact is required for easy detection of the device, the same large artifact inherently distorts the local anatomy and reduces the obtainable accuracy. Indeed, not only does the artifact increase the apparent size of the device but, at least for cylindrical geometries such as biopsy needles, there is an associated shift of the artifact center away from the physical center of the device (KUGEL et al. 1996; LADD et al. 1996; Fig. 4.2). The size of the artifact and the accompanying shift place limits on the accuracy of needle tip placement (KUGEL et al. 1996).

The orientation and pulse sequence dependencies can be ameliorated by using shapes other than cylindrical. Spherical objects, for example, show less dependency owing to their symmetry. This fact has been exploited in catheters by incorporating multiple rings of diamagnetic material along the catheter tip, allowing the catheter to be consistently visualized independent of orientation to B_0 (BAKKER et al. 1996).

4.5
Contrast Agents

Both the signal void and susceptibility artifact techniques rely on negative contrast. The instrument is visualized as a domain of signal drop-out immersed in the signal-producing spins of the surrounding anatomy. An appealing alternative would be to render the instrument brighter than its surroundings.

Paramagnetic contrast agents can be used in MR to shorten the longitudinal relaxation time, T1, of fluids and tissues. Normally, as the repetition time of an imaging sequence is decreased, the longitudinal magnetization becomes saturated and the available signal decreases. By decreasing T1 and allowing the longitudinal magnetization to recover more quickly, the signal of the contrast-enhanced material is maintained.

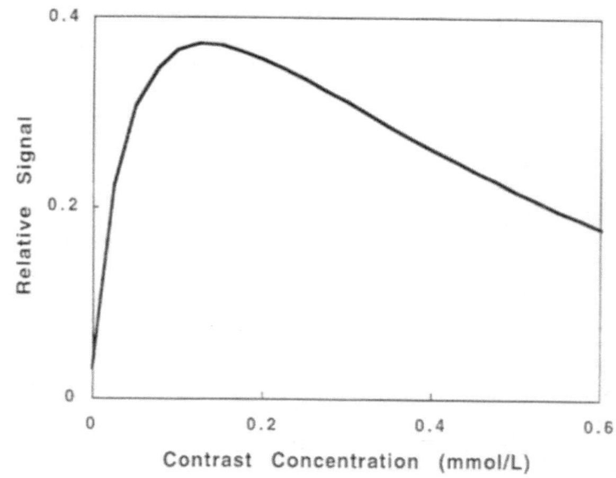

Fig. 4.5. Plot of signal versus contrast agent concentration for a hypothetical contrast agent using a spoiled gradient-echo sequence with TR 10/TE 4, and flip angle 40°. Native T1 was assumed to be 800 ms, i.e. roughly blood. As concentration increases, T1 decreases, leading to a signal increase. T2* also decreases, however, leading to a signal decrease at high concentrations

Unfortunately, the concentration of the contrast agent can not be increased arbitrarily to reduce the T1 relaxation time. The T2* is simultaneously reduced with increasing concentration. For a given sequence with fixed echo and repetition times, there will be an optimum concentration, beyond which the signal starts to decrease because of intra-voxel dephasing caused by T2* effects (HOHENSCHUH and WATSON 1997; Fig. 4.5). The contrast effect can be put to use by filling a device with a contrast-doped solution and imaging with a short repetition time and relatively high flip angle. This combination saturates the longitudinal magnetization in the non-contrast-enhanced tissue outside the device. In the resultant images, the device is displayed with high contrast relative to the background.

Figure 4.6 shows the balloon of a 5-F PTA catheter imaged with a spoiled gradient-echo sequence with TR 150 ms and flip angle 60°. The balloon has been inflated with saline doped with 20 mmol/l gadolinium-DTPA (Magnevist, Schering, Berlin). The location of the balloon is clearly visualized because of the signal-rich solution.

This approach to instrument visualization has two drawbacks. First, an extra lumen must be incor-

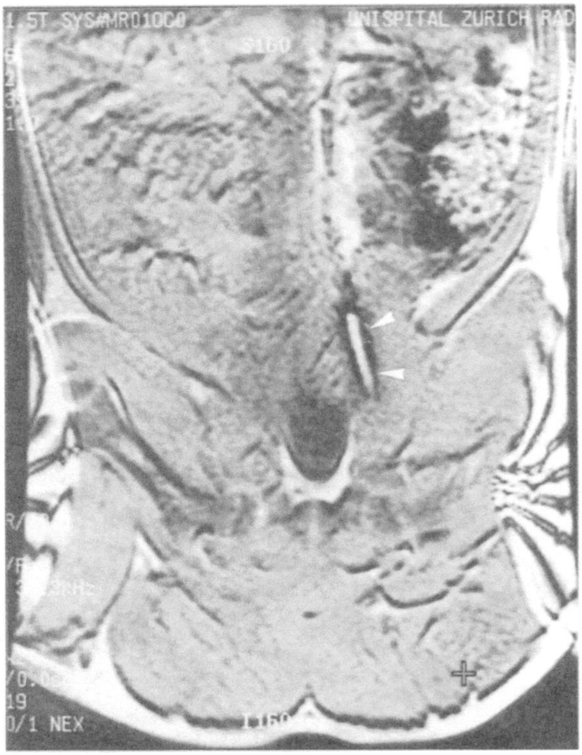

Fig. 4.6. A 6-mm balloon catheter (*arrows*) imaged with a spoiled gradient-echo sequence. The balloon is inflated with a saline solution doped with 20 mmol/l gadolinium-DTPA paramagnetic contrast agent

porated into the device, increasing its size. Second, the contrast is again highly dependent on image resolution, as well as section thickness. For thicker sections, the contrast decreases. The technique does, however, make the device visible even in air-filled regions of the body, and might be suitable for larger catheters or laparoscopic instruments.

4.6 Alternatives

The greatest challenge to passive visualization is creating enough contrast so that an interventional device can be readily and reliably seen in the MR image. Unlike X-ray projections, the device rapidly disappears as the MR section thickness is increased. Since the device position is frequently impossible to predict, the thin sections required for device localization must be balanced with the rapid imaging updates required for interactive guidance. A series of contiguous images must be searched for the device, and often an oblique slice is most suitable for seeing a significant length of the device. During the course of an intervention, the plane of the device can change, and the search process must be begun anew.

The susceptibility artifact can be used to increase the apparent size of the device, making it better visible in the MR image. Unfortunately, it also distorts signal from surrounding tissues, resulting in a tradeoff between device visualization and morphologic accuracy.

Because of the difficulties encountered with purely passive approaches, several alternatives have been developed to actively visualize devices. One allows direct control over the severity of the susceptibility artifact (Glowinski et al. 1996). Two other techniques rely on the incorporation of miniature radiofrequency (RF) coils into the device (Dumoulin et al. 1993; Ladd et al. 1997; Leung et al. 1995). The local sensitivity of the RF coil provides a robust signal, identifying the device location with high contrast.

For rigid objects such as biopsy needles, the position inside the body can be projected based on the position and orientation of the object outside the body. One system uses a hand-piece with infrared light-emitting diodes to triangulate the object position, and overlays the predicted trajectory onto the MR image (Silverman et al. 1995).

Given the challenges involved with passive imaging, it is likely that a combination of active and passive approaches will find application in the MR interventional suite of the future.

References

Bakker CJG, Bhagwandien R, Moerland MA, Fuderer M (1993) Susceptibility artifacts in 2DFT spin-echo and gradient-echo imaging: the cylinder model revisited. Magn Reson Imaging 11:539–548

Bakker CJG, Bhagwandien R, Moerland MA, Ramos LMP (1994) Simulation of susceptibility artifacts in 2D and 3D Fourier transform spin-echo and gradient-echo magnetic resonance imaging. Magn Reson Imaging 12:767–774

Bakker CJG, Hoogeveen RM, Weber J, van Vaals JJ, Viergever MA, Mali WP (1996) Visualization of dedicated catheters using fast scanning techniques with potential for MR-guided vascular interventions. Magn Reson Med 36:816–820

Callaghan PT (1991) Principles of nuclear magnetic resonance in microscopy. Oxford University Press, New York

Dumoulin CL, Souza SP, Darrow RD (1993) Real-time position monitoring of invasive devices using magnetic resonance. Magn Reson Med 29:411–415

Farahani K, Sinha U, Sinha S, Chiu LCL, Lufkin RB (1990) Effect of field strength on susceptibility artifacts in magnetic resonance imaging. Comput Med Imaging Graph 14:409–413

Frahm C, Gehl HB, Melchert UH, Weiss HD (1996a) Visualization of magnetic resonance-compatible needles at 1.5 and 0.2 Tesla. Cardiovasc Intervent Radiol 19:335–340

Frahm C, Gehl HB, Weiss HD, Rossberg WA (1996b) Technik der MRT-gesteuerten Stanzbiopsie im Abdomen an einem offenen Niederfeldgerät: Durchführbarkeit und erste klinische Ergebnisse. Rofo Fortschr Geb Roentgenstr Neuen Bildgeb Verfahr 164:62–67

Glowinski A, Adam G, Bücker A, Neuerburg J, van Vaals JJ, Günther RW (1996) Catheter visualization for interventional MR by actively controlled locally induced field inhomogeneities. (abstract) Proceedings of Fourth Scientific Meeting and Exhibition of International Society for Magnetic Resonance in Medicine, New York, p 51

Hohenschuh E, Watson AD (1997) Contrast media: theory and mechanisms of contrast-enhancing agents. In: Higgins CB, Hricak H, Helms CA (eds) Magnetic resonance imaging of the body, 3rd edn. Lippincott-Raven, Philadelphia, pp 1439–1464

Köchli VD, McKinnon GC, Hofmann E, von Schulthess GK (1994) Vascular interventions guided by ultrafast MR imaging: evaluation of different materials. Magn Reson Med 31:309–314

Kugel H, Langen HJ, Krahe T, Heindel W, Lackner K (1996) Precision of MR-guided needle placement - experimental results. MAGMA 4(2)[Suppl]:143–144

Ladd ME, Erhart P, Debatin JF, Romanowski BJ, Boesiger P, McKinnon GC (1996) Biopsy needle susceptibility artifacts. Magn Reson Med 36:646–651

Ladd ME, Erhart P, Debatin JF, Hofmann E, Boesiger P, von Schulthess GK, McKinnon GC (1997) Guidewire antennas for MR fluoroscopy. Magn Reson Med 37:891–897

Lenz G, Drobnitzky M, Dewey C (1996) MR-visible catheters for intra-vascular interventional MRI procedures. (abstract) Proceedings of Fourth Scientific Meeting and Exhibition of International Society of Magnetic Resonance in Medicine, New York, p 901

Leung DA, Debatin JF, Wildermuth S, McKinnon GC, Holtz D, Dumoulin CL, Darrow RD, Hofmann E, von Schulthess GK (1995) Intravascular MR tracking catheters: preliminary experimental evaluation. AJR 164:1265–1270

Lewin JS, Duerk JL, Jain VR, Petersilge CA, Chao CP, Haaga JR (1996) Needle localization in MR-guided biopsy and aspiration: effects of field strength, sequence design, and magnetic field orientation. AJR 166:1337–1345

Lüdeke KM, Röschmann P, Tischler R (1985) Susceptibility artefacts in NMR imaging. Magn Reson Imaging 3:329–343

Lufkin RB, Teresi L, Hanafee WN (1987) New needle for MR-guided aspiration cytology of the head and neck. AJR 149:380–382

Marshall SV, Skitek GG (1987) Electromagnetic concepts and applications, 2nd edn. Prentice-Hall, New Jersey

Mueller PR, Stark DD, Simeone JF, Saini S, Butch RJ, Edelman RR, Wittenberg J, Ferrucci JT (1986) MR-guided aspiration biopsy: needle design and clinical trials. Radiology 161:605–609

Orel SG, Schnall MD, Newman RW, Powell CM, Torosian MH, Rosato EF (1994) MR imaging-guided localization and biopsy of breast lesions: initial experience. Radiology 193:97-102

Rubin DL, Ratner AV, Young SW (1990) Magnetic susceptibility effects and their application in the development of new ferromagnetic catheters for magnetic resonance imaging. Invest Radiol 25:1325–1332

Schenck JF (1996) The role of magnetic susceptibility in magnetic resonance imaging: MRI magnetic compatibility of the first and second kinds. Med Phys 23:815–850

Silverman SG, Collick BD, Figueira MR, Khorasani R, Adams DF, Newman RW, Topulos GP, Jolesz FA (1995) Interactive MR-guided biopsy in an open-configuration MR imaging system. Radiology 197:175–181

van Sonnenberg E, Hajek P, Gylys-Morin V, Varney RA, Baker L, Casola G, Christensen R, Mattrey RF (1988) A wire-sheath system for MR-guided biopsy and drainage: laboratory studies and experience in 10 patients. AJR 151:815–817

5 Passive Visualization of Needles

H.-B GEHL and C. FRAHM

CONTENTS

5.1 Introduction

Today, two forms of visualization of needles or any other interventional device are possible: active visualization and passive visualization. The first is a technically ambitious procedure owing to the need for equipment, such as a second high-frequency channel, and special hard- and software for superimposing the actively visualized device on an MR image. The second method is the traditional way of performing intervention in radiology by using the direct depiction of the device itself in an X-ray beam or of the artifact it causes in sonography or computed tomography (DUCKWILER et al. 1989; FISCHER et al. 1994; LUFKIN et al. 1987). The advantage of this concept is its straightforwardness, because no specialized hardware or software is necessary. In passive visualization of needles in MRI some difficulties can be encountered. The main factors influencing the size of the artifact caused by a needle are manifold and more complicated than in CT or sonography: field strength, sequence type, echo time, alloy or composition of the needle, needle diameter and angle of needle orientation in relation to the main magnetic field and the read-out gradient (MUELLER et al. 1986; WESBEY et al. 1990; HENDRICK et al. 1993; LUFKIN et al. 1988). The latter factor is of minor importance in CT and sonography and radiologists have hitherto been unaware of it. The ferromagnetic (stainless steel) CT needles cannot be used in MRI because the field nonuniformities resulting from the very large magnetic susceptibility differences between needle and surrounding tissue cause both strong geometric and signal intensity distortion. The purpose of this chapter is to describe the influence of the different factors on the visualization of needles from a clinical point of view without being too "physical."

5.2 Factors Influencing Passive Needle Visualization in MRI

To give an impression of the possible variation in needle artifacts (Fig. 5.1) two "extremes" are demonstrated (all needles shown are called "MR compatible" by the manufacturer). In Fig. 5.1a the "worst case" of needle visualization is given, where even a 25-G needle produces an artifact several centimeters wide. The other "extreme" is given in Fig. 51.b, where the same needles become partly invisible or only faintly appreciable just by changing the sequence, the angle to B_0 and the field strength. Figure 5.1c demonstrates that a small change in the angle of the needle to the main magnetic field B_0 renders all needles visible. Thus, to of the most important factors in depiction of needles in MRI are the angle of the needle to B_0 and the sequence type used. Figure 5.2a-d gives a systematic view of the interdependence of these factors with needle artifact size.

H.-B. GEHL, MD, C. FRAHM, MD, Im Institute of Radiology, Lübeck Medical University, Ratzeburger Allee 160, D-23538 Lübeck, Germany

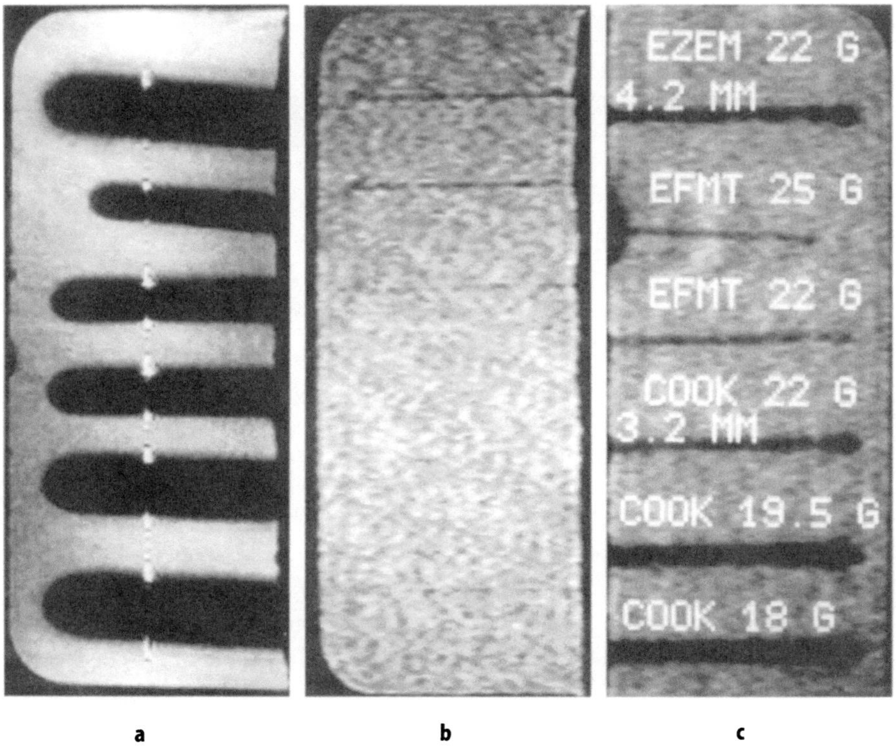

Fig. 5.1a-c. The variability of needle artifact size at different settings. **a** At 1.5 T using a spoiled gradient echo and an angle of 90° to the main magnetic field B_0 the artifacts of all needles are of several centimeters diameter and too large for exact visualization of the needle for biopsy purposes. **b** The other extreme can be observed when, at 0.2 T, a turbospin echo is used at an angle of 0° to B_0, where some needles become invisible. **c** At low angles to B_0 and 0.2 T, changing the echo type to a spoiled gradient echo renders the needles shownin **a** and **b** visible with an acceptable size of susceptibility artifact

5.2.1 Needle Orientation to the Main Magnetic Field (B_0)

The size and shape of the area of local disruption of B_0 caused by the magnetic polarization of the needle obviously depend on the needle orientation relative to B_0. At a given field strength the needle angle to B_0 was evidently the main factor influencing artifact size. A greater angle produces larger artifacts (Fig. 5.2a-d). An especially steep increase in artifact diameter is observed in the range of 30° to 50° for the spin echo (SE) and the turbo spin echo (TSE) at 1.5 T, resulting in an obviously nonlinear curve (Fig. 5.2c). At 0.2 T no such steep increase was observed (Fig. 5.2d).

5.2.2 Field Strength

At any given angle, larger needle artifacts were generally found at 1.5 T than at 0.2 T (Fig. 5.2).

5.2.3 Pulse Sequence

Employing gradient echo (GE) produces significantly larger artifacts than employing SE or TSE (Fig. 5.2). We found no significant differences in artifact diameter between TSE and SE (Frahm et al. 1996).

5.2.4 Echo Time

Increasing echo time (TE) within the given range for the GE (at 0.2 T 9–20 ms, at 1.5 T 6–20 ms) results in a significantly increased artifact diameter (Frahm et al. 1996).

5.2.5 Needle Orientation in Relation to Phase- and Frequency-Encoding Axis

Using SE and TSE at 0.2 T, the artifact diameter was diminished at an angle of 90° by a factor of approximately 0.4–0.5 (at 1.5 T artifact diameter is diminished at an angle of 90° by a factor of 0.3–0.5) if the gradient was swapped to gain orientation parallel to the needle (Frahm et al. 1996). Applying SE and TSE at an angle of 0°, no definite influence on artifact diameter or visibility was observed at 0.2 T and 1.5 T. With GE, swapping the phase-encoding and frequency-encoding axes has had no major effect on artifact diameter and visibility either at 0° or at 90°.

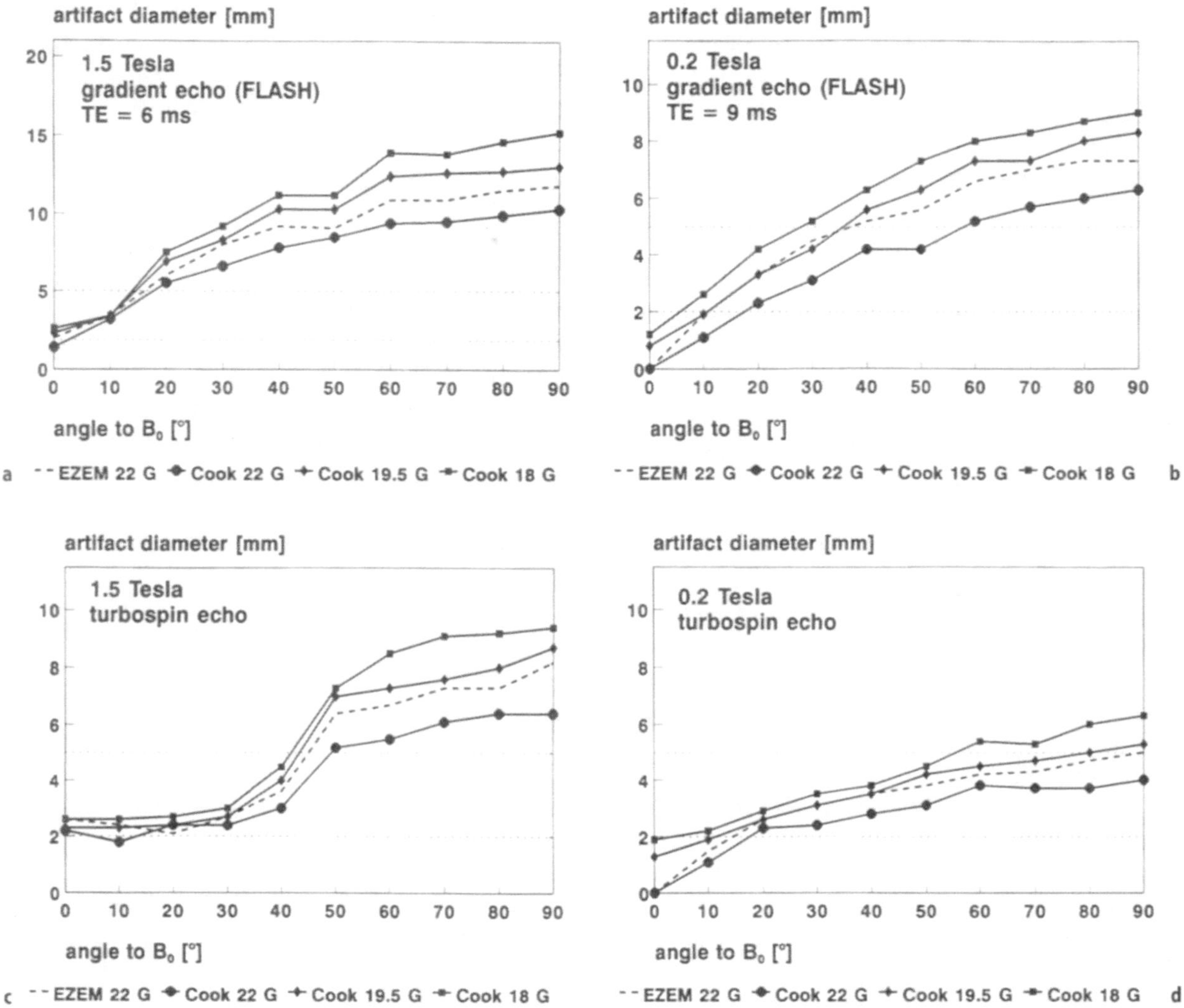

Fig. 5.2a-d. The relationship between needle artifact diameter and needle angle to the static field B_0. **a** Employing spoiled gradient echoes at 1.5 T (TR 200/TE 6) and at low angles of more than 20°, all needles show artifacts larger than 5 mm, which was subjectively chosen as the upper tolerable limit. **b** Employing spoiled gradient echoes (flip angle 80°, TR 200/TE 9) at 0.2 T, artifact size is distinctly smaller than at 1.5 T, but at larger angles the upper limit of 5 mm is surpassed as well. **c** Employing turbospin echoes at 1.5 T (TR 351/TE 19), very similar curves (not shown) are found using simple spin echoes. At needle angles to B_0 greater than 40° the needle artifact size sharply increases and becomes too large for exact localization, although 180° refocusing high-frequency pulses are used. **d** Employing turbospin echoes (TR 350/TE 24) at 0.2 T, optimal or nearly optimal artifact sizes, even at a 90° needle angle to B_0, become possible. For small angles the artifact is too small to allow safe visualization of all needles. For needle depiction at small angles on a low-field scanner gradient echoes are recommended (see Fig. 5.1c, 5.2b)

5.2.6 Alloy

Normal, ferromagnetic stainless steel needles for biopsy purposes with CT cannot be readily used in MRI because of field inhomogeneity resulting from the difference in magnetic susceptibility between the needle and the surrounding tissue. This inhomogeneity leads to strong geometric distortion and signal-intensity changes in the MR image. Several manufacturers have tried to solve the problem by using nonferromagnetic alloys. Needles made of these alloys cause lower disruption of the local field homogeneity and produce a linear local signal loss. These artifacts allow visualization of the needle path. A comparison of the artifact diameters of the 22-G Cook and the 22-G E-Z-EM Chiba needles shows that the Cook alloy produces significantly smaller artifacts (Fig. 5.2). At 0.2 T field strength all needles show artifacts of acceptable size.

5.3 Practical Application of Passive Visualization

The passive visualization of needles in MRI for interventional purposes has been a problem in the era of high-field scanners and non-MR-compatible alloys. Following the introduction of MRI scanners of lower field strength and a more open design a few years ago, the idea of MRI-guided intervention was immediately taken up. The problem with 1.5-T scanners in MRI-guided intervention is the combination of the tube design and the craniocaudal (horizontal) direction of B_0. Large needle angles to B_0 are especially practical for punctures, since access will mostly be in the axial plane. The axial plane in high-field scanners implies that a wide angle of the needle of almost 90° must be employed, resulting in large artifacts. To obtain needle artifacts of suitable size at wide angles and 1.5 T, TSE or SE have to be applied. T1-weighted TSE are not widely used because only a few slices can be obtained by this technique using a short TR. In TSE and SE imaging, the diameter of the needle artifact may be decreased additionally by swapping the phase- and frequency-encoding gradient to gain parallel or nearly parallel orientation of the read-out gradient and the needle. Geometric distortion (and associated signal attenuation or compression) related to susceptibility artifacts is pronounced along the frequency-encoding axis when echo refocusing by a 180° pulse is employed (HENDRICK et al. 1993). By swapping the gradients, the geometric and signal intensity distortion caused by the local nonlinearity of the frequency-encoding gradient remains, but the signal loss from spin dephasing promoted by the local field inhomogeneities is counteracted by the 180° refocusing pulse. Nevertheless, most artifact diameters are still much greater than acceptable at 1.5 T, in spite of SE sequences and gradient swapping.

In contrast, when low-field scanners are used the visibility of the needle artifacts becomes critically diminished or insufficient (except for very large core needles) when the angle of the needle to B_0 becomes smaller than 20°. B_0 of low-field scanners is in anterior-posterior direction (vertical), thus, all needle angles to B_0 in low-field imagers are of practical interest. Generally, when the angle of 0° cannot be avoided, the poor visualization of needles can be counteracted by using GE sequences. These are, on the whole, more sensitive to spin dephasing promoted by the local field inhomogeneities occurring around the needles because they lack a 180° refocusing pulse (Hendrick et al. 1993). Thus, employing GE produces larger artifacts than employing SE or TSE. Signal loss from spin dephasing can be reduced with an earlier signal read-out (shorter TE) and vice versa. This manipulation can be applied effectively to GE without essentially changing the kind of image contrast or weighting. Therefore, at angles of from 0° up to 90° suitable compromises in artifact diameter may be obtained if the effect of needle angling to B_0 is counterbalanced by proper selection of pulse sequence type and echo time. Generally, we recommend GE sequences especially for angles of 10°–60° and SE or TSE sequences for an angle of 40°–90°. Furthermore, GE are more interesting for interventional purposes at low-field strength than SE or TSE because imaging can be performed in breath-hold.

Overall, all needles tested proved more appropriate for low-field scanners. The Cook alloy seems to be more suitable for thicker needles than the alloy of E-Z-EM. Differences in artifact size with the two alloys may be explained by the different nickel content, which is significantly higher in the Cook alloy than in the E-Z-EM alloy. Adding nickel changes the highly magnetic alpha iron to gamma iron, which is much less magnetic (NEW et al. 1983), resulting in smaller magnetic susceptibility differences between needle shaft and the surrounding tissue.

In conclusion, the concept of passive visualization is appealing for so-called open low-field scanners. Although this procedure is also possible with high-field scanners, the advantage of the low-field environment is apparent. Furthermore, taking into account the "low" cost of a low-field scanner, the passive visualization of needles is appropriate, since no further costly "high-tech" equipment is necessary. Therefore, in performing simple biopsies under MRI guidance, passive visualization with low-field scanners represents a good, clinically feasible alternative to other guiding modalities.

References

Duckwiler G, Lufkin RB, Teresi L, Spickler E, Dion J, Vinuela F, Bentson J, Hanafee W (1989) Head and neck lesions: MR-guided aspiration biopsy. Radiology 170:519–522

Fischer U, Vosshenrich R, Keating D, Bruhn H, Döler W, Oestmann JW, Grabbe E (1994) MR-guided biopsy of suspect breast lesions with a simple stereotaxic add-on device for surface coils. Radiology 192:272–273

Frahm C, Gehl HB, Melchert UH, Weiss HD (1996) Visualization of magnetic resonance compatible needles at 1.5 and 0.2 Tesla. Cardiovasc Intervent Radiol 19:335–340

Hendrick RE, Russ PD, Simon JH (1993) MRI: principles and artifacts. Raven Press, New York, pp 144-179

Lufkin R, Teresi L, Hanafee W (1987) New needle for MR-guided aspiration cytology of the head and neck. AJR 149:380–382

Lufkin R, Teresi L, Chiu L, Hanafee W (1988) A technique for MR-guided needle placement. AJR 151:193–196

Mueller PR, Stark DD, Simeone JF, Saini S, Butch RJ, Edelman RR, Wittenberg J, Ferrucci JT (1986) MR-guided aspiration biopsy: needle design and clinical trials. Radiology 161:605–609

New PFJ, Rosen BR, Brady TJ, Buonanno FS, Kistler JP, Burt CT, Hinshaw WS, Newhouse JH, Pohost GM, Taveras JM (1983) Potential hazards and artifacts of ferromagnetic and non-ferromagnetic surgical and dental materials and devices in nuclear magnetic resonance imaging. Radiology 147:139–148

Wesbey G, Edelman RR, Harris R (1990) Artifacts in MR-imaging: description, causes, and solutions. In: Edelman RR, Hesselink JR (eds). Clinical magnetic resonance imaging. WB Saunders, Philadelphia, pp 74–108

6 Susceptibility-Based Catheter Visualization

H.F.M. Smits and C.J.G. Bakker

CONTENTS

6.1 Introduction

The visualization of the devices is the first step in making MR a useful tool for monitoring and guiding endovascular interventions. Basically there are three approaches to achieving this aim: active tracking, passive tracking, and the technique of locally induced field inhomogeneities (see Chaps. 7 and 8). In active tracking, a small receiver coil is built into the tip of the catheter or guidewire so as to actively identify its spatial position (Ackermann et al. 1986; Dumoulin et al. 1993; Wildermuth et al. 1997). Active tracking allows localization of the tip of a device in tens of milliseconds. The three-dimensional (3D) coordinates can be used to display the tip of the device as a white or colored dot on any previously acquired MR image. Also, the 3D coordinates can be used to steer the image acquisition. In passive tracking, the attempt is made to directly visualize a device on MR images on the basis of its associated signal voids and susceptibility artifacts or on the basis of susceptibility inhomogeneities that were deliberately incorporated into the device (Bakker et al. 1996). The main problems with this approach are inconsistent visualization of susceptibility artifacts and inadequate temporal resolution. These items will be discussed in this chapter.

The high temporal resolution together with the possibility to use the 3D coordinates to steer the scan plane are the main advantages of active tracking over passive tracking. However, the positioning of a small receiver coil in the tip of a device can degrade its mechanical properties, e.g., steerability and robustness. The introduction of conductive materials in the scanner can provoke electrical currents and radiofrequency (RF) heating.

H.F.M. Smits, MD, Department of Radiology, University Hospital Utrecht, Huispostnr E.01.1.32, Heidelberglaan 100, 3584 CX Utrecht, The Netherlands
C.J.G. Bakker, PhD, Department of Radiology, University Hospital Utrecht, Huispostnr E.01.1.32, Heidelberglaan 100, 3584 CX Utrecht, The Netherlands

6.2 Susceptibility Artifacts

Susceptibility artifacts are artifacts produced by local inhomogeneities of the static magnetic field, B_0, and are predominantly caused by the presence of diamagnetic or paramagnetic materials. The local field inhomogeneities cause intravoxel phase dispersion and, hence, signal loss. The appearance of the resultant artifact depends on multiple parameters (Bakker et al. 1994): the shape, size and susceptibility distribution of the object, as well as multiple imaging and acquisition parameters. Typically, the configuration of the artifact is related to the orientation of the object within the main magnetic field B_0. Cylindrical nonuniformities are best visualized when perpendicular to the main magnetic field. When aligned with B_0, the severity of the artifact is very much reduced. Whenever a device is homogeneously doped with a paramagnetic material so as to make it visible on MR, the visualization will depend on its orientation to the main magnetic field. As a consequence some parts of the device will be highly visible, while those parts that are aligned with B_0 will barely be visualized. The visualization of uniformly doped devices will be inconsistent and the position of the device might be misregistered. This orientational dependency of the susceptibility artifact is demonstrated in Fig. 6.1.

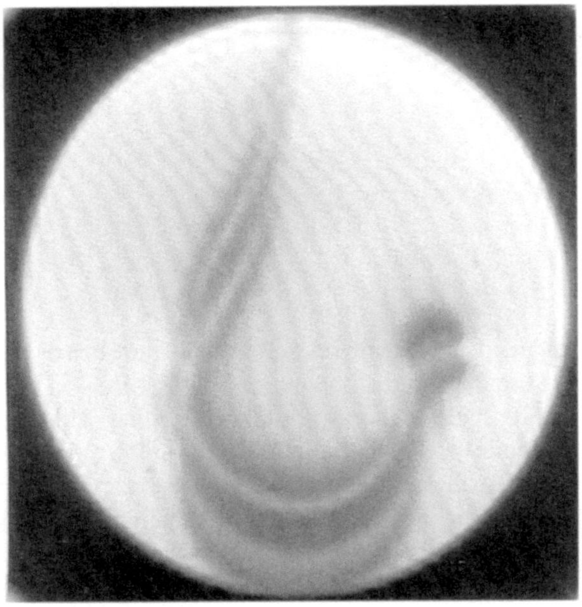

Fig. 6.1. A J-shaped catheter that is uniformly doped with a paramagnetic substance. The orientation of the main magnetic field is from south to north (vertically). Aligned with B_0 the catheter is barely visible. Perpendicular to B_0 the susceptibility artifact enlarges

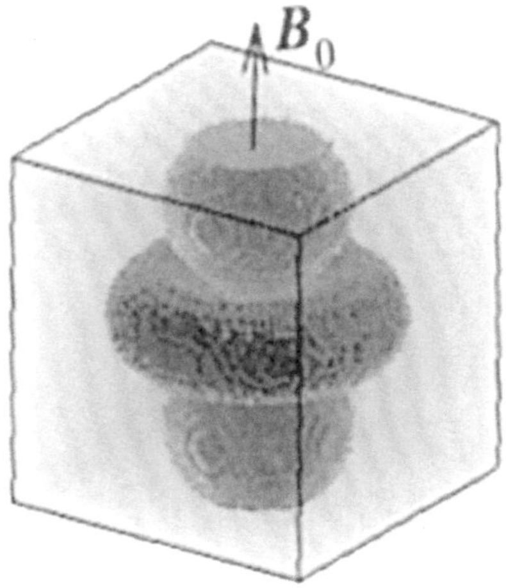

Fig. 6.2. An iso-intensity plot of the magnetic field of a dot of paramagnetic substance in an external static field B_0

Most interesting is the appearance of the field of a dot of paramagnetic material. It has the shape of a horizontally oriented biconcave linear structure with two teardrops perpendicular to its center. The field of a dot can be calculated, and this calculation is displayed in Fig. 6.2 (Bhagwandien 1994). In normal MR interventional circumstances the shape is more or less round and, what is more important, is unrelated to the orientation with respect to the main magnetic field (Fig. 6.3). In the resultant MR image, the center of gravity of the artifact reflects the exact position of the dot. Thus, with the construction of dot-shaped deposits of paramagnetic material in the devices that have to be visualized, the problem of inconsistent visualization can be solved.

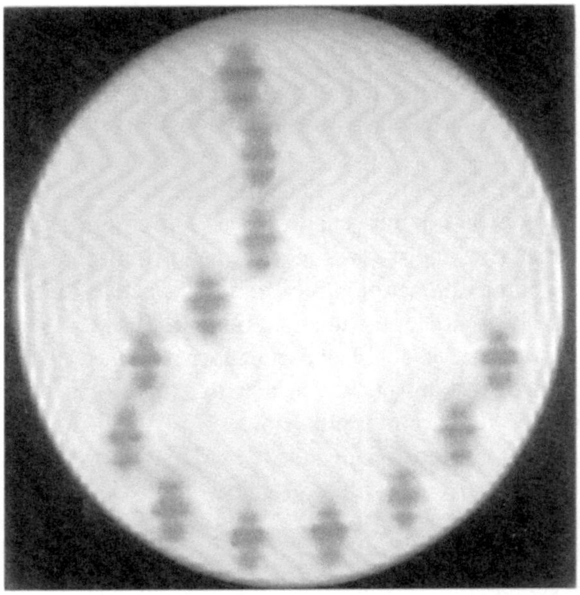

Fig. 6.3. A J-shaped catheter that is prepared with dysprosium rings. The orientation of the main magnetic field is from south to north (vertically). Aligned with B_0 and perpendicular to B_0 the susceptibility artifact remains constant

6.3 Catheter Design

To preserve the good and well-known mechanical properties of standard catheters, these devices best serve as a basis for developing interventional MR equipment. Although some devices are MR compatible, i.e. nonferromagnetic, most catheters are braided with stainless steel. These catheters produce a large susceptibility artifact and inconsistent visualization (Koechli et al. 1994). An MR-compatible device should be void of any ferromagnetic components, be visible on MR images, and should not produce image artifacts, for instance due to RF artifacts (Camacho et al. 1995). Susceptibility-based catheter visualization can be achieved by locally impregnating the wall with a paramagnetic substance. Like gadolinium, dysprosium oxide (Dy_2O_3) has high magnetic susceptibility and is suitable for embedding in the wall of a catheter without affecting its mechanical properties. In this way, rings of enhanced susceptibility can be created to demarcate the tip segment of a catheter or the margins of a balloon. These tiny rings give an almost dot-shaped artifact, independent of the orientation to B_0. When a ring is tilted 90° to B_0, the shape will still be round and the created susceptibility artifact will be constant. The number of rings to be incorporated depends on what part of the device is to be visualized. A concentration of the paramagnetic substance of 10% by weight, a length of the ring of 1 mm and an interspacing of 10–20 mm gave satisfactory results in phantom experiments (Bakker et al. 1996) and preliminary volunteer work (Bakker et al. 1997). If desired, the configuration of the rings can be altered, i.e., a higher concentration of dysprosium or a different interspacing near the tip, to improve the visualization of the tip segment of a catheter or the margins of a balloon. For a balloon catheter two rings just proximal and distal to the balloon are sufficient for visualization without disturbance of the lumen of the inflated balloon (Fig. 6.4).

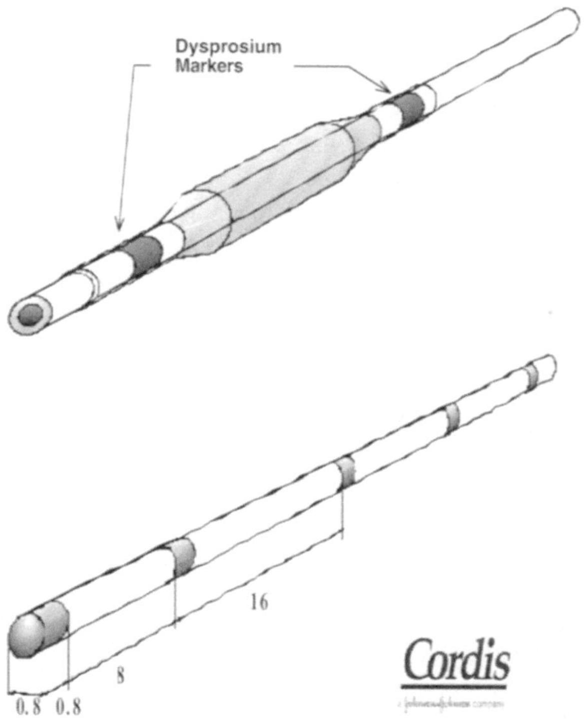

Fig. 6.4. Drawings of a 6-mm balloon catheter with two dysprosium markers (*top*) and a 0.035-in. (0.89-mm) fiberglass guidewire with five markers (*bottom*)

6.4 Guidewire Design

The design of an MR-compatible catheter is relatively simple, for it is an adaptation of a standard catheter. For guidewires it is more difficult. Most standard guidewires have a stainless steel ferromagnetic core, which are forcefully drawn into the scanner and are thus not MR compatible. Nitinol guidewires are nonferromagnetic and called MR compatible, but they cause an image degradation due to RF artifacts, visible as a grid of noise over the source images and subtraction images (Camacho et al. 1995; Koechli et al. 1994). The artifact of the wire itself is barely visible. The introduction of conductive materials into the scanner presents a safety risk to patients. In vitro it is not difficult to coagulate a piece of meat between the two ends of a copper wire, spirally positioned in the scanner. The safety risk associated with the use of metals can partly be overcome by splitting the metal components into smaller parts so as to reduce conductivity. A possible way to avoid metals in guidewires is to use ultrastrong superfibers. This is all experimental work and has not yet led to the development of products for clinical use. Although some devices are MR compatible, i.e., nonferromagnetic, there clearly is a need for special MR-dedicated, nonmetallic guidewires with some kind of markers for susceptibility-based visualization. With non-metallic materials, however, it is difficult to construct a wire with the robustness and steerability of standard guidewires.

For experimental work 0.035-in. (0.89 mm) fiberoptic guidewires have been developed. The fiberglass core gives an excellent torque, is not conductive, and produces neither susceptibility nor RF artifacts. For susceptibility-based visualization paramagnetic rings are embedded in the tip segment. The distal markers have a different interspacing to indicate curving of the wire. This arrangement is still under development and has not yet been approved for human application.

6.5 MR Fluoroscopy

In passive tracking, a new image is required each time new information about the actual position of the device becomes necessary. Hence, during passive tracking the acquisition time must be short. Time-consuming pulse sequences and options like presaturation slabs and 3D sequences must be avoided. Prior to the interventional procedure reference scans are made in the three orthogonal planes. Three-dimensional angiographic sequences can be acquired before the introduction of the devices and used as a "roadmap". The endovascular intervention itself is guided by dynamic 2D gradient-echo techniques. The prepared part of the device is monitored best by a dynamic subtraction technique, i.e., by computing the device-induced difference in signal intensity between images obtained prior to and during insertion of the device. Useful tools for increasing tracking speed are a reduced field of view (Frederickson and Pelc 1996; Hu and Parrish 1994) and keyhole imaging (van Vaals et al. 1993). With the use of "on-the-fly" subtraction, the field of view can be greatly reduced because artifacts due to aliasing are subtracted. Moving structures outside the field of view but within the area of image wrap-around are not subtracted and have to be avoided (e.g., bowel movement). In order to be able to track the device through tortuous vessels a relatively thick slice is required. With the standard gradient capability of 15 mT/m, a field strength of 1.5 T, a reconstruction time of 0.1 s per 256^2 image, TR 15/TE 9, a field of view of 128 × 256 mm, matrix 128 × 256, flip angle of 10°, and first order flow compensation, imaging times of 0.5 s are possible. With MR interventions it is necessary to obtain the images in the MR suite. The time between scanning and display in the scanning room is called the delay time. The delay time of about 0.5 s has to be added to the scan time. This results in MR fluoroscopy with one frame per second. In this way it is possible to manipulate guidewires through artificial stenoses in phantoms and to properly position balloon catheters. It then is possible to follow the deployment of the balloon (Fig. 6.5).

For most clinical indications a tracking speed of 1 frame per second is not sufficient and faster scan techniques have to be developed. One must keep in mind that every pulse sequence influences the visualization of susceptibility artifacts. New fast scan techniques, such as radial and spiral scanning, are promising but their usefulness for interventional MR has still to be evaluated.

6.6 Postprocessing

The subtraction technique described in Sect. 6.5 only visualizes the part of the device where the markers are located. The information provided by the dynamic subtraction images can be projected onto corresponding MR angiograms or other reference images. This supercomposition produces an image comparable to a roadmap in the angiosuite and indicates the position of the prepared part of the device with respect to the vasculature. With computer-aided pattern recognition it might be possible to calculate the spatial position of the device and to use this information to steer image acquisition.

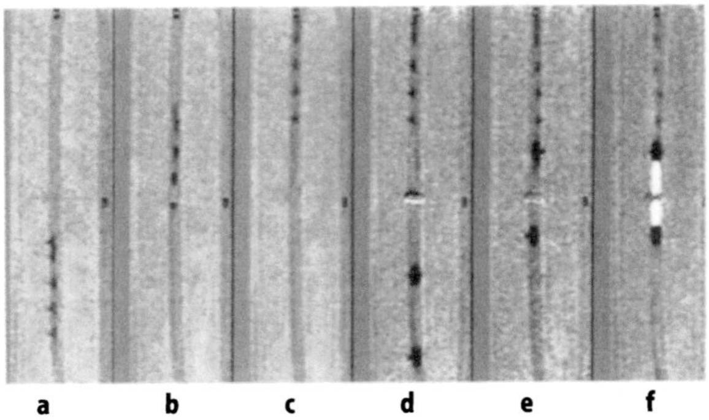

Fig. 6.5a-f. Six selected frames from a dynamic series of coronal two-dimensional gradient-echo subtraction images of a flow phantom with a locally constricted 6-mm plastic tube. From left to right: the fiberoptic guidewire (five dysprosium rings 10% by weight, interspacing 16 mm, near the tip 8 mm) is negotiated through the stenosis (**a–c**); a balloon catheter (diameter 6 mm, length 4 cm) is introduced (**d**) and positioned over the stenosis (**e**); the balloon is inflated with Gd-DTPA-doped water (**f**)

6.7 Discussion

Results obtained so far demonstrate excellent and consistent visualization of properly prepared fiberoptic guidewires and polyethylene catheters in near real-time 2D gradient echo images. The paramagnetic markers cause local signal losses which clearly show up in dynamic (subtraction) images. Visualization with respect to the vessels of interest is readily achieved by mapping these subtraction images onto a previously acquired roadmap. With the help of the described tools the entire interventional procedure, from the introduction and placement of a guidewire to the positioning of a catheter across the stenosis, the inflation of the balloon and the dilatation of the stenotic region can be performed under MR guidance in phantoms.

Obviously, the reported phantom experiments merely constitute a first step toward introduction of MR-guided vascular interventions in clinical practice. Many difficulties have yet to be overcome. Remaining issues include the improvement of the steerability of fiber-optic guidewires so as to make them suitable and safe for clinical application, the development of a complete armature of MR-dedicated interventional devices, the extension of the capabilities of the MR system with regard to real-time image processing and display, the realization of faster scan techniques, the development of functional tests and the development of gating or motion compensation strategies to reduce gross motion artifacts.

A very important issue is the flexibility of the MR system. With the first conventional X-ray tubes it was not possible to perform interventional procedures. It took years to develop dedicated X-ray fluoroscopy systems to perform the interventions that we take for granted today. Likewise, it will take some time to reshape the current inflexible MR equipment, which is optimized to make high quality diagnostic images, into a system that provides images just good enough for guiding interventions with maximal speed and flexibility. To enhance the flexibility of the system, interactive modification of scan parameters during scanning and intermittent execution of MR fluoroscopy, angiography or flow measurements are being developed.

Passive tracking as proposed in this chapter has several appealing properties which make it a promising alternative or adjunct to active tracking (Chap. 8) or to the concept of field inhomogeneity catheters (Chap. 7). It allows visualization of the entire prepared part of the device, the mechanical properties and steerability of the device are virtually unaffected by the markers, even for microcatheters, and passive tracking does not pose serious safety problems. On the other hand, active tracking offers higher tracking speeds and provides 3D coordinates which can be projected onto any MR image and which can be used to steer image acquisition. Passive and active visualization seem complementary, and it is not unlikely that an integrated approach will provide the ultimate solution.

References

Ackerman JL, Offut MC, Buston RB, Brady TJ (1986) Rapid 3D tracking of small RF coils (abstract) Fifth. Annual meeting of Society of Magnetic Resonance in Medicine, Montreal, p 1131

Bakker CJG, Bhagwandien R, Moerland MA, Ramos LMP (1994) Simulation of susceptibility artifacts in 2D and 3D Fourier transform spin-echo and gradient-echo magnetic resonance imaging. Magn Reson Imaging 12:767–774

Bakker CJG, Hoogeveen RM, Weber J, et al (1996) Visualization of dedicated catheters using fast scanning techniques with potential for MR-guided vascular interventions. Magn Reson Med 36:816–820

Bakker CJG, Hoogeveen RM, Hurtak WF, et al (1997) MR-guided endovascular interventions: susceptibility-based catheter and near-real-time imaging technique. Radiology 202:273–276

Bhagwandien R (1994) Object induced geometry and intensity distortions in magnetic resonance imaging. Thesis, Utrecht University, Utrecht, The Netherlands

Camacho CR, Plewes DB, Henkelman RM (1995) Non-susceptibility artifacts due to metallic objects in MR imaging. J Magn Reson Imaging 5:75–88

Dumoulin CL, Souza SP, Darrow RD (1993) Real-time position monitoring of invasive devices using magnetic resonance. Magn Reson Med 29:411–415

Fredrickson JO, Pelc NJ (1996) Temporal resolution improvement in dynamic imaging. Magn Reson Med 35:621-625

Hu X, Parrish T (1994) Reduction of field of view for dynamic imaging. Magn Reson Med 31:691–694

Koechli VD, McKinnon GC, Hofmann E, von Schulthess GK (1994) Vascular interventions guided by ultrafast imaging: evaluation of different materials. Magn Reson Med 31:309–314

van Vaals JJ, Brummer ME, Dixon WT, et al (1993) "Keyhole" method for accelerating imaging of contrast agent uptake. J Magn Reson Imaging 3:671–675

Wildermuth S, Debatin JF, Leung DA, et al (1997) MR imaging-guided intravascular procedures: initial demonstration in a pig model. Radiology 202:578–583

7 Field Inhomogeneity-Based Catheter Visualization

A. GLOWINSKI

CONTENTS

7.1 Introduction

With the growing interest in interventional MRI (JOLESZ and BLUMENFELD 1994), the visualization of catheters under MR control has become a field of intense research. Compared to conventional catheterization under fluoroscopy, MR-guided catheterization has several advantages and disadvantages. The two primary advantages of MR guidance are the lack of X-ray exposure for the patient and medical staff and the good soft tissue contrast, which allows excellent depiction of the anatomy. Unfortunately, excellent anatomic contrast is also a disadvantage during catheterization since the contrast between the background and catheter is very low compared to conventional X-ray fluoroscopy. An additional disadvantage is that MRI has lower spatial and temporal resolution. In this chapter, a new method for visualizing catheters via MRI using locally induced, interactively adaptable field inhomogeneities is presented.

A. GLOWINSKI, MS, Department of Diagnostic Radiology, University of Technology Aachen, Pauwelsstrasse 30, 52057 Aachen, Germany

7.2 Catheter Visualization Under MR Control: Other Techniques

Passive catheter visualization means that the catheter is directly visualized in the acquired image by its effect on the spins in the area of the catheter. Active visualization means that the catheter itself is not imaged, but a receiving coil is incorporated into the tip of the catheter and its position determined by a three-dimensional analysis of the fields immediately surrounding the tip (ACKERMAN et al. 1986; DUMOULIN et al. 1993; LEUNG et al. 1995; MCKINNON et al. 1996; Chaps. 8, 9). For passive catheter visualization, different effects are used. Generally, the catheter appears dark in an MR image, due either to the typical signal void associated with the catheter material or to susceptibility changes between the catheter material and the background tissue. In order to increase conspicuity using the signal void effect, one would like to have a signal from the background in contrast to the dark appearance of the catheter. However, to ensure that the catheter is within the imaged slice, slice thickness must be large enough to include the full width of the vessel into which the catheter has been placed. Due to this constraint, the use of a pure signal void for catheter visualization is not beneficial, since the relatively small catheter suppresses only a part of the vascular signal in the slice and the partial volume effect renders the catheter signal void invisible. Especially in tortuous vessels, where slice thickness has to be increased even further in order to cover the entire vessel, this method is not feasible. One solution to this problem is to use susceptibility effects for catheter visualization (KÖCHLI et al. 1994; LENZ et al. 1996). The region of intravoxel dephasing at the point of susceptibility change extends the "edge" of the catheter material, so that the catheter appears much larger in the image than it actually is. The effect is strongly dependent on the employed pulse sequence. Spin echo sequences are less sensitive to susceptibility effects than gradient echo sequences. The effect also varies with the echo time in gradient echo sequences. Unfortunately, the susceptibility effect is strongly dependent on the orientation of the catheter with respect to B_0. A method to reduce this orientation dependency is described in Chap. 6 (BAKKER et al. 1996). Unfortunately, this method no longer allows visualization of the entire length of the catheter. The following sections describe a method that allows visualization of the entire length of the catheter on the basis of electrically induced field inhomogeneities. The effects used for visualization can be adjusted online during the procedure. This allows adjustment of the catheter appearance to suit the imaging sequence, as well as the slice thickness.

7.3 Catheter Visualization Based on Field Inhomogeneity

7.3.1 The Basic Concept

In order to achieve visualization of the entire catheter, a wire loop is incorporated into the catheter (GLOWINSKI et al. 1997). If a small current is sent through this wire, an electromagnetic field is established locally around the catheter. This local field is superimposed on the field of the MR scanner and produces local B_0 field inhomogeneities. As in the case of the susceptibility effect, these B_0 field inhomogeneities lead to intravoxel dephasing and, hence, to signal suppression and a catheter-associated signal void.

7.3.2 Current-Induced Magnetic Fields

When a direct current is sent through a straight wire, the magnetic field that is established by this current has a circular, concentric shape around the wire. Figure 7.1a depicts the field in a plane perpendicular to the wire. The field strength B at a distance r from the wire can be described by the equation

$$B \propto \frac{I}{2 \cdot \pi \cdot r},$$

where I is the current strength.

As magnetic fields are additive, more complicated cases can be derived from this simple model by

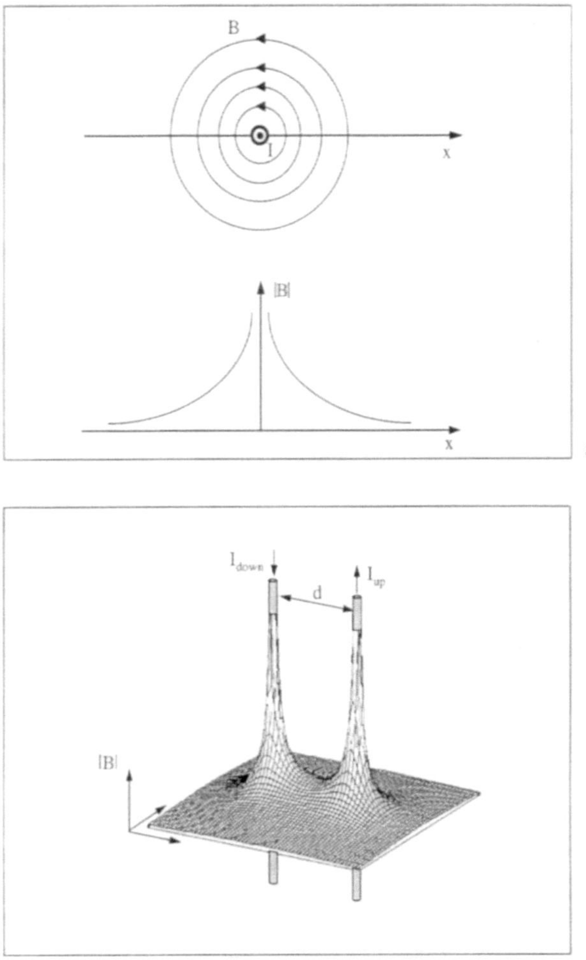

Fig. 7.1a, b. Magnetic fields established by **a** a single current and **b** two currents with opposite directions. **B**, magnetic field; B, field strength; I, current; d, distance

superimposing the fields induced by several currents.

Catheter visualization using this technique requires a closed wire loop that covers the entire catheter and has two connectors at the hub end for the current source (Fig. 7.2). In the simplest case, the catheter is constructed with a wire that starts at the hub, leads straight to the tip, and then returns directly to the hub (Fig. 7.3a). Such a wire configuration can be represented as two parallel wires, separated by a constant distance equal to the diameter of the catheter, with the current in both wires of equal strength but in opposite directions. The electromagnetic field established by such a configuration can be derived from the previous case of a single, straight wire. Figure 7.1b shows the strength of the magnetic field induced by a pair of parallel and oppositely directed currents in a plane perpendicular to the two wires. The distance between the two

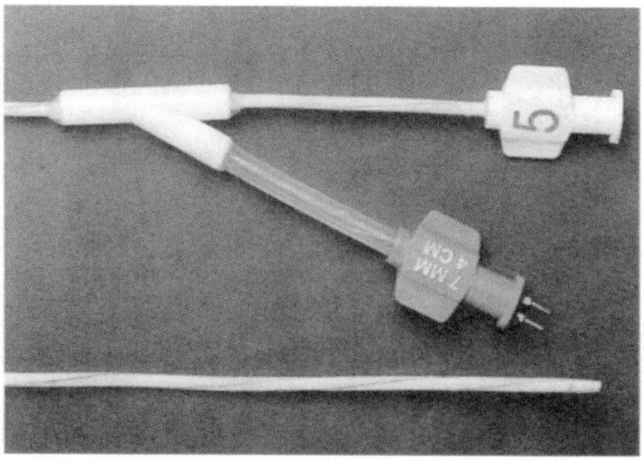

Fig. 7.2. The catheter is equipped with a copper wire (in this case not covered by the catheter wall in order to show the principle). The wire starts at one connector at the distal end of the catheter, leading to the tip and then back to the second connector. This wire setup defines a closed wire loop along the catheter

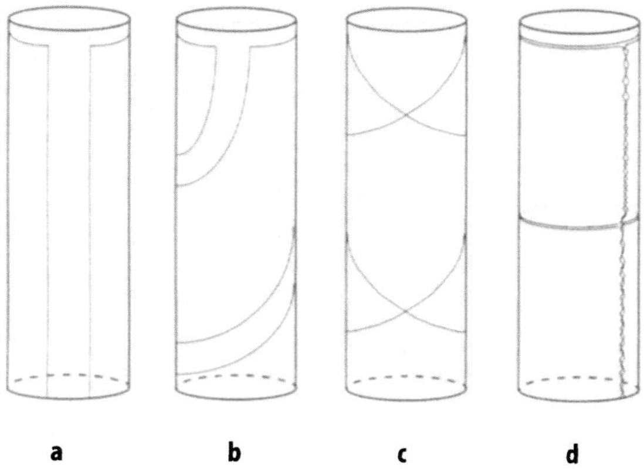

Fig. 7.3a-d. Different wire configurations. **a** Straight antiparallel, **b** double helix, **c** opposed double helix, **d** local markers

wires is d and the current strength is I. The height of the surface indicates the strength of the magnetic field. The field has its maximum close to the wires. Between the two wires, the field components from the two wires add, while they subtract outside the wires. This ensures that only local fields are established, which produce only local signal suppression in the image.

7.3.3 Catheter Design

Generally, any modern catheter material and shape is compatible with the above method. In order to introduce the current, a wire must be incorporated into the catheter wall. The wire has to be nonmagnetic

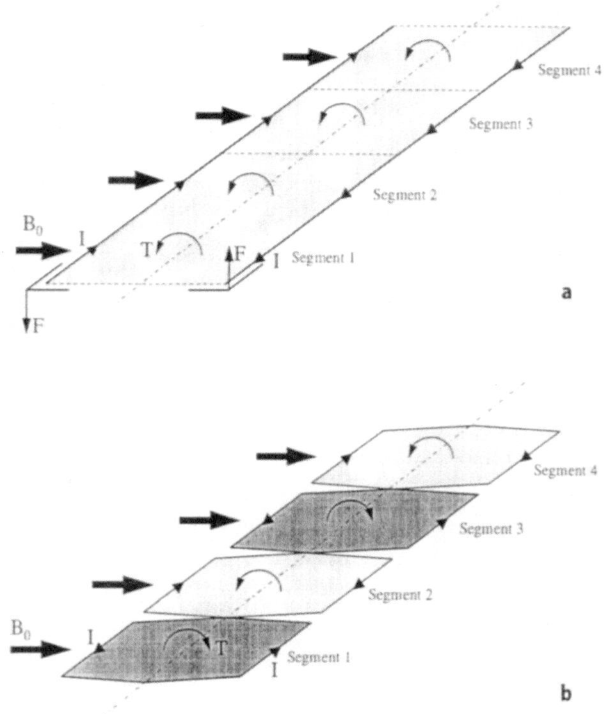

Fig. 7.4a, b. Forces on pairs of wires; **a** Straight parallel configuration; **b** modified configuration. B_0, magnetic field; **F**, force; **I**, current; **T**, torque (curved vector)

and should be thin enough to avoid visible susceptibility artifacts when the current is switched off. The wire may have an additional thin layer of insulation. Thin transformer wires made of copper with a diameter of approximately 50–80 μm fulfill all of these criteria.

Figure 7.3 shows four different wire configurations. The simplest configuration – a straight pair of parallel wires – is depicted in Fig. 7.3a. However, the two helical configurations have proven to be more useful.

Theoretically, a wire with a current within a magnetic field is subject to a force perpendicular to both the magnetic field (in this case the B_0 magnetic field of the scanner) and the direction of the current. This force is proportional to the field strength and the current. Therefore, even a small current of less than 150 mA can induce a strong force due to the strength of the B0 magnetic field. Because of the "symmetrical and opposite" wire configuration, we have two currents of the same strength, yet opposite directions. Assuming sufficient field homogeneity of the main magnetic field, both wires are subject to the same force, yet in opposite directions. These two forces counteract each other, so that the catheter does not undergo any "translational" movement. However, both forces always establish a torque with oppositely directed currents, wherever the two wires are straight and parallel.

Assuming a configuration of two parallel but oppositely directed wires, the two wires can be virtually split into segments, such as the four segments depicted in Fig. 7.4a. The force **F** on the wires acts perpendicular to both the direction of the current I and the direction of the magnetic field **B**. The forces on the wires act to flip each segment into a position perpendicular to the external field as indicated by the curved vector **T**. In order to avoid this torque, the loop can be divided into actual segments, with each wire changing sides from one segment to the next as shown in Fig. 7.4b. Each of the segments is subject to a torque of the same strength as before, but the direction changes for each segment. Therefore, the force on each segment is counteracted by that on the adjoining segments. In order to prevent catheters from turning, the latter configuration is preferred. Figure 7.3b shows a wire configuration in which the oppositely directed wires are wrapped around the catheter in a variation of a double helix. The result is a configuration similar to that depicted in Fig. 7.4b. Such a catheter avoids movement as well as torquing.

There is another interesting benefit of this helical configuration. The effect of the locally induced fields depends on the orientation of the wires in the B_0 magnetic field. The effect is weaker if the wire is oriented parallel to the B_0 field, and becomes stronger as the angle between the wire and B_0 increases. With the helical configuration, the angle between the wires and B_0 continuously changes along the catheter, so that there are always well-visualized segments alternating with poorly visualized segments. This results in a typical "beaded" appearance of the catheter which is insensitive to the orientation of the catheter in the B_0 magnetic field. A second helical configuration is shown in Fig. 7.3c. In this case, the helical course of the oppositely directed wires is offset, so that they cross at certain points. This means that the distance between the two wires is no longer constant along the catheter, which changes the visualization pattern of the catheter.

Under certain circumstances, it might be useful to mark only a part of the catheter. Instead of visualizing the whole catheter, one can also apply local markers, in order, for instance, to mark the beginning and end of an angioplasty balloon (Fig. 7.3d). In this case, the two wires are wrapped closely around each other in areas where no local field is desired.

Wherever the wires are very close to each other, the two induced magnetic fields essentially cancel each other. Only the ring-like regions induce a visible local field.

7.3.4 Sequences for Catheter Imaging

Field inhomogeneity catheters produce local signal loss in the vicinity of the catheter when the current is switched on. To detect this loss, the signal from the surrounding blood must be bright. This restricts the choice of sequences to those based on gradient echo techniques. These sequences allow short image-acquisition times.

There are two ways to visualize the catheter: direct imaging and subtraction methods with superimposed, false colors used to designate the catheter position.

7.3.4.1 Direct Imaging

Obviously, the easiest way to use a catheter for direct imaging is to switch it on constantly during image acquisition. Figure 7.5 shows a 5-F multipurpose catheter with a double helical wire configuration at three different levels of current. This image clearly shows the increasing conspicuity resulting from an increase in current. It also demonstrates that the pure signal void of the catheter alone does not result in adequate contrast between catheter and background for a 5-F catheter in a 10-mm-thick slice. Even with no current, however, one can see the tiny artifacts arising from the susceptibility effect of the copper wire. The effect of the local field of the wire reaches beyond the catheter and, hence, allows better depiction of the catheter. During in vivo experiments, current strength can be adapted to the desired catheter. The bright signal from flowing blood is achieved, as mentioned above, by the use of gradient echo-based sequences. Figure 7.6 shows a catheter in a preliminary pig study. The use of coronal slices allows visualization of the vessel over a length of several centimeters, providing good orientation. A T1-weighted gradient echo sequence (TR = 17 ms, TE = 4.1 ms, $\alpha = 15°$) with a rising flip angle has been used for imaging. A slice-selective presaturation pulse suppresses the stationary tissue and enhances the vessel. If one operates in big vessels like the aorta, the slice thickness needs to be large enough to cover

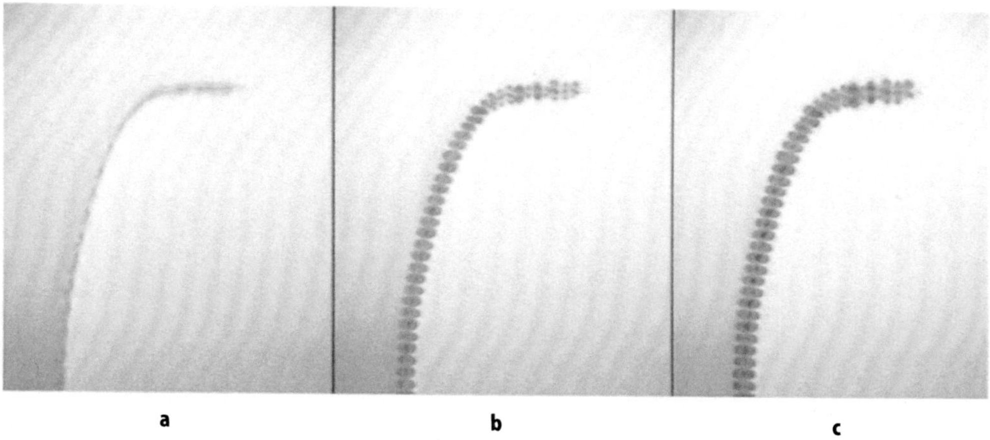

Fig. 7.5a-c. Multipurpose catheter in a waterbath experiment at **a** 0 mA, **b** 80 mA, **c** 150 mA

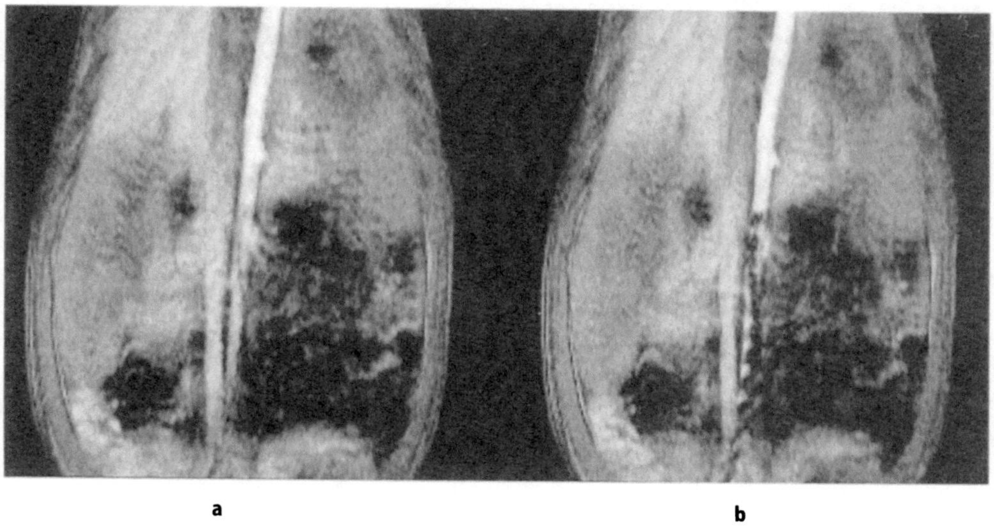

Fig. 7.6a, b. Results of a preliminary pig study using direct imaging at **a** 0 mA and **b** 150 mA

the diameter of the vessel. This ensures that the catheter will be in the imaged slice. Therefore, the current strength must be high in order to override the partial volume effect that reduces the visibility of the catheter. This effect is shown in Fig. 7.6. On the left side, a 5-F catheter is imaged without any current in a 15-mm-thick slice. On the right side, the current has been switched on at 150 mA. Comparison of the two images shows that the 5-F catheter is difficult to detect by exploring only the intrinsic signal void of the catheter and wire. The local inhomogeneities induced by the current, however, allow good visualization of the entire length of the catheter. If during a procedure thinner vessels are entered and slice thickness is reduced to achieve better resolution, the current should be reduced as well.

Figure 7.7 shows the use of a field inhomogeneity-based balloon catheter, where two local markers indicate the beginning and end of the balloon (length = 35 mm, diameter = 5 mm). The pulse sequence used for this image is the same as that used for the image in Fig. 7.6.

7.3.4.2 Subtraction Imaging

The benefit of direct imaging is that any sequence that provides good visibility of the vessel can be used for catheter imaging. No additional connections between the MR scanner and the catheter are needed. Unfortunately, problems can arise if the catheter is close to a vessel wall which itself is located near a dark background. Under these circumstances, the effect may not be sufficiently obvious to allow secure differentiation between contrast changes due to the catheter and those due to changes in the background. A computed image that shows only the catheter superimposed on an anatomic image can be created with dedicated pulse sequences. In principle, two images are acquired, one with the current switched on and one with the current switched off. Subtraction of these two images yields an image in which only the catheter and its local field appear while addition of the two images yields an anatomic image. Compared to the direct imaging discussed in

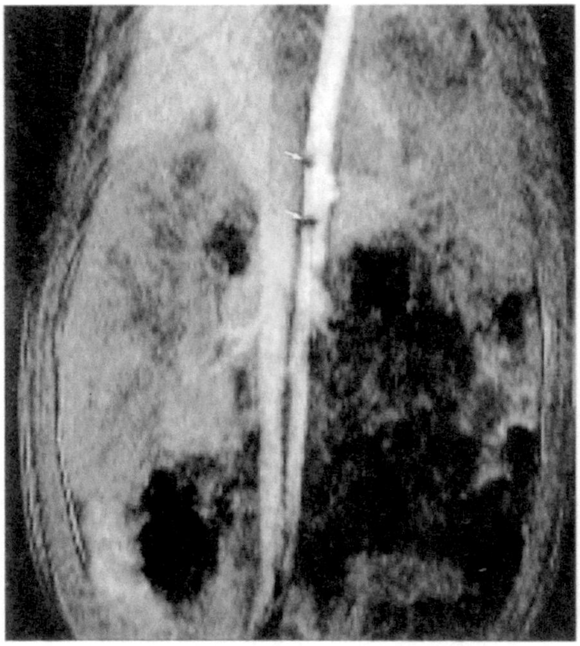

a

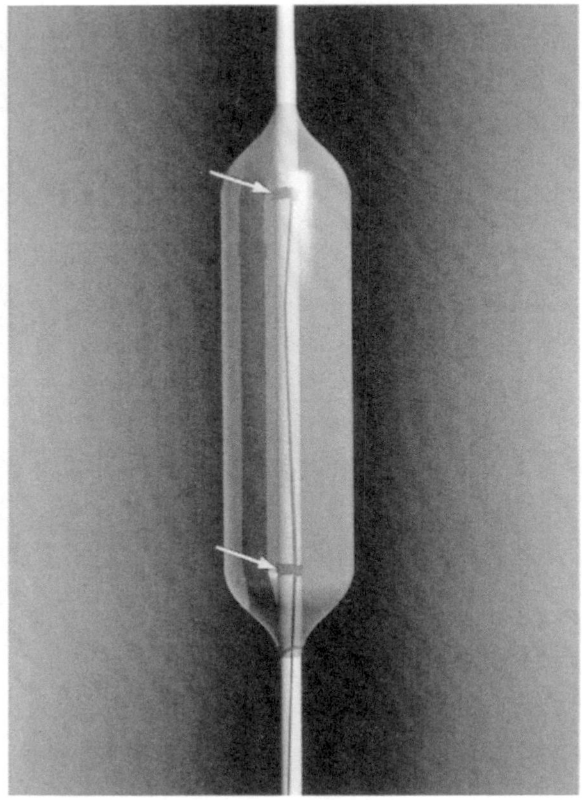

b

Fig. 7.7. **a** Local inhomogeneities mark beginning and end (*arrows*) of the balloon. **b** The two markers (*arrows*) establish the local fields that mark the balloon

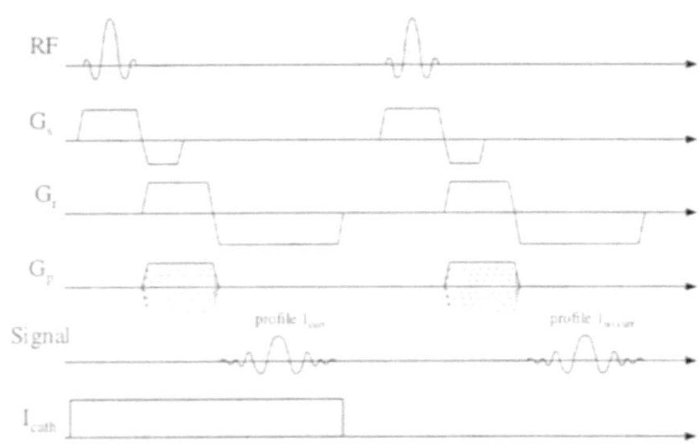

Fig. 7.8. Timing diagram of a gradient echo sequence used for subtraction imaging. The additional line at the *bottom* indicates when the current in the catheter is switched on or off. Two subsequent TRs scan the same line in k-space

the previous section, the anatomic image has the same quality as a scan with two signal averages. Although the catheter will be less well displayed in the anatomic image, one signal average contains the signal void while the other does not, so the subtracted catheter image that was acquired simultaneously can be superimposed on that image. During in vivo experiments, the movement of the tissue has to be taken into account. Therefore, the time between the two echoes that scan the same profile in k-space must be minimized. It is no longer possible to scan both images separately. Instead, the two profiles must be scanned immediately one after another. This requires a little more effort during the designing of the power supply, since the catheter has to be triggered by the MR scanner. Figure 7.8 shows the pulse sequence of a gradient echo sequence. For the first echo, the current in the catheter is switched on. For the second echo, it is switched off. Both echoes scan the same line in k-space. The time between two adjacent profiles is determined by the TR of the sequence. Short TRs prevent artifacts in the subtraction image arising from movement of the background. Figure 7.9 shows images from a pig experiment using the subtraction method with a gradient echo sequence (TR = 9.9 ms, TE = 5.1 ms, $\alpha = 25°$).

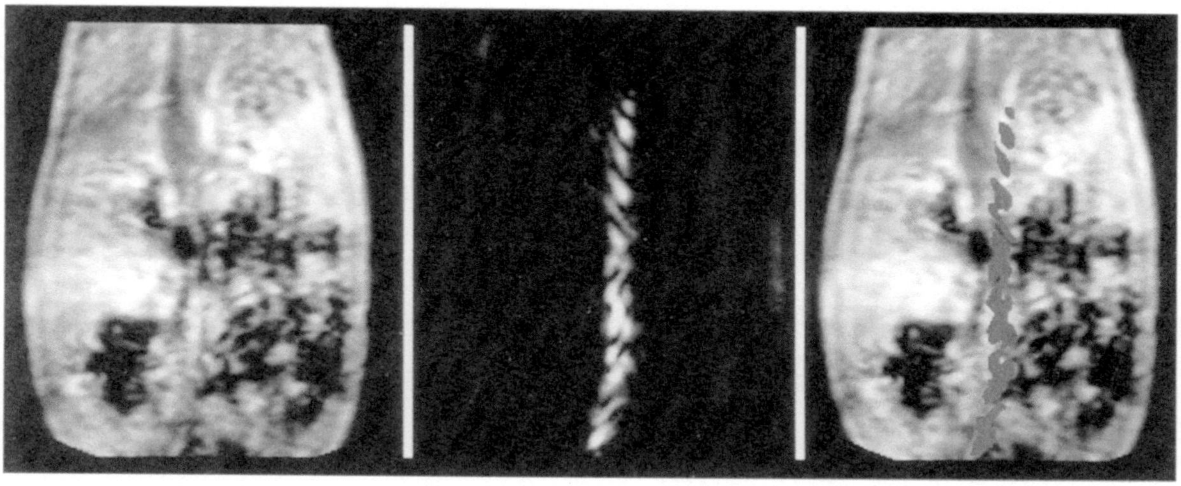

a b c

Fig. 7.9. Subtraction imaging in a pig experiment. The anatomic image (*left*) and the catheter image (*middle*) are acquired with the same scan. The *right* image shows the computed image, where the catheter image is superimposed on the anatomic image

References

Ackerman L, Offutt MC, Buxton RB, Brady TJ (1986) Rapid 3D tracking of small RF coils. In: Proceedings, SMRM, 5th Annual Meeting, Montreal, p 1131

Bakker CJ, Hoogeveen RM, Weber J, van Vaals JJ, Viergever MA, Mali WP (1996) Visualization of dedicated catheters using fast scanning techniques with potential for MR-guided vascular interventions. Magn Reson Med 36:816–820

Dumoulin L, Souza SP, Darrow RD (1993) Real-time position monitoring of invasive devices using magnetic resonance. Magn Reson Med 29:411–415

Glowinski A, Adam G, Bücker A, Neuerburg J, van Vaals JJ, Günther RW (1977) Catheter visualization using locally induced, actively controlled field inhomogeneities. Magn Reson Med 12 (in press)

Jolesz FA, Blumenfeld SM (1994) Interventional use of magnetic resonance imaging. Magn Reson Q 10:85–96

Köchli D, McKinnon GC, Hofmann E, von Schulthess GK (1994) Vascular interventions guided by ultrafast MR imaging: evaluation of different materials. Magn Reson Med 31:209–314

Lenz G, Drobnitzky M, Dewey C (1996) MR-visible catheters for intravascular interventional devices. In: Proceedings, ISMRM, 4th Annual Meeting, New York, p 901

Leung DA, Debatin JF, Wildermuth SW, et al (1995) Intravascular MR tracking catheter; preliminary experimental evaluation. AJR Am J Roentgenol 164:1265–1270

McKinnon GC, Debatin JF, Leung DA, Wildermuth S, Holtz DJ, von Schulthess GK (1996) Towards active guidewire visualization in interventional magnetic resonance imaging. MAGMA 4:13–18

8 Active Visualization – MR Tracking

C.L. Dumoulin

CONTENTS

8.1 Introduction

Magnetic resonance imaging (MRI) is well established in diagnostic radiology and has become the method of choice for diagnosing many disease states. The use of MRI during therapeutic procedures, however, is still in its infancy. Among the many challenges facing interventional magnetic resonance (MR) are: patient access, patient monitoring, MR compatibility of therapeutic devices and the need for real-time visualization. Nevertheless, interventional MRI shows great promise (Jolesz et al. 1988; Bleier et al. 1991; Darkazanli et al. 1992; Kahn et al. 1992; Gewiese et al. 1992; Matsumoto et al. 1992) and is likely to become an important tool in clinical medicine in the future.

Methods for the real-time visualization of invasive devices in an MR scanner can be categorized as either passive or active. Passive methods employ MRI for the visualization of the device within the patient and are typically performed without any special scanner hardware (Lufkin et al. 1987; Koechli et al. 1994; Bakker et al. 1996). Active visualization procedures, on the other hand, require the creation of a signal which is selectively detected or emitted by the device. Active visualization techniques in which light acts as the locating signal have been described (Schenck et al. 1995). Since the body is not transparent to light, however, optical methods can only be applied to devices outside the body. Optical tracking of devices inside the body is possible, but only with the assumption that a fixed geometric relationship exists between the optical markers and the unseen portions of the device.

Active device tracking methods based on radiofrequency (RF) signals have also been described (Dumoulin et al. 1993a, 1995). These methods are not restricted to rigid devices since an RF signal can be easily carried over a flexible cable within the device. Although both optical and RF tracking methods can be used within an MR scanner, use of either technique requires a calibrated mapping of tracking coordinates into MRI coordinates since the distortions of an MR image are unrelated to the spatial distortion of an optical or RF tracking system.

8.2 Principles of MR Tracking

The active visualization method described in this chapter employs magnetic resonance signals which are excited within the entire patient and are detected by the device. Although active visualization methods in which MR signals are detected along the entire

C.L. Dumoulin, General Electric Research and Development Center, P.O. Box 8, Schenectady, NY 12301, USA length of the device have been reported (McKinnon et al. 1994), this chapter will focus on a method in which small receive coils built into the device are tracked (Ackerman et al. 1986; Dumoulin et al. 1993). The method uses the same instrumentation and physical phenomena as MRI and thus can be well registered with an MR image. Unlike most MRI methods, however, MR tracking can be performed at rates as high as 20 frames per second over the entire three-dimensional volume of the patient.

8.2.1 The Sensitivity of a Small Coil

MR tracking of a device relies on the following fundamental principle: if the magnetic field within a volume is made to vary monotonically with position (e.g., in the presence of a field gradient) the Larmor frequency of the sample varies with position. Unlike conventional MRI, however, the MR signal in an MR tracking procedure is detected by a small receive coil which has a limited sensitive volume. Consequently, when the received MR signal is subjected to frequency analysis (using a Fourier transform) a single sharp peak is observed in the power spectrum. The frequency of this peak is indicative of the location of the coil within the sample.

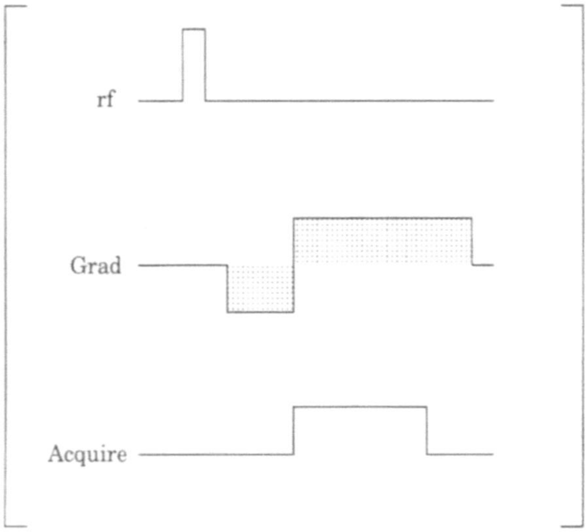

Fig. 8.1. A simple pulse sequence for locating a small coil. A spatially nonselective (RF) pulse is used to excite all nuclear spins within the excitation coil. Data is then acquired in the presence of a magnetic field gradient

8.2.2 The Simplest MR Tracking Pulse Sequence

Several pulse sequences for the localization of a small coil within a sample have been described (Ackerman et al. 1986; Dumoulin et al. 1993). The simplest of these pulse sequences is shown in Fig. 8.1. This sequence employs a spatially non-selective RF pulse which excites all nuclear spins within the volume of the excite RF coil, which is generally positioned outside the body. A gradient-recalled echo is generated with a read-out gradient pulse applied on a single axis. The MR signal is detected in the presence of this magnetic field gradient and a Fourier transform is performed to compute the location of the coil along the axis of the applied gradient, as shown in Fig. 8.2. The entire process is repeated for the two remaining orthogonal gradient axes to render a set of three-dimensional coordinates of the coil.

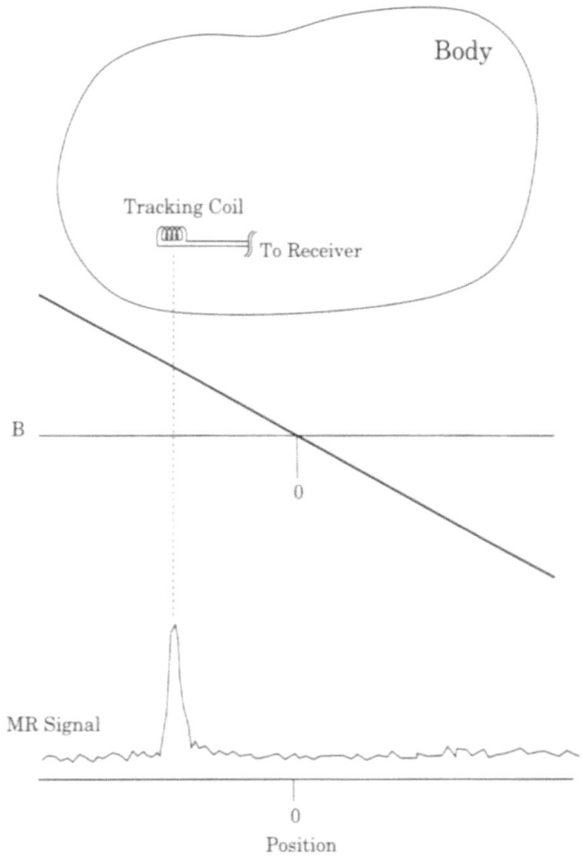

Fig. 8.2. MR signals detected by a small coil are Fourier transformed to give a frequency spectrum. Because the data is acquired in the presence of a magnetic field gradient, the frequency of the signal is proportional to the position of the coil along the gradient

The peak is easily located within the power spectrum by identifying the point having the greatest signal intensity. This method is insensitive to the phase of the peak and works well even when the signal-to-noise ratio is relatively low.

8.2.3 Compensation of Resonance Offset Errors

With the simple pulse sequence shown in Fig. 8.1, any phenomenon which changes the resonance frequency of the detected nuclear spins will create an offset in the detected location of the coil. Potential sources of unwanted offsets include: (1) offset of the transmitter and receiver frequency from the Larmor frequency of the spins, (2) inhomogeneities in the static magnetic field and (3) local inhomogeneities of the magnetic field created by magnetic susceptibility differences of materials within the sensitive volume of the coil. Magnetic susceptibility differences in particular can cause undesired behavior during tracking since the device itself may not have a magnetic susceptibility which exactly matches the surrounding tissue.

Resonance offset errors can be effectively removed during MR tracking if the localizing process is multiplexed. This can be done using the generic pulse sequence shown in Fig. 8.3. Two modulation schemes which can locate a coil with four excitations are possible. In the first scheme, one excitation is performed without a localizing gradient to provide a reference. The other excitations provide positional information for the three orthogonal directions. The X, Y and Z coordinates of the coil are determined by computing the locations as in the simple tracking sequence, but the offset computed from the reference data is subtracted from each location.

The second modulation scheme uses Hadamard multiplexing in which three orthogonal localizing gradient pulses are simultaneously applied during each of the four excitations. The polarity of each gradient pulse is made to vary with each excitation as given in Table 8.1.

Table 8.1. Hadamard modulation of gradient polarities

	Gradients		
Excitation	X	Y	Z
1	–	–	–
2	+	+	–
3	+	–	+
4	–	+	+

The X, Y and Z locations can be easily computed using the following equations where P(ex 1), P(ex 2), P(ex 3) and P(ex 4) are the coil positions determined in the first, second, third and fourth excitations, respectively.

$$X = -P(\text{ex } 1) + P(\text{ex } 2) + P(\text{ex } 3) - P(\text{ex } 4) \quad (8.1)$$

$$Y = -P(\text{ex } 1) + P(\text{ex } 2) - P(\text{ex } 3) + P(\text{ex } 4) \quad (8.2)$$

$$Z = -P(\text{ex } 1) - P(\text{ex } 2) + P(\text{ex } 3) + P(\text{ex } 4). \quad (8.3)$$

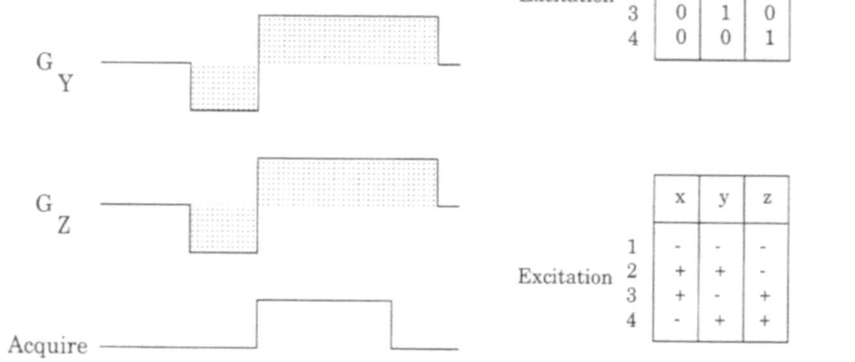

Fig. 8.3 A multiplexed pulse sequence for locating a small coil. As with the simple pulse sequence shown in Fig. 8.1, a spatially nonselective RF pulse is used. During data acquisition, however, magnetic field gradients are applied on all axes. The polarity (or amplitude) of these gradients is varied in each acquisition. With the appropriate modulation scheme, resonance offset artifacts can be removed from the positional data

As with the first modulation scheme, the Hadamard modulation scheme provides X, Y and Z locations in which offset errors have been removed. The Hadamard multiplexing scheme has the additional advantage of providing identical behavior for all three coordinate axes when there are positional changes (i.e., movement) during the acquisition of the four excitations.

8.2.4 Uses of MR Tracking

An MR tracking system such as the one described here is capable of creating a continuous stream of three-dimensional coordinates from the MR tracking coil, which can be incorporated into various instruments used for minimally invasive procedures (Fig. 8.4). These coordinates can be used in a number of ways and present several opportunities for use in medicine (Leung et al. 1995a; Wildermuth et al. 1997a; Steiner et al. 1997). For example, the stream of coordinates can be used to provide a real-time representation of the location of the coil. This representation can be a numeric output, or it can be a graphic symbol superimposed on an image. With a graphic representation, movement of the coil is instantaneously reflected as a change of position of a cursor or icon displayed upon a reference image (Fig. 8.5). It is important to note that any image can be used as a reference. The image could be a conventional spin-echo or gradient- echo MR image, an MR angiogram, a CT image or even a live video image of the patient.

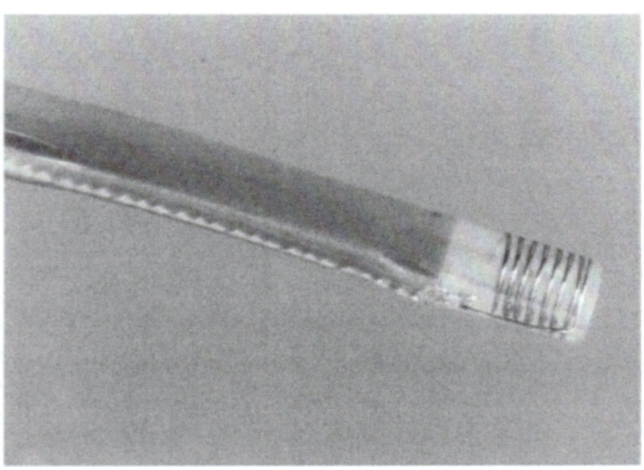

Fig. 8.4. A close-up of a catheter tip, equipped with a tracking coil. The coil is made of copper and has a diameter of 1.2 mm. It is coated to prevent exposure of the toxic copper to body fluids. The coil can be seen to be connected to a coaxial cable, which carries the tracking signal to the scanner

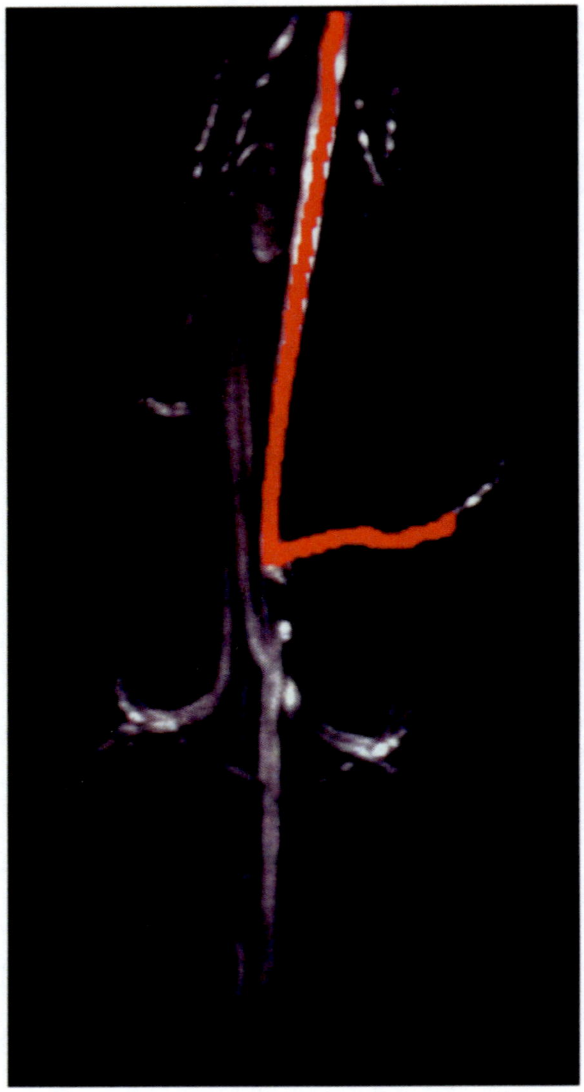

Fig. 8.5. The tip of an MR tracking catheter, introduced through the carotid artery of a fully anesthetized pig, has been tracked through the descending aorta into the splenic artery. A coronal MR angiogram served as the "road map" image. The course of the catheter tip has been marked in red

A second way in which the coordinate stream provided by an MR tracking system can be used combines the imaging and tracking functions of the MR scanner. With this approach the MR scanner identifies the location of the coil and then uses that location to position a subsequent MR image. The entire process can be repeated continuously so that as the tracked coil is moved within the body, MR images of the patient containing the device are always available. This "guided-scan" mode of operation may be particularly useful for biopsy-needle placement and for imaging of moving joints (Daniel et al. 1997).

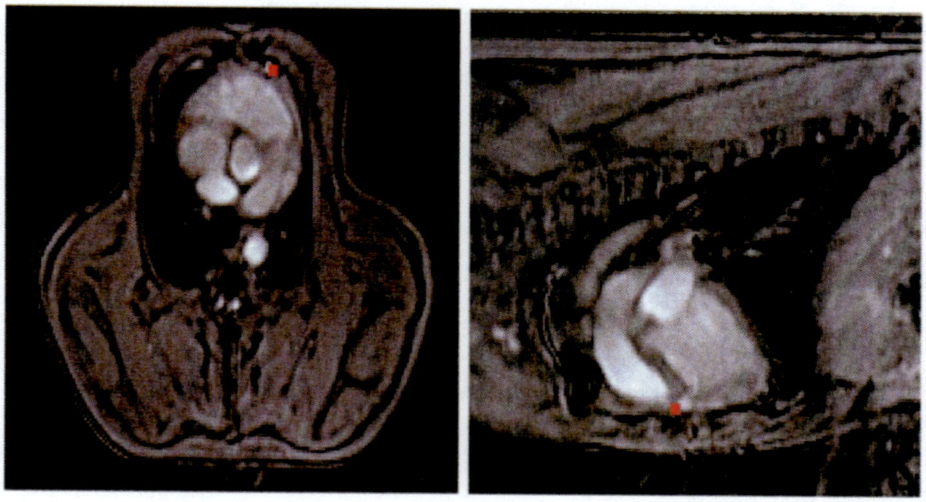

Fig. 8.6a,b. A coil-tipped MR tracking catheter has been intoduced into the left anterior descending coronary artery of a fully anesthetized pig. The catheter tip position is visualized both on EKG-gated gradient-echo images (cine-mode) in both **a** the axial and **b** the sagittal plane

8.2.5 Biplane and Three-Dimensional Display

It has been noted previously in this chapter that MR tracking can be employed using any image as a reference. One method which exploits the arbitrary image plane capability of MRI is to superimpose the tracking icon on two independent images. Since MR tracking provides a stream of three-dimensional coordinates, relatively little computation is needed to superimpose an icon on as many image planes as desired, even if the images are oblique to one another. Biplane formats similar to those used in X-ray fluoroscopy are relatively straightforward. For example, interventional vascular procedures in which orthogonal maximum pixel projection images from three-dimensional MR angiograms are used as reference images have been demonstrated (Leung et al. 1995b) (Fig. 8.6) .

8.2.6 Tracking Multiple Devices

In the tracking pulse sequences described above, a nonselective RF pulse is employed to create the MR signal. This ensures that an MR signal will be detected by the tracking coil regardless of it location within the RF excitation coil. Because the location of the tracked coil is not restricted within the volume of the excitation coil, and since small RF coils do not interact unless they are very close to each other, simultaneous tracking of multiple coils is possible. Multiple coils can be tracked by time multiplexing a single receiver channel between the tracked receive coils, or by employing a full receiver chain for each coil. Also, tracking of multiple coils can be used to monitor multiple positions within a single device, or to monitor the location of multiple devices (Fig. 8.7).

8.3 Characteristics of an MR Tracking Device

Many factors go into the design and construction of an invasive device. For example, careful consideration should be given to the choice of materials used in the construction of the device. Materials must be bio-compatible and sufficiently durable to prevent breakage during normal use. The materials must also withstand the rigors of sterilization.

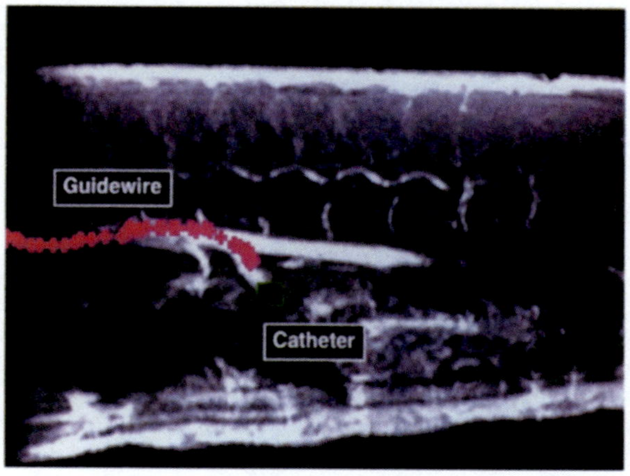

Fig. 8.7. The tips of a coil-tipped tracking guidewire and a catheter are tracked simultaneously in the descending aorta of a fully anesthetized pig. The vascular anatomy is displayed in the sagittal plane. The tip of the catheter has been placed in the superior mesenteric artery. While the catheter was left in position, the guidewire was slowly withdrawn. The course of the guidewire is marked

In addition to the factors which are normally considered for the construction of an invasive device, an MR tracking device must have certain attributes. For proper operation it must not only be compatible with MRI but must also have the appropriate characteristics for MR tracking.

8.3.1 MR Compatibility

Perhaps the most obvious aspect of an MRI-compatible invasive device is that it cannot be ferromagnetic. Devices which are constructed with ferromagnetic materials will exhibit an attraction to the static magnetic field of the MRI system. This attraction can occur with a substantial amount of force and can result in serious injury to the patient.

Ferromagnetism, however, is not the only magnetic property which renders an invasive device unsuitable for use in an MR scanner. Devices constructed with materials which are not ferromagnetic, but have a magnetic susceptibility which is different from that of human tissue, can create large signal voids in MR images. The effect is exacerbated at higher field strengths and with longer echo times, particularly for gradient-recalled echo imaging sequences.

Another consideration for the construction of an invasive device to be used during MR scanning is the geometry of the device. Devices which contain an electrically conducting loop have the potential to couple with the RF excitation coil of the MR scanner. The consequence of this coupling can be a localized change in signal intensity in the image or, in some cases, a "focusing" of RF power into a small region within the patient with the corresponding generation of heat. It should be noted that an electrically conducting loop need not be entirely composed of the device since biological tissue is itself conducting.

In light of the potential for problems with metallic materials, it is prudent to choose nonmetallic materials for device construction whenever possible. Many plastic and ceramic materials have been demonstrated to be suitable for use in an MR environment. Nevertheless, the potential for magnetic susceptibility induced artifacts should be considered when constructing a device. Since the severity of a susceptibility-induced artifact is influenced by the size and shape of the material, as well as the strength of the magnetic field, evaluation of a new material for device construction should be performed carefully.

8.3.2 MR Tracking Compatibility

In addition to all the attributes which make a device suitable for use in an MR scanner, MR tracking devices contain several that are unique. Since an MR tracking device must propagate an RF signal from one or more receive coils to the MRI system, it must contain some electrically conducting material. Fortunately, non-ferromagnetic miniature coaxial cables having a minimum of susceptibility-induced artifacts are readily available.

An important consideration in the construction of an MR tracking device is the sensitivity of the receive coil. Unfortunately, many invasive devices are by necessity small and it is difficult to incorporate tuning and matching elements into the device. The lack of these elements makes it difficult to achieve an impedance match between the coil and the MR system's preamplifier which in turn results in a decrease in the signal-to-noise ratio of the tracking signal. Nevertheless, simple coils constructed without tuning and matching elements can have been shown to have sufficient sensitivity for MR tracking.

Since the MR tracking method described in this chapter requires the detection of signal from the local neighborhood surrounding a small coil, any other signal source in the device has the potential to disturb tracking. For example, if a twisted pair cable is used to carry the MR signal from the tracking coil to the MR system, MR signals present along the length of the cable may be unintentionally received and sent to the preamplifier. If these corrupting signals exceed the signal detected by the tracking coil,

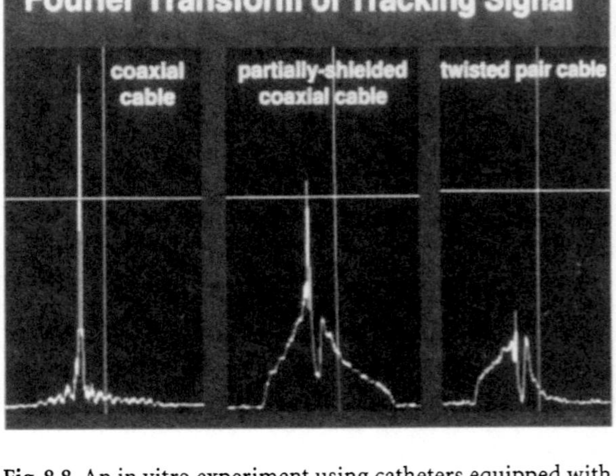

Fig. 8.8. An in vitro experiment using catheters equipped with various cables. Only the fully shielded coaxial cable permits tracking on a well-defined frequency peak with a sufficiently high signal-to-noise ratio.

tracking of the device becomes impossible. Coaxial cables provide greater shielding than twisted-pair cables and typically perform much better for MR tracking (Fig. 8.8).

8.3.3 Multiple Coils

MR guidance of more complex procedures may necessitate tracking of multiple coils. This may be incorporated into a single device for better determination of its orientation or, in the case of a flexible device, such as a catheter, the curvature of the device can be made visible.

In an invasive device having multiple tracking coils, it is necessary to propagate the detected MR signals to the MR system for detection and display. The designer of such a device might be tempted to combine the signals from multiple coils into a single receiver channel, rather than send the signals detected at each coil to a separate receiver. While this may make construction of the device easier and reduce the overall cost of the tracking system, it presents severe, and perhaps insurmountable barriers to safe use. Signals from multiple coils which are detected with a single receiver cannot be guaranteed to be always differentiated by the tracking software. For example, if a two-coil device is constructed such that the coils are placed in series, the Fourier transform of the detected MR signal for tracking will have two peaks. These two peaks will overlap, however, whenever the tracking magnetic field gradient is orthogonal to the line formed by the two coils. Consequently, it is possible that as the device orientation changes during an interventional procedure, the two peaks will coalesce causing the identification of each peak to become ambiguous. Schemes in which the sensitivity of each coil is made different (e.g., by constructing each coil with a different number of turns) may help somewhat, but do not guarantee correct identification of the peaks all the time.

Tracking of multiple devices, each equipped with a tracking coil, is also possible (Fig. 8.8). Since the signal of each coil is fed into a separate receiver, multi-device tracking can be performed simultaneously, without loss in temporal resolution. The number of devices that can be tracked simultaneously is limited by the number of receivers available on the MR system (Fig. 8.7).

8.4 Safety Considerations for Interventional MRI

The most important consideration in the design and use of any diagnostic or therapeutic system is the safety of the patient. While the safety issues of active MR visualization are not unique, the use of invasive devices with an MR scanner is novel enough that a full analysis of safety concerns is warranted prior to the routine use of invasive devices with an MR scanner.

8.4.1 Registration of Tracking Data with an MR Image

The inherent registration of MR tracking data with an MR image is typically very good. This is because the same physical process and instrumentation are used for both imaging and tracking. Nonlinearities in the magnetic field gradients of the MRI system are reflected both in the image and the tracking data. Care should be taken, however, to guarantee that any correction for spatial non-linearities is applied to both the tracking and the imaging data.

While the uses of MR tracking parallel those of an X-ray fluoroscope, there is one important distinction between the two methods. An X-ray fluoroscope provides a real-time image of both the patient and the invasive device, whereas current MR tracking systems do not provide simultaneous tracking and imaging. Consequently, a user of the methods described in this chapter always performs the procedure with a "road map" image rather than one which reflects the immediate condition of the patient.

Although not a serious limitation for most clinical applications, the use of a road map image does present some restrictions, just as it does when used in X-ray fluoroscopy. For example, care must be taken to minimize patient motion during the procedure to ensure that the viewed image is registered with the tracked data. Often, patient cooperation is sufficient to maintain tracking registration with the image.

In some MR tracking applications, physiological motion must be compensated. For example, breathing displaces many of the organs in the abdomen by several centimeters. This displacement can be monitored using a variety of methods, including navigator echoes (Ehman and Felmlee 1989). These navigator echoes provide a one-dimensional image of the patient's anatomy and can be acquired in real-time. If the RF excitation pulses are properly placed so that the one-dimensional image contains both the liver and lung of the patient, the location of the diaphragm can be easily monitored. This one-dimensional image can be used to provide a numeric value corresponding to the location of the diaphragm, which in turn can be used to translate either the image or the tracking icon in real-time. Conversely, the one-dimensional data can be displayed in real-time to provide the operator with an instantaneous representation of the patient's diaphragm.

Cardiac motion can also be monitored by navigator echoes, but a potentially more useful method employs the acquisition of a dynamic road map image. With this method, the road map image is actually a cine loop which is synchronized to the heartbeat of the patient. This method presents certain technical challenges, particularly for a patient with cardiac arrhythmia.

8.4.2 Isolation of the Patient from the MRI System

An important safety consideration in the construction of every interventional system is the electrical isolation of the patient from the system's hardware. A prudent design is robust and will provide full protection to the patient, even if two or more simultaneous failures in the system hardware occur. For example, in an interventional MR system, a properly designed isolation circuit will prevent harm to a patient, even if there is an exposed conductor in one of the coronary arteries and a system failure has placed full-line voltage on the nonisolated side of the circuit.

Two specifications are typically used when designing a patient isolation circuit. These specifications place limits on the current and voltage that a patient can be exposed to in the event of a system failure. While safe limits of current and voltage may vary from tissue to tissue within the patient, in general, the most stringent and widely used safety criterion applies to electrical exposure to the heart. Various regulatory agencies have established a number of criteria. In general, however, any isolation circuit which can protect the patient from at least 4000 V AC and limits the maximum leakage current to 10 μA will meet these criteria.

8.4.3 Heating

Whenever conducting structures are placed in a region which contains changing magnetic and electric fields, transfer of energy into the structure and the generation of heat is possible. An MR scanner generates such changing fields with both its gradient and RF subsystems. In principle, these changing fields can create electrical currents (and hence heat) within the human body and in interventional devices placed within the body.

8.4.3.1 Gradient-Induced Heating

The gradient subsystem creates spatially dependent, changing magnetic and electric fields whenever a magnetic field gradient pulse is applied. Significant heating in patients due to gradient pulses has not been observed, but high gradient switching speeds are known to cause peripheral nerve stimulation.

8.4.3.2 RF-Induced Heat

The RF excitation subsystem also creates changing magnetic and electric fields within the patient, but at a much higher frequency than the gradient subsystem. At these high frequencies, the human body is somewhat lossy (i.e., not perfectly transparent to the RF energy), and some of the energy in the RF pulse is converted to heat. Limits on the amount of heat which can be delivered to the body, head and local tissue have been established by regulatory agencies. The most commonly used measure for heat deposition with an MR scanner is the "specific absorption rate" (SAR), which is given in watts per kilogram of tissue. One commonly used limit for local tissue heating is "8 W/kg in any gram of tissue" (International Electrotechnical Commission IEC 601-2-33).

While much is known about the deposition of heat in the human body during an MR scan, relatively little is known about the generation of heat in or near interventional devices. Nevertheless, some experiments have been performed (Maier et al. 1995; Wildermuth et al. 1997b) which suggest that, under certain conditions, the RF pulses of an MR scanner can induce high electric fields at the tip of a device, which in turn can cause heating of the surrounding tissue.

In one set of experiments, deliberate actions were taken to generate as much heat as possible at the tip of a copper wire placed in saline solution. These experiments were performed with the body coil of a 1.5-T scanner. The transmitter amplifier gain was set to maximum and a very aggressive fast spin-echo pulse sequence was used. Heat generation was monitored with a fiber optic temperature probe and was found to be localized at the tip of the device. Several different locations and orientations of the copper wire were investigated and the configuration yielding the most heat was used in subsequent measurements.

In one representative experiment, an initial temperature rise of 1.44°C/s was observed as the temperature of the saline was raised 20°C. Using the value of 4200 W s/°C as the heating capacity of saline, the SAR can be computed as

$$\begin{aligned} \text{SAR} &= (\text{temperature rise/s})(4200\ \text{W s/°C}) \quad (8.4)\\ &= 6048\ \text{W/kg} \end{aligned}$$

While this number greatly exceeds every regulatory limit, it must be put in the proper context. It is important to note that the heat observed in these experiments was highly localized and appeared to be deposited in a region approximately 1 mm^3 in volume. Thus, only approximately 1 mg of saline was heated. If one considers the 1 g of saline containing this "hot spot," then the observed SAR is actually

6 W/kg

and falls below the IEC specification of "8 W/kg in any gram of tissue." Despite being within the regulatory SAR limit, in this experiment some portion of the saline was excessively heated. Clearly, the traditional guidelines for SAR are not appropriate when the source of heating is highly localized.

A more useful safety limitation for the deposition of heat in a small region is the maximum local temperature rise. In general, human tissue can survive a local temperature rise of 4°C without difficulty. Using this limit and the assumption that the temperature rise is proportional to the power of the RF pulse, the relationship between RF power and maximum temperature rise can be expressed as

$$\text{temperature rise} = K\,\alpha^2/\text{TR} \quad (8.5)$$

where α is the flip angle, TR is the repetition time and K is constant of proportionality. If the maximum temperature rise is measured under worst-case conditions, then K can be empirically determined. Once K is known, then the maximum acceptable flip angle and minimum acceptable TR of any pulse sequence can be calculated.

8.4.3.3 RF Heating as a Function of Field Strength

It is important to note that the heating reported above was observed at 1.5 T under extreme conditions. Several factors exist which greatly reduce the amount of heating observed under identical conditions, but at lower fields. The first factor is that the power of an RF pulse used for MR imaging is proportional to the square of the magnetic field. Consequently, using this consideration alone, an imaging procedure will generate 1/9 as much heat at 0.5 T as it does at 1.5 T. The second factor is the wavelength of the radiofrequency. For example, at 0.5 T the wavelength of the RF is three times longer than it is at 1.5 T. Consequently, devices appear to be shorter from an electrical point of view and there is less efficient coupling to the excitation coil.

The heating observed in these experiments is not a consequence of active MR visualization of a device. Rather it is the consequence of applying MR pulses in the presence of a long conducting structure. The long conducting structure could be a guidewire, EKG lead or endoscope. Based on the experiments reported so far, it appears that RF-induced heating of interventional devices will only be an issue at the higher field strengths.

8.5 A Comparison of Active and Passive Visualization Techniques

8.5.1 Temporal Resolution

Active visualization of invasive devices during interventional MR procedures has certain advantages and disadvantages with respect to passive methods. For example, only four MR signals are acquired for each localization in an MR tracking procedure. Consequently, tracking rates as rapid as human perception (approximately 20 frames per second) are easily achieved. The temporal resolution of passive methods, on the other hand, is limited to the temporal resolution of the imaging scheme used to visualize the device. While very fast imaging methods, such as spiral scanning and echo-planar imaging, are becoming available, a significant computational challenge remains for the real-time reconstruction and display of these two-dimensional images.

While the MR tracking method provides the location of one or more points within a device, passive visualization methods can provide an image of a large portion of the device. To obtain acceptable temporal resolution, however, passive visualization methods require the collection of two, rather than three dimensions of data. Consequently, procedures employing passive visualization require the invasive device to be manipulated within the confines of the imaging slice.

8.5.2 Spatial Resolution

The spatial resolution of passive and active visualization methods arises from entirely different considerations. The spatial resolution of passively visualized devices is limited by the spatial resolution of the imaging scheme used in the procedure. To make a device visible in a relatively thick image slice, however, it is frequently necessary to intentionally create an artifactual void in the image by doping the device with a substance having a magnetic susceptibility different from that of human tissue. Unfortunately, the size of a susceptibility-induced void varies with the orientation of the device and the direction of the imaging gradient pulses. The dependency on voids decreases the accuracy of device localization while disturbing the visualization of the tissue surrounding the device.

With MR tracking, on the other hand, the limit of spatial resolution is determined by the strength of the localizing magnetic field gradient (as it is in passive methods), as well as the size of the tracked coil. Since it is the most intense signal source within the sensitive volume of the tracked coil which is located, factors which cause the location of the maximum signal within the coil to change will cause a loss in spatial precision and accuracy. In general, the spatial resolution limit of a tracked coil is approximately equal to the coil size, but if the tracked coil incorporates its own MR signal source (Erhart et al. 1997), and if that signal is made to be stronger than the signal arising from the tissue surrounding the coil, then the spatial accuracy limit is determined by the sample size and not the coil size.

8.6 Conclusion

Active visualization of a device using the MR tracking technique described in this chapter is currently being evaluated in several institutions. To date, MR tracking has been used to follow biopsy needles, catheters and external anatomic markers. Almost any device can be made MR trackable by incorporating one or more miniature receive coils. The MR tracking technique uses the MR signal detected by these coils to locate each coil in three dimensions. The location of these coils can be represented in real-time as an icon superimposed upon one or more reference images. Alternatively, the coordinates of the tracked coil can be used to control the imaging plane of the scanner.

The ultimate role of MR and MR device tracking in interventional radiology remains poorly defined. Nevertheless, it is becoming increasingly clear that the use of MRI systems for interventional procedures offers unique possibilities.

References

Ackerman JL, Offutt MC, Buxton RB, et al (1986) Rapid 3D tracking of small RF coils. Proceedings of the 5th Annual Meeting of the Society of Magnetic Resonance in Medicine, Montreal p 1131

Bakker CJ, Hoogeveen RM, Weber J, et al (1996) Visualization of dedicated catheters using fast scanning techniques with potential for MR-guided vascular interventions. Magn Reson Med 36:816–820

Bleier AR, Jolesz FA, Cohen MS, et al (1991) Real-time magnetic resonance imaging of laser heat deposition in tissue. Magn Reson Med 21:132–137

Daniel BL, Norbash AM, Butts K, et al (1997) Active scan plane registration during dynamic musculoskeletal MR imaging using an external MR-tracking coil. Proceedings of the 5th Annual Meeting of the Society of Magnetic Resonance, Vancouver, 1927

Darkazanli A, Hynynen K, Damianou C, et al (1992) MRI guided ultrasonic surgery. Proceedings of the 11th Annual Meeting of the Society of Magnetic Resonance in Medicine, Berlin p 591

Dumoulin CL, Souza SP, Darrow RD (1993b) Real-time position monitoring of invasive devices using magnetic resonance. Magn Reson Med 29:411–415

Dumoulin CL, Darrow RD, Schenck JF, et al (1995) Tracking system to follow the position and orientation of a device with radiofrequency fields. US patent 5,377,678. US Patent and Trademark Office, Department of Commerce, Arlington, Va

Dumoulin CL, Darrow RD, Schenck JF, et al (1993a) Tracking system to follow the position and orientation of a device with radiofrequency field gradients. US patent 5,211,165. US Patent and Trademark Office, Department of Commerce, Arlington, Va

Ehman RL, Felmlee JP (1989) Adaptive technique for high-definition MR imaging of moving structures. Radiology 173:255–263

Erhart P, Ladd ME, Steiner P, et al (1997) Tissue-independent MR tracking of invasive devices with an internal signal source. Magn Reson Med (in press)

Gewiese B, Beuthen J, Fobbe F, et al (1992) MRI-controlled laser-induced interstitial thermotherapy (MR-LITT). Proceedings of the 11th Annual Meeting of the Society of Magnetic Resonance in Medicine, Berlin, p 793

Jolesz FA, Bleier AR, Jakab P, et al (1988) MR imaging of laser-tissue interactions. Radiology 168:249–253

Kahn T, Ulrich F, Bettag M, et al (1992) MR guided laser interventions in cerebral gliomas. Proceedings of the 11th Annual Meeting of the Society of Magnetic Resonance in Medicine, Berlin, p 731

Koechli VD, McKinnon GC, Hofmann E, et al (1994) Vascular interventions guided by ultrafast MR imaging: evaluation of different materials. Magn Reson Med 31:309–314

Lufkin RB, Teresi L, Hanafee WN (1987) New needle for MR-guided aspiration cytology of the head and neck. Am J Radiol 149:380–382

Leung DA, Debatin JF, Wildermuth S, et al (1995a) Real-time biplanar needle tracking for interventional MR imaging procedures. Radiology 197:485–488

Leung DA, Debatin JF, Wildermuth S, et al (1995b) Active visualization of intravascular catheters with MRI: in-vitro and in-vivo evaluation. Am J Radiol 164:1265–1270

Maier SE, Wildermuth S, Darrow RD, et al (1995) Safety of MR tracking catheters Proceedings of the 3rd Annual Meeting of the Society of Magnetic Resonance, Nice, p 497

Matsumoto R, Selig AM, Colucci VM, et al (1992) Real-time MR monitoring of cryoablation in the liver: predictability of the histological outcome. Proceedings of the 11th Annual Meeting of the Society of Magnetic Resonance in Medicine, Berlin, p 794

McKinnon GC, Debatin JF, Leung DA, et al (1994) Towards visible guide wire antennas for interventional MRI. Proceedings of the 2nd Annual Meeting of the Society of Magnetic Resonance, San Francisco, p 429

Schenck JF, Jolesz FA, Roemer PB, et al (1995) Superconducting open-configuration MR imaging system for image guided therapy. Radiology 195:805–814

Steiner P, Erhart P, Heske NL, et al (1997) Active biplanar tracking for biopsies in humans. Am J Radiol (in press)

Wildermuth S, Debatin JF, Leung DA, et al (1997a) MR-guided percutaneous intravascular interventions: evaluation of preliminary catheter design. Radiology 202:578–583

Wildermuth S, Dumoulin CL, Pammatter T, et al (1997b) MR-guided percutaneous angioplasty: assessment of tracking safety, catheter handling and functionality. Cardiovasc Intervent Radiol (in press)

9 Active Visualization – MR Profiling

M.E. Ladd

CONTENTS

9.1 Introduction

Reliable visualization of instruments inside the body is essential for safe and successful execution of interventional procedures. The device should be easy to identify in the MR image and should be visible throughout the procedure under various imaging conditions. An ideal method would provide some form of high contrast signature for the device, along with high resolution for accurate placement. An additional requirement is speed, to provide the real-time feedback necessary for interactive guidance.

The simplest and most elegant method of visualizing an instrument is to make it visible in the MR image itself. Unfortunately, attempts to visualize instruments as part of the image have encountered several problems due to poor contrast (Bakker et al. 1996; Köchli et al. 1994). The instrument is hard to pick out from the ambient tissue, and thin instruments are particularly difficult to image. Flexible instruments, such as catheters or guidewires, add complexity, since their position is impossible to predict and may lie outside the imaging plane.

"MR profiling" is based on the incorporation of a radiofrequency (RF) coil into the device under consideration. The diameter of the coil is very small; however, the length can be extended over several centimeters. When an image is acquired using this RF coil as the receive antenna, the localized sensitivity of the coil results in an outline of the coil. The surroundings are essentially black (Fig. 9.1a).

Various coil geometries are possible. One approach is to use electrically coupled antennas (McKinnon et al. 1996). The other is to use magnetically coupled antennas, which have been traditionally applied to MR imaging (Burl and Young 1996; Ladd et al. 1997).

Incorporation of RF coils for device visualization has also been used in the "MR tracking" technique (Ackerman et al. 1986; Dumoulin et al. 1993; Leung et al. 1995a,b). In contrast to MR tracking, which enables visualization of the antenna position as a single point in real time, MR profiling allows depiction of the entire length of the device at the cost of reduced temporal resolution. If the profiling coil is incorporated into a flexible device, the complete position and orientation of the device along the axis of the coil can be visualized.

9.2 Example: Vascular Guidewire

Profiling was originally conceived for visualization of vascular interventional devices such as catheters and guidewires. For guidewires, it is especially critical that the entire course of the distal tip be seen. Curves and loops must be fully visible to selectively target small vessels.

A 0.035-in. (0.89-mm) guidewire was constructed with a 6-cm long RF coil integrated into its distal tip (Schneider Europe, Bülach, Switzerland; Fig. 9.2). The coil was attached to the surface coil input port of the MR scanner via a 40-G coaxial cable running through the center of the guidewire. The coil consisted of a loosely wound solenoid in two layers, with approximately 60 total turns. The coil was 0.6 mm in diameter and was covered with a layer of fluoroethylenepropylene, making the tip flexible. The coaxial

M.E. Ladd, MSEE, Department of Medical Radiology, MRI Center, University Hospital Zürich, Rämistraße 100, CH 8091 Zürich, Switzerland

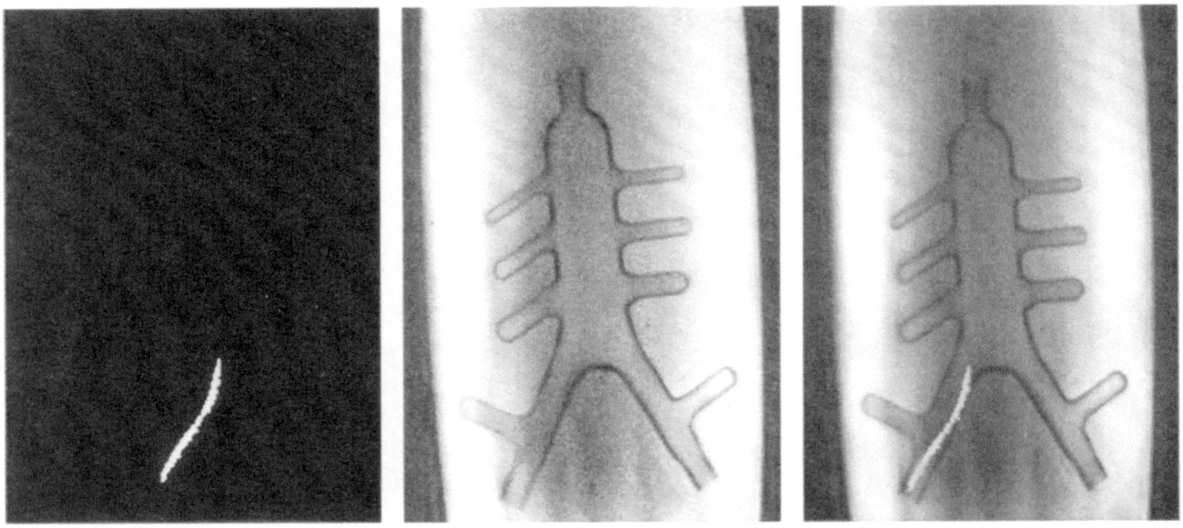

Fig. 9.1. **a** An image acquired with a profiling RF coil. **b** Phantom representing the abdominal aorta and its branches. **c** Superposition of **a** and **b** showing the position of the profiling coil in the phantom

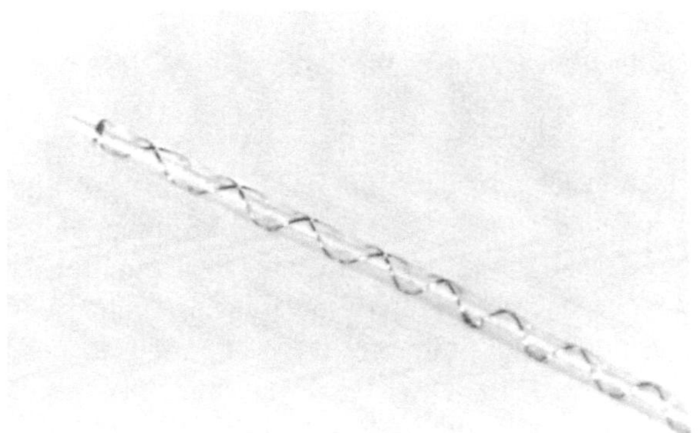

Fig. 9.2. A close-up of the guidewire tip showing the windings of the RF coil. The outer diameter is 0.75 mm (0.035-in. guidewire)

cable was covered with polyetheretherketone, a more rigid plastic, to provide the torque control and mechanical stability necessary for controlling the guidewire during insertion.

The guidewire was tuned and matched with a pair of capacitors at the coaxial cable/scanner interface. Although the quality factor, Q, of the resulting tuned circuit was less than could be obtained with tuning and matching at the RF coil/coaxial cable interface, space saving was an overriding factor.

9.3 Morphology "Roadmap"

Only signal from spins very close to the coil are received and imaged, so the surrounding anatomy is not visualized. To visualize the device in relation to the surrounding tissue morphology, a "roadmap" image, acquired with a separate, conventional RF coil, is required (Fig. 9.1b). The profiling image is superimposed on the roadmap image (Fig. 9.1c).

Since the roadmap acquisition is independent of the profiling acquisition, any imaging sequence showing desired functional or morphologic information can be used as an underlying roadmap image. For example, a high-quality angiogram, requiring an acquisition time of several tens of seconds, can be used for vascular interventions. For intracranial interventions, the use of functional maps could be considered.

The device outline can be superimposed on the roadmap in any desired color. Typically, a simple threshold is performed on the profiling image. All the pixels above the threshold are assigned a color and overlaid on the roadmap. Unique colors allow easy identification when multiple devices are in use, especially if they are being manipulated close to one another.

Breathing or patient motion can lead to misregistration of the profiling image and the roadmap. Patient restraints, some form of respiratory compensation, as well as periodic roadmap updates may be necessary.

9.4 Projection Imaging

For flexible devices, it is important that a visualization technique be capable of following the device as it changes planes and orientation during the course of the intervention. MR profiling accomplishes this by turning off the slice selection gradient when the profiling image is acquired. The result is a projection through the entire body, similar to conventional X-ray. The localized sensitivity of the coil ensures that the device is still imaged with high contrast, regardless of the profiling section thickness.

The projection of the device is superimposed onto the roadmap image. It is not necessary that the device position be at the same level as the roadmap image, and even maximum intensity projection images, covering substantial depths of anatomy, can be used as roadmaps. Biplanar profiling, in which two separate roadmaps are used in orthogonal planes and a profiling projection is collected in both planes, can be used to resolve any device position ambiguities.

9.5 Fast Imaging

To interactively guide a profiling device, image updates, displaying the outline of the device, need to be acquired and reconstructed in real time. With the newer, high-strength gradient systems now commercially available, repetition times of 4-10 ms can be achieved with a standard gradient-echo sequence. For a 256 × 256 matrix size, this implies update times of 1–2.6 s. Several strategies have been developed to allow fast image updates on systems equipped with slower gradient systems, or for increasing the update rate without sacrificing spatial resolution. A sampling of approaches is presented here.

One technique, commonly referred to as, "keyhole imaging" (Duerk et al. 1995; van Vaals et al. 1993), is to acquire a high-resolution map of k-space first, then subsequently sample only the low-frequency lines for the updates. The new k-space lines are combined with the high-frequency lines from the original, high-quality acquisition. The high-frequency lines can also be updated in an interleaved manner, such that all lines are replaced after several acquisitions. Since the low-frequency k-space lines determine image contrast and contain the most important information for a moving device, the resulting images may indeed be adequate for guidance.

A second technique is also based on reduced k-space sampling (Ladd et al. 1996). The largest dimension of the interventional device is known a priori. For the guidewire example above, the largest dimension of the profiling coil is 6 cm. If a 28-cm field of view (FOV) is used for image acquisition, the FOV in the phase direction can be reduced to 7 cm without risk of any part of the device wrapping onto another part of the device. Hence, only 25% of the k-space lines need to be collected, reducing the data acquisition time by 75%. Of course, there is an associated signal-to-noise penalty. When the image is reconstructed, it can be properly unwrapped using the information from a single MR experiment with the frequency-encoding gradient along the phase direction of the image.

A third technique uses wavelet encoding (Wendt et al. 1996). Whereas key-hole imaging is based on updating a selected region in k-space, this technique allows updates of a selected region in image space. A region of interest can be selected around the interventional device, and only that part of the image is updated. Since the device typically represents only a small fraction of the total image area, the required acquisition time is greatly reduced.

Other techniques for fast image acquisition include spiral or ring k-space trajectories and sharing of views for increasing the reconstruction frame rate over the acquisition frame rate (Kerr et al. 1995).

9.6 Safety

9.6.1 Whole-Body RF Exposure

A major safety concern relates to the whole-body RF exposure required to follow a device with regular updates throughout an MR-guided interventional procedure. Various governmental agencies have set limits on the allowable exposure (FDA 1988; NRPB 1991). Most of the limits are expressed as specific absorption rate (SAR), i.e., W/kg, or as a permissible temperature rise. Limits have been specified for whole-body exposure, part-body exposure, length of exposure, etc. Since it is difficult to measure temperature rises in individual patients, the usual approach taken in diagnostic imaging has been to limit SAR.

MR for diagnostic imaging has been in widespread use for over a decade, and no detrimental effects associated with the current limits have been observed. In fact, the SAR limits are probably conservative (Simunic et al. 1996). Exposure during an interventional procedure may be much higher than during a diagnostic examination, reflecting the need for continuous imaging. As long as current SAR guidelines are followed, however, there is little reason to expect negative repercussions.

9.6.1.1 Transmit-Receive Versus Receive-Only

Most surface coils are used for reception only. Another coil, typically the body coil of the scanner, is used for RF transmission. If surface coils are used for transmission, their inhomogeneous excitation fields create non-uniform flip angles across the image, leading to artifacts (Edelstein et al. 1986). For profiling coils, however, homogeneity is not a dominant criterion. The goal is simply to outline the device. Therefore, these coils can be used for both transmission and reception. Usually, transmit-receive delineates the coil better, since the excitation field falls off radially away from the coil. Spins distant from the coil are not excited, so they contribute no signal to the image.

The whole-body RF exposure can be drastically reduced if the coil is used for both transmission and reception. Only a small amount of energy is required to excite spins very near to the coil. For the guidewire example above, the RF transmit power was reduced 70 dB when the profile coil was used for transmission.

9.6.2 Local Tissue Heating

An additional concern arises due to the integration of an RF coil into the device itself. Because of currents induced during transmit, local tissue heating could potentially occur around the coil or along the coaxial cable used to connect the coil to the scanner. If the body coil is used for transmit, part of the energy can be coupled into the cable and coil. The coupling to the coil itself can be reduced by detuning the coil during transmission. If the decoupling fails, it has been demonstrated that, for conventional, external surface coils, the increased SAR can induce significant local heating (Buchli et al. 1989). The coupling to the coaxial cable is more difficult to reduce.

Significant temperature increases have been demonstrated around MR tracking coils when using RF-intensive imaging sequences such as fast spin echo (Maier et al. 1995). These experiments were conducted at 1.5 T under worst-case scenarios, i.e., no heat conduction or convection, catheter perpendicular to the static field of the imager, etc. At smaller field strengths, RF heating is less problematic because of the lower RF transmit power required (Maier et al. 1995). These experiments also demonstrated that most of the heating was due to coupling to the coaxial cable, not to the coil itself.

With regard to possible heating effects, MR profiling coils are similar to MR tracking coils. Thus, the same precautions for safe use should be observed. When used in the receive-only mode, no RF-intensive imaging should be conducted. Since gradient-echo sequences with moderate flip angles are typically used for guiding interventional procedures, this is not a significant handicap. If an RF-intensive imaging sequence, such as a fast spin-echo scan, is desired, the interventional device should be removed prior to acquisition of the data.

As mentioned before, MR profiling coils can be used in the transmit-receive mode rather than the receive-only mode. Although the RF transmit power is significantly lower than when the body coil is used for transmission, and although significant coupling to the coaxial cable is unlikely, possible heating effects due to transmission along the coaxial cable have not been investigated to date.

These safety concerns will have to be addressed more thoroughly prior to any use of these interventional devices in patients. The fact that no adverse effects have been documented in numerous in vivo experiments with MR tracking or MR profiling coils must be considered encouraging.

9.7 In Vivo Results

The profiling technique, implemented with the vascular guidewire as described above, has been successfully evaluated in a rabbit model. Figure 9.3a shows the guidewire inserted into the left renal artery. A maximum intensity projection image generated from a two-dimensional time-of-flight angiogram (TR 33/TE 10, flip angle 30°, NEX 2, section thickness 4 mm, matrix 256 × 192, FOV 16 cm) is used as the underlying roadmap image. The profiling images were acquired with a gradient-echo sequence (TR 12.7/TE 5.9, flip 30°, receive bandwidth ±16 kHz, no slice selection, matrix 256 × 128, FOV 16

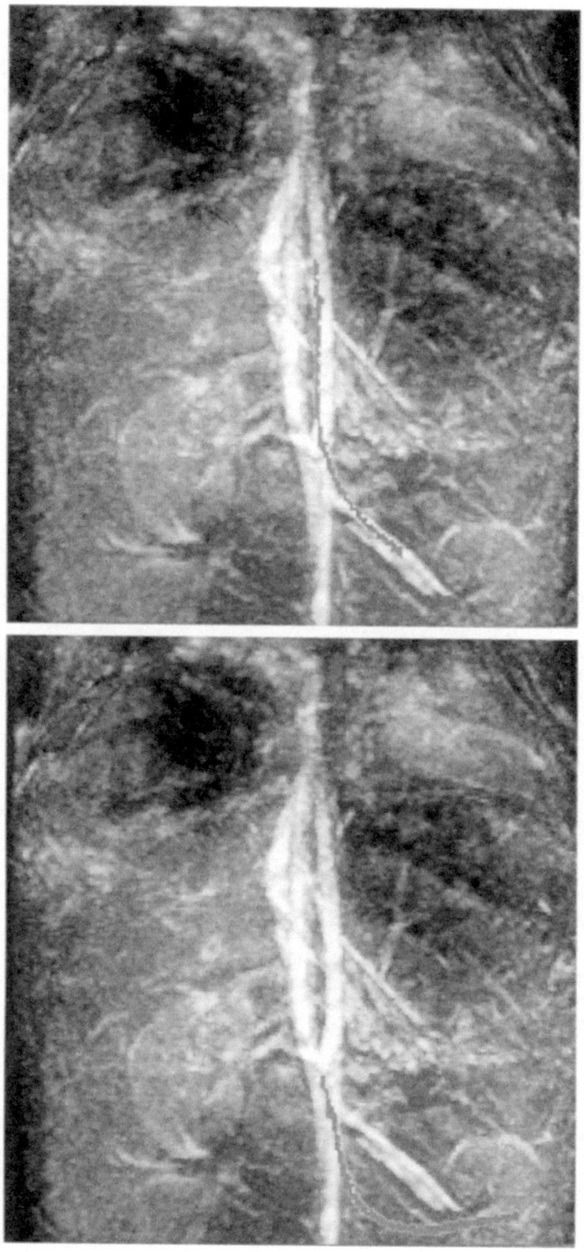

a

b

Fig. 9.3. a A profiling guidewire inserted into the left renal artery of a rabbit. b Curvature of the guidewire after further insertion. Misregistration between the guidewire and the roadmap image demonstrates displacement of the renal artery

cm). The profiling images were updated every 1.6 seconds, reconstructed, and superimposed on the roadmap.

Figure 9.3b displays the guidewire in an inferiorly curved position, indicating that the left renal artery has been forced from its relaxed position by applying too much force to the guidewire. This example illustrates the importance of visualizing the entire length of the guidewire tip, as opposed to merely a single point at its tip.

9.8 Conclusion

MR profiling provides a robust means for visualizing thin, flexible devices, including catheters and guidewires. A long, slender RF coil, integrated into the tip of the device, provides a high-contrast signal. For easy delineation from surrounding tissues, any desired color can be applied to the outline of the device, permitting the simultaneous display of multiple devices. Above all, the ability to visualize the position and curvature of the device along its entire length considerably enhances the capabilities of MRI for guidance of intravascular procedures.

References

Ackerman JL, Offutt MC, Buxton RB, Brady TJ (1986) Rapid 3D tracking of small RF coils. (abstract) Proceedings of the 5th Annual Meeting of the Society for Magnetic Resonance in Medicine, Montreal, p 1131

Bakker CJG, Hoogeveen RM, Weber J, van Vaals JJ, Viergever MA, Mali WP (1996) Visualization of dedicated catheters using fast scanning techniques with potential for MR-guided vascular interventions. Magn Reson Med 36:816–820

Buchli R, Saner M, Meier D, Boskamp EB, Boesiger P (1989) Increased RF power absorption in MR imaging due to RF coupling between body coil and surface coil. Magn Reson Med 9:105–112

Burl M, Young IR (1996) A novel coil for catheters or guide wires. (abstract) Proceedings of the 4th Scientific Meeting and Exhibition of the International Society for Magnetic Resonance in Medicine, New York, p 403

Duerk JL, Lewin JS, Wu DH (1995) Application of keyhole imaging to interventional MRI: a simulation study to predict sequence requirements. (abstract) Proceedings of the 3rd Scientific Meeting and Exhibition of the Society for Magnetic Resonance, Nice, p 492

Dumoulin CL, Souza SP, Darrow RD (1993) Real-time position monitoring of invasive devices using magnetic resonance. Magn Reson Med 29:411–415

Edelstein WA, Hardy CJ, Mueller OM (1986) Electronic decoupling of surface-coil receivers for NMR imaging and spectroscopy. J Magn Reson 67:156–161

FDA (Food and Drug Administration) (1988) Guidance for content and review of a magnetic resonance diagnostic device 510(k) application – safety parameter action levels. FDA, Rockville, Maryland

Kerr AB, Pauly JM, Meyer CH, Nishimura DW (1995) New strategies in spiral MR fluoroscopy. (abstract) Proceedings of the 3rd Scientific Meeting and Exhibition of the Society of Magnetic Resonance, Nice, p 99

Köchli VD, McKinnon GC, Hofmann E, von Schulthess GK (1994) Vascular interventions guided by ultrafast MR imaging: evaluation of different materials. Magn Reson Med 31:309–314

Ladd ME, Erhart P, Debatin JF, Hofmann E, Boesiger P, von Schulthess GK, McKinnon GC (1997) Guidewire antennas for MR fluoroscopy. Magn Reson Med 37:891-897

Ladd ME, Erhart P, Göhde SC, Debatin JF, Boesiger P, McKinnon GC (1996) Faster image acquisition for visualizing vascular guidewire tips. MAGMA 4 [Suppl]:305

Leung DA, Debatin JF, Wildermuth S, Heske N, Dumoulin CL, Darrow RD, Hauser M, Davis CP, von Schulthess GK (1995a) Real-time biplanar needle tracking for interventional MR imaging procedures. Radiology 197:485–488

Leung DA, Debatin JF, Wildermuth S, McKinnon GC, Holtz D, Dumoulin CL, Darrow RD, Hofmann E, von Schulthess GK (1995b) Intravascular MR tracking catheters: preliminary experimental evaluation. AJR 164:1265–1270

Maier SE, Wildermuth S, Darrow RD, Watkins RD, Debatin JF, Dumoulin CL (1995) Safety of MR tracking catheters. (abstract) Proceedings of the 3rd Scientific Meeting and Exhibition of the Society of Magnetic Resonance, Nice, p 497

McKinnon GC, Debatin JF, Leung DA, Wildermuth A, Holtz DJ, von Schulthess GK (1996) Toward active guidewire visualization in interventional magnetic resonance imaging. MAGMA 4:13–18

NRPB (National Radiological Protection Board) (1991) Documents of the NRPB, vol II/1. NRPB, Chilton, UK

Simunic D, Wach P, Renhart W, Stollberger R (1996) Spatial distribution of high-frequency electromagnetic energy in human head during MRI: numerical results and measurements. IEEE Trans Biomed Eng 43:88–94

van Vaals JJ, Brummer ME, Dixon WT, Tuithof HH, Engels HE, Nelson RC, Gerety B, Chezmar JL, den Boer JA (1993) 'Keyhole' method for accelerating imaging of contrast agent uptake. J Magn Reson Imaging 3:671–675

Wendt M, Busch M, Lenz G, Bornstedt A, Seibel R, Groenemeyer D (1996) Dynamic tracking algorithm for interventional MRI using wavelet-encoding in 3D gradient-echo sequences. (abstract) Proceedings of the 4th Scientific Meeting and Exhibition of the International Society of Magnetic Resonance in Medicine, New York, p 497

10 External Referencing Systems

R.W. Newman, E.A. Penner

CONTENTS

10.1 Introduction

The value of MR, CT or other diagnostic imaging modalities in assisting in surgical procedures has long been recognized. To extend the clinical utility of these images, stereotactic frames were introduced to allow the spatial information from the computer-based "image space" to be translated back into patient-based "physical space", allowing for increased precision in the planning of interventional procedures. Several computer workstation systems are in clinical use for common stereotactic procedures, such as brain biopsies and, the introduction of stents, lasers, or radiotherapy devices into critical areas. The process is rather complex, however, as it is first necessary to attach a set of fiducials to the patient prior to MR/CT imaging (i.e., a mechanical head frame, implanted markers, skin markers, etc.). A complete volume of images is subsequently collected including the fiducials. These are then transferred to a computer for display. A path for the interventional device is planned on the computer, and calculations are performed for later use. During the interventional procedure it is necessary to accurately locate the fiducials and use them to reference a physical interventional device back into the patient space. This allows the workstation images to be used as a basis to calculate a planned trajectory or show a calculated location of a device.

However, this method has several well-recognized drawbacks:

- The attachment of the fiducials or stereotactic frame to the patient may involve a minor surgical procedure of its own.
- The assumption that, following the generation of the images and the surgical plan, the anatomy will not be altered relative to the fixed external references and that the intraoperative registration of the two volumes can be maintained, is not always fulfilled.
- The "image" displayed on the workstation during the interventional procedure can only show the likely position of the device relative to anatomical features as shown on the pre-operative images. It is not possible to positively demonstrate the position of an interventional device in the actual patient.

With the exception of the head, stereotactic approaches are not possible because intraoperative motion cannot be controlled by patient immobilization, mechanical frames, or other means. Examples of this type of involuntary intraoperative motion are respiratory or cardiac motion and tissue motion following a resection or other means of treatment. Even in the head, where stereotactic frames, or external fiducial markers are commonly used, brain swelling or anatomic shifts following resection can render the spatial information from previously acquired images useless within minutes following the start of the procedure. With the availability of intraoperative MR imaging, it is possible to eliminate the uncertainty resulting from dynamic changes in anatomy and to identify the positive location of devices within the

R.W. Newman, M.S., General Electric Company, P.O.B. 414, Milwaukee, WI 53201-0414, USA
E.A. Penner, PhD, GE Medical Systems, Gregorstrasse 32, D-52066 Aachen, Germany

body. This requires the acquisition of conventional "diagnostic" type images within the operating room during the actual procedure.

Modifications to the MR scanner can allow the physician to use an interactive scan plane pointer system that tracks the position and orientation of a hand-held device to directly acquire images in any scan plane, including multi-angle obliques. This pointer feature can be incorporated into common interventional devices (e.g., biopsy needles, suction tips, and endoscopes). Thus, the interventional device itself becomes a scan plane pointer, similar to the use of an intraoperative ultrasound transducer. The choice of MR imaging parameters and scan protocols is the same as available on current MR systems. The contrast and quality of these interactively acquired MR images are identical to those possible with more conventional scan prescriptions. With the scan plane pointer the interventionalist can rapidly select an MR imaging plane orientation relative to the device and insure maximal control during the procedure. This type of guidance can provide a global view of the total operative field, allowing the physician to move more quickly through areas of complex anatomy while staying oriented to the perspective of the surgical approach.

Several types of pointer system are available, each with its own advantages and disadvantages:

- Mechanical arm systems. These provide accurate spatial mapping of a volume. However, the system itself must be physically mounted at a single point, limiting its working volume. Also, because of the mechanical linkages, it has certain limitations on its movement and access to all points within the imaging volume (Sipos et al. 1996)
- Passive detection systems. These video-based systems use computer analysis from an overhead observation camera to detect a uniquely shaped or colored object that is attached to the interventional device. From these images, the system computes the actual location of the object and calculates the axis and tip of the interventional device. This type of system has the advantage that the pointer can move freely within the observation volume. The limitation is that the tracked object has to remain within the line of sight of the video observation camera and it must be totally unique from any other object that may come into the operative field (Smith et al. 1994)
- Active detection systems. These are systems where the hand-held pointer has an active element that sends a unique radiofrequency, magnetic, or optical pattern that is detected and translated into physical coordinates. As with the passive detection system, the pointer is free to move throughout the observation volume, providing a great deal of flexibility during the procedure.

Because of the metallic cryostat and the magnetic field of the imaging system, the optical systems are the most practical to use in the MR environment at this time. This type of system does have the limitation that it is necessary to maintain line of sight between the pointer and the observation cameras.

10.2 System Description

Belonging to the category of active optical detection systems, the infrared light-emitting diode-(LED)-based Flashpoint tracking system is one of the key features of the Signa SP (General Electric Medical Systems, Milwaukee, Wis.; Schenck et al. 1995; Silverman et al. 1995; Silverman 1996; Steiner et al. 1996; Moriarty et al. 1996). It may be used for the following purposes:

- Scan plane pointer
- Instrument localization and visualization
- Intraoperative guidance

The Flashpoint tracking system consists of a camera system that determines the position and the angular orientation of a custom-built hand-held device within the scanning volume. It provides an intuitive, interactive means to control the scan plane in addition to localizing the tip of an instrument anywhere within the imaging volume. To select the desired scan plane it may be used very similar to an ultrasound probe. Hence, it provides an intuitive means for rapid selection of oblique or double-oblique sections with respect to the instrument.

The tracking system may be used in conjunction with common interventional devices and allows the user to directly acquire an MR image that is aligned with the axis of the interventional device. The operator may select a feature that will apply annotation on top of the MR image to indicate the path and tip of the device.

10.2.1 Principle of Operation

Figure 10.1 shows the principle of operation and how the system has been integrated in the Signa SP (see

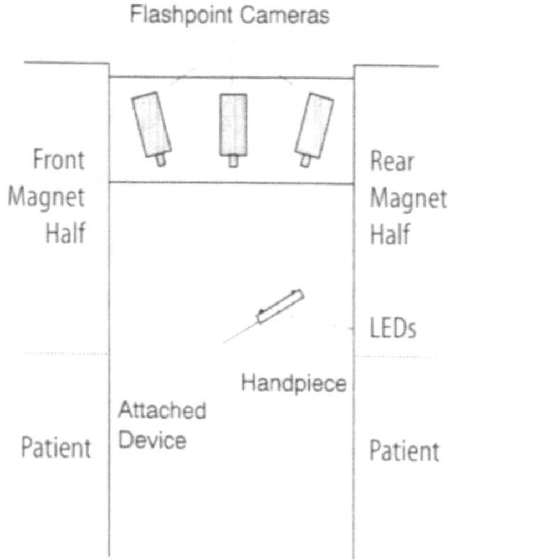

Fig. 10.1. Principle of operation: infrared light-emitting diodes (LEDs), mounted on a handpiece, are tracked by three cameras mounted in the upper magnet bridge connecting the two magnet halves

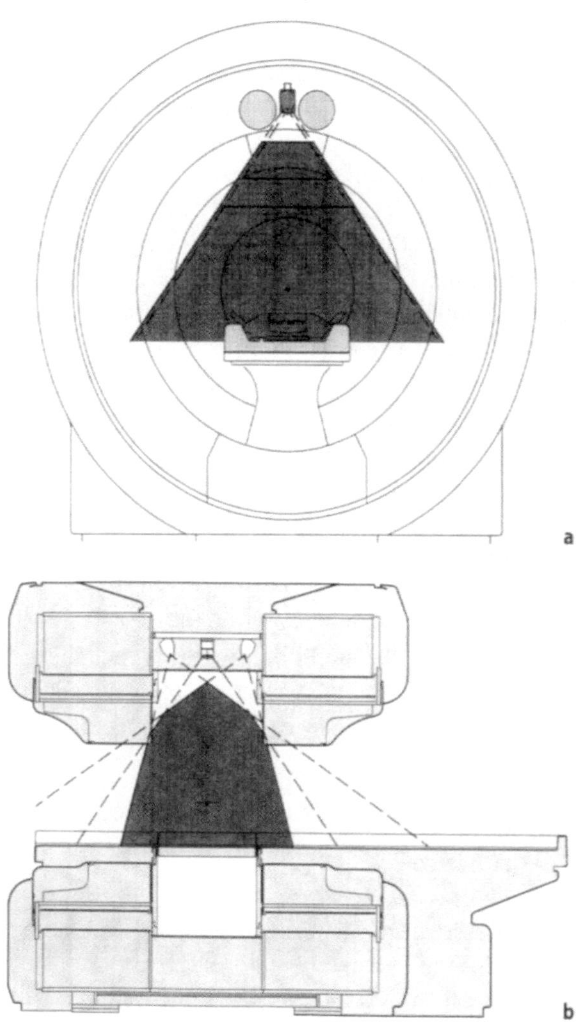

Fig. 10.2. Area of coverage of the Flashpoint cameras: **a** front and **b** side view.

description in Chap. 2). The upper bridge connecting the two magnet halves contains three one-dimensional cameras which track the position of an array of infrared LEDs mounted on a Flashpoint handpiece. Because of the vertical gap design of the magnet, the field of view of the Flashpoint cameras includes and extends beyond the MR imaging volume of the system (Fig. 10.2). Given the positions of the LEDs in three-dimensional (3D) space it is possible to calculate the position and angular orientation of the Flashpoint handpiece. If a device with known mechanical dimensions is attached to the handpiece, it is possible to calculate the position and orientation of the tip of the device. Of course, this type of tracking method is restricted to rigid devices only. A typical example of such an attached and fairly rigid device would be a biopsy needle.

10.2.2 Block Diagram

In Fig. 10.3 a block diagram of the Flashpoint 5000 system and the interconnection to the MR scanner are shown. The Flashpoint handpieces, as well as the camera array have been designed by Image Guided Technologies (Boulder, Colo.; Image Guided Technologies 1996). As shown, the PC is controlling the handpiece-mounted LEDs, which are flashing at different rates to make them distinguishable. The position and angular orientation of one or more Flashpoint handpieces relative to the sensor array is determined by evaluating the corresponding outputs from the cameras mounted directly above the imaging

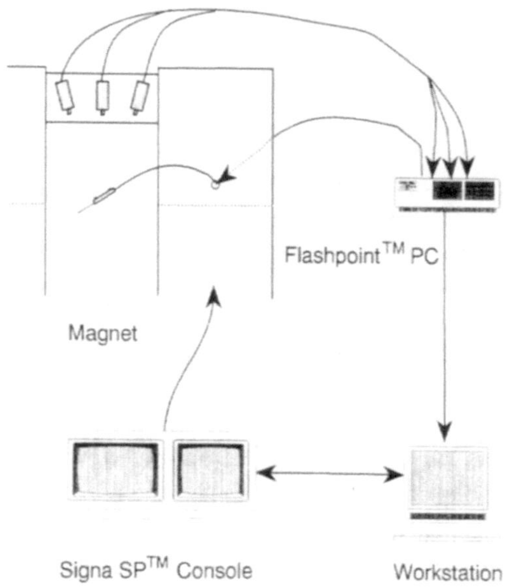

Fig. 10.3. Block diagram and system interconnections.

volume. The locations of the handpieces are transmitted to the workstation. Based on programmed information about the geometrical properties of the interventional device, the instrument's tip position and orientation can be calculated. As part of the process, corrections for geometrical distortions of the MR imaging system are applied. The operator subsequently selects the desired scan plane relative to the interventional device being used. Based on the most recent pointer position detected, the position of the next MR scan to be acquired is transmitted from the workstation to the scanner. Once acquired and reconstructed, the image is displayed with annotations indicating the calculated tip position as well as the projected path of the interventional device. These images are displayed both on the workstation monitor and on the in-bore liquid crystal display monitors in direct view of the physician. The Flashpoint tracking system operates completely independent of the scanning process. Hence there is no compromise in the selection of MR imaging parameters when this type of tracking is in use.

10.2.3 Spatial Accuracy

During system installation, all standard MR system calibration and image quality tests are performed. Following this, the scan plane pointer system is calibrated to align its optical center, the *x*-, *y*-, and *z*-axes, and distance measurements with the imaging isocenter and the *x*-, *y*-, and *z*-axes of the imaging gradients throughout the imaging volume. This first involves a mechanical alignment of the Flashpoint camera system with the center of the imaging volume. During the second step a correlation between the geometry of points in the field of view of the pointer system with those of the MR imaging volume is established. With this correlation, the location in the MR imaging volume corresponding to the physical location of the tip of any pointer device selected by a physician is calculated. It is by this method that the very linear sampling space of the pointer system can be mapped into the characteristic spatial distortions inherent in MR image acquisition. Thus, the physician is provided with the most accurate localization of physical points within the patient as depicted on the MR image.

Following calibration, a final verification of the accuracy of the pointer system is made. It utilizes a special-purpose combination of a pointer device and an attached imaging phantom. The pointer is positioned at isocenter and at 12 registered points around the surface of a 28-cm sphere centered about isocenter. Images are collected for each of these 13 points. An automated image analysis package locates the center point location of each MR image created and compares this with the position reported by the scan plane pointer. The errors are reported and retained as a permanent record of the total pointer system performance. This provides the physician with a quantitative indication of the accuracy of the pointer system in a clinical setting.

In Table 10.1 a summary is given of data compiled from ten Signa SP systems when they were installed at clinical sites. The average error for the pointer system at isocenter was 0.67 mm. The average error for any of the points in a 28-cm sphere was 0.98 mm. The standard deviation for any pointer error was 0.46 mm. The maximum error for any of the points on any of the systems was 2.50 mm.

10.3 Tracking and Guidance

10.3.1 Available Handpieces

In Fig. 10.4 some of the currently available handpieces are shown. The two-LED instrument holder shown in Fig. 10.4a is formed like a pen. It may be used to perform freehand punctures, like body biopsies or percutaneous laser fiber placement. The three-LED guide is shown in Fig. 10.4b. There is a 5-mm hole at the center of the handpiece. The handpiece can either be mounted directly onto an instrument or small adapters may be used (see figure) with varying inner diameters providing guidance for needles or other cannulas passed perpendicular to the LED array. In the latter case, the handpiece can be fixed in position by attaching it to a mechanical positioning arm. Other handpiece configurations are possible to allow a wide range of interventional or surgical devices to be used as scan plane pointers.

10.3.2 Definition of Scan Planes

As mentioned above, the position of the Flashpoint handpiece, or – to be more accurate – the position of the tip and the orientation of the interventional device, determines the position and orientation of the next image which will be acquired by the Signa SP.

Table 10.1. Scan plan pointer calibration results (all distances in millimeters)

Isocenter	Site 1 0.55	Site 2 0.31	Site 3 0.48	Site 4 0.73	Site 5 0.73	Site 6 1.26	Site 7 0.95	Site 8 0.40	Site 9 0.83	Site 10 0.47
Points on 28 cm sphere										
1	0.33	1.19	0.57	0.37	0.66	1.81	1.95	0.38	1.04	0.49
2	0.57	0.91	0.67	0.46	1.13	1.82	1.58	0.41	1.35	0.73
3	1.15	0.52	0.94	2.04	0.65	1.17	1.61	0.76	1.40	0.61
4	0.57	0.63	0.54	1.08	0.45	1.06	1.46	1.00	1.02	0.55
5	1.20	1.26	0.75	0.72	1.32	1.91	1.04	0.43	0.43	0.49
6	0.62	1.05	1.04	1.85	1.20	1.36	2.50	1.61	1.36	0.57
7	1.58	1.27	1.46	0.37	1.05	1.36	1.47	0.44	0.84	0.50
8	1.04	0.74	0.43	1.28	0.33	1.96	0.60	0.52	1.64	0.53
9	1.06	1.32	0.58	1.29	0.50	0.61	0.97	0.80	0.95	0.81
10	0.95	1.32	0.96	0.99	0.76	0.87	0.46	0.65	0.99	0.76
11	0.55	1.75	1.47	0.41	0.77	1.14	0.93	0.77	1.15	0.94
12	0.96	0.61	0.56	1.42	1.13	1.10	2.25	1.04	0.61	0.58
Minimum error	0.33	0.31	0.43	0.37	0.33	0.61	0.46	0.38	0.43	0.47
Maximum error	1.58	1.75	1.47	2.04	1.32	1.96	2.50	1.61	1.64	0.94
Mean error[a]	0.86	0.99	0.80	1.00	0.82	1.34	1.37	0.71	1.05	0.62
Standard deviation[b]	0.35	0.41	0.35	0.56	0.32	0.42	0.62	0.35	0.34	0.15

[a]Mean error for all isocenters, 0.67, for all points on a 28-cm sphere, 0.98; for all points
[b]Standard deviation for all points 0.46; 95% confidence interval 1.87

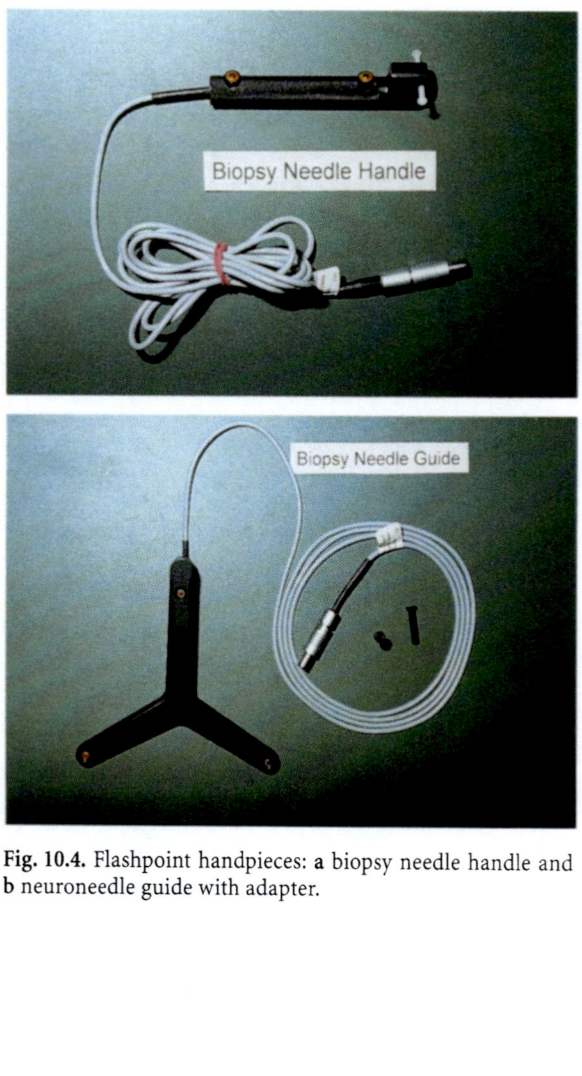

a
b

Fig. 10.4. Flashpoint handpieces: **a** biopsy needle handle and **b** neuroneedle guide with adapter.

The system allows three basic choices of image plane (GE Medical Systems 1997):

1. Conventional axial, coronal, or sagittal planes: the position of the tip of the interventional device determines the center of the next image to be acquired. Therefore, the center of the image will be located at the very tip of the interventional device.
2. Single axis obliques: again, the tip of the interventional device determines the center of the next image to be acquired. In addition, the orientation of the image is selected in such a way that the whole length of the interventional device will be visible in the image. This is achieved by rotating the image plane around the *x*-, *y*-, or *z*-axis, depending on the selections made at the workstation. Hence, the resulting images can either be in the axial-coronal (but never sagittal), in the axial-sagittal (but never coronal), or in the coronal-sagittal (but never axial) plane. On the display monitors the images are depicted in the familiar orientation for axial, coronal, or sagittal images, with the pointer annotation overlaid at an oblique angle, reflecting the current pointer position.
3. Double axis obliques: as above, the tip of the interventional device determines the center position of the next image. The orientation of the image is defined solely with respect to the interventional device in such a way that, once again, the whole

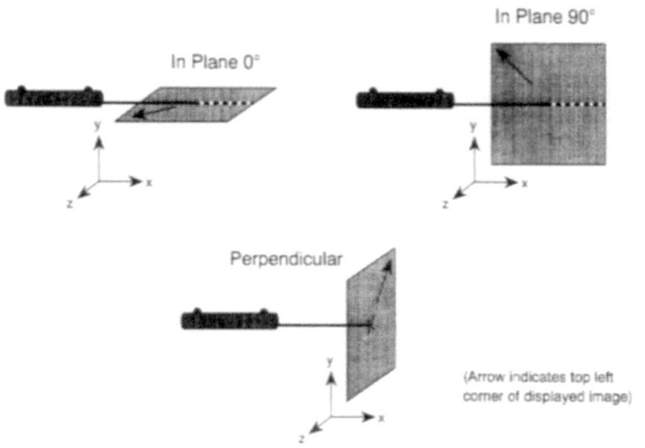

Fig. 10.5. Definition of scan planes relative to the interventional device: **a** In-plane 0°, **b** in-plane 90° and **c** perpendicular.

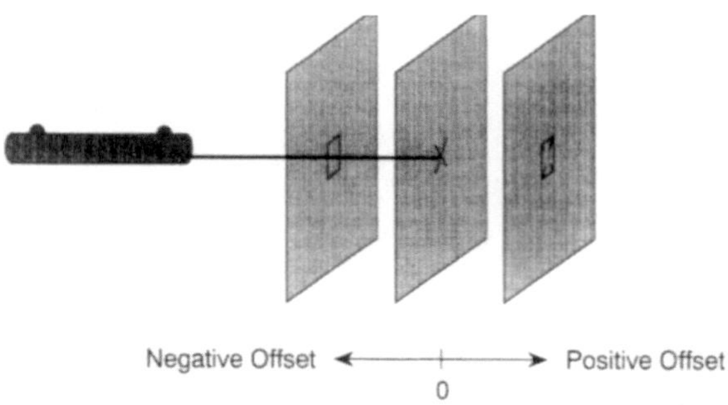

Fig. 10.6. Adding a positive or negative offset shifts the image along the axis of the interventional device, here shown for a perpendicular image. The proximal location is indicated by a *rectangle*, the center position by *X*, and the distal location by a *rectangle* with *X* inside it.

length of the interventional device will be visible in the next image to be acquired. In contrast to the single axis obliques described above, the pointer annotation will be overlaid in a fixed position from the top to the bottom of the image, and the image underneath will move, reflecting the changes in pointer position. This mode is very similar to using an ultrasound probe. Because of its intuitiveness, it has become the most frequently used mode for clinical purposes. For the double axis oblique mode, Fig. 10.5 illustrates three choices of image plane relative to the interventional device: "in-plane 0°," "in-plane 90°," and "perpendicular.". As shown, the perpendicular image will be perpendicular to the axis of the interventional device, with the tip of the device defining the center of the image plane as indicated by the cross in the center of the image. The "in-plane 90°" image contains the axis of the interventional device and is perpendicular to the floor; the representation for the "in-plane 0°" image is rotated 90° to the previously described image acquisition. An arbitrary selection of other angles is also possible. In the in-plane images, the interventional device itself is represented by a line with long dashes, whereas the projected path of the instrument is projected as short dashes onto the current MR image. The tip of the device corresponds with the end of the last long dash in the center of the image. Fig. 10.8 shows an example of such an image with overlaid pointer annotation.

All of the imaging modes described above can be modified by adding a positive or negative offset along the axis of the interventional device. This is shown in Fig. 10.6 for perpendicular images. A typical application would be to position the imaging plane a little bit ahead of the current tip position of the interventional device, for example, prior to penetrating a highly sensitive region. By using a combination of the different imaging modes it is possible to confirm the position of the tip of the instrument with high accuracy. Positive confirmation may be achieved by checking the position of the artifact: typically, the in-plane resolution and hence the accuracy is around 1 mm. The uncertainty resulting from the much larger slice thickness (typically 3–10 mm) can be resolved by checking a second and even a third image acquired in a plane orthogonal to the first image. It is thus possible to positively demonstrate the position of the tip of the interventional device in 3D space with an accuracy around 1 mm relative to the surrounding lesion or anatomy in any direction.

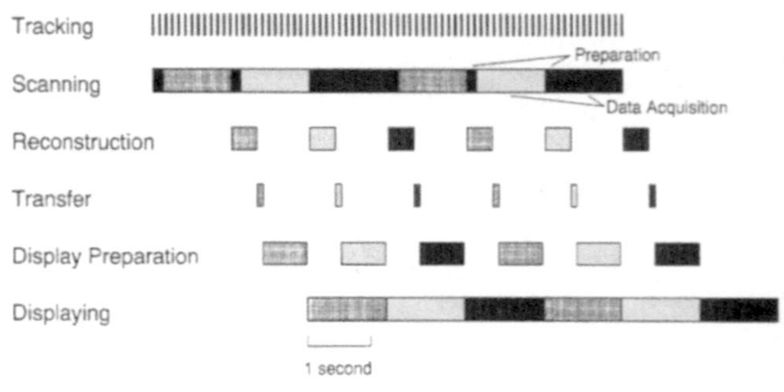

Fig. 10.7. Timing diagram.

10.3.3 Fast Graphics

Owing to basic MR imaging limitations, the speed of the Flashpoint system with a tracking rate of up to ten localizations per second is considerably higher than the approximately 1 s minimum scan time of the Signa SP. In Fig. 10.7 the timing is shown in detail. The upper row shows the tracking information calculated by the Flashpoint system and mapped onto magnet space by the workstation at a rate of ten tracking events per second. When a new scan is prepared, the latest tracking information available will determine the next plane to acquire. The actual image scan time will depend on the necessary MR image contrast and the desired image quality. Following completion of the scan, some time is needed to reconstruct the image [(≈) 0.4 s], to transfer the image to the workstation [(≈) 0.2 s], for display preparation including annotation, and for the projection of the instrument [(≈) 0.6 s] on top of the anatomic image. In total, this adds up to a delay of 1.2 s in addition to the actual MR scan time before the image corresponding to the initial tracking event will be shown on the monitors.

It is possible to accelerate this process considerably by using all of the available tracking information instead of only the information from the very last tracking event prior to the next scan. This option is called "fast graphics" and allows one of two choices:

1. "Freeze" mode: the scanner continues to acquire data in a plane previously selected by the physician. On this frozen, but continuously updated image plane the current position of the interventional device is depicted at a rate of up to ten updates per second.
2. "Tracking" mode: tracking mode may be considered as a combination of the standard mode and the freeze mode. The position of the scan plane is updated with the standard delay of 2–3 s. In addition, as in the freeze mode the actual position of the interventional device is depicted on the image acquired earlier with almost no delay. The fast graphics option is especially useful and helps to minimize total procedure time when high quality scans, requiring longer imaging times, are requested.

10.4 Applications

As described above, there are several types of scan plane pointers that are currently available. Because of the flexibility of the LED-based system being used, it is possible to design additional pointers to support new intraoperative MR procedures as they are developed.

10.4.1 Clinical Accuracy

When using interventional devices with the scan plane pointer, the computed trajectory of the device is displayed on the image as a computer generated icon (Fig. 10.8). The trajectory computation is based on the assumption that the device is introduced in a straight line. Any aberration from a straight course will thus inevitably result in a discrepancy between the calculated and true device position. The probability of the instrument deviating from a straight line is increased if thin instruments are used or if firm tissues need to be penetrated. This is the case in most abdominal and pelvic biopsies (Fig. 10.9). Here it is of particular importance to rely on a second means of instrument visualization, reflecting the true device position. Once the device penetrates the body, it is usually visible on the MR images because of at least one of two effects. The first is independent of the type of material used. It reflects a displacement

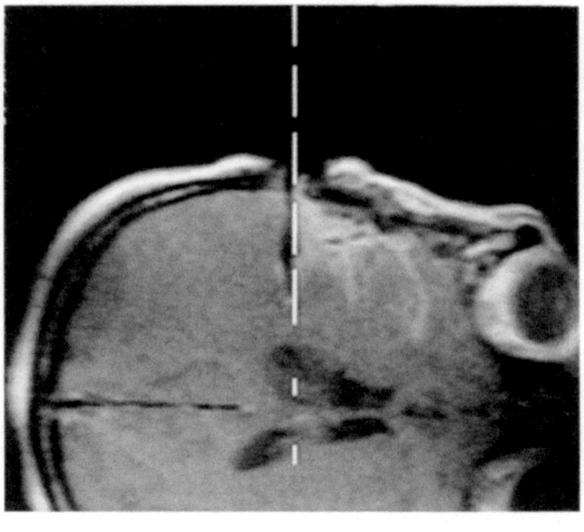

Fig 10.8. Neurobiopsy showing the computer generated icon of the needle trajectory (*long dashed lines*), the extended centerline of the needle trajectory (*short dotted lines*), and the artifact of the needle (black signal void beneath needle icon).

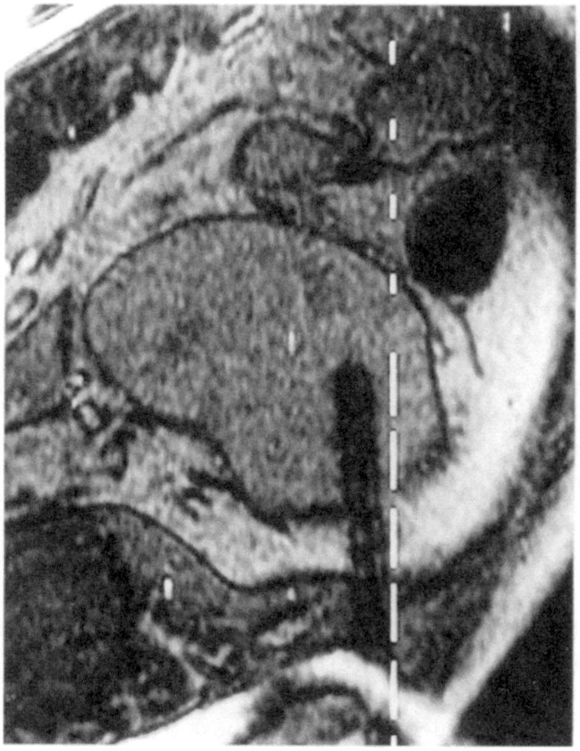

Fig. 10.9. Oblique image of the upper abdomen in a patient undergoing biopsy of a small liver lesion. The calculated needle trajectory (*dashed white line*) is different from the true needle path (*black signal void*).

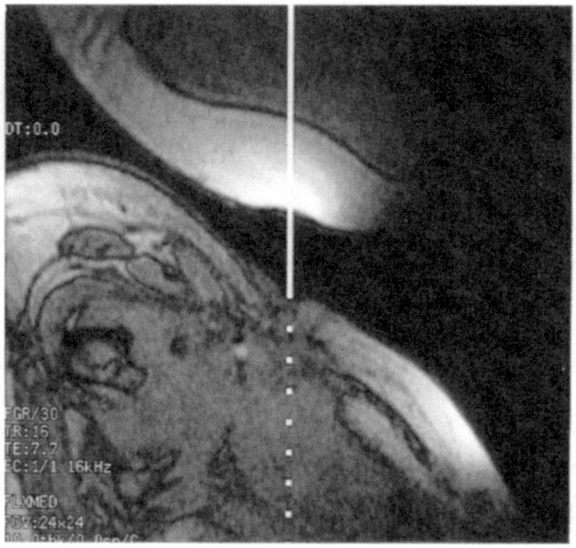

Fig. 10.10. Liver biopsy prior to needle penetration of the skin. The *short dotted line* shows the computed path the needle will take given its current position outside the body.

of protons as the device moves through the tissue, resulting in a dark line. Another contrast effect is also possible. It is caused by the difference in magnetic susceptibility between the device and surrounding tissues. This combination of computer generated icon and instrument artifact presentation of the information with the Signa SP system allows the physician to first predict the path of an interventional device as it is held outside the body for approach planning, and then to confirm its actual location with the real-time image by observing its position (Fig. 10.10). By this method, it is always possible to maintain positive control of interventional devices within the body.

To evaluate the accuracy of the intraoperative scan plane pointer and its ability to predict the location of interventional devices, we retrospectively analyzed 27 clinical cases (i.e., body biopsies, endoscopic sinus procedures, neurobiopsies). In all cases, the interventionalist was using the scan plane pointer in an interactive manner. Using software available on the operator console, 43 measurements of the distance between the location of the tip of the actual interventional device and the tip as indicated by the scan plane pointer were performed (Table 10.2).

The resulting average error distance for any of the measurements was 2.3 mm. Divided into body and neurological applications the average error distance found for body applications was 3.5 mm, and 1.8 mm for neurological cases. The three images with the greatest distances between the tip of the scan plane pointer annotation and the actual device were a prostate biopsy and two liver biopsies. When viewing an in-plane scan from each of these cases, while the scan pointer annotation correctly indicated the distance from the skin surface to the tip of the needle, the actual needle was displaced laterally relative to the indicated path of the pointer. In these cases, the biopsy needle was bent as it passed through tissue. Respiratory and voluntary patient motion may have been other likely contributors to these misregistrations during intraoperative imaging. It is important to note that these cases only occurred in the abdomen and pelvis. In all neurobiopsy cases the scan plane pointer annotation correctly indicated the alignment of the trajectory of the biopsy needle. However, in two cases, the actual needle tip was shown to be slightly short or long of the computed tip. Since the entire needle course was clearly depicted in the image, this did not represent a problem. During the neurobiopsy procedures, it was common to biopsy first the proximal margin and then the central area or distal margin of the tumor by later extending the needle further through the biopsy

Table 10.2. Clinical accuracy (27 cases)

Total number of points	43
Mean error distance (all cases)	2.3 mm
Mean error distance (body)	3.5 mm
Mean error distance (neurological)	1.8 mm
Maximum error distance (1 case)	9.0 mm
Minimum error distance (19 cases)	0.0 mm
Median error distance	2.1 mm

needle holder without moving the actual scan plane pointer device itself. Real-time MR guidance permitted visualization the actual location of the sample window of the needle and deliberate selection of these targets during the procedure. This approach was found to be very helpful in optimizing diagnostic yield, as corroborated by the pathology reports.

In all of the clinical cases examined, the scan plane pointer clearly represented the actual path of an interventional device relative to surrounding anatomy within the patient. By looking at a single image, it was always possible to visualize the entire tract of the device from entry at the patient's skin surface to the tip of the device. Thus, the scan plane pointer was able to align the imaging plane of the MR system with the device held by the interventionalist with sufficient accuracy to permit full control of the interventional devices throughout the procedure.

10.5 Summary

Moving all of the capability of diagnostic MR imaging into an interventional or operative environment promises to be of great clinical benefit. These benefits are based on the ability to see beneath the surface and in allowing what was previously "post-operative" MR imaging to be carried out during the procedure and prior to closing the operative field. However, it is the ability of the physician to quickly direct the MR scan plane with common surgical/radiological devices that makes this type of system truly interactive. Intraoperative scanning will continue to grow in importance as the development of minimally invasive procedures continues.

Acknowledgements. All images courtesy of The Brigham and Women's Hospital, Boston, and University Hospital, Zurich.

References

Image Guided Technologies (1996) Flashpoint™ Model 5000 3D localizer user's and programmer's manual. Image Guided Technologies, Inc., Boulder, Colo.

GE Medical Systems (1997) GE Signa SP™ Optional Accessories Operators Manual. GE Medical Systems, Milwaukee, Wis.

Moriarty TM, Kikinis R, Jolesz FA, Black PM, Alexander E (1996) Magnetic resonance imaging therapy – intraoperative MR imaging. Neurosurg Clin N Am 7:323–331

Schenck JF, Jolesz FA, Roemer PB, et al (1995) Superconducting open-configuration MR imaging system for image guided therapy. Radiology 195:805–814

Silverman SG, Collick BD, Figueira MR, Khorasani R, Adams DF, Newman RW, Topulos GP, Jolesz FA (1995) Interactive MR-guided biopsy in an open-configuration MR imaging system. Radiology 197:175–181

Silverman SG (1996) Percutaneous abdominal biopsy: recent advances and future directions. Semin Interv Radiol 13:3–15

Sipos EP, Tebo SA, Zinreich SJ, Long DM, Brem H (1996) In-vivo accuracy testing and clinical experience with the ISG viewing wand. Neurosurgery 39:194–202

Smith KR, Frank KJ, Bucholz RD (1994) The Neurostation – a highly accurate, minimally invasive solution to frameless stereotactic neurosurgery. Comput Med Imaging Graph 18:247–56

Steiner P, Schoenenberger AW, Penner EA, Erhart P, Debatin JF, von Schulthess GK, Kacl GM (1996) Interaktive, stereotaktische Interventionen im supraleitenden, offenen 0,5-Tesla-MR-Tomographen. Rofo Fortschr Geb Röntgenstr Neuen Bildgeb Verfahr 165:276–280

Safety and Imaging Aspects in Interventional MRI

11 Safety Issues in the MR Environment

J.F. Schenck

CONTENTS

11.1 Introduction

Although precise data are difficult to obtain, it is worthwhile to attempt to quantify the safety experience so far obtained with MRI. Using market research data it can be inferred that more than 100 000 000 diagnostic MR studies have been performed worldwide between the introduction of clinical MRI in the early 1980s and the end of 1996. The number of reported serious complications resulting from these studies is relatively small. A brief literature review finds reports of seven deaths attributed to MR scanning - one during examination for cerebral infarction (Gangarosa et al. 1987), one involving a ferromagnetic cerebral aneurysm clip (Klucznik et al. 1993; Kanal and Shellock 1993) and five related to inadvertent scanning of patients with cardiac pacemakers (Gimbel et al. 1996a). Anaphylactoid reactions to intravenous MR contrast agents have been estimated to occur in the range of 1:100 000 to 1:500 000 (Shellock and Kanal 1996).

Underreporting of serious adverse events and difficulty confirming MRI as the proximate cause of death in many of the reported cases make precise numerical evaluation of MRI-induced deaths impossible. It appears likely, however, that death occurs less than once in five million scans. For comparison, death from the use of high osmolality vascular contrast material in X-ray angiography is estimated to be in the range of 1:60 000 to 1:100 000 studies (Parker and Bettman 1996). Other serious complications during MRI, such as radiofrequency burns, have been reported at a rate of perhaps 1: 100 000 studies. The types of serious injuries reported for MRI appear to be preventable in the sense that their incidence does not depend on intrinsic aspects of the scanning procedure, such as hypothetical effects of high magnetic fields on human tissues. Instead, they can be reduced by developing improved techniques for the application of radiofrequency coils, by limiting the presence of ferromagnetic materials, and by preventing contraindicated procedures, such as the uncontrolled imaging of pacemaker patients.

The large number of trouble-free studies attests to the high level of achievable safety in this modality; the much smaller number of serious complications reminds us of the need for continued vigilance. Naturally, the safety protocols now under development for interventional MRI are an extension of those that have worked well for diagnostic MRI. However, certain differences between diagnostic and interventional MRI require additional considerations and emphasis in order that interventional MRI can be expected to continue, and hopefully even improve upon, the excellent safety record of diagnostic MRI.

11.1.1 History of MRI Safety Regulations

From the inception of MRI research in the late 1970s it was recognized that MRI units required patients to be immersed in a variety of intense electromagnetic fields. This unfamiliar environment posed potentially dangerous levels of electromagnetic exposure of

J.F. Schenck, MD, PhD, General Electric Company, Corporate Research and Development Center, Research Circle, Schenectady, NY 12309, USA various types. As a consequence, the Food and Drug Administration (FDA) was involved in regulating the use of MRI in the United States of America from the very beginning of clinical MRI research. Parallel regulatory activity was carried out by the National Radiological Protection Board (NRPB) in the UK (National Radiological Protection Board 1980; National Radiological Protection Board 1982; Saunders and Smith 1984) and the International Electrotechnical Commission (International Electrotechnical Commission 1995) in the European Union. Although the regulations promulgated by these three agencies differ somewhat in detail, the major aspects are quite similar. As the field of MRI has matured, the role of the FDA with regard to MRI regulation in the USA has gone through several stages.

In 1976, in order to protect human subjects during the development and use of medical devices, the US Congress amended the Food, Drug and Cosmetic Act of 1938 to govern the introduction of new medical devices. In response to this legislation in January 1980 the FDA issued regulations that applied to manufacturers of new medical devices and to researchers using these devices. These regulations were designed in a manner analogous to those governing the introduction of new drugs, they required the recording of data regarding the safety and efficacy of any new devices prior to the granting of permission to market them.

There was widespread criticism of the initial proposals both from the medical device industry and from health researchers. In response to these criticisms the FDA revised their regulations (Goyan 1980; Richmond 1981). As these regulations were not retroactive, X-ray computed tomography (CT) scanners, which had been introduced prior to 1980, were not subject to them, and MRI became the first major imaging modality to apply the newly developed requirements on safety and efficacy. Requirements specifically designed for MRI were soon published (Randolph 1982; Villforth 1982; Gundaker 1982).

During the 1980s several manufacturers successfully sought approval to market MR scanners. With the availability of substantial clinical experience, the FDA reclassified MR scanners operating below 2.0 T as non-significant risk devices in 1987 (Young 1988; US Food and Drug Administration 1988). Further experience led the FDA in 1996 to extend the range of non-significant risk for main magnetic fields to 4.0-T systems. Exposure of research subjects to experimental conditions that go beyond the parameters of non-significant risk require the informed consent of the patients and the approval of the proposed protocol by an institutional review board (IRB; Greenwald et al. 1982).

11.2 Standard Safety Practices in Diagnostic MRI

MR scanners place the patient in an environment that is quite different from that of any other medical instrument. Possible physiological of metabolic changes in response to strong magnetic fields are the most obvious concern with regard to MRI and drew much of the initial attention with regard to the safety profile of this modality. However, in hindsight, it appears that biological effects induced by static magnetic fields are either absent altogether or of a very limited and generally benign nature even up to the strongest fields for which whole-body imaging is currently feasible (Schenck 1992; Schenck et al. 1992; Erhard et al. 1995).

11.2.1 Classsical Safety Issues in MRI

The classical safety issues (Table 11.1) associated with MRI have been related to the strength of the static field; the specific absorption rate (SAR; in W/kg) associated with the energy deposition and tissue heating produced by the radiofrequency (RF) transmitter field; the possibility of peripheral nerve, cardiac or central nervous system excitation by the time-dependent gradient fields (dB/dt); and acoustic noise (Budinger 1979; Budinger 1981; Schaefer 1988). The regulations for each of these factors as of early 1996 were summarized by the FDA (Letter from L. Yin to Dr. Charles Springer, Brookhaven National Laboratory, 1996) as paraphrased below:

- Static field: the use of 4.0 T or less for imaging or spectroscopy of human subjects is considered non-significant risk.
- RF power deposition (SAR): RF power deposition insufficient to cause a core temperature increase in excess of 1° C and localized heating to greater than 38° C in the head, 39° C in the trunk and 40° C in the extremities, or otherwise adverse effect.
- Gradient switching rates: switched gradients insufficient to produce peripheral nerve stimulation or other adverse effects.
- Acoustic noise: acoustic noise levels meeting the requirements of the American Conference of

Table 11.1. Classical safety issues in MRI

Effect	Possible mode of action	Comments
Static field (B_0)	Possible physiological effects; twisting or acceleration of ferromagnetic objects; projectile danger	From a physiological standpoint field strengths up to 4.0 T are considered a non-significant risk by the US FDA Forces on ferromagnetic objects are a potential hazard at all field strengths Sensory effects seen at high field strengths do not appear to be harmful
Gradient switching (dB/dt)	Potential for excitation of electrically excitable nerve or cardiac tissue	Peripheral nerve excitation has been observed at very high slew rates. Excitation of central nervous system and cardiac tissue requires a higher threshold and has not been reported
Radiofrequency power deposition (SAR)	Tissue damage from excessive heating	Proximity to conducting portions of radiofrequency transmitter coils can be dangerous. The effect is reduced in systems using transmit surface coils rather than whole-body coils for transmission The possibility of heating of indwelling metallic devices, such as catheters and coils, should be carefully considered
Audiofrequency noise	Potential hearing loss	Safe levels of acoustic energy decrease with duration of exposure

Governmental Industrial Hygienists (ACGIH) for exposure up to 1 h or the permissible time-averaged and peak noise exposure given by the Occupational Safety and Health Administration (OSHA). OSHA currently permits occupationally necessary individual exposure of 105 dBA for 1 h sound level slow response, where the ACGIH permits 100 dBA for 1 h exposure. The ACGIH has indicated that, in the future, the 1 h exposure limit may be reduced to 94 dBA and states that this is a more conservative value intended to protect workers who may experience a lifetime of occupational exposure.

In this letter the FDA recognized alternative approaches to meeting the switched gradient requirements based on the duration of the switching pulse. It also stated that the agency had become convinced that mild peripheral stimulation is not harmful to the subject or patient. The FDA also recognized surrogates to temperature rise, based on SAR, which manufacturers or investigators may use in determining the RF power deposition.

The above summary is provided to give a sense of the regulatory situation, but because of the intricacy of these regulations, investigators with protocols approaching the significant risk levels should consult the relevant FDA or IEC documents directly.

11.2.2 Hazards Associated with Magnetic Materials

The greatest risk associated with practical scanning has turned out to be of forces and torques exerted on ferromagnetic materials that are present inside the patient or that are inadvertently brought near to the scanner. These forces arise from strong magnetic fields within the central region of the scanner and from the weaker, but still treacherous, fringing field which surrounds it. Many objects commonly present in hospitals (e.g., oxygen bottles, stethoscopes, mops, fans, pens, paper clips, and hairpins) are sufficiently magnetic that they can be drawn rapidly and forcefully into the magnet, thus striking or entrapping the patient within it. Figure 11.1 illustrates an extreme example of this danger. In this case an RF transmitter containing a substantial amount of ferromagnetic material was inadvertently moved too close to a 1.5-T superconducting magnet. The strong fringing magnetic field and the large mass of ferromagnetic materials overcame the ability of the staff to restrain it and it was forcefully drawn into the magnet, causing it to quench. To prevent such accidents it is common practice to scrupulously limit access to rooms where MR scanning is taking place (Karlik et al. 1988). The risk associated with forces on ferromagnetic objects is present to some extent in all MR systems, but this risk is reduced in lower field systems, in permanent magnet systems, and in those

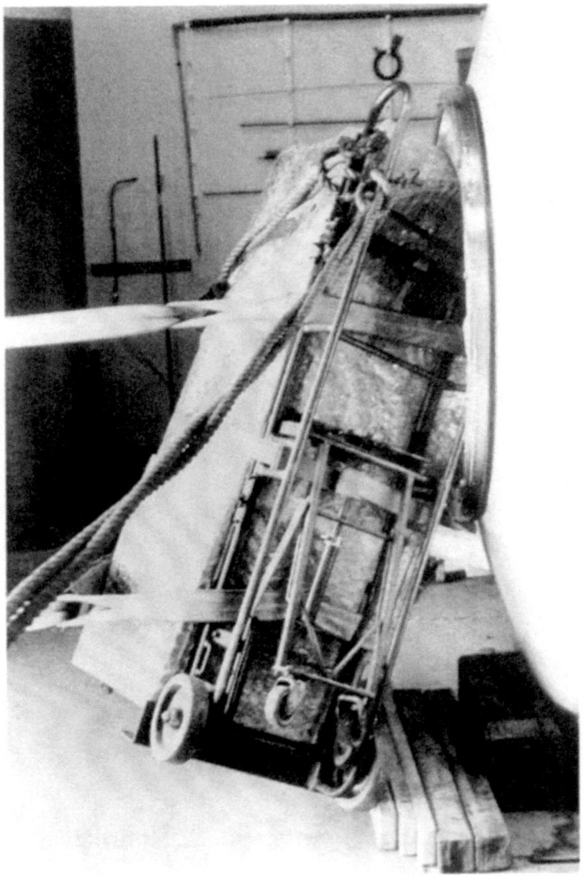

Fig. 11.1. A radiofrequency transmitter accidentally drawn into a superconducting magnet. (Courtesy of Dr. W.A. Edelstein; from SCHENCK 1996 with permission)

superconducting systems that are magnetically shielded.

Another aspect of this problem occurs when patients have ferromagnetic prostheses or ferromagnetic materials embedded within their bodies (e.g., NEW et al. 1983; SHELLOCK 1988; TEITELBAUM et al. 1988; BECKER et al. 1988; SHELLOCK and CURTIS 1990; CLAYMAN et al. 1990; KAGETSU and LITT 1991; SMITH et al. 1991; YUH et al. 1991; KLUCZNIK et al. 1993; SHELLOCK et al. 1993; HARMATI et al. 1994). While the presence of metallic objects is usually related to surgical procedures, such as the clamping of an arterial cerebral aneurysm, in some cases iron fragments (e.g., shrapnel) are present within patients, often without their knowledge, as a result of accidental exposure to flying metal fragments. When the patient's history suggests the possibility of such exposure, X-ray examination to rule out such fragments is often performed, although there is some disagreement as to the proper indications for this precaution (WILLIAMSON et al. 1993; SHELLOCK and KANAL 1993). Particular care should be taken if the metal fragment is positioned in the brain, the eyes or close to other critical body structures.

11.2.3 Hazards Associated with Cardiac Pacemakers

A variety of the potentially serious consequences of exposing pacemaker-dependent patients to the static magnetic field and RF have been described. These include physical motion or twisting of the pacemaker itself, uncontrolled changes in programming, inhibition of output, episodic asynchronous pacing, and reed switch malfunction. Because of these risks (PAVLICEK et al. 1983; POHOST et al. 1992; INBAR et al. 1993; GIMBEL et al. 1996b), the presence of an implanted pacemaker is very close to being an absolute contraindication to MR scanning (BAROLD and ZIPES 1997, p 729). However, strategies for scanning pacemaker patients have been advanced and, using a carefully controlled protocol and with the informed consent of patients, successful scanning of a series of six pacemaker-dependent patients with a specific model of pacemaker has been reported (GIMBEL et al. 1996b). However, the wide variation in pacemaker models in use makes generalization with regard to acceptable scan procedures impossible. Electromagnetic interference (EMI) associated with the RF transmitter field of the MR scanner provides a more serious challenge to MR-compatibility of cardiac pacemakers than do the magnetic forces and torques associated with the static magnetic field, as these can be controlled by proper choice of materials.

11.3 Safety Considerations in Interventional MRI

For the first decade of its clinical use MRI was virtually exclusively performed for the purposes of diagnostic imaging. However, in the late 1980s and the 1990s a number of groups began to report the use of MRI-guided surgical interventions (e.g., LUFKIN et al. 1988; JOLESZ and SHTERN 1992; LEWIN et al. 1995; SCHENCK et al. 1995; ABELE et al. 1995; VOGL et al. 1995; WILDERMUTH et al. 1995). In diagnostic MR imaging, standard safety procedures have usually required the exclusion from the scan room of all extraneous materials and all personnel other than the patient and the scan operator. With the advent of interventional MRI the presence in the scan room of additional personnel – e.g., surgeons, interventional radiologists, anesthesiologists, and their assistants

– and new devices – e.g., surgical implements, catheters, and anesthesia stations – has become necessary. This has been the cause for new safety considerations.

11.3.1 Exposure of the Operating Team

Whereas patients are generally subject to a single exposure, lasting, in most cases, less than 1 h, the operating team involved in performing interventional MRI-guided procedures can be expected to be exposed repeatedly to the MRI environment as an occupational necessity. This brings about a new aspect of MR safety for which there is not a great deal of accumulated direct experience. Although measurements (PHILLIPS 1990) and guidelines for chronic magnetic field exposure have not identified (e.g., MILLER 1987) any reproducible health effects, the available data remain scant. At this time there appears to be no scientific basis for attributing a health hazard to prolonged field exposure.

In interventional MRI there are a number of ameliorating factors that tend to reduce the likelihood of serious safety hazards associated with chronic exposure to the scanner environment. These include the relatively low magnetic field strength (0.2-0.5 T) used in most interventional systems and the use of small area surface coil transmitters rather than RF body coils. Most interventional systems are designed to keep dB/dt and SAR exposures of the operating team within FDA guidelines. These guidelines are designed to prevent peripheral nerve stimulation and excessive tissue heating. A cumulative effect to subthreshold stimuli is not expected. Nonetheless, it is highly desirable that a means be found of recording exposure information on the staff involved with interventional MRI to provide a scientific basis to verify the occupational safety of these procedures.

11.3.2 Locally Enhanced Radiofrequency Energy Deposition

Careful calculations of the fields produced by the RF transmitter coils (e.g., JIN et al. 1996) can ordinarily predict energy deposition patterns. This can be used to assure compliance with SAR guidelines and protect patients and staff from thermal injury. However, it should be remembered that a large amount of RF power (up to several kilowatts) is involved in MRI, and in certain situations excessive energy deposition and severe local heating can occur. An analogous situation occurs in unipolar electrocautery, where the RF current from the cauterizing electrode flows through the patient's body and is returned through a large area electrode located, for example, on the patient's back. If for some reason the contact to the return electrode is inadequate, an undesired current concentration may occur at some point on the patient's body which is accidentally grounded, leading to a burn at this site (GEDDES and BAKER 1989). A recently described case (KNOPP et al. 1996) involved a body coil image in which a current loop of mostly large cross-sectional area within a patient contained a small region of very small cross-sectional area at a point of contact between the medial calves of the lower leg. The heating associated with the greatly increased current density at the point of current concentration produced a significant local burn during an otherwise routine MRI scan.

The presence of metallic conductors within the region of strong RF fields leads to the possibility of high induced currents in closed loop situations (CAMACHO et al. 1995) or high induced voltages if narrow gaps between otherwise closed conducting paths are present. If a metallic conductor, such as a metal-containing guidewire catheter or biopsy needle, is oriented parallel to the electric field of the RF coil and at least one end is embedded within the patient's tissues, the possibility of local tissue excitation (PEDEN et al. 1993) or heating at the metallic tip needs to be considered (see Chap. 8; CHOU et al. 1997). It is also necessary that the patient and the clinical staff be protected from coil locations, such as series capacitors in surface transmitter coils, which are associated with locally high electric field strengths. This can generally be accomplished by providing a sufficiently thick layer of electrical insulation to cover these locations.

11.3.3 Stereotactic Positional Accuracy

One function often utilized during MRI-guided interventional procedures is the ability of the MR image to provide stereotactic positional information (e.g., KONDZIOLKA et al. 1992). Theoretically, MR imaging is able to provide positional information with an accuracy limited only by the voxel size – that is by the slice thickness and the pixel size in the imaging plane. However, a number of factors, such as inhomogeneity in the main magnetic field and nonlinearity in the gradient fields, can reduce this accuracy and must be taken into account to avoid potentially harmful positional errors. A particular form of this potential error arises when foreign bodies, such as surgical instruments, are introduced into the patient or into other regions close to the imaging field of view. If these objects do not have magnetic susceptibility closely matching that of air, for objects outside the patient, or that of human tissues, for objects located within the patient, they will produce an induced magnetic field that will distort the applied magnetic field. The distortion can lead to considerable errors in positional coordinates derived from the images (LÜDEKE et al. 1985; DEROSIER et al. 1991; CHANG and FITZPATRICK 1992; BHAGWANDIEN et al. 1992, 1994; BAKKER et al. 1993; BUEF et al. 1993; SUMANAWEERA et al. 1993, 1994, 1995; BHAGWANDIEN 1994; LEWIN et al. 1995; SCHENCK 1996; CONDON and HADLEY 1997). The extent of these positional errors depends on many factors, including the magnetic susceptibility, as well as the size, orientation, and location of the magnetized body. They should be taken into account whenever precise positional data is being inferred from an MR image.

11.4 MR Compatibility

Interventional MRI, unlike diagnostic MRI, requires the presence of many additional objects, in addition to the patient, within the imaging volume. Therefore, the issue of compatibility of materials and devices with the MRI environment is far more significant in the interventional applications of MRI. The most obvious form of MR incompatibility involves ferromagnetic materials, which are absolutely unacceptable in the MRI suite (Fig. 11.1). Somewhat less obvious is the fact that materials normally thought to be "non-magnetic" may produce significant distortions in MR images and be unacceptable for this reason as well. It is also becoming clear that the EMI produced by interactions between the RF transmitter and instruments of various types is also a major consideration in MRI compatibility. Ideally, a material introduced into the imaging region would have a perfect magnetic susceptibility match, as described in Sect. 11.4.1, and zero electrical conductivity. These criteria tend to discriminate against metal objects and favor instruments constructed from thermoplastic or ceramic materials. However, there are many additional practical considerations, including strength and reliability, tissue biocompatibility, sterilizability, and the ability to hold a cutting edge, that must be considered in the design of instrumentation for use in interventional MRI.

11.4.1 Magnetic Susceptibility

The magnetic susceptibility, χ, is yet another important material property that determines magnetic compatibility. This parameter is the proportionality factor relating the induced magnetization, M, to the magnetic field strength, H. That is, $M = \chi H$. Some materials can be permanently magnetized and have a magnetization, M_0, even in the absence of an applied magnetic field. The magnetic susceptibility of materials varies over many orders of magnitude (TEITELBAUM et al. 1988; LENZ and DEWEY 1995; GEHL et al. 1995; LEWIN et al. 1995; SCHENCK 1996). Most common materials are slightly repelled by a magnetic field: these materials are called diamagnetic and have negative values of χ. Water has $\chi = -9.05\times10^{-6}$. Human tissues are also diamagnetic with a susceptibility within a few parts per million (ppm) of that of water (SCHENCK 1996). Paramagnetic materials are attracted by a magnetic field and have positive values of χ. Because of the presence of oxygen, air is very slightly paramagnetic with $\chi = +0.36\times10^{-6}$. Paramagnetic materials can have relatively large values of susceptibility, and it is not uncommon for a small amount of a paramagnetic impurity, such as an iron oxide, to overwhelm the diamagnetism of a much larger object.

Table 11.2 introduces two kinds of magnetic compatibility with MRI. Magnetic compatibility of the first kind requires that an object is not permanently magnetized or does not become so strongly magnetized by the MR magnet as to be dangerous. Magnetic compatibility of the second kind implies that the object does not significantly interfere with the quality and usefulness of the MR image.

A magnetized object produces a magnetic field of its own, and, when the object is present in the imaging region, the induced magnetic field distorts the field of the main magnet. For ideal magnetic compatibility, the introduction of an object into the imaging region would not cause any change in the pre-existing field. Thus, for an object present outside the patient the ideal susceptibility of the object would be that of air, $+0.36\times10^{6}$, and for an object inside the body the ideal susceptibility would be that

Table 11.2. Proposed classification for the MRI magnetic compatibility of materials. The magnetic susceptibility of water, $\chi_{water} = -9.05\times10^{-6}$, is very close to that of human tissues. The precise susceptibility boundaries between the classes is approximate and will depend to some extent on the application. In theory, if M_0 is very small but not precisely zero, a material may exhibit magnetic field compatibility of the first kind ($M_0 \leq 10^4$ A/m) or of the second kind ($M_0 \leq 10$ A/m). (Modified from SCHENCK 1996 with permission)

Classification	Conditions on the magnetization and susceptibility	Examples	Comments
MRI magnetic incompatibility	$M_0 \neq 0$ and/or $\lvert\chi\rvert \geq 10^{-2}$	Iron, cobalt, magnetic stainless steel, nickel	In a magnetic field these materials experience strong, and potentially dangerous forces and torques and create image distortion and degradation far from their immediate vicinity
MRI magnetic compatibility of the first kind	$10^{-5} \leq \lvert\chi\rvert \leq 10^{-2}$	Titanium, bismuth, "non-magnetic" stainless steel	In a magnetic field these materials do not experience obvious magnetic forces and torques, but they produce marked image distortion and degradation in their immediate vicinity
MRI magnetic compatibility of the second kind	$\lvert\chi - \chi_{water}\rvert \leq 10^{-5}$	Teflon, Plexiglas, quartz, copper, zirconia	The susceptibilities of these materials are within 10 ppm of those of water and human tissues. These materials experience no easily detected forces or torques and produce very limited or no image distortion even when they are located within the imaging field of view

of human tissues, -9.05×10^{-6}. Such that small distinctions are often insignificant; however, because of the sensitivity of MRI to magnetic field variations, susceptibility variations of a few ppm can easily be demonstrated in MR images. Table 11.3 provides a list of materials which have good susceptibility matches to human tissues. In general terms, those materials with susceptibilities within 3 ppm of human tissues will produce no detectable distortion in MR images; those with susceptibility variation of less than 10 ppm will produce a demonstrable, but often insignificant, image distortion; and those with a susceptibility variation of less than 200 ppm will produce a readily apparent, but often acceptable image distortion in their vicinity.

Materials with very good matches to tissue susceptibility will produce very little image distortion. In some circumstances, some degree of image distortion may be desirable to identify the position of an object, such as a biopsy needle, in an MR image. This is particularly true in lower field systems and systems using thick scan slices. However, it should be remembered that a degree of positional accuracy is lost when this method of localization is employed.

Stainless steel is an important material as many surgical instruments and medical implants are constructed from it. Many varieties of stainless steel are strongly magnetic and hazardous in magnetic fields. Other forms are much less magnetic and are commonly referred to as non-magnetic stainless steels. However, all so-called non-magnetic stainless steels have a relatively strong paramagnetic susceptibility and can cause significant distortion in MR images. Also, it is important to realize that, when cold-worked, it is possible for non-magnetic steels to revert to the strongly magnetic form (KANAL et al. 1996; SCHENCK 1996).

11.5 Conclusion

Since the beginning of clinical MR imaging in the early 1980s the field has maintained a good safety record. This record is being improved by increasing knowledge of techniques for excluding ferromagnetic materials and in the safe use of RF transmitter coils. Close attention to safety issues should make it possible to maintain and improve on this record as interventional MRI takes its place alongside diagnostic MRI.

Acknowledgements. It is a pleasure to acknowledge helpful conversations with Drs. E. Kanal, F.G. Shellock, J.R. Gimbel, and C.L. Dumoulin.

References

Abele MG, Jensen JH, Rusinek H (1995) Open permanent magnet for surgical applications. (abstract) Proceedings of Society of Magnetic Resonance, Berkeley, Calif., p 1154

Bakker CJG, Bhagwandien R, Moerland MA (1993) 3D analysis of susceptibility artifacts in spin-echo and gradient-echo magnetic resonance imaging. (abstract) Proceedings of Society of Magnetic Resonance, Berkeley, Calif., p 746

Barold SS, Zipes DP (1997) Cardiac pacemakers and antiarrhythmic devices. In: Braunwald E (ed) Heart disease: a textbook of cardiovascular medicine. Saunders, Philadelphia, pp 705, 741

Becker RL, Norfray JF, Teitelbaum GP, Bradley WG Jr, Jacobs JB, Wacaser L, Rieman RL (1988) MR imaging in patients with intracranial aneurysm clips. Am J Neuroradiol 9:885–889

Bhagwandien R (1994) Object induced geometry and intensity distortions in magnetic resonance imaging. PhD thesis, University of Utrecht, Utrecht, The Netherlands

Bhagwandien R, Van Ee R, Beermsa R, Bakker CJG, Moerland MA, Lagendijk JJW (1992) Numerical analysis of the magnetic field for arbitrary magnetic susceptibility distributions in 2D. Magn Reson Imaging 10:299–313

Bhagwandien R, Moerland MA, Bakker CJG, Beermsa R, Lagendijk JJW (1994) Numerical analysis of the magnetic field for arbitrary magnetic susceptibility distribution in 3D. Magn Reson Imaging 12:101–107

Buef O, Crémillieux Y, Briguet A, Lissac M, Coudert JL (1993) Correlation between magnetic susceptibility and image disturbances caused by prosthetic materials. (abstract) Proceedings of Society of Magnetic Resonance, Berkeley, Calif., p 805

Budinger TF (1979) Threshold for physiological effects due to rf and magnetic fields used in NMR imaging. IEEE Trans Nucl Sci 26:2821–2825

Budinger TF (1981) Nuclear magnetic resonance (NR) in vitro studies: known thresholds for health effects. J Comput Assist Tomogr 5:800–811

Camacho CR, Plewes DB, Henkelman RM (1995) Nonsusceptibility artifacts due to metallic objects in MR imaging. J Magn Reson Imaging 5:75–78

Chang H, Fitzpatrick JM (1992) A technique for accurate magnetic resonance imaging in the presence of field inhomogeneities. IEEE Trans Med Imaging 11:319–329

Chou C-K, McDougall JA, Chan KW (1997) RF heating of implanted spinal fusion stimulator during magnetic resonance imaging. IEEE Trans Biomed Eng 44:367–373

Clayman DA, Murakami ME, Vines FS (1990) Compatibility of cervical spine braces with MR imaging: a study of nine nonferrous devices. Am J Neuroradiol 11:385–390

Condon B, Hadley D (1997) Errors in MRI stereotaxy due to undetected extraneous metal objects. (abstracts) Proceedings of International Society for Magnetic Resonance in Medicine, Berkeley, Calif., p 260

Derosier C, Delegue G, Munier T, Pharboz C, Cosnard G (1991) IRM, distorsion géométrique de l'image et stéréotaxie (MRI, geometric distortion of the image and stereotaxy). J Radiol 72:349–353

Erhard P, Chen W, Lee J-H, Ugurbil K (1995) A study of effects reported by subjects at high magnetic fields. (abstracts) Proceedings of Society of Magnetic Resonance, Berkeley, Calif., p 1219

Gangarosa RE, Minnis JE, Nobbe J, Praschan D, Genberg RW (1987) Operational safety issues in MRI. Magn Reson Imaging 5:287–292

Geddes LA, Baker LE (1989) Principles of applied biomedical instrumentation, 3rd edn. Wiley, New York, pp 848–872

Gehl H-B, Frahm C, Melchert UH, Weiss H-D (1995) Suitability of different MR-compatible needles and magnet designs for MR-guided punctures. (abstracts) Proceedings of Society of Magnetic Resonance, Berkeley, Calif., p 1156

Gimbel JR, Lorig RJ, Wilkoff BL (1996a) Survey of magnetic resonance imaging in pacemaker patients. HeartWeb 1 (1) http://webaxis.com/heartweb/

Gimbel JR, Johnson D, Levine PA, Wilkoff BL (1996b) Safe performance of magnetic resonance imaging on five patients with permanent cardiac pacemakers. PACE Pacing Clin Electrophysiol 19:913–919

Goyan JE (1980) Medical devices: procedures for investigational device exemptions. Fed Regist 45:3732–3759

Greenwald RA, Ryan MK, Mulvihill JE (1982) Human subjects research: a handbook for institutional review boards. Plenum, New York

Gundaker WE (1982) Guidelines for evaluating electromagnetic risks for trials of clinical NMR systems. US Food and Drug Administration, Rockville, Md.

Haramati N, Penrod B, Staron RB, Barax CN (1994) Surgical sutures: MR artifacts and sequence dependence. J Magn Reson Imaging 4:209–211

International Electrotechnical Commission (1995) International standard. Part 2, Particular requirements for the safety of magnetic resonance equipment for medical diagnosis. CEI/IEC 601-2-33. International Electrotechnical Commission, Geneva, Switzerland

Inbar S, Larson J, Burt T, Mafee M, Ezri MD (1993) Case report: nuclear magnetic resonance imaging in a patient with a pacemaker. Am J Med Sci 305:174–175

Jin JM, Chen J, Chew WC, Gan H, Magin RL, Dimbylow PJ (1996) Computation of electromagnetic fields for high-frequency magnetic resonance imaging applications. Phys Med Biol 41:2719–2738

Jolesz FA, Shtern F (1992) The operating room of the future: report of the National Cancer Institute Workshop – imaging-guided stereotactic tumor diagnosis and treatment. Invest Radiol 27:326–328

Kagetsu NJ, Litt AW (1991) Important considerations in measurement of attractive force on metallic implants in MR imagers. Radiology 179:505–508

Kanal E, Shellock F (1993) MR imaging of patients with intracranial aneurysm clips. Radiology 187:612–614

Kanal E, Shellock FG, Lewin JS (1996) Aneurysm clip testing for ferromagnetic properties: clip variability issues. Radiology 200:576–578

Karlik SJ, Heatherley T, Pavan F, Stein J, Lebron F, Rutt B, Carey L, Wexler R, Gelb A (1988) Patient anesthesia and monitoring at a 1.5-T MRI installation. Magn Reson Med 7:210–221

Klucznik PA, Carrier DA, Pyka R, Haid RW (1993) Placement of a ferromagnetic intracerebral aneurysm clip in a magnetic field with a fatal outcome. Radiology 187:855–856

Knopp MV, Essig M, Debus J, Zabel H-J, van Kaick G (1996) Unusual burns of the lower extremities caused by a closed conducting loop in a patient at MR imaging. Radiology 200:572–575

Kondziolka D, Dempsey PK, Lunsford LD, Kestle JRW, Dolan EJ, Kanal E, Tasker RW (1992) A comparison between magnetic resonance imaging and computed tomography for stereotactic coordinate determination. Neurosurgery 30:402–407

Lenz G, Dewey C (1995) Study of new titanium alloys for interventional MRI procedures. (abstracts) Proceedings of Society of Magnetic Resonance, Berkeley, Calif., p 1159

Lewin JS, Duerck JL, Haaga JR (1995) Needle localization in MR guided therapy: effect of field strength, sequence design, and magnetic field orientation. (abstracts) Proceedings of Society of Magnetic Resonance, Berkeley, Calif., p 1155

Lüdeke KM, Röschmann P, Tischler R (1985) Susceptibility artifacts in MR imaging. Magn Reson Imaging 3:329-343

Lufkin R, Teresi L, Chiu L, Hanfee W (1988) A technique for MR-guided needle placement. Am J Roentgenol 151:193–196

Miller G (1987) Exposure guidelines for magnetic fields. Am Ind Hyg Assoc J 48:957-968

National Radiological Protection Board (NRPB) (1980) Exposure to nuclear magnetic resonance clinical imaging. Radiography 47:258-260

National Radiological Protection Board (NRPB) (1982) Revised guidance on acceptable limits of exposure during nuclear magnetic resonance clinical imaging. Br J Radiol 56:974–977

New PFJ, Rosen BR, Brady TJ, Buonanno FS, Kistler JP, Burt CT, Hinshaw WS, Newhouse JH, Pohost GM, Traveras JM (1983) Potential hazards and artifacts of ferromagnetic and non-ferromagnetic surgical and dental materials and devices in nuclear magnetic resonance imaging. Radiology 147: 139–148

Parker JE, Bettman MA (1996) Angiographic contrast media. In: Taveras M, Ferrucci JT (eds) Radiology: diagnosis-imaging-intervention. (Vascular Radiology, vol 2) Lippincott-Raven, Philadelphia

Pavlicek W, Geisinger M, Castle L, Borkowski GP, Meaney TF, Bream BL, Gallagher JH (1983) The effects of nuclear magnetic resonance on patients with cardiac pacemakers. Radiology 147:149–153

Peden CJ, Collins AG, Butson PC, Whitwam JG, Young IR (1993) Induction of microcurrents in critically ill patients in magnetic resonance systems. Crit Care Med 21:1923–1928

Phillips ML (1990) Industrial hygiene investigation of static magnetic fields in nuclear magnetic resonance facilities. Appl Occup Environ Hyg 5:353-358

Pohost GM, Blackwell GG, Shellock FG (1992) Safety of patients with medical devices during application of magnetic resonance methods. In: Magin RL, Liburdy RP, Persson B (eds) Biological and safety aspects of nuclear magnetic resonance imaging and spectroscopy. (Proceedings of the New York Academy of Science, vol 649) New York Academy of Sciences, New York, pp 302–312

Randolph WF (1982) Guidelines for evaluating electromagnetic exposure risk for trials of clinical NMR systems: availability. Fed Regist 47:11972–11973

Richmond JB (1981) Final regulations amending basic HHS policy for the protection of human research subjects. Fed Regist 46:8366–8392

Saunders RD, Smith H (1984) Safety aspects of NMR clinical imaging. Br Med Bull 40:148–154

Schaefer DJ (1988) Safety aspects of magnetic resonance imaging. In: Wehrli FW, Shaw D, Kneeland JB (eds) Biomedical magnetic resonance imaging: principles, methodology, and applications. VCH Verlagsgesellschaft, Weinheim, pp 553–578

Schenck JF (1992) Health and physiological effects of human exposure to whole-body four-tesla fields during MRI. In: Magin RL, Liburdy RP, Persson B (eds) Biological and safety aspects of nuclear magnetic resonance imaging and spectroscopy. (Proceedings of the New York Academy of Sciences, vol 649) New York Academy of Science, New York, pp 285–301

Schenck, JF (1996) The role of magnetic susceptibility in magnetic resonance imaging: magnetic field compatibility of the first and second kinds. Med Phys 23:815–850

Schenck JF, Dumoulin CL, Redington RW, Kressel HY, Elliott RT, McDougall IL (1992) Human exposure to 4.0 tesla magnetic fields in a whole-body scanner. Med Phys 19:1089–1098

Schenck JF, Jolesz FA, Roemer PB, et al (1995) Superconducting open-configuration MR imaging system for image-guided therapy. Radiology 195:805–814

Shellock FG (1988) MR imaging of metallic implants and materials: a compilation of the literature. Am J Radiol 151:811-814

Shellock FG, Curtis JS (1990) MR imaging and biomedical implants. Materials, and devices: an updated review. Radiology 180, 541–550

Shellock FG, Kanal E (1993) Re: metallic foreign bodies in the orbits of patients undergoing MR imaging: prevalence and value of radiography and CT before MR. Am J Radiol 162:985–986

Shellock FG, Kanal E (1996) Magnetic resonance: bioeffects, patient safety, and patient management, 2nd edn. Lippincott-Raven, Philadelphia, pp 102–11

Shellock FG, Morisoli S, Kanal E (1993) MR procedures and biomedical implants, materials, and devices: 1993 update. Radiology 189:587–599

Smith AS, Hurst GC, Duerk JL, Diaz PJ (1991) MR of ballistic materials - imaging artifacts and potential hazards. Am J Neuroradiol 12:567–572

Sumanaweera T, Napel S, Glover G, Song S (1993) A new method to quantify the geometric accuracy of MRI in tissue using MRI itself. (abstract) Proceedings of Magnetic Resonance, Berkeley, Calif., p 745

Sumanaweera T, Glover G, Song S, Adler J, Napel S (1994) Quantifying MRI geometric distortion in tissue. J Magn Reson 31:40–47

Sumanaweera TS, Glover GH, Hemler PF, van den Elsen PA, Martin D, Adler JR, Napel S (1995) Geometric distortion correction for improved frame-based stereotaxic target localization accuracy. Magn Reson Med 34:106–114

Teitelbaum GP, Bradley WG Jr, Klein BD (1988) MR imaging artifacts, ferromagnetism, and magnetic torque of intravascular filters, stents, and coils. Radiology 166:657–664

US Food and Drug Administration (1988) Guidance for content and review of a magnetic resonance diagnostic device 510(k) application. Silver Spring, Md.

Villforth JC (1982) Guidelines for evaluating electromagnetic exposure risk for trials of clinical NMR systems. US Food and Drug Administration, Rockville, Md.

Vogl TJ, Mack MG, Müller P, et al (1995) Recurrent nasopharyngeal tumors: preliminary clinical results with interventional MR imaging-controlled laser-induced thermotherapy. Radiology 196:725–733

Wildermuth S, Debatin JF, Leung DA, et al. (1995) MR-guided percutaneous intravascular interventions: in vivo assessment of potential applications. (abstracts) Proceedings of Society of Magnetic Resonance, Berkeley, Calif., p 1161

Williamson MR, Espinosa MC, Boutin RD, Orrison WW Jr, Hart BL, Kelsey CA (1994) Metallic foreign bodies in the orbits of patients undergoing MR imaging: prevalence and value of radiography and CT before MR. Am J Radiol 162:981-983

Young FE (1988) Magnetic resonance diagnostic device: panel recommendation and report on petitions for MR reclassification. Fed Regist 53:7575-7579

Yuh WTC, Hanigan MT, Nerad JA, Ehrhardt JC, Carter KD, Kardon RH, Shellock FG (1991) Extrusion of eye socket magnetic implant after MR imaging: potential hazard to patient with eye prosthesis. Magn Reson Imaging 1:711-713

12 Patient Monitoring in the MR Environment

J. FELBLINGER and C. BOESCH

CONTENTS

12.1 Introduction

During routine diagnostic MR, patient monitoring is required for sedated or anesthetized patients as well as for those with instable vital functions (BOESCH 1995; SHELLOCK and KANAL 1993). Patient monitoring during an MR examination is complicated since the MR system is an extremely hostile environment for other electronic devices and sensors, and at the same time a very sensitive receiver, making the images prone to artifacts. Before devices were commercially available, many monitoring devices were developed by adaptation of existing systems (BOESCH 1995 and references therein; KANAL and SHELLOCK 1992 and references therein). The constant evolution of MR techniques (e.g., interventional MR or echo planar imaging) has necessitated adaptation and evolution of the existing systems.

For interventional MR procedures, patient monitoring is essential, and the MR compatibility of monitoring devices is even more demanding than during conventional MR. Since multiple electronic devices are used at the same time, the mutual interaction between the MR system and these devices increases. At the moment, some solutions for patient monitoring are commercially available, but new developments for monitoring systems are still inevitable. An increasing number of applications and progress of new MR techniques require a continuous evolution of monitoring devices to maintain complete MR compatibility.

12.2 Patient Monitoring

12.2.1 Adapted Strategies for Patient Monitoring

Generally, the MR system is located in closed, radiofrequency-shielded (RF-shielded) room, referred to as a "Faraday cage" (Fig. 12.1). Opening of the door during MR scans can result in degradation of image quality. This makes it necessary to adapt and change patient monitoring as we know it from the intensive care unit or from classical surgical interventions. Patient monitoring during diagnostic MR is somewhat different from monitoring during interventional MR. A standard diagnostic MR examination takes about 30-60 min and can be stopped if necessary. An MR-guided intervention, however, can take longer and has to be completed without any delay or interruption. We can distinguish three main groups of patients needing different levels of monitoring during MR examination (BOESCH 1995):

1. Patients with stable vital functions needing monitoring at a low level or just to provide a trigger for synchronization of the MR sequence (for example ECG). In this case surveillance can be done from outside by the MR operator (Fig. 12.1a).

C. BOESCH, MD, PhD, MR Center 1, University and Inselspital, CH-3010 Bern, Switzerland
J. FELBLINGER, PhD, MR Center 1, University and Inselspital, CH-3010 Bern, Switzerland

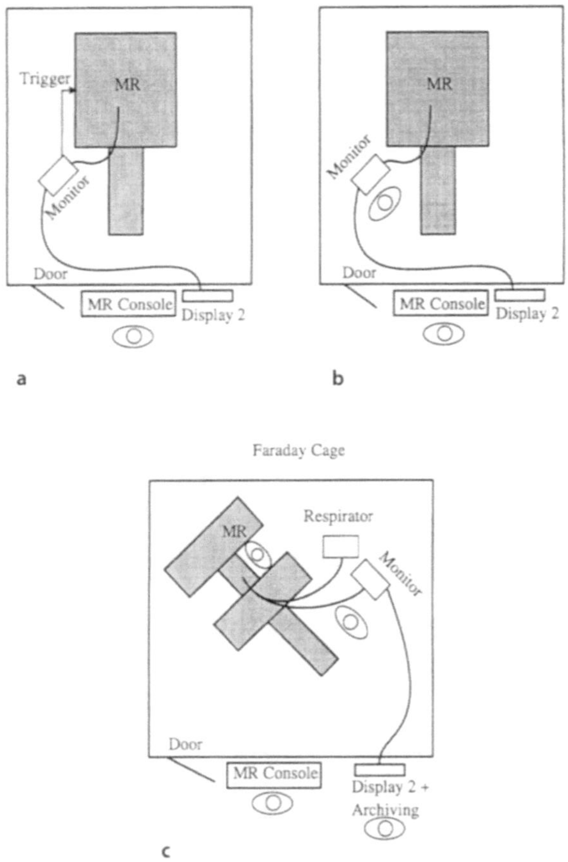

Fig. 12.1a-c. A comparison of different strategies for patient monitoring during conventional and interventional MR examinations. In both cases, the MR system is placed in a radiofrequency-shielded room (i.e., in a Faraday cage). Opening of the door during MR scans can cause image artifacts and degradation of image quality. **a, b** For diagnostic MRI, patient monitoring and life support management depend on the level of patient consciousness and anesthesia. Patients with stable vital functions (**a**) can be monitored at a low level, or trigger-signals for synchronization of MR sequences can be acquired. High-risk patients (**b**; sedated or anesthetized) need strict surveillance. The survey team and the monitoring devices should be positioned near the patient. Outside the Faraday cage, an optional second display (Display 2) may aid the supervision of the examination. **c** For interventional MR, the anesthetist and part of the survey team should be located close to the patient, i.e., near the magnet. Several other devices have to be placed inside the Faraday cage in addition to the monitoring system (e.g., respirator, surgical equipment, laser). A satellite display of the monitoring screen outside the MR cabinet, as well as an archiving system for documentation of the procedure are recommended (Display 2 and archiving)

2. High risk patients (e.g., sedated or anesthetized patients), where the survey team and the monitoring device should be placed near the patient in the Faraday cage (Fig. 12.1b). Optionally, a second display (Fig. 12.1b) can be placed outside the examination room for supervision.
3. Patients undergoing an interventional MR procedure. In this case, the MR room is transformed into a surgical unit (Fig. 12.1c) and it is obvious that the anesthetist(s) should be positioned close to the patient. The monitoring device, the respirator and other devices are placed close to the patient, reducing the available space and increasing the mutual interaction between these devices and the MR system. During interventional MR, a second monitoring display (Fig. 12.1c) may be helpful for the continuous information of the staff outside, as well as for computerized archiving.

12.2.2 Monitoring Parameters

Depending on the type of patient, the survey team needs continuous control of different vital parameters:

- The electrocardiogram gives information about the electrical activity of the heart. An undisturbed ECG signal can indicate different forms of arrhythmia and is altered through ischemia or infarction of the heart muscle.
- The pulse oximeter (SaO_2 or SpO_2) shows the heart rate and the oxygen saturation in an extremity (e.g., finger, toe, or foot of a neonate).
- The transcutaneous PO_2 and PCO_2 give the partial pressure of O_2 and CO_2 mainly in neonates.
- The body or skin temperature.
- The non-invasive blood pressure (NIBP) and the invasive blood pressure (IBP) reflect the cardiovascular functions.
- The capnograph analyzes the expired air using a sampling tube in the airflow. The respiration rate and apnea can be monitored. For an intubated patient with a closed ventilation circuit, capnography determines absolute concentrations of end-expiratory CO_2 (end-tidal CO_2) and some anesthetic gases.

More details of the physical underlying these parameters are given by Boesch (1995) and Kanal and Shellock (1992) and in biomedical engineering handbooks (Mendelson 1995). The adaptations of these parameters to achieve MR compatibility are shown in detail below.

12.2.3 Training the Survey Team

Influences of the MR system on patient monitoring devices and readings may be strong, and special sensors are used which are unfamiliar to most anesthetists. For example, the ST segment of an ECG recorded in the MR magnet could be misrepresented as ischemia due to the distortion of the signal by the main magnetic field (see Sect. 12.5.1). It is obvious that all paramagnetic tools should be kept outside the MR environment. Even following thorough investigation some magnetic properties remain hidden (e.g., a magnetic battery in a nonmagnetic laryngoscope). Furthermore, in emergency situations paramagnetic devices are used (e.g., a defibrillator). The staff responsible for monitoring during MR examinations must be appropriately trained: (a) to know the particular situation of an MR environment, (b) to manage the special and unfamiliar devices used for patient monitoring and life support, (c) to distinguish normal from abnormal readings of all parameters under these uncommon conditions and (d) to know which tools and technical devices can be used - and to remember this information even in emergency situations.

12.3 Interaction in the MR Environment

12.3.1 The MR Environment

To obtain images of the body, a strong magnetic field (termed B_0), ranging typically between 0.2 and 1.5 T, is used. Most open magnets used for interventional MR work with lower fields (e.g., 0.2 or 0.5 T). The static magnetic field B_0 of supraconductive magnets is always present. Depending on the type of MR magnet (shielded vs unshielded, open vs closed), the fringe field decays within several meters outside the magnet's bore.

To obtain a localization of the MR signal, i.e., to form an image, additional magnetic fields are added to the very homogeneous magnetic field B_0. These "gradients" are switched with high slew rates and vary along the three spatial coordinates linearly with typically 10 mT/m. Switched gradients are a source of strong audio noise and induce potentials in conducting objects.

The observed tissue is excited by RF generated by powerful (up to 20 kW) transmitters and emitted by antennas ("RF coils"). Following these excitation pulses, extremely weak MR signals are emitted by the tissue and have to be picked up by the receiver RF coil. MR sequences consist of a simultaneous combination of switching RF pulses, switching gradients and a selection between RF transmission and reception mode. All this occurs in fractions of a millisecond.

12.3.2 Influences of the MR System on Patient Monitoring Devices

All three physical effects used in MRI, i.e., the static magnetic field B_0, gradients and RF, may interact with patient monitoring devices (Boesch 1995) and interfere with their proper function. Multiple physical laws are involved at the same time:

- Mechanical forces due to the static magnetic field B_0. They transform magnetic instruments into projectiles, provoke sticking of electromagnetic devices (e.g., pumps and electrovalves) and sautration of the transformers and inductances used in electronic circuits.
- Mechanical forces (Lorentz force) produced by the motion of charged particles in a magnetic field. These forces prohibit the use of cathode ray tubes and introduce distortion of the ECG curve due to the motion of blood in the magnetic field (see Sect. 12.5.1).
- Induced voltages (Faraday's law) generated by gradients and RF. These interfering voltages are generated in any conducting loop (e.g., acquisition wires) when the magnetic field or the surface of the enclosed area changes. This effect can saturate an ECG signal completely when long acquisition wires are used (Fig. 12.2; Felblinger et al. 1994). The artifacts produced cover the frequency range from several hertz up to some kilohertz. Since the ECG bandwidth lies in this range, reduction of these influences by filtering is difficult or impossible. The powerful RF pulses used can also saturate the first stage of amplifiers.

Every extended conductive structure (e.g., wires) can act as an RF antenna. In addition to artifacts which may be produced, this effect can focus RF

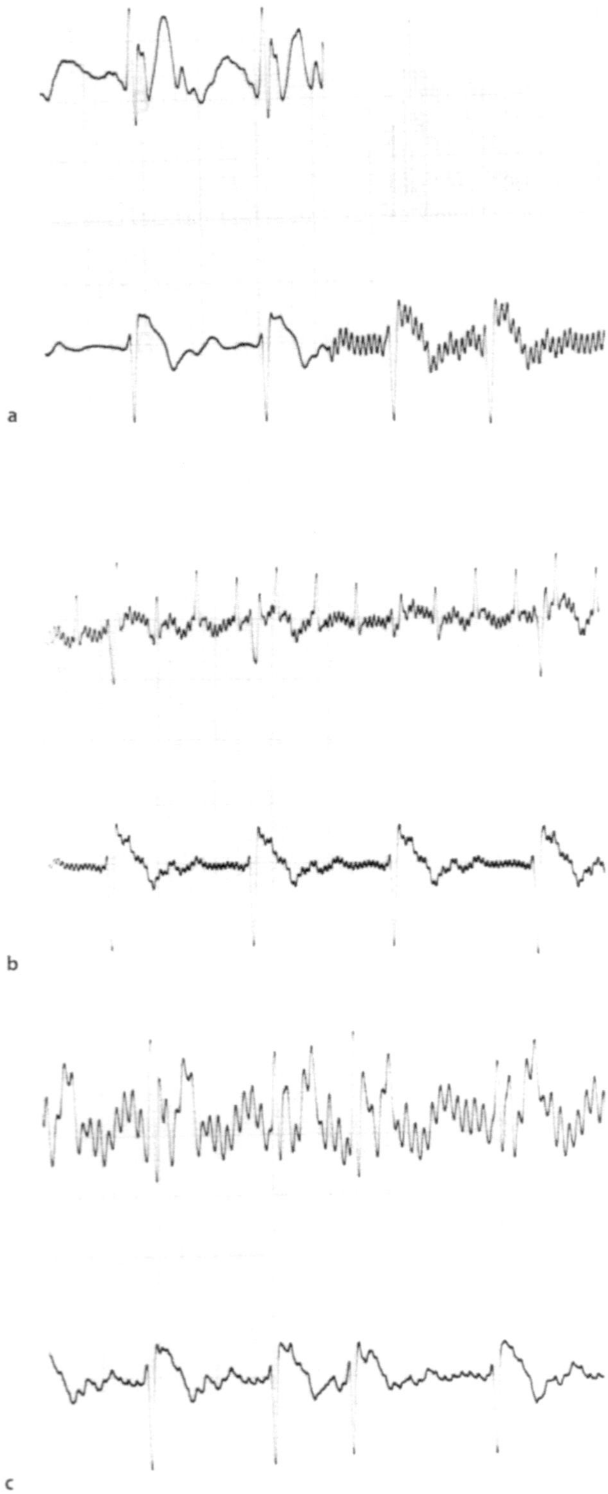

Fig. 12.2a-c. An illustration of the possible interactions on ECG signals obtained from the same patient (age 31 years, weight 88 kg) with three different configurations of coils and sequences. The *top row* of all panels shows an ECG signal acquired by long carbon wires. The *bottom row* of all panels shows an ECG signal obtained by amplification and conversion into optical signals directly on the patient (Felblinger et al. 1994). Coils and sequences of the different panels were: **a** body coil, spin-echo, field of view (FOV) = 20cm, **b** surface coil, fast spin-echo/rapid acquisition with relaxation enhancement, FOV = 22cm; and **c** body coil, gradient-echo, FOV = 48 cm. The MR sequence in **a** starts halfway during the acquisition of the ECG signal, while the sequences in the other panels run for the entire acquisition window. Acquisition of the ECG by long wires show in a complete saturation of the signal, in **b** possible misinterpretation of the pulses generated by the sequence as QRS complexes and in **c** strong artifacts which prevent even a simple judgement of the cardiac rhythm. The comparison with the 'optical' ECG amplifier shows that signals acquired by this device can be used for monitoring purposes even under these extreme conditions

energy, causing heating or burning hazards to the patient (Bashein and Syrovy 1991; Felmee et al. 1995). For the same reason use of tracking catheters in interventional MR (Maier et al. 1995) may generate potential dangers. The analysis of these artifacts is often complicated by the fact that even strong effects are not reproducible and that they depend strongly on the exact position of the sensors, the patient and the coil and the MR sequence used (Fig. 12.2). Different interactions occur simultaneously on a time scale of several milliseconds (Boesch 1995), making separation of the various effects difficult. This renders interpretation of such artifacts difficult.

12.3.3 Influences of Patient Monitoring Devices on MR Systems

An MR system is an exceptionally sensitive RF receiver. To isolate it from all RF noise, the MR system is placed in a Faraday cage (i.e., a wall-integrated RF shield). Monitoring and life support devices placed inside the Faraday cage (Fig. 12.1) are full of digital electronics emitting considerable amounts of electromagnetic fields. These RF fields can be picked up by the MR receiver and can provoke image degradation (Boesch 1995; Jorgensen et al. 1994; Shellock and Kanal 1993). Again, multiple factors influence the level of interaction (e.g., position of the sensors, the patient or the coils used, magnetic field strength B_0 and design of the magnet).

The static magnetic field has to be very homogeneous for imaging purposes (in the order of 1 part per million). Sensors placed in the region of interest can affect homogeneity and introduce imaging artifacts. Fast imaging techniques such as gradient-echo or echo-planar sequences are more prone to artifacts due to field inhomogeneity than standard spin-echo sequences.

12.3.4
Interventional MR

Special designs, techniques and procedures have been developed for interventional MR, which complicate patient monitoring additionally. Open MR systems without active B_0 shielding produce a considerable fringe field. This requires an increased distance between magnet and monitoring device or enhanced magnetic shielding for electromagnetic components. A standard magnet design has an inherent Faraday shielding effect by the dewar and coils, which is not the case in open magnets. For these magnets, residual RF noise generated by the devices in the Faraday room can be picked up by the receiver coils more easily and affect the signal-to-noise ratio. During critical steps of intervention procedures, continuous image acquisition may be necessary. Since monitoring must not be interrupted during these periods, completely artifact-free readings are required. A growing number of electronic devices built by different manufacturers is placed in the Faraday cage at the same time. This increases possible interactions and the possibility of image quality deterioration. As a consequence, monitoring devices used in interventional MR have to be even more robust and reliable than for standard diagnostic imaging.

12.4
Current Solutions for Patient Monitoring

12.4.1
MR-Compatible Monitoring Devices

Many adaptations of existing monitoring devices have been published (Boesch 1995 and references therein; Kanal and Shellock 1992 and references therein). Some MR-compatible devices are now commercially available; examples of complete monitoring systems are given in Table 12.1. These devices allow patient monitoring in a conventional MR system where interactions are reduced to an acceptable level. However, MR methods are in the process of evolution, and devices which are currently MR-compatible may fail if new MR techniques, such as increased gradient slew rates, larger fringe fields, or different RF coils are introduced. It is important that users of MR-compatible monitoring devices are

Table 12.1. Examples of commercially available MR-compatible, complete monitoring systems (data according to manufacturers; for devices with fewer parameters, see Kanal and Shellock 1992)

Name	Manufacturer	Parameters available	Remarks
Model 9500 vital signs multigas monitor	Magnetic Resonance Equipment (Bay Shore, N.Y.)	ECG (optically encoded), SaO_2 (optically encoded), noninvasive blood pressure, invasive blood pressures (2), anesthetic agents (5), FiO_2, $EtCO_2$, NO_2, respiration rate, optical temperature[a]	Optional display and control outside; remote archiving (paper) and trends
Maglife	Odam-Bruker (Wissembourg, France)	ECG, SaO_2 (optically encoded) noninvasive blood pressure, invasive blood pressure $EtCO_2$, NO_2, respiration rate	Optional display and control outside; remote digital archiving
Maglife C		ECG (optically encoded), SaO_2 (optically encoded), noninvasive blood pressure, invasive blood pressures (4), anesthetic agents (5), FiO_2, $EtCO_2$, NO_2, respiration rate, optical temperature[a]	Optional display and control outside; remote digital archiving[a]
Omni-Trak 3100	In Vivo Research, (Orlando, Fla.)	ECG, SaO_2, noninvasive blood pressure, $EtCO_2$, NO_2, respiration rate	Different devices placed inside and outside the Faraday cage
Omni-Trak 3150(a)		ECG, SaO2, noninvasive blood pressure, invasive blood pressure, EtCO2, NO2, respiration rate	Compact device using telemetry system for communications, archiving (paper)

[a]According to the manufacturer, these options should be available end of 1997

aware of the current limitations for patient monitoring.

The common principle used for these monitoring devices is to RF-shield all parts containing digital or switching electronics. Different solutions exist for a communication between the inside and outside of the RF shield, depending on the tape of parameter. Eventually, all physiological signals have to be converted into electrical signals for treatment and visualization. Some parameters are inherently electrical signals (ECG) or depend on transducers which have to be placed near or on the patient (temperature, PO_2, PCO_2 and SaO_2). Other parameters are measured pneumatically (NIBP and gases) or hydraulically (IBP). These transducers may be placed far away from the patient.

Nonelectrical parameters may be forwarded through RF-penetration guides in the RF shield to bring the signal into the monitoring device. Electrical signals need to be filtered or – preferably – converted into optical signals which can be fed through the RF shield without additional effort.

Ferromagnetic and electromagnetic components have to be avoided in the MR environment. However, this is not possible for all electronic components used in patient monitoring devices (e.g., motors, pumps, printers, valves, transformers and inductances). These devices have to be magnetically shielded to work properly, or the distance to the magnet needs to be increased. Cathode-ray tubes have to be replaced by liquid-crystal displays of electro-luminiscent screens.

12.4.2 Acquisition of Nonelectrical Signals

For measuring blood pressure, it is possible to elongate the tubes such that the electronic circuits and sensors (pressure transducer, valves and pumps) can be located outside the magnetic field. The same applies for the pump and analyzing chamber for breathing gases (end-tidal CO_2 and NO_2), which can be located far away from the magnet if longer sampling tubes are used. A resulting registration delay – up to 10 s for expired gases – is acceptable for patient monitoring. The resistance and the additional volume of the longer tubes can cause difficulties for measurements in small children. Standard sensors for anesthesia gases can be placed directly at the respirator. Immediate conversion into optical signals is desirable to avoid long wires which can act as RF antennas. The IBP sensor can be placed far away from the magnetic and RF fields if extension tubes are used.

12.4.3 Acquisition of Electrical Signals

If long wires are used for the acquisition of electrical parameters, heating or burning hazards are of concern. RF pulses (Bashein and Syrovy 1991; Felmee et al. 1995) and voltages can be induced by the gradients, the RF and the motion of the wires in the main magnetic field. Several conventional means have been proposed to reduce artifacts on ECG recordings: use of high-resistance electrodes and wires (van Genderingen et al. 1989), positioning of the electrodes in a small precordial area (Dimick et al. 1987), addition of strong filters, as well as postprocessing. However, these methods do not work for all combinations of sequences, patients and coils (Fig. 12.2), and the possibility of heating or burning hazards remains real. For these reasons, only devices which permit an immediate conversion of the electrical into an optical signal promise to be safe and permit acquisition of reliable signals. This has been realized for the registration of the ECG signal (Felblinger et al. 1994), where the length of the wires has been drastically reduced by a small RF-shielded box. The box is placed on the patient's chest. Here, the signal is amplified and converted into optical pulses which can be transmitted by fiberoptics. This method prevents not only problems arising from large changes of the enclosed area (Fig. 12.2) but also burning hazards.

Traditional SaO_2 sensors work with two diodes and one phototransistor placed on each side of the finger or toe, or foot of the neonate (Mendelson 1995). In commonly used MR-compatible pulse-oximeters, the light-emitting diodes and the photodetector are placed outside the magnet and transmission of the light is made by optical fibers (Shellock et al. 1992). This optical method prevents burning hazards, but precaution is necessary since all pulse-oximeters – electrical or optical – may produce false alarms and wrong saturation values (Mendelson and Yocum 1991; Barker et al. 1993). Because "cold light" is used in optical SaO_2 sensors, no warming of the emitting diodes is achieved which could increase the capillary flow. Additionally, the opening angle is very small in optical fibers, making measurement of the SaO_2 more difficult than in conventional electrical systems. As a consequence, it is important to have a correct pulse curve prior to

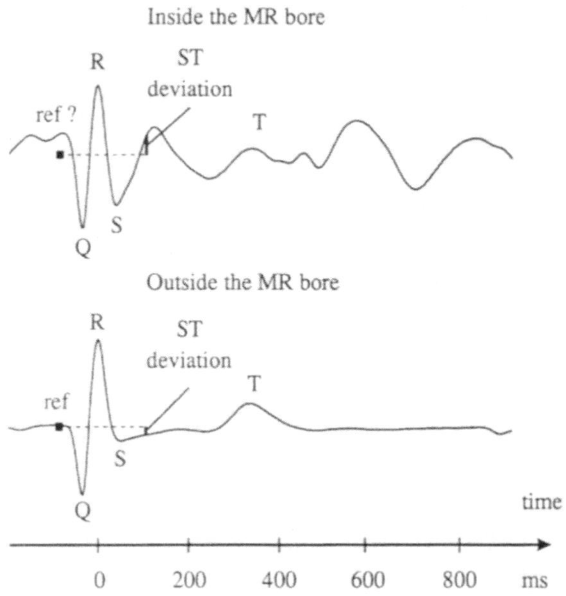

Fig. 12.3. An example of a current problem of patient monitoring in the MR environment. The *bottom row* shows an ECG cycle acquired outside the MR magnet. The *top row* shows the same signal but obtained after the volunteer was brought into the magnet of a 1.5-T MR system. The ST segment of an ECG signal changes during ischemia or infarction of the heart. However, in the magnetic field the ST segment is completely distorted, preventing diagnosis of heart ischemia and causing possible misinterpretation. For automatic estimation of the ST deviation, the voltage difference between the middle of the ST segment and a reference is calculated. This computation is almost impossible since both the ST segment and the reference point are affected by the magnetic field

interpretation of the data shown by the optical pulse-oximeter.

The measurement of body or skin temperature with conventional devices is also prone to burning hazards and should therefore be replaced by optical temperature registration (Taber and Hyman 1992). These optical sensors are currently not widely used due to their expense and the insufficient adaptation of the sensors for medical use.

12.5 Development of Future Tools for Patient Monitoring

12.5.1 Improvement of Patient Monitoring

As described above, motion of electrically charged particles (e.g., ions of the blood) in the static magnetic field leads to a magnetohydrodynamic effect (Balcavage et al. 1996; Keltner et al. 1990). The moving blood produces extra-voltages (known as Hall effect in conductors) which are added to all electrophysiological signals (Felblinger et al. 1994; Tenforde et al. 1983), mainly during the systolic period of the ventricular action (Fig. 12.3). This additional signal occurs during the ST segment of the ECG which is commonly used for diagnosis of ischemic or infarcted heart muscle. Detection of a deviation of the ST segment requires an extension of the signal bandwidth to frequencies to 0.05 Hz. Because these low frequencies are susceptible to motion artifacts and the measurement of the ECG signal is additionally complicated by the uncommon precordial position of the electrodes, the diagnostic interpretation of an ST deviation is difficult. At present, no calculation of the ST deviation is commercially available or published in the literature. Nevertheless, estimation of ST elevation remains highly desirable during interventional MR procedures.

Optical SaO_2 sensors are now standard in MR monitoring devices. As mentioned above some problems remains (e.g., too low oxygen saturation) due to malpositioning or insufficient capillary flow (Mendelson and Yocum 1991; Barker et al. 1993). Misinterpretation can be reduced when other monitoring parameters are used simultaneously (e.g., the heart rate by SaO_2 and ECG) and the pulsatile saturation curve is displayed (e.g., indicating signal-to-noise ratio and periodicity).

Only optical temperature sensors should be used (especially for rectal measurements). Currently available sensors seem not to be robust enough and need extensive calibrations. New methods or adaptations of optical temperature transducers for medicine are necessary.

12.6 Conclusions and Perspectives

Proper patient monitoring is fundamental to the success of interventional MR procedures. Although limitations still do exist, most vital parameters can be safely monitored in an MR environment. Just as important as the proper equipment is adequate training of the patient survey team.

References

Balcavage WX, Alvager T, Swez J, Goff CW, Fox MT, Abdullyava S, King MW (1996) A mechanism for action of extremely low frequency electromagnetic fields on biological systems. Chem Biophys Res Commun 222: 374–378

Barker SJ, Hyatt J, Shah NK, Kao YJ (1993) The effect of sensor malpositioning on pulse oximeter accuracy during hypoxemia. Anesthesiology 79: 248–254

Bashein G, Syrovy G (1991) Burns associated with pulse oximetry during magnetic resonance imaging. Anesthesiology 75: 382–383

Boesch C (1995) Patient life support and monitoring facilities for whole body MRI. In: Grant DM, Harris RK (eds) Encyclopedia of nuclear magnetic resonance, Wiley, Chichester, pp 3467–3475

Dimick RN, Hedlund LW, Herfkens RJ, Fram EK, Utz J (1987) Original investigations: optimizing electrocardiograph electrode placement for cardiac-gated magnetic resonance imaging. Invest Radiol 22: 17–22

Felblinger J, Lehmann C, Boesch C (1994) Electrocardiogram acquisition during MR examinations for patient monitoring and sequence triggering. Magn Reson Med 32: 523–529

Felmee J, Hokanson D, Zink F, Perkins W (1995) Real time evaluation of EKG electrode heating during MRI at 1.5 T. (abstract) Proceedings of the 3rd annual meeting of the Society of Magnetic Resonance, Nice, p 1226

Jorgensen NH, Messick JM, Gray J, Nugent M, Berquist TH (1994) ASA monitoring standards and magnetic resonance imaging. Anesth Analg 79: 1141–1147

Kanal E, Shellock FG (1992) Patient monitoring during clinical MR imaging. Radiology 185: 623–629

Keltner JR, Ross MS, Brakeman PR, Budinger TF (1990) Magnetohydrodynamics of blood flow. Magn Reson Med 16: 139–149

Maier SE, Wildermuth S, Darrow RD, Watkins RD, Debatin JF, Dumoulin CL (1995) Safety of MR tracking catheters. (abstract) Proceedings of the 3rd annual meeting of the Society of Magnetic Resonance, Nice, p 497

Mendelson Y (1995) Optical sensor. In: Bronzino JD (ed) The biomedical engineering handbook. CRC Press, Florida, pp 764–778

Mendelson Y, Yocum BL (1991) Noninvasive measurement of arterial oxyhemoglobin saturation with heated and a non heated skin reflectance pulse oximeter sensor. Biomed Instrum Technol 25: 472–480

Shellock FG, Myers SM, Kimble KJ (1992) Monitoring heart rate and oxygen saturation with a fiber-optic pulse oximeter during MR imaging. AJR Am J Roentgenol 158: 663–664

Shellock FG, Kanal E (1993) Magnetic resonance in bioeffects, safety, and patient management. Raven, New York, pp 61–79

Taber KH, Hayman LA (1992) Temperature monitoring during MR imaging: comparison of fluoroptic and standard thermistors. J Magn Reson Imaging 2: 99–101

Tenforde TS, Gaffey CT, Moyer BR, Budinger TF (1983) Cardiovascular alterations in macaca monkeys exposed to stationary magnetic fields: experimental observations and theoretical analysis. Bioelectromagnetics 4: 1–9

van Genderingen HR, Sprenger M, de Ridder JW, van Rossum AC (1989) Carbon-fiber electrodes and leads for electrocardiography during MR imaging. Radiology 171: 872

13 Fast Imaging Techniques for MR-Guided Biopsies

A. Bücker

CONTENTS

13.1 Introduction

The development of MR-compatible biopsy needles (Lufkin et al. 1987; Mueller et al. 1986; van Sonnenberg et al. 1988) has made it possible to exploit the high contrast and the multiplanar imaging capabilities of MR (Fig. 13.1) for MR-guided biopsy procedures of all kinds (Adams et al. 1997; Duckwiler et al. 1989; Hathout et al. 1992; Mueller et al. 1989; Pitt et al. 1993). A growing understanding of the artifacts induced by these devices when used with different sequences (Ladd et al. 1996) will help to make this a routinely performed procedure in the near future. Besides sophisticated and expensive methods like active tip tracking (Leung et al. 1995), the inherent susceptibility artifact of MR-compatible needles can be used for depiction and localization of the needle itself. Furthermore, doping with paramagnetic substances may prove effective not only for catheters, but also for needles (see Chap. 6). The shape and size of the needle artifact are dependent on the needle's orientation relative to the main magnetic field and the phase-encoding direction and, in addition, on the pulse sequence and the sequence parameters (Ladd et al. 1996; see Chap. 4). The author's experience has been gained on a 1.5-T system. The principles stated here can be easily transferred to other high-field systems. For field strengths below 1 T, two main differences have to be taken into account. Firstly, the lower the field strength, the more the acquisition

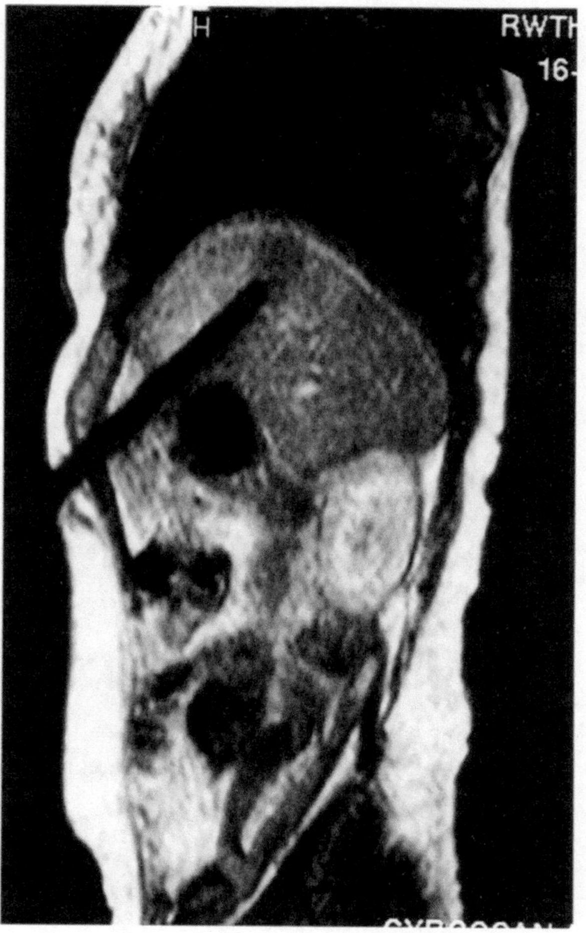

Fig. 13.1. An image showing a lesion histologically proved to be a hepatocellular carcinoma, just below the dome of the diaphragm. The sagittal orientation allowed for easy planning of the angulated needle tract. A 14-G needle was guided between the costophrenic angle and the gallbladder. Sequence parameters are given in Table 13.1 (page 117)

A. Bücker, MD, Department of Diagnostic Radiology, University of Technology Aachen, Pauwelsstrasse 30, D-52057 Aachen, Germany time will need to be prolonged or the signal-to-noise ratio will be decreased for any given resolution. Secondly, susceptibility artifacts will be less pronounced. While it has been shown that MR-guided biopsies are possible on low- and mid-field systems (Chaps. 1–3), the demands for sequence optimization are more crucial than with high-field systems in order to circumvent the disadvantages of a lower signal-to-noise ratio and decreased imaging speed.

13.2 MR Imaging and Needles: General Considerations

13.2.1 Choice of Sequence

The ideal sequence for MR-guided biopsies has to fulfill four requirements: firstly, for obvious reasons it has to be quick. But "quick" is, of course, a relative term, and the demand for image speed depends among other factors on the region to be biopsied and the patient's compliance. In general, the acquisition of a single image should at least not take much longer than that of a conventional CT slice. Secondly, the needle artifact should be big enough to be easily detected, but not so big as to obscure the lesion to be punctured (Sinha et al. 1989). Thirdly, there must be sufficient contrast between the lesion and the adjacent tissue, such as between the lesion and the needle artifact. As the needle artifact will tend to be black whichever sequence is used, and as most pathology is brighter on T2- than on T1-weighted sequences, one might, in general, expect T2-weighted sequences to be advantaged. Fourthly, vulnerable structures along the puncture tract have to be clearly depicted by the ideal sequence. This implies that there must be conspicuity of vessels, whether they flow perpendicular to or within the imaging plane. Delineation of other anatomic structures, such as bowel, kidneys or lung parenchyma, is of interest depending on the location of the lesion and the biopsy pathway.

There is no doubt that it is impossible to fulfill all four demands perfectly with one single sequence. Therefore, compromises will have to be accepted, and it might be advisable to use more than one sequence for planning the biopsy procedure, and maybe even during the monitoring of biopsy itself.

13.2.2 Temporal Versus Spatial Resolution

A prerequisite for any standard MR-biopsy sequence is that it is easy to perform during a breath-hold. Although, in principle, it is possible to apply sequences with a longer duration for biopsies outside the abdomen, this would significantly lengthen the procedure itself. Speed adds considerably to patient comfort because it shortens the biopsy procedure itself. Furthermore, the use of fast or ultrafast sequences reduces the risk of accidental displacement of the needle by breathing, coughing or other movements. The lesion to be punctured will usually be at least 10 mm in size and the artifact caused by the needle will be in the range of 5–10 mm. Correspondingly, spatial resolution can be sacrificed for temporal resolution either through a reduction of phase-encoding steps, which will reduce the matrix and resolution proportionally, or by applying a spin-echo sequence with a high turbo factor, which will cause widening of the point spread function and blurring in the image (Mulkern et al. 1990; Vlaardingerbroek and den Boer 1996). Both methods are feasible to reduce the acquisition time of a sequence, but they should be applied in such a way that a robust, standard sequence is created which can be employed in all kinds of cases without the need for modifications. This allows the physician to become familiar with the contrast and size of the needle artifact.

Another way to save time is to measure only part of k-space and invoke its hermitian symmetry to calculate the unmeasured part. While this leaves resolution unaffected, it lowers the signal-to-noise ratio (Mezrich 1995).

13.2.3 Needle Artifacts

Artifacts can be divided into those related to and those unrelated to the sequence and sequence parameters. System-dependent effects of field-strength differences or due to variation of needle orientation in relation to the main magnetic field B_0 have already been discussed in Chap. 5.

The material a needle is made of will influence the size of its artifact. To date, the commercially available MR-compatible needles have been constructed of different metal alloys, and before utilizing a particular brand, one should perform in vitro tests in order to determine the needle's imaging characteristics for different sequences.

Apart from the material, the main parameter influencing the size of a needle artifact is the choice of either a gradient-echo or a spin-echo sequence (Fig. 13.2). The 180° pulses applied during spin-echo sequences will re-establish the spin dephasing which had been caused by constant magnetic field inhomogeneities. This gives rise to the well-known T2 as opposed to T2* weighting of spin-echo sequences compared to gradient-echo sequences. Consequently, needle artifacts are, in general, smaller when spin-echo sequences are applied instead of gradient-echo sequences.

When using gradient-echo sequences, the echo time is one of the prime determinants for the size of the needle artifact. The more it can be reduced, the smaller the artifact will be. Care has to be taken, however, when the echo time is shortened by sampling an asymmetric echo. The shape of the needle artifact will change so that the point of maximum signal extinction will no longer be positioned in the center of this artifact. If the needle is oriented perpendicular to the frequency-encoding direction and asymmetric echo sampling is performed, part of the susceptibility artifact created by the needle will be shifted from one side of the needle to the other. The amount of shifting depends on the degree of asymmetry which is applied during scanning. A similar effect can be observed when only part of k-space is sampled, but this time the needle has to be oriented perpendicular to the phase-encoding direction in order to show the change in the artifact shape described above and the relative shift of the dark, center artifact of the needle.

Even if neither asymmetric sampling of the echo nor partial k-space sampling is used, the orientation of the needle in relation to the frequency-encoding direction is an important factor which can be easily exploited to manipulate the artifact size. A needle oriented parallel to the frequency-encoding direction will generally show a smaller artifact than a needle perpendicular to the frequency-encoding direction. Although one might expect the smallest needle artifact to be the best, this is not true for all sequences. Even on a high-field system, spin-echo sequences can show artifacts too small to be easily detected. Therefore, orientation of the frequency-

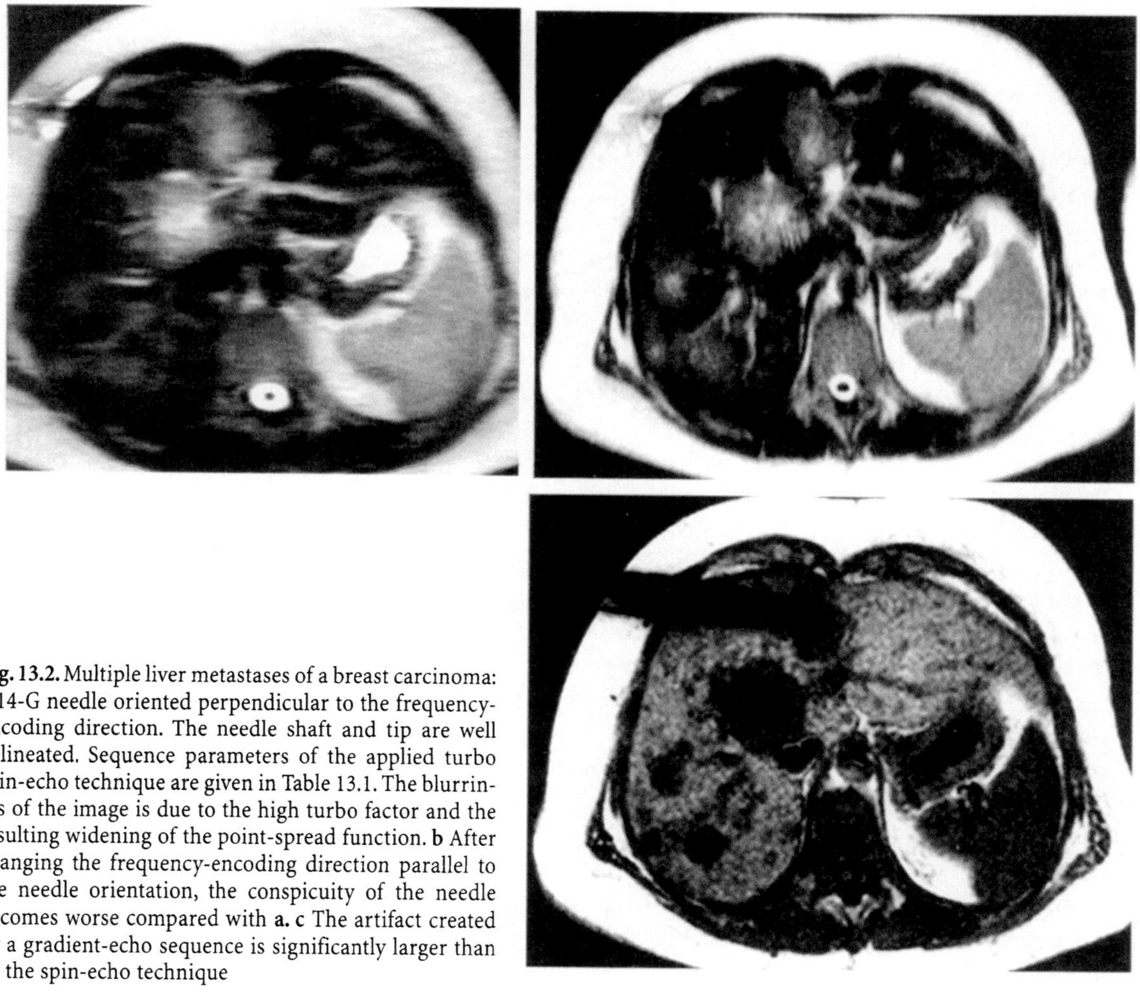

a b c

Fig. 13.2. Multiple liver metastases of a breast carcinoma: **a** 14-G needle oriented perpendicular to the frequency-encoding direction. The needle shaft and tip are well delineated. Sequence parameters of the applied turbo spin-echo technique are given in Table 13.1. The blurriness of the image is due to the high turbo factor and the resulting widening of the point-spread function. **b** After changing the frequency-encoding direction parallel to the needle orientation, the conspicuity of the needle becomes worse compared with **a**. **c** The artifact created by a gradient-echo sequence is significantly larger than by the spin-echo technique encoding direction perpendicular to the needle is sometimes more suitable for needle localization (Fig. 13.2a, b). Depending on the type of needle, its size and orientation to B_0, and the different sequence parameters, one has to keep in mind this possibility to change the artifact size without manipulating the other sequence parameters.

It has been reported that the needle tip itself can be localized more precisely when the frequency-encoding direction is perpendicular to the needle shaft (Langen et al. 1996). This might produce an inacceptable size of the susceptibility artifact around the needle shaft when gradient-echo sequences are applied. For spin-echo sequences, the orientation of the frequency-encoding direction perpendicular to the needle axis usually yields better delineation of the needle shaft, together with more precise needle tip localization (Fig. 13.2a, b). Voxel size has also been shown to have an effect on susceptibility artifacts (Young et al. 1988), but this can be neglected in the clinical setting of biopsies.

13.2.4 Image Contrast and Vessel Conspicuity

For lesion detection, contrast is at least as crucial as spatial resolution. However, when a biopsy is to be performed, the diagnosis of a suspicious lesion has invariably been made already and, therefore, the demands on the biopsy sequence are not as great as on a diagnostic scan. As the biopsy needle will cause a black artifact, it is easier to exactly localize the needle tip in a bright lesion. In general, these requirements favor the use of T2-weighted sequences. However, this is accompanied by the drawback that T2-weighted images normally take longer than T1-weighted sequences of comparable resolution.

T1-weighted gradient-echo sequences yield a flat contrast which is not well suited to biopsy procedures. Therefore, a prepulse should be added to create sufficient contrast. The prepulse delay time can be varied, which influences lesion visibility. With image contrast appropriately determined, it is possible to create an image which will delineate the lesion with the needle tip inside it.

Accurate anatomic information is needed to choose the safest needle path to the target. As vessels are of major concern, it should be possible to identify them independent of their orientation to the slice. Unfortunately, this is not easily accomplished with a single sequence. Gradient-echo sequences will show vessels running perpendicular to the slice as bright spots due to the inflow effect of blood. The prepulse has to be slice selective in order not to destroy this useful characteristic. In-plane flow will usually not express high signal intensity on gradient-echo sequences. This does not necessarily mean that it is impossible to detect vessels with a course parallel to the slice, but it is undoubtedly more difficult. The T2-weighted spin-echo sequences discussed below will depict slow in-plane flow as relatively high signal intensity. Therefore, the combination of these two techniques yields an accurate delineation of the vascular anatomy.

13.3 MR Imaging and Needles: Specific Sequence Considerations

13.3.1 Fast Gradient-Echo Sequences

Initially, a fast gradient-echo sequence was the workhorse of MR-guided biopsies on our high-field system. An additional slice-selective inversion prepulse with a prepulse delay time of about 1000 ms yielded good contrast characteristics without the need for adaptation in most cases. The precise sequence parameters are given in Table 13.1. This sequence renders reliable contrast and a good anatomical overview without restrictions in the field of view (FOV). Signal strength is adequate and the number of acquisitions can be varied in order to acquire images of higher resolution with a similar signal-to-noise ratio. The sequence parameters given in Table 13.1 are just one possible example (Figs. 13.1, 13.2c). They can be altered significantly without losing their usefulness for the biopsy procedure. For example, the echo time can be further shortened when gradients above 10 mT/m and faster slew rates are available on a system. It is advisable to use a sequence which will be applicable to almost all biopsy procedures without the need for a change of sequence parameters. This practice helps the operator to become familiar with the expected contrast and decreases the chance of needing to stop the scan to prepare a new sequence, with the corresponding loss of time.

Table 13.1. Examples of sequence parameters of a fast gradient-echo sequence without (Figs. 13.1, 13.3c), and with segmented EPI technique (Fig. 13.4), of a fast spin-echo sequence (Fig. 13.3a, b), and of an ultrafast spin-echo sequence with the LoLo technique (Fig. 13.5)

Gradient-echo sequence	
	FOV 450 mm × 450 mm
	Matrix 256 × 256
	Slice thickness 10 mm
	TR 8 ms
	TE 3.6 ms
	Flip angle 25°
	Slice selective inversion prepulse with a delay time of 1052 ms
	No k-space segmentation
	Number of acquisitions 2
	Acquisition time per image 4.1 s
Gradient-echo sequence with segmented EPI technique	
	FOV 375 mm × 275 mm
	Matrix 128 × 128
	Slice thickness 7 mm
	TR 246 ms
	TE 4.6 ms
	Flip angle 80°
	EPI factor (number of echoes per excitation) 3
	Number of acquisitions 2
	Adjacent slices 16
	Acquisition time for 16 slices 15 s
Fast spin-echo sequence	
	FOV 375 mm × 275 mm
	Matrix 256 × 187
	Slice thickness 10 mm
	TR (minimum) 576 ms
	TE (effective) 100 ms
	Echo spacing 7.2 ms
	Flip angle 90°
	Half scan 0.6
	Turbo factor 79
	Number of acquisitions 2
Ultrafast spin-echo sequence: Local Look (LoLo)	
	FOV 250 mm × 125 mm
	Matrix 256 × 256
	Slice thickness 10 mm
	TR (minimal) 592 ms
	TE (effective) 104 ms
	Echo spacing 7.5
	Flip angle 90°
	Half scan 0.6
	Turbo factor 77
	Number of acquisitions 1

EPI, echo planar imaging; FOV, field of view; LoLo, local look; TE, echo time; TR, repetition time

13.3.2 Segmented Echo Planar Imaging (Multishot EPI)

In terms of speed, echo planar imaging (EPI) is a most favorable technique. After the initial excitation pulse, multiple echoes are created by quickly switching the readout gradient. Additionally, short gradient blips are applied for phase encoding. The original version described by Mansfield collected all echoes necessary to fill k-space after one single excitation pulse (single shot; MANSFIELD 1977). However, EPI will not yield a sufficiently high signal-to-noise ratio together with an acceptable resolution when applied as a single-shot technique. This is due to the accompanying long effective echo time when long echo trains are applied. This effective echo time is a major determinant for the dimensions of geometric distortions introduced by EPI. One way to reduce the geometric distortion artifacts is to segment k-space and thereby shorten the effective echo time. This technique is also referred to as multishot EPI, which has been shown to render image quality far superior to single shot EPI (WELTER et al. 1995). Only a few echoes are collected per excitation pulse. The inherent speed of EPI makes this a tempting technique, especially when coverage of multiple slices in a breath-hold is needed. Although good contrast and sufficient signal strength can be achieved with gradient-echo EPI and k-space segmentation, one has to be aware of the possible illusions created by geometric distortion artifacts (Fig. 13.3); besides the distortion of the needle itself, nonferromagnetic material can cause artifacts degrading the whole imaging procedure (Fig. 13.3b). Therefore, EPI techniques should not be applied for biopsy procedures without final verification of the needle tip position by another imaging sequence. Nonetheless, an example of a multishot EPI sequence is given in Table 13.1. Sixteen slices are acquired in a single breath-hold of 15 s. The number of slices can be decreased, but one has to remember that this will shorten the repetition time and, thereby, alter the contrast.

13.3.3 Fast Spin-Echo Sequences

Fast spin-echo sequences apply more than one 180°-pulse per excitation pulse. Therefore, similar to EPI, more than one profile in k-space is collected during one repetition time. The echo-train length, also called the turbo factor, describes the number of echoes sampled after one single excitation pulse. Acquisition times will be shortened substantially, especially for sequences with a long TR. T2-weighted images with a reasonable resolution can be acquired in a breath-hold. The main difference between fast spin-echo and conventional T2-weighted spin-echo sequences is the high signal intensity from fatty

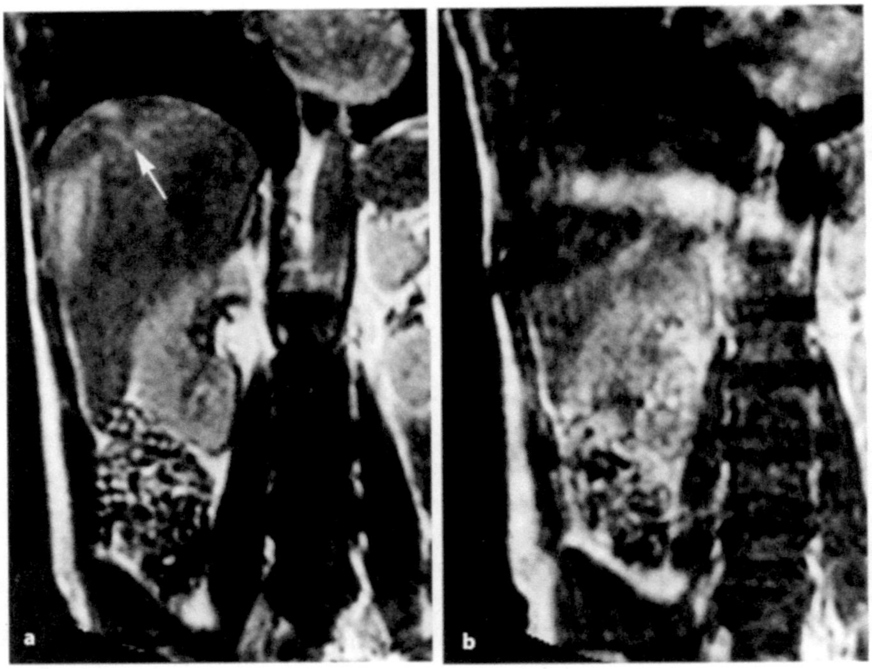

Fig. 13.3. One of 16 coronal slices of a gradient-echo image by the echo planar imaging technique acquired in a single breath-hold of 15 s (for sequence parameters; see Table 13.1). **a** Without the biopsy needle there is good anatomical orientation, but the small liver abscess below the dome of the diaphragm is not well visualized (*arrow*). **b** After insertion of the 14-G biopsy needle, artifacts are introduced into the image, degrading even the anatomical information. The needle itself appears to be bent at the tip. A subsequently acquired gradient-echo image proved this to be due to a distortion artifact

tissue and the introduction of blurring into the image. This blurriness increases as the echo-train lengthens (MULKERN et al. 1990). As with EPI, the fastest spin-echo sequences are achieved when all echoes are sampled in one TR. Due to T2 decay this causes a continuous loss of signal for those echoes acquired further away from the excitation pulse, and the resulting images usually suffer from low signal-to-noise ratios. Another way to shorten the imaging time is to collect only slightly more than half of the full number of profiles. Due to the symmetry of k-space, it is possible to calculate one half of raw data from the other. It is necessary to sample more than 50% of the profiles in order to be able to correct for phase errors occurring during the collection of the first half of k-space. As the second part of the raw data is calculated and not just supplemented by zero-filling, the resolution will be maintained, but the signal-to-noise ratio will be lower. The sequence parameters given in Table 13.1 are meant as a guideline and not a strict rule for a T2-weighted fast spin-echo sequence (Fig. 13.2a, b).

One has to be aware of the fact that there are complex correlations between the number of phase-encoding steps (determining resolution and FOV), echo-train length, echo time and repetition time for fast spin-echo sequences. As it is not easy to quickly change sequence parameters, two standard, fast spin-echo sequences should be developed which are universally applicable to biopsy procedures in different locations. The difference between the two versions should "only" be the orientation of the phase-encoding direction. This allows one to vary the needle artifact size by simply exchanging the frequency and phase-encoding directions. As the anatomic area to be biopsied is not usually square, the use of a rectangular FOV necessitates the implementation of two different sequences to optimally exploit the advantage of a reduced FOV without creating backfolding artifacts (Fig. 13.2a b).

13.3.4
Ultrafast Spin-Echo Sequence: Local Look

As described above, acquisition of all profiles in k-space after a single excitation will yield a significant drop in the signal-to-noise ratio of the image due to the T2 decay experienced by the profiles sampled late after the excitation pulse. A reduction in the number of phase-encoding steps will circumvent this problem. The so-called local look or LoLo technique is a specially designed single-shot spin-echo technique which allows use of a small FOV together with a corresponding reduction of phase encoding steps (N; VAN VAALS et al. 1994). As the pixel size is defined by FOV/N, diminishing both the FOV and the number of phase-encoding steps will not lead to a bigger pixel size and will not decrease the resolution. Further phase-encoding steps are saved by reducing the rectangular field of view (RFOV). This will result in a rectangular image, where the phase-encoding direction gives the orientation along which the FOV is reduced. Both measures, reduction of

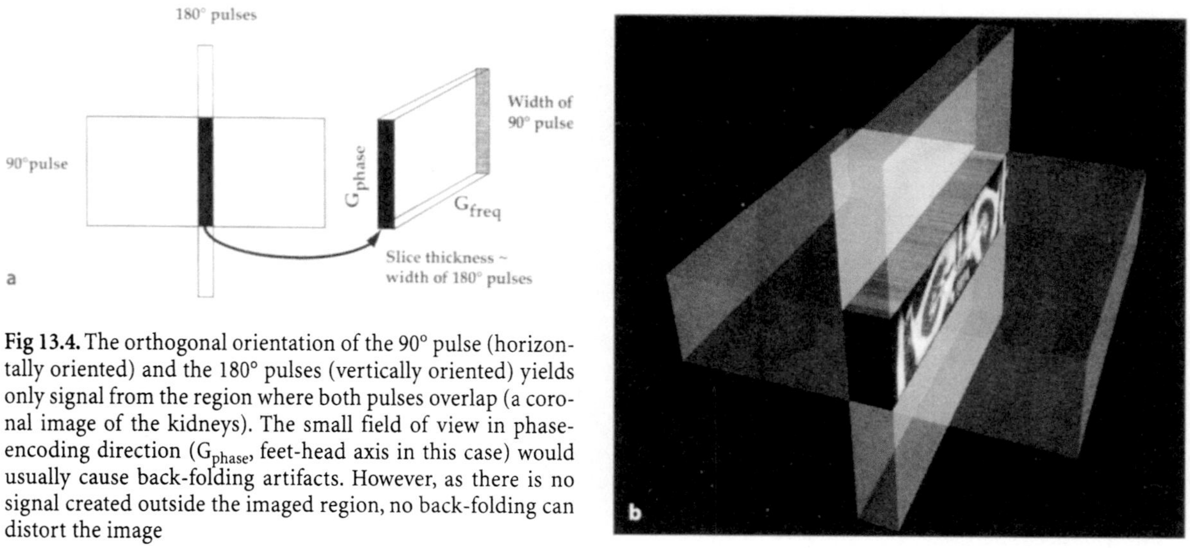

Fig 13.4. The orthogonal orientation of the 90° pulse (horizontally oriented) and the 180° pulses (vertically oriented) yields only signal from the region where both pulses overlap (a coronal image of the kidneys). The small field of view in phase-encoding direction (G_{phase}, feet-head axis in this case) would usually cause back-folding artifacts. However, as there is no signal created outside the imaged region, no back-folding can distort the image

FOV and of RFOV, can cause back-folding artifacts if the imaged object exceeds the boundaries of the FOV in the phase-encoding direction. Therefore, the phase-encoding direction is also called the fold-over direction. Unfortunately, the saving of phase-encoding steps will reduce the FOV along this fold-over direction and thereby create back-folding artifacts unless the object to be imaged is correspondingly small. To avoid this kind of artifact, a dedicated technique is exploited which applies the 90° excitation pulse orthogonally rotated to the following 180° refocusing pulses (FEINBERG et al. 1985). Inherent to spin-echo techniques, only the spins first excited by the 90° pulse and then refocussed by the 180° pulse will give signal to the image. If these pulses are oriented perpendicular to each other, only the area which is hit by the excitation and refocussing pulses will give rise to signal (Fig. 13.4). Consequently, no fold-over artifacts from outside this region can occur. Thereby, it is possible to obtain a small FOV in the frequency-encoding direction together with a further reduction of the FOV in the phase-encoding direction.

The resulting high resolution images are not degraded by back-folding artifacts. The overall reduction of phase-encoding steps makes it possible to acquire single-shot images with a good signal-to-noise ratio. With these thoughts in mind, we have developed a T2-weighted sequence for biopsy procedures, the parameters of which are given in Table 13.1. This sequence yields a T2-weighted image with an in-plane resolution of 1 mm × 1 mm in 600 ms (Fig. 13.5). The small needle artifact caused by this spin-echo method allows also biopsy of small lesions because the needle artifact itself will not obscure the lesion to be punctured.

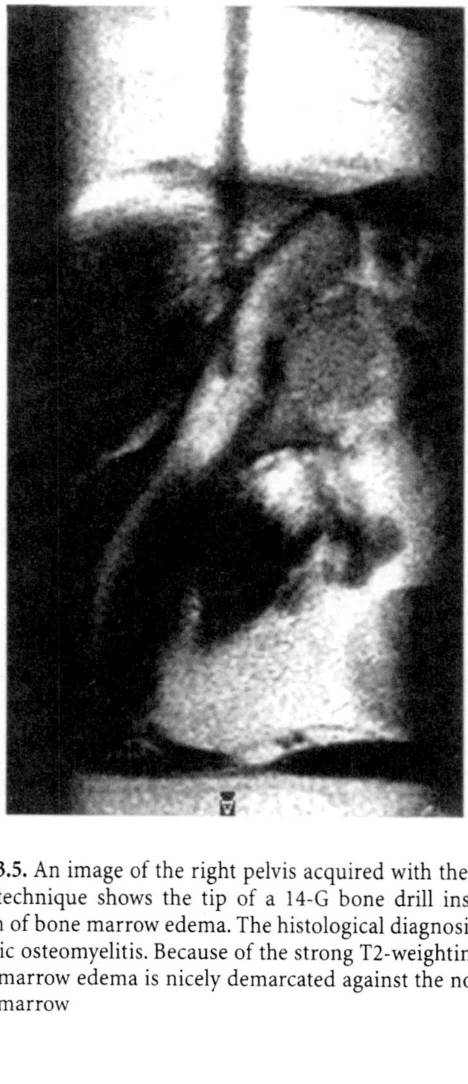

Fig. 13.5. An image of the right pelvis acquired with the local look technique shows the tip of a 14-G bone drill inside a region of bone marrow edema. The histological diagnosis was chronic osteomyelitis. Because of the strong T2-weighting the bone marrow edema is nicely demarcated against the normal bone marrow

References

Adam G, Neuerburg J, Bücker A, et al (1997) Interventional magnetic resonance: initial clinical experience with a 1.5-tesla magnetic resonance system combined with C-arm fluoroscopy. Invest Radiol 23(4):191–197

Duckwiler G, Lufkin RB, Hanafee WN (1989) MR-directed needle biopsies. Radiol Clin North Am 27:255–263

Feinberg DA, Hoenninger JC, Crooks LE, Kaufman L, Watts JC, Arakawa M (1985) Inner volume MR imaging: technical concepts and their application. Radiology 156:743–747

Hathout G, Lufkin RB, Jabour B, Andrews J, Castro D (1992) MR-guided aspiration cytology in the head and neck at high field strength. J Magn Reson Imaging 2:93–94

Ladd ME, Erhart P, Debatin J, Romanowski BJ, Boesiger P, McKinnon GC (1996) Biopsy needle susceptibility artifacts. Magn Reson Med 36:646-651

Langen HJ, Kugel H, Krahe T, Heindel W, Gieseke J, Lackner K (1996) Precision of MR imaging-guided needle placement: experimental results. Radiology 201:358

Leung DA, Debatin JF, Wildermuth S, Heske N, Dumoulin CL, Darrows RD, Hauser M, Davis CP, von Schulthess GK (1995) Real-time biplanar needle tracking for interventional MR imaging procedures. Radiology 197:485–488

Lufkin R, Teresi L, Hanafee W (1987) New needle for MR-guided aspiration cytology of the head and neck. AJR Am J Roentgenol 149:380–382

Mansfield P (1977) Multi planar image formation using NMR spin-echoes. J Phys Chem 10:55–58

Mezrich R (1995) A perspective on k-space. Radiology 195:297–315

Mueller PR, Stark DD, Simeone JF, Saini S, Butch RJ, Edelman RR, Wittenberg J, Ferrucci JT (1986) MR-guided aspiration biopsy: needle design and clinical trials. Radiology 161:605–609

Mueller PR, Stark DD, Simeone JF, Saini S, Hahn PF, Steiner E, Beaulieu P, Wittenberg J, Ferrucci JT (1989) Clinical use of a nonferromagnetic needle for magnetic resonance-guided biopsy. Gastrointest Radiol 14:61–64

Mulkern RV, Wong STS, Winalski C, Jolesz FA (1990) Contrast manipulation and artifact assessment of 2D and 3D RARE sequences. Magn Reson Imaging 8:557–566

Pitt AM, Fleckenstein JL, Greenlee RG, Burns DK, Bryan WW, Haller R (1993) MRI-guided biopsy in inflammatory myopathy: initial results. Magn Reson Imaging 11:1093–1099

Sinha S, Sinha U, Lufkin R, Hanafee W (1989) Pulse sequence optimization for use with a biopsy needle in MRI. Magn Reson Imaging 7:575–579

van Sonnenberg E, Hajek P, Gylys-Morin V, Varney RA, Baker L, Casola G, Christensen R, Mattrey RF (1988) A wire-sheath system for MR-guided biopsy and drainage: laboratory studies and experience in 10 patients, AJR Am J Roentgenol 151:815–817

Welter DR, McKinnon GC, Debatin JF, v. Schulthess GK: Cardiac Echo-Planar MR Imaging 1995: Comparison of Single and Multiple-shot Techniques. Radiology 194:765-770

Young IR, Cox IJ, Bryant P, Budder GM (1988) The benefits of increasing spatial resolution as a means of reducing artifacts due to field inhomogeneities. Magn Res Imaging 6:585–590

van Vaals JJ, van Yperen GH, de Boer RW (1994) Real-time MR imaging using the LoLo (local look) method for interactive and interventional MR at 0.5 T and 1.5 T. Proceedings, Second Meeting of Society of Magnetic Resonance, San Francisco, p 421

Vlaardingerbroek MT, den Boer JA (1996) Magnetic resonance imaging, 1st edn. Springer, Berlin Heidelberg New York, pp 224-227

Transcutaneous MR-Guided Interventions

14 MR-Guided Biopsy of the Abdomen

C. Frahm and H.-B. Gehl

CONTENTS

14.1 Introduction

The excellent soft tissue contrast of MRI, its multiplanar imaging capabilities, and detailed delineation of anatomic features gave rise to the concept of MR-guided biopsy. The first attempt to realize this idea was reported by Mueller et al. (1986), who described phantom trials for needle visualization, as well as MR-guided aspiration biopsies of liver masses. Other groups followed with applications in the head and neck, but also in the abdomen, musculoskeletal system, and breast (Lufkin et al. 1987, 1988; Lufkin and Layfield 1989; van Sonnenberg et al. 1988; Duckwiler et al. 1989; Pitt et al. 1993; Greenstein Orel et al. 1994). The first specially designed commercially available aspiration biopsy needle was developed and introduced by Lufkin et al. in 1987.

However, the practicability of the procedure, especially for the body, is essentially affected by the closed, tube-shaped magnet design of conventional MR imagers with their long and narrow magnet bores. The access to the patient and to the puncture site is hindered considerably, and it may be difficult to maintain sterile conditions at the puncture site. Thus, MR-guided biopsy did not become a widely established method in clinical practice. In recent years, the activities in the field of MR-guided percutaneous procedures for the body have been stimulated again by the widespread introduction of new, open configuration low-field and mid-field scanners (Schenck et al. 1995; Silverman et al. 1995; Frahm et al. 1996; Gehl et al. 1996; Steiner et al. 1996; Lee et al. 1996; Lewin et al. 1996). In this chapter, we will deal with the state of the art in MR-guided abdominal biopsies in general and on low-field units in particular.

C. Frahm, MD, Institute of Radiology, Medical University of Lübeck, Ratzeburger Allee 160, D-23538 Lübeck, Germany
H.-B. Gehl, MD, Institute of Radiology, Medical University of Lübeck, Ratzeburger Allee 160, D-23538 Lübeck, Germany

14.2 Patient Accessibility in Open-Configuration MR Imagers

Up to now, only one open-configuration imager has been presented which is dedicated to MR-guided interventions (Signa Advantage SP, General Electric Medical Systems, Milwaukee, Wis., with 0.5 T and horizontal field axis). This superconductive magnet was designed with two cryostats with a vertical gap in between (Chapter 2) (Schenck et al. 1995). With regard to the access of the puncture site, the magnet design is not the only point of concern. If a surface coil has to be used, its shape must be taken into consideration too. In this unit a suitable open transmit/receive surface coil is applied for abdominal procedures, thus, the radiologist's freedom of movement is affected neither by the magnet nor by the surface coil, and patient repositioning is not necessary.

Conversely, there is the group of horizontally open, low-field and mid-field units with a vertical field axis – primarily designed and offered for low-budget imaging and secondarily discovered to be useful for interventional purposes (Magnetom Open, Siemens Medical Engineering, Erlangen, Germany, 0.2 T; Outlook, Picker International, Cleveland, Ohio, 0.23 T; Airis, Hitachi Medical Corporation, Tokyo, Japan, 0.3 T; Signa Profile, General Electric Medical Systems, Milwaukee, Wis., 0.2 T; Opart, Toshiba Medical Systems, San Francisco, Calif., 0.35 T). Despite the broad access in various horizontal directions, the vertical access from above the patient is limited by the upper magnet pole. The maximum (vertical) distance between the upper pole face and the scanner table (without table pad) is around 40 cm, with differences of a few centimeters. For an abdominal biopsy this means that some manipulations at the puncture site may have to be performed outside the magnet, depending on the localization of the entry point. Nevertheless, these units are much more suitable for abdominal interventions than a conventional unit: a number of manipulations can be performed inside the magnet, continuous immediate visual and voice contact, as well as manual contact to the patient are possible, and there are no difficulties in maintaining sterile conditions at the puncture site.

For body imaging on these units, a receive surface coil is required. Owing to the vertical field axis, the problem of a surface coil suitable for percutaneous procedures can be solved relatively simply by using a slim, beltlike, linear polarized coil, which is wrapped around the patient's body a few centimeters away from the entry site and does not affect access.

14.3 MR-Compatible Biopsy Instruments

All of the commercially available MR-compatible biopsy needles were designed for passive visualization, i.e., the needle is localized and visualized by its susceptibility artifact appearing as a signal loss of linear shape (see Chap. 5). Several manufacturers offer suitable nonferromagnetic aspiration needles, as well as core biopsy devices of various diameters (Table 14.1). Furthermore, after initial MR-guided placement and localization of a suitable nonferromagnetic needle, common ferromagnetic (non-MR-compatible) biopsy needles can be introduced in coaxial fashion through the MR-compatible needle to sample the target lesion.

14.4 Puncture Technique

14.4.1 The Basic Technique

The basic technique performed step by step is very similar to the technique of CT-guided biopsy and does not require extensive hardware modifications or complicated accessories. At our institution, MR-guided abdominal biopsies are carried out on a horizontally open low-field imager (Magnetom Open, Siemens Medical Engineering, Erlangen, Germany).

Instead of the standard body receive coils we apply a slim ring coil (a large, linear polarized, flexible multi-purpose coil with a circumference of 107 or 94 cm) which is wrapped like a belt around the patient's body near the probable puncture site. A radiofrequency(RF)-shielded slave monitor

Table 14.1. Commercially available MR-compatible biopsy needles and devices

Manufacturer	Needle device	Design	Alloy
E-Z-EM, Inc., Westbury, NY, USA Fax +516 333 8278	Lufkin biopsy needle MRI histology needle MRI Biogun	Aspiration; 22 G Aspiration; 20 G, 18 G Disposable, automated, side-cutting gun; 18 G, 14 G	Nonferromagnetic nickel-chromium alloy
William Cook Europe, Bjaeverskov, Denmark Fax +45 53 67 14 96	MReye Chiba biopsy needle	Aspiration; 21 G, 19.5 G, 18 G	Nonferromagnetic nickel-chromium alloy
Daum GmbH, Schwerin, Germany Fax +49 385 6344 152	PunctureNeedle BiopsyNeedle	Aspiration; 20 G, 18 G Side-cutting needle (Tru-Cut type); 18 G, 14 G	Titanium alloy
Somatex GmbH, Berlin, Germany Fax +49 30 625 30 47	Chiba Needle Ultra Rotating biopsy needle Soma-Cut	Aspiration; 21 G, 19.5 G, 18 G Side-cutting needle (Tru-Cut type); 18 G, 14 G	Titanium alloy
C.R. Bard GmbH, Karlsruhe, Germany Fax +49 721 9445100	Magnum Core High Speed	High-speed biopsy device for non-MR-compatible side-cutting biopsy needles (16 G), with MR-compatible coaxial needles (14 G)	Coaxial needle of titanium alloy Biopsy needle of ferromagnetic stainless steel

(1024×1024, liquid crystal display) and a second mouse console are installed near the scanner so that imaging can be directed by the interventional team within the scanning room. As in CT-guided procedures, the in-room monitor is a very helpful and desirable tool.

Two-dimensional (2D) FT spoiled gradient echo images (for example, FLASH, TR 80–154/TE 7–9, flip 70–80°, one excitation, matrix 128×256, field of view (FOV) 350 mm×350 mm) or 2D FT steady-state gradient echos (for example FISP, single slice technique, TR 18 TE 7-8, flip 80-90 °, one excitation, matrix 128 x 256, FOV 350 mm x 350 mm) are suitable to visualize both the intended approach and the needle position. For scanning with transverse or sagittal slice orientation, a rectangular FOV may be used to reduce acquisition time. The imaging protocol should enable acquisition of a package of five to seven slices in a single breath-hold.

To determine the entry point, a localization grid visible in MRI is placed on the skin. At first, we employed surface markers made of glycerol trinitrate or nifedipine capsules; later, we developed a special tube grid made of welded plastic foils and filled with a highly diluted gadolinium chelate (Targogrid, Daum, Schwerin, Germany; Fig. 14.1). While advancing the needle to the target lesion, the puncture angle is checked with a simple three-dimensional laser guidance system (TargoBeam, Daum, Schwerin, Germany; Frahm et al. 1995).

As a rule, we use either a 14-G Tru-Cut-type needle (BiopsyNeedle; Table 14. 1 and Fig. 14.2) or a coaxial biopsy system consisting of an MR-compatible 14-G coaxial needle and an automated high-speed device with 16-G biopsy needles made of stainless steel (Magnum Core High Speed, Table 14.1 and Fig. 14.2).

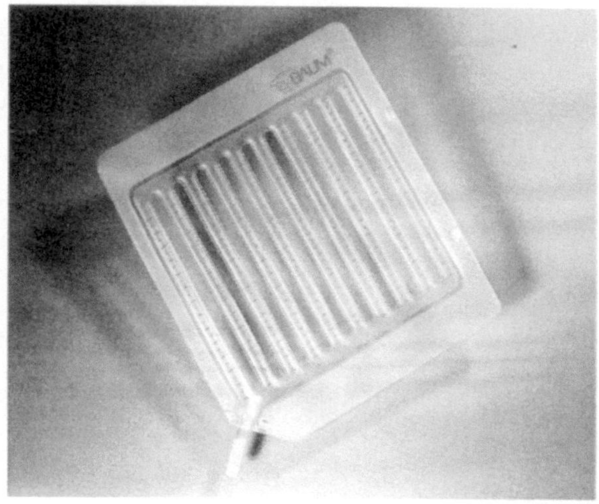

Fig. 14.1. A localization grid for MR-guided biopsy (Targogrid, Daum, Schwerin, Germany). A flexible grid of tubes is formed by two welded plastic foils and filled with a highly diluted solution of a gadolinium chelate. The broad margins are for fixation with adhesive tape on the skin

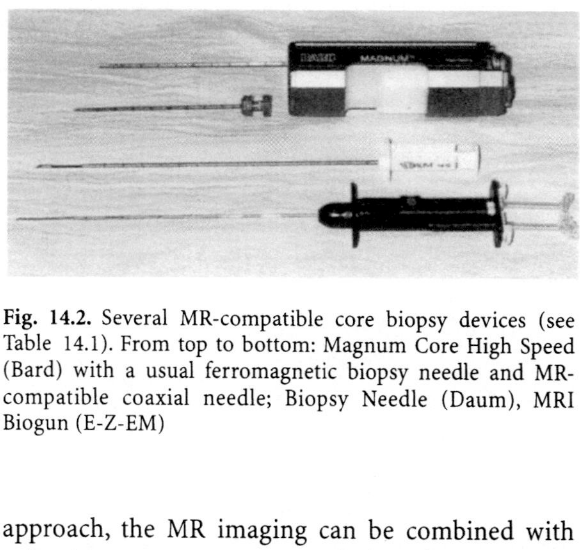

Fig. 14.2. Several MR-compatible core biopsy devices (see Table 14.1). From top to bottom: Magnum Core High Speed (Bard) with a usual ferromagnetic biopsy needle and MR-compatible coaxial needle; Biopsy Needle (Daum), MRI Biogun (E-Z-EM)

Procedure Steps

Imaging of the target lesion and the surrounding structures is performed in axial and/or sagittal slice direction using packages of five or seven slices (Fig. 14.3a). After having fixed the localization grid or surface markers upon the skin, new scans are obtained using a slice direction along the intended approach with the lesion centered in the middle slice (Fig. 14.3b). If the approach appears complex or requires double oblique angulation, the intended biopsy path is visualized by additional scans in a second plane (Fig. 14.3c). In case of an intercostal or subcostal approach, the MR imaging can be combined with palpation to ensure proper choice of entry point (Fig. 14.4).

Based on these images, the length, angulation, and entry point of the puncture path are determined. The entry point is marked with an indelible-ink pen and the localization device is removed.

If necessary the receive coil can be repositioned now to achieve an optimal distance to the entry point (3–8 cm). The skin is cleaned, draped, and anesthetized in the standard sterile fashion. The sterile drape covers the surface coil too. A small incision is made with a scalpel and the needle is inserted.

In advancing the needle, a guidance device (such as Targobeam) can be valuable, especially for difficult approaches (for example, angled, long or narrow approaches and small target lesions). In cases of long puncture paths, a stepwise needle insertion with

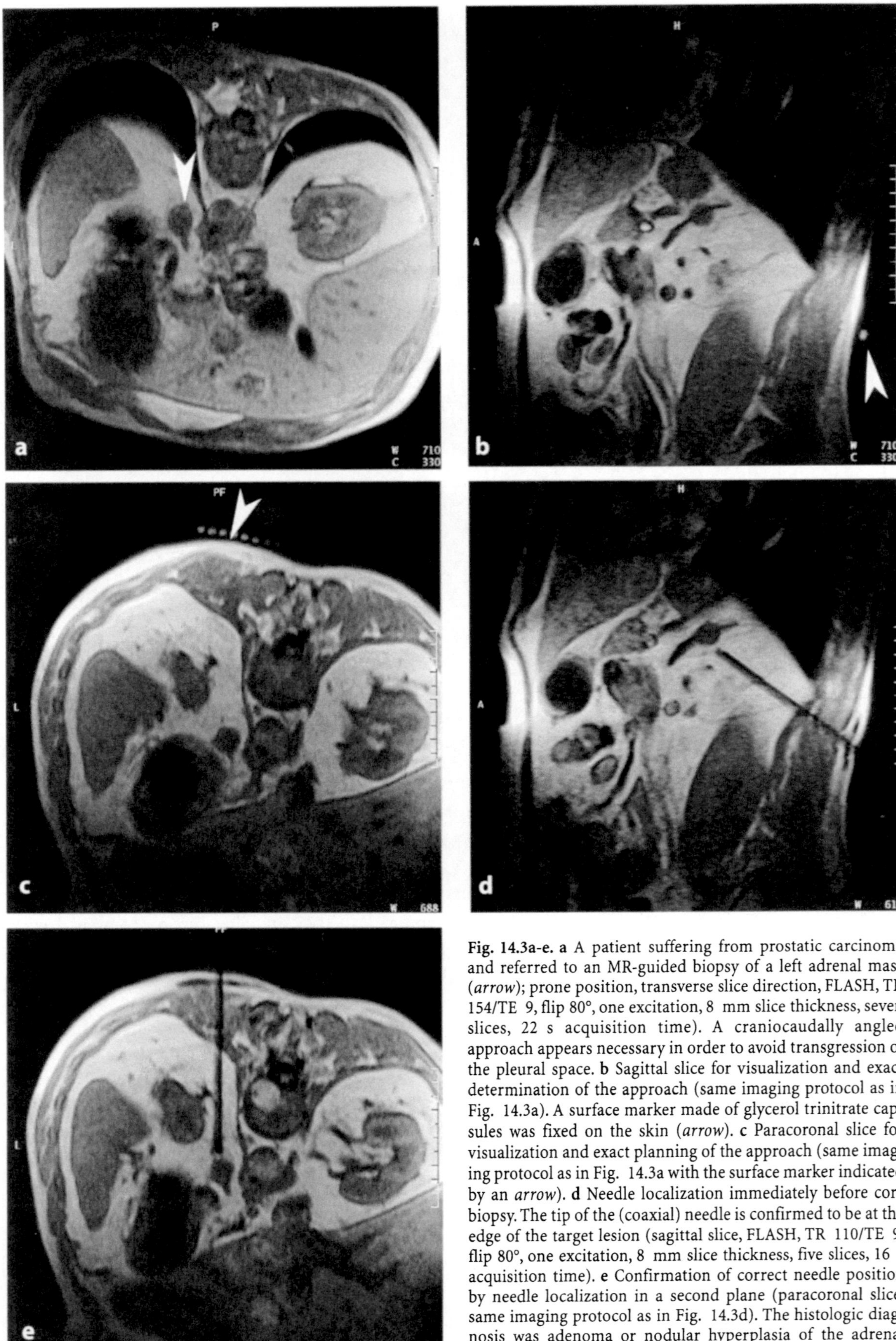

Fig. 14.3a-e. **a** A patient suffering from prostatic carcinoma and referred to an MR-guided biopsy of a left adrenal mass (*arrow*); prone position, transverse slice direction, FLASH, TR 154/TE 9, flip 80°, one excitation, 8 mm slice thickness, seven slices, 22 s acquisition time). A craniocaudally angled approach appears necessary in order to avoid transgression of the pleural space. **b** Sagittal slice for visualization and exact determination of the approach (same imaging protocol as in Fig. 14.3a). A surface marker made of glycerol trinitrate capsules was fixed on the skin (*arrow*). **c** Paracoronal slice for visualization and exact planning of the approach (same imaging protocol as in Fig. 14.3a with the surface marker indicated by an *arrow*). **d** Needle localization immediately before core biopsy. The tip of the (coaxial) needle is confirmed to be at the edge of the target lesion (sagittal slice, FLASH, TR 110/TE 9, flip 80°, one excitation, 8 mm slice thickness, five slices, 16 s acquisition time). **e** Confirmation of correct needle position by needle localization in a second plane (paracoronal slice, same imaging protocol as in Fig. 14.3d). The histologic diagnosis was adenoma or nodular hyperplasia of the adrenal cortex

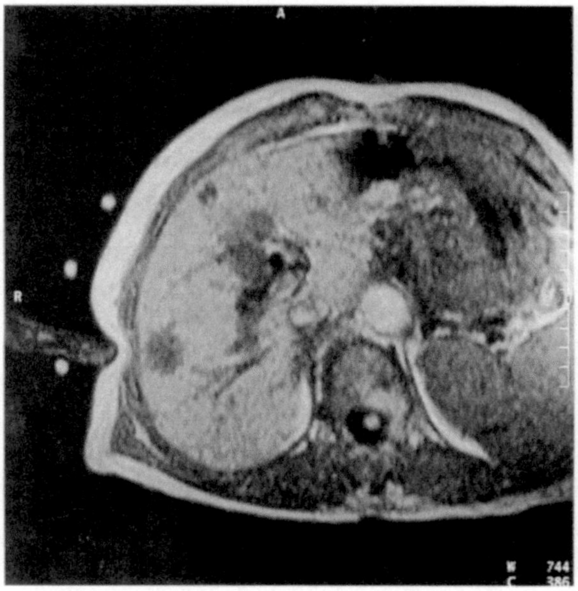

Fig. 14.4. Combined application of surface markers and palpation to determine the entry point for an intercostal approach (transverse slice, same imaging parameters as in Fig. 14.3d; metastasis of a pancreatic carcinoma)

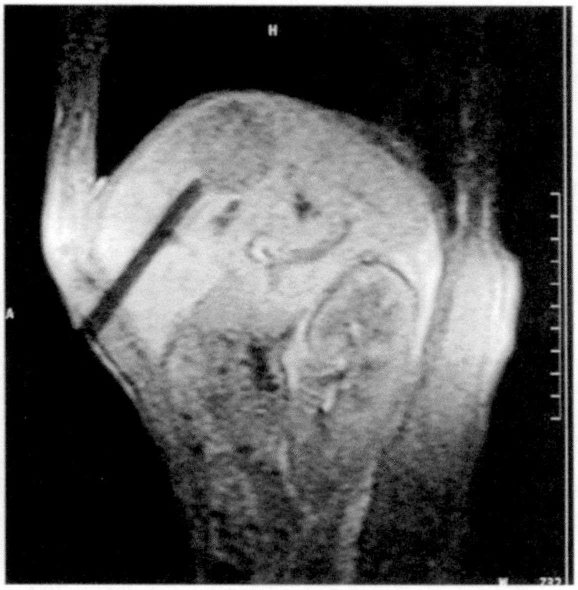

Fig. 14.5. MR-guided biopsy of a relatively large subphrenic lesion in the hepatic dome using an anterior, subcostal, and craniocaudally angled approach (sagittal slice direction, TR 80/TE 9, flip 70°, one excitation, slice thickness 8 mm, three slices, acquisition time 12 s; metastasis of a bronchial carcinoma)

Table 14.2. Data from MR-guided abdominal biopsies performed at our institution (n = 32, 11 female/21 male patients)

Biopsy characteristics	Mean	Minimum	Maximum
Age of patients (years)	57	27	83
Lesion diameter (cm)	3.5	1.2	12.5
Pathway length (cm)	7.5	2.5	15
Time patient on table (min)	49	20	84
Needle passes	2	1	5

repeated imaging for needle localization is recommended enabling the puncture angle to be corrected several times if necessary. Prior to cutting or aspirating the specimen, the final needle position is confirmed by MR imaging along the needle course in two planes (Fig. 14.3d, e); for simple approaches and/or relatively large target lesions, one plane is sufficient (Fig. 14.5). We prefer packages of only three slices for needle localization to minimize the time intervals in breath-hold needed for the image data acquisition.

In each case of abdominal biopsy (Table 14.2), we could position the biopsy instrument accurately and sufficient material was obtained (20 liver lesions, 5 adrenal masses, 4 pelvic masses, 3 soft tissue masses). The target lesion was hit on first or second attempt in most cases. In 13 cases, craniocaudally angled approaches were necessary to avoid transgression of the pleural space. Using sagittal or parasagittal and coronal or paracoronal slice orientation even these approaches could be realized safely because in each case it was possible to generate an image along the course of the approach and the needle. Two complications occurred (shock, pneumothorax); however, both incidents were unrelated to image guidance or needle visualization.

14.4.2
Interactive MR-Guided Biopsy

There are reports of biopsies guided by interactive and nearly-real-time imaging performed on open-configuration interventional 0.5-T systems (Silverman et al. 1995; Steiner et al. 1996), as well as on a horizontally open 0.2-T scanner (Lewin et al. 1996). "Interactive" means that the image plane is determined by (and therefore includes) the puncture needle and changes automatically with the needle position. The MR imager is integrated with a frameless, optically linked stereotaxy system (Flashpoint, Pixsys, Boulder, Colo.).

Optical tracking of the needle is performed using three video sensors to localize two light-emitting diodes (LEDs) mounted on a hand-held probe attached to the biopsy needle. The biopsy probe position is calculated from the spatial location of the two LEDs and translated into the coordinate system of the MRI system to define the imaging plane for subsequent image acquisition. Following target localization, the needle is advanced under a continuous imaging mode consisting of automated sequential acquisition, reconstruction, and display employing a fast gradient-echo sequence. The time involved for image data collection, reconstruction, and display of a single slice on the in-room monitor is about 3–4.5 s, and a new image is presented every 1.5–2 s.

14.5 Clinical Value

The multiplanar imaging capabilities form the most advantageous feature in MR-guided biopsies of the abdomen. Long and difficult craniocaudally angled approaches can be easily accomplished. Visualization of any desirable approach in multiple plane enhances safety and reduces procedure times. Despite the fact that sonography is also multiplanar and, furthermore, well tried for image-guided biopsies, sonographic image guidance is problematic in cases of long and/or intercostal approaches – such as the angled infrapleural "posterior" approach to upper abdominal masses (van Sonnenberg et al. 1981). For example, all of our patients referred to MR-guided biopsy of adrenal masses were referred by experienced sonographers in the department of internal medicine who considered sonographic guidance as insufficient. Unfortunately, a pneumothorax cannot be proved by MRI – though MRI shares this disadvantage with sonography. In experienced hands, the procedure times needed for MR-guided biopsies performed on open-configuration magnets appear generally comparable to the times involved for CT-guided biopsies in cases of similar complexity.

Although the high soft tissue contrast of MRI was an important argument for attempting MR-guided biopsies, we have not taken significant advantage of this. Among our biopsy patients, there was no case of an abdominal target lesion visible only on MRI. However, others have reported a number of cases of MR-guided biopsies of liver lesions not visible on CT or ultrasound (Mack et al. 1997).

A slight drawback of MR-guided biopsy is the fact that the susceptibility artifact, which indicates the needle position, may obscure the target area. Even in a 0.2-T system, a 14-G titanium needle causes an artifact with a width up to 10 mm. In this setting, a lower limit of 1.5 cm is recommended for the diameter of the target lesion to ensure a safe and successful procedure. Moreover, the spatial resolution is considerably lower than by CT because a relatively low matrix (recommended: 128×256) combined with a large field of view which has to be chosen to achieve a sufficient signal/noise ratio within as short a time interval as possible. However, in our patients no procedure was hampered by the limited spatial resolution. Overall, the studies published so far suggest that MR-guided abdominal biopsy is a safe and accurate method with results comparable to those of biopsy series using CT or sonography.

At present, the number of clinical indication for the MR-guided abdominal biopsy remains limited. MR-guided biopsies of abdominal structures can be performed safely.

References

Duckwiler G, Lufkin RB, Teresi L, Spickler E, Dion J, Vinuela F, Bentson J, Hanafee W (1989) Head and neck lesions: MR-guided aspiration biopsy. Radiology 170:519–522

Frahm C, Kloess W, Gehl HB, Weiss HD (1995) Ein neues Laser-Punktionsvisier für CT- und MRT-gesteuerte Punktionen des Körperstamms. Rofo Fortschr Geb Rontgenstr Neuen Bildgeb Verfahr 163:73–76

Frahm C, Gehl HB, Weiss HD, Rossberg WA (1996) Technik der MRT-gesteuerten Stanzbiopsie im Abdomen an einem offenen Niederfeldgerät: Durchführbarkeit und erste klinische Ergebnisse. Rofo Fortschr Geb Rontgenstr Neuen Bildgeb Verfahr 164:62–67

Gehl HB, Frahm C, Schimmelpenning H, Weiss HD (1996) Technik der MRT-gesteuerten abdominellen Drainage an einem offenen Niederfeldmagneten: Durchführbarkeit und erste Ergebnisse. Rofo Fortschr Geb Rontgenstr Neuen Bildgeb Verfahr 165:70–73

Greenstein Orel S, Schnall MD, Newman RW, Powell CM, Torosian MH, Rosato EF (1994) MR imaging-guided localization and biopsy of breast lesions: initial experience. Radiology 193:97–102

Lee H, Lu DSK, Farahani K, Krasny RM (1996) Biopsies of hepatic dome lesions: semi-real time coronal MR guidance technique. (abstract) Proceedings of the 4th Scientific Meeting and Exhibition of the International Society for Magnetic Resonance in Medicine, New York, p 889

Lewin JS, Duerk JL, Petersilge CA, et al (1996) Interactive MRI for procedure guidance on a clinical c-arm system: A pilot biopsy study. (abstract) Proceedings of the 4th Scientific Meeting and Exhibition of the International Society for Magnetic Resonance in Medicine, New York, p 53

Lufkin R, Layfield L (1989) Coaxial needle system of MR- and CT-guided aspiration cytology. J Comput Assist Tomogr 13:1105–1107

Lufkin R, Teresi L, Hanafee W (1987) New needle for MR-guided aspiration cytology of the head and neck. Am J Roentgenol 149:380–382

Lufkin R, Teresi L, Chiu L, Hanafee W (1988) A technique for MR-guided needle placement. Am J Roentgenol 151:193–196

Mack MG, Vogl TJ, Balzer JO, Hammerstingl R, Pegios W, Lobbeck H, Felix R (1997) MR-guided biopsies of soft tissue tumors on a conventional high-field MR-system. (abstract) Eur Radiol 7 [Suppl]: S188

Mueller PR, Stark DD, Simeone JF, Saini S, Butch RJ, Edelman RR, Wittenberg J, Ferrucci JT (1986) MR-guided aspiration biopsy: needle design and clinical trials. Radiology 161:605–609

Pitt AM, Fleckenstein JL, Greenlee RG, Burns DK, Bryan WW, Haller R (1993) MRI-guided biopsy in inflammatory myopathy: initial results. Magn Reson Imaging 11:1093–1099

Schenck JF, Jolesz FA, Roemer PB, et al (1995) Superconducting open-configuration MR imaging system for image-guided therapy. Radiology 195:805–814

Silverman SG, Collick BD, Figueira MR, et al (1995) Interactive MR-guided biopsy in an open-configuration MR imaging system. Radiology 197:175–181

Steiner P, Schoenenberger AW, Penner EA, Erhart P, Debatin JF, von Schulthess GK, Kacl GM (1996) Interaktive stereotaktische Interventionen im supraleitenden, offenen 0,5-Tesla-MR-Tomographen. Rofo Fortschr Geb Rontgenstr Neuen Bildgeb Verfahr 165:276–280

van Sonnenberg E, Wittenberg J, Ferrucci JT, Mueller PR, Simeone JF (1981) Triangulation method for percutaneous needle guidance: the angled approach to upper abdominal masses. Am J Roentgenol 137:757–761

van Sonnenberg E, Hajek P, Gylys-Morin V, et al (1988) A wire-sheath system for MR-guided biopsy and drainage: laboratory studies and experience in 10 patients. Am J Roentgenol 151:815-817

15 MR-Guided Biopsy of the Bone

J.-M. Neuerburg

CONTENTS

15.1 Introduction

Before starting any specific treatment of musculoskeletal disease, confirmation of the diagnosis is considered mandatory. As an alternative to surgical biopsy procedures, the diagnosis can be confirmed percutaneously in many situations. Accurate positioning of biopsy needles within bone lesions has been greatly facilitated by the improvements in imaging techniques in recent years. Biopsy guidance by multi-angle fluoroscopy, computed tomography (CT), a combination of an integrated X-ray fluoroscopy C-arm and CT and, more recently, magnetic resonance imaging (MRI) has enabled us to obtain cytologic or histologic specimens from sites previously thought to be inaccessible using a percutaneous approach.

15.2 Radiologic Guidance Modalities

Fluoroscopic guidance for percutaneous biopsy of musculoskeletal lesions is readily available and allows permanent control of the path of the biopsy needle into the lesion. Biplane fluoroscopy or a C-arm fluoroscopic unit allows control of the needle position in two perpendicular planes without changing the position of the patient. However, percutaneous biopsy under fluoroscopic guidance is restricted to those lesions which can be clearly visualized by fluoroscopy without delineation of vulnerable structures within the chosen biopsy path.

CT guidance can provide an intermittent, reliable three-dimensional (3D) control of the biopsy needle path. In contrast to fluoroscopy, CT guidance allows discrimination of associated soft-tissue masses and delineation of vital anatomic vascular and neural structures. Thus CT guidance is recommended in small bone lesions not clearly depicted by fluoroscopy and bone lesions with an additional suspected soft tissue mass, as well as lesions located in high-risk areas.

Installation of a mobile fluoroscopic C-arm between the gantry of the CT unit and the examination table allows alternative use of the two imaging modalities for guidance of percutaneous biopsy procedures for musculoskeletal lesions. This concept combines the advantages of both methods, while diminishing their limitations.

Over the past few years technical innovations and clinical needs have prompted an expansion of MRI to a host of applications throughout the entire body and central nervous system. There is an increasing interest in using MRI to guide and monitor various interventional procedures. Recently, MR-guided percutaneous bone biopsy has been introduced into clinical routine (Neuerburg et al. 1996). Advantages of MR-guidance over the other imaging modalities include lack of irradiation, high soft-tissue contrast, and ability to obtain multiplanar and 3D imaging. The use of MRI to control percutaneous bone biopsies may be complementary to CT and advantageous in lesions not visible with other imaging modalities. However, compared with CT, disadvantages of MR-guidance are evident: additional requirements for MR-compatible patient monitoring (e.g., magnetic field and radiofrequency shielding), limited spatial and temporal resolution, limited access to the site of

J.-M. Neuerburg, MD, PhD, Department of Diagnostic Radiology, University of Technology Aachen, Pauwelsstr. 30, D-52057 Aachen, Germany intervention, and difficulty in locating instrumentation-based passive image artifacts within the lesion.

15.3 Equipment and Instrumentation

15.3.1 Requirements for the MR Scanner

Compared with the conventional MR-imaging magnets, there are three different types of "interventional MR scanner" suitable for MR guided biopsies: open 0.5-T superconducting magnets constructed in a "double doughnut" configuration with access to the patient between two vertical magnets; partially open horseshoe (0.2 T) and temple-like (0.064 T) low-field magnets; and modified conventional superconducting high-field (1.5 T) MR scanners with an integrated X-ray fluoroscopy C-arm (see Chaps. 1–3).

The technique of percutaneous bone biopsy procedures under MR guidance using a modified conventional superconducting high-field (1.5 T) MR scanner is similar to the CT-guided technique. In both instances the procedure is performed outside the gantry; by moving the examination table, alternative, intermittent use of MR imaging and fluoroscopy is possible.

15.3.2 Requirements for MR Accessories

Biopsy procedures under MR guidance require MR-compatible low-artifact interventional instruments which can be visualized by MRI. However, the visualization of instrumentation-based passive image artifacts depends on the susceptibility and configuration of the instrument, pulse-sequence parameters, the field strength B_0, and the orientation of the instrument to B_0.

According to the composition of the bone lesion, biopsy needles are required for osteolytic bone lesions or adjacent soft tissue masses and bone trephine needles for osteosclerotic lesions.

15.3.2.1 Biopsy Needles for Sampling of Osteolytic Bone Lesions

A variety of MR-compatible biopsy needles is presently available for cytologic or histologic sampling of soft tissue masses or osteolytic bone lesions. Table 15.1 provides a survey of MR-compatible percutaneous biopsy needles. In general, configuration, handling, and cutting properties of the MR-compatible biopsy needles are similar to those needles used for fluoroscopic or CT-guided percutaneous procedures. Ferromagnetic materials are exchanged for nonferromagnetic components (e.g., titanium, tantalum, and tungsten alloys with aluminum/vanadium).

Table 15.1. Instruments for MR-guided biopsy of osteolytic bone lesions (selection)

MReye Spinal needle 22, 19.5 or 18 G; MReye Chiba biopsy needle 22, 19.5 or 18 G (William Cook Europe, DK-4632 Bjaeverskov, Denmark)
mrt biopsy needle 14 or 18 G (Daum Medical, D-19061 Schwerin, Germany)
Lufkin biopsy needle 22 G; biopsy needle 18 or 20 G (E-Z-EM, Westbury, N.Y.; distributed by Guerbet, D-65843 Sulzbach, Germany)
Soma-Cut MR tool 14 or18 G (Somatex, Berlin, Germany)

A "side-slit" type of biopsy needle allows multiple sampling, with the outer cannula kept in place, while the inner cannula with the specimen is taken out and replaced. Other types of needle are completely withdrawn together with the cytologic or histologic specimen.

15.3.2.2 Biopsy Needles for Sampling of Osteosclerotic Bone Lesions

Percutaneous penetration of intact, thick cortical bone or osteosclerotic bone lesions (e.g., osteoid osteomas, osteoplastic metastasis, etc.) carried out by means of cutting needles or sharpened cannulas can cause considerable discomfort to the patient and may be time consuming or even impossible. To this purpose, a new hand-driven or, optionally motor-driven MR- and CT-compatible percutaneous bone biopsy system (Fig. 15.1) has been developed (Neuerburg et al. 1996). At the moment, this system is under clinical evaluation but not yet commercially available. The coaxial bone biopsy system (Cook Europe) consists of a 12-G guiding cannula with a trocar, a 14-G drill with a 16-G trocar, a plastic handle with a Luer-Lok for manual use and a pneumatic turbine with a Luer-Lok and a foot panel for infinitely variable motor-assisted drilling (10–250 rotations/min at 6 bar compressed air).

Alternatively, an 8-G guiding cannula with a 10-G trocar and 10-G drill with a 12-G trocar can be used.

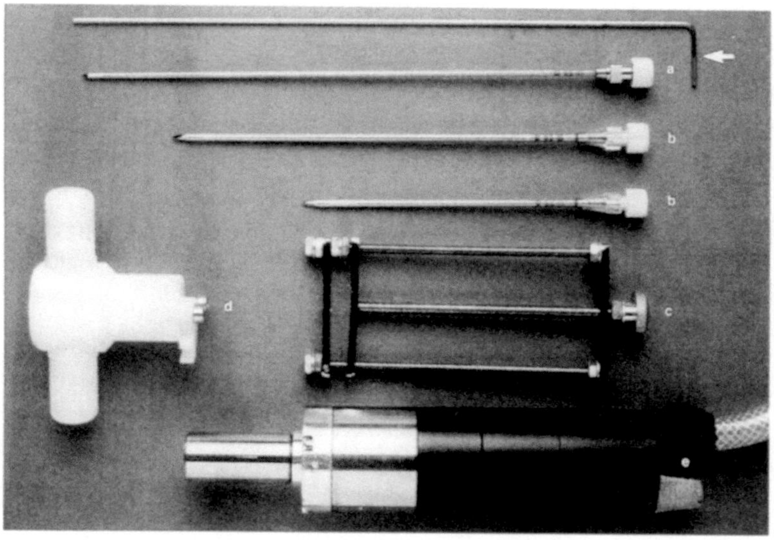

Fig. 15.1. Prototype hand-driven or, optionally, motor-driven MR-compatible percutaneous coaxial bone biopsy system: 14-G drill with a sharp trocar and a blunt-edged obturator (*arrow*; *a*), 12-G outer guiding cannulas with trocars (*b*), a specimen pusher (*c*), plastic handle with a Luer-Lok for manual drive (*d*), and a pneumatic turbine with a Luer-Lok for motor-assisted drilling (*e*)

The guiding cannulas and the drills are available in two different lengths. Similar to the "side-slit" type of needle, the coaxial bone biopsy system allows multiple sampling with one penetration while maintaining the outer guiding cannula in place.

15.4 Technique

15.4.1 Anesthesia

In general, biopsies may be performed on an outpatient basis with local anesthesia. Compared with neuroleptanalgesia or general anesthesia, local anesthesia offers the advantage of patient cooperation in informing the physician of radiating pain due to nerve impingement by the biopsy needle. However, in the case of some lesions, such as osteoid osteomas (drilling of the nidus is extremely painful! Adam et al. 1995), neuroleptanalgesia or even general anesthesia is recommended. Furthermore, general anesthesia is required for young children and for restless and/or uncooperative patients.

15.4.2 Location of the Puncture Site

Several aspects have to be analyzed prior to selection of the percutaneous approach to the bone lesion:

- Review of the available imaging modalities with regard to selecting a representative part of the bone lesion (e.g., edema, necrosis, inflammation, vascularity, etc.).
- Areas with cortical destruction or soft tissue components are easier to biopsy than osteosclerotic areas.
- The percutaneous approach should take potential surgical access into account (coordination with the surgeon).

15.4.3 Puncture

For MR-guided biopsies using an open MR scanner, the chosen puncture site on the skin can be located under MR-imaging control by compression with the finger tip. With a conventional MR imager, a grid is stuck to the skin to allow location of the puncture site on the skin and to determine the correct puncture depth and angle. We apply two different grids: for T1-weighted sequences, we use 9-F plastic tubes filled with an aqueous Gd-DTPA solution and, for T2-weighted sequences, 9-F plastic tubes filled with tap water.

The puncture site is marked on the skin using a permanent marker and sterile conditions are created. Local anesthetic is applied using a long thin spinal needle all the way down to the periosteum. Liberal application of local anesthetics is recommended as penetration of the periosteum is frequently very painful. According to Schweitzer et al. (1995), the use of lidocaine does not affect culture of percutaneous bone biopsy specimens obtained to diagnose osteomyelitis. A small skin incision is usually made. The biopsy needle including the stylet or the guiding cannula of the coaxial bone biopsy set with its trocar is inserted as far as the periosteum (NB: Remove ferromagnetic instruments to avoid dislocation by magnetic field!).

In osteolytic lesions the biopsy needle can be forced into the lesion using moderate axial pressure. In penetration by means of the coaxial bone biopsy system the guiding cannula is held against the periosteum and the trocar is exchanged for the 14-G drill and its trocar. The trocar is removed and the plastic handle is Luer-Loked to the drill. The drill is rotated manually clockwise using slight axial pressure until the target lesion is reached.

The needle path can be controlled by intermittent MR scans, either within the open MR system or by moving the patient into the (modified conventional) magnet (Fig. 15.2). Using an MR system with an integrated mobile C-arm fluoroscopy unit, the procedure can be performed alternatively under fluoroscopic guidance: while the procedure has been planned under MR guidance, fluoroscopy can be used to show the position of the drill.

While drilling through thick cortical or osteosclerotic bone the drill might become occluded and the specimen hard-packed within the hollow drill. In this situation the drill has to be removed and cleaned or exchanged. This improves the drilling properties and avoids hard-packing of the specimen and alterations in the specimen's architecture. During this exchange, the guiding cannula has to be firmly pressed against the periosteum to allow a second passage of the drill into the same hole! In addition, we use a pneumatic turbine with a Luer-Lok for variable motor-assisted drilling. Connected to 6-bar compressed air (anesthesia equipment!), rotations may be varied in the range of 10–250 rotations per minute using a foot panel.

The specimen obtained with the drill has to be ejected by inserting the obturator into the Luer-Lok opening and passing it out the drilling end. However, the specimen may become firmly fixed within the hollow drill. To facilitate removal, we use a specimen pusher (Fig. 15.1).

Core biopsies are fixed in 10% formalin, whereas cytologic specimens are smeared on glass slides. Further fixation has to be carried out as advised by the pathologist. When infection is suspected, additional bacteriologic cultures are acquired.

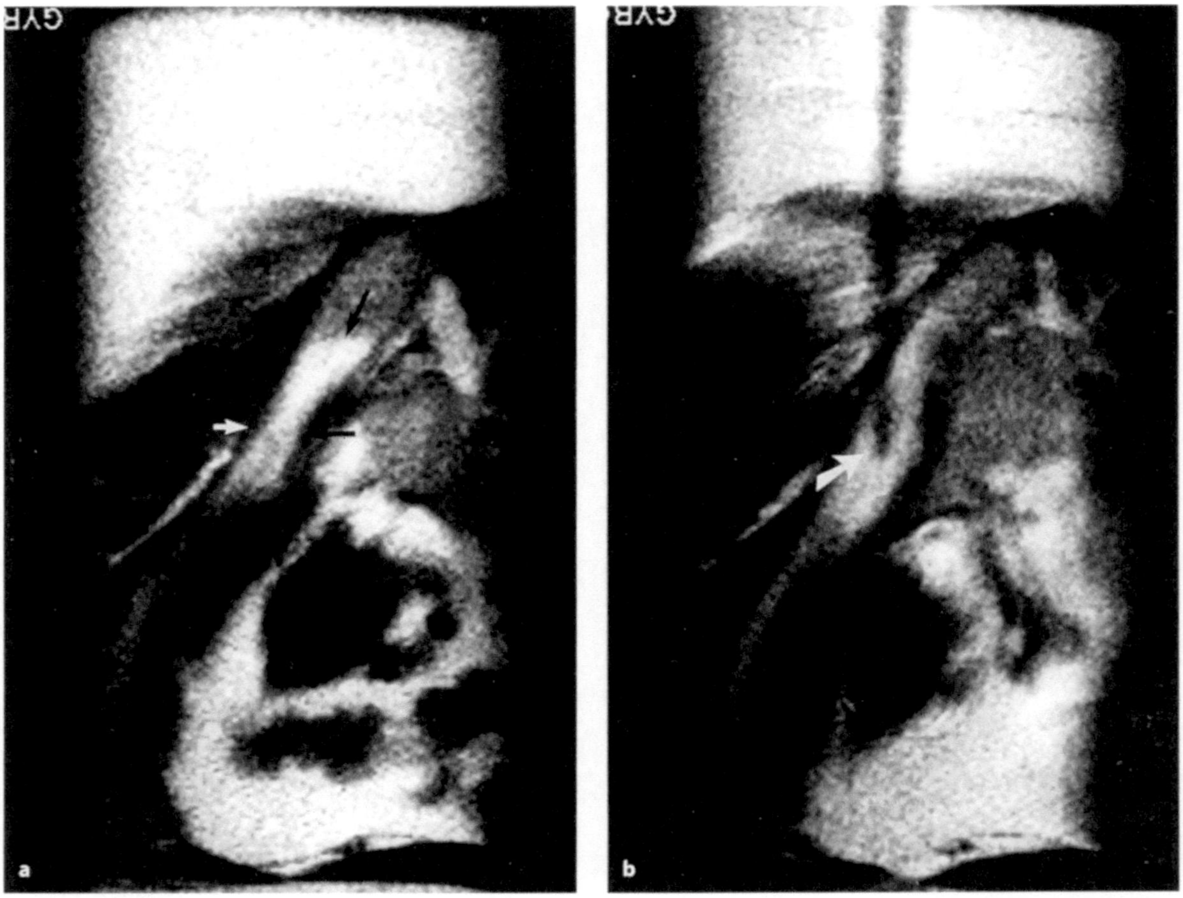

Fig. 15.2a, b. Percutaneous MR-guided biopsy of an abacterial chronic sacroiliitis using a dorsal approach (33-year-old woman, prone position, transaxial T2-weighted "local look" sequence): **a** Circumscribed edema of the medullary space within the left os ilium (*arrows*). **b** The tip of the low-signal 14-G drill can be delineated within the bone marrow edema (*arrow*)

15.5 Indications

Indications for percutaneous bone biopsies include cytologic or histologic confirmation of primary and secondary bone lesions with an unknown etiology and/or demonstration of the infectious agent in suspected osteomyelitis (LAREDO et al. 1994; LOGAN et al. 1996; WHITE et al. 1995). MR-guided percutaneous bone biopsy can be used as an alternative to the CT-guided technique, indications for both modalities are similar. The MR-guided bone biopsy technique is advantageous for lesions not visible with other imaging tools and in young patients to avoid irradiation. Several biopsy techniques and their indications have been described elsewhere (AHLSTROM and ASTROM 1993; ARCA et al. 1995; LAREDO et al. 1994; REUTHER 1994; TIKKAKOSKI et al. 1992).

Percutaneous skeletal aspiration and core biopsies are complementary techniques (SCHWEITZER et al. 1996; TIKKAKOSKI et al. 1992). In small soft-tissue masses and small osteolytic bone lesions, fine-needle aspiration techniques may be recommended, and in large soft-tissue masses and large osteolytic bone lesions, histologic samples by means of a "side-slit" needle (TruCut) should be obtained (LOGAN et al. 1996). For osteosclerotic bone tumors and osteosclerotic tumor-like lesions, as well as for osteolytic bone tumors covered with an intact bony shell, trephine needles are more suitable. In very dense lesions use of a (pneumatic) drill may be necessary (LOGAN et al. 1996; LAREDO et al. 1994).

In general, MR guidance is appropriate for lesions located in low-risk areas (e.g., the peripheral skeleton or pelvis). However, for lesions in high-risk areas (e.g., the spine) CT guidance is recommended (NEUERBURG et al. 1996).

15.6 Results and Complications

Within a time interval of 10 months we performed a total of 20 percutaneous biopsies on bone lesions, of which 16 could be finalized within the MR unit (Table 15.2). However, in four patients we preferred to work under CT guidance: As the entire MR-compatible monitoring equipment to control general anesthesia during percutaneous removal of osteoid osteomas is not yet available for our interventional MR scanner and as visualization of the nidus of osteoid osteomas by CT is superior to MRI, we performed this procedure within the CT unit. In one case of a transpedicular biopsy approach to osteomyelitis of a lumbar vertebra we shifted from the MR unit to the CT unit because of the superior delineation of the drill and the local anatomy by CT.

Table 15.2. MR-guided percutaneous biopsy of bone: patient population (Department of Diagnostic Radiology, University of Technology Aachen, January to October 1996; $n = 20$)

Indications	*n*	*Location of lesions*	*n*
Unknown etiology of bone lesions	12	Pelvis	9
		Femur	5
Demonstration of the infectious agent in suspected osteomyelitis	4	Tibia	3
		Lumbar spine	1
		Humerus	1
Core decompression (AVascularNecrosis of the femoral head)	1	Sternum	1
Removal of an osteoid osteoma	3		

MR-guided percutaneous biopsy yielded a diagnosis in 13 out of 16 cases (Tab.15.3). There was one incorrect histologic diagnosis of the core biopsy revealing osteomyelitis in a patient with surgically proven low-grade osteosarcoma of the femur. In two patients the specimens obtained by the 14-G coaxial bone biopsy set proved insufficient. One of the patients underwent subsequent surgery. In the other, the percutaneous biopsy was repeated to confirm the diagnosis of a hemangiopericytoma. Data concerning the accuracy of skeletal MR-guided percutaneous bone biopsy obtained in this limited series of patients are comparable with the data reported for the CT-guided technique (LAREDO et al. 1994).

The reported complication rate of percutaneous bone biopsy is low (LAREDO et al. 1994; MURPHY et al. 1981). Procedure-related complications did not occur in our small series of MR-guided percutaneous bone biopsies. Rare but typical complications of percutaneous bone biopsy include sequelae due to nerve or vessel injury, infections, and/or breakage of the needle or drill.

Table 15.3. MR-guided percutaneous biopsy of bone: results (Department of Diagnostic Radiology, University of Technology Aachen, January to October 1996; $n = 20$)

Adequate biopsy	
Metastasis	3
Osteoid osteoma	3[a]
Aneurysmatic bone cyst	2
Chondromyxoidsarcoma	1
Fibrosis	1
Sterile osteomyelitis	3[b]
Salmonellosis	1
Avascular necrosis	1
Transient osteopenia	1
Postomerative hemorrhage	1
Total	17
Inaccurate biopsy	
Histologic diagnosis of percutaneous bone biopsy material: osteomyelitis	
Postoperative histologic diagnosis: sarcoma and inflammation	
Total	1
Inadequate biopsy	
Postoperative histologic diagnosis: solitary bone cast	
Second percutaneous biopsy: hemangiopericytoma	
Total	2

[a] Three osteoid osteomas were removed under CT guidance
[b] One biopsy of a lumbar vertebra was performed under CT guidance

15.7 Conclusion

Percutaneous biopsy of bone lesions of unknown origin is considered a safe and accurate procedure to establish the diagnosis unless there is a primary indication for surgery. MRI may be used as an alternative guidance modality to CT. However, for lesions located in high-risk areas CT guidance remains the imaging modality of choice.

References

Adam G, Keulers P, Vorwerk D, Heller KD, Fuzesi L, Günther RW (1995) Perkutane CT-gesteuerte Behandlung von Osteoidosteomen: kombiniertes Vorgehen mit einem Hohlbohrer und nachfolgender Äthanolinjektion. Fortschr Röntgenstr 162:232-235

Ahlstrom KH, Astrom KG (1993) CT-guided bone biopsy performed by means of a coaxial biopsy system with an eccentric drill. Radiology 188:549-552

Arca MJ, Biermann JS, Johnson TM, Chang AE (1995) Biopsy techniques for skin, soft-tissue, and bone neoplasms. Surg Oncol Clin North Am 4:157-174

Laredo JD, Bellaiche L, Hamze B, Naouri JF, Bondeville JM, Tubiana JM (1994) Current status of musculoskeletal interventional radiology. Radiol Clin North Am 32:377-398

Logan PM, Connell DG, O'Connel JX, Munk PL, Janzen DL (1996) Image-guided percutaneous biopsy of musculoskeletal tumors: an algorithm for selection of specific biopsy techniques. AJR Am J Roentgenol 166:137-141

Murphy WA, Destouet JM, Gilula LA (1981) Percutaneous skeletal biopsy: a procedure for radiologists. Results, review and recommendations. Radiology 139:545-549

Neuerburg J, Adam G, Schmitz-Rode T, Katterbach FJ, Bücker A, Zilkens KW, Rasmussen E, van Vaals JJ, Günther RW (1996) Neues MR-kompatibles Knochenbiopsiesystem. Fortschr Röntgenstr 165:316

Reuther G (1994) CT-kontrollierte Biopsien des Achsenskeletts. Zugangswege und Ergebnisse. Fortschr Röntgenstr 160:78-83

Schweitzer ME, Deely DM, Beavis K, Gannon F (1995) Does the use of lidocaine affect the culture of percutaneous bone biopsy specimens obtained to diagnose osteomyelitis? An in vitro and in vivo study. AJR Am J Röntgenol 164: 1201-1203

Schweitzer ME, Gannon FH, Deely DM, O'Hara BJ, Juneja V (1996) Percutaneous skeletal aspiration and core biopsy: complementary techniques. AJR Am J Röntgenol 166:415-418

Tikkakoski T, Lahde S, Puranen J, Apaja-Sarkkinen M (1992) Combined CT-guided biopsy and cytology in diagnosis of bony lesions. Acta Radiol 33:225-229

White LM, Schweitzer ME, Deely DM, Gannon F (1995) Study of osteomyelitis: utility of combined histologic and microbiologic evaluation of percutaneous biopsy samples. Radiology 197:840-842

16 MR-Guided Lesion Localization and Biopsy of the Breast

C.K. KUHL

CONTENTS

16.1 Introduction

Breast cancer continues to represent the leading cause of cancer death among women in the western hemisphere (American Cancer Society 1996). In spite of well-developed screening programs, diversified therapeutic options with modified surgical strategies and adjuvant therapies, and in spite of the considerably increased public awareness of the need for early diagnosis, the incidence of breast cancer is still increasing.

The importance of early diagnosis of breast cancer has been documented in numerous studies. It is an established fact that early diagnosis is the only means of reducing breast cancer mortality because tumor stage is the most important factor contributing to the overall prognosis (HURLEY and KALDOR 1992).

Mammography, particularly if combined with ultrasound in dense breasts, is an effective tool in the fight against breast cancer (TABAR et al. 1989). So far, only routine mammography has been demonstrated to significantly reduce the mean size of breast cancer at the time of detection, thus implying its potential to improve overall and/or disease-free survival.

C.K. KUHL, MD, Department of Radiology, University of Bonn, Sigmund-Freud-Straße 25, D-53105 Bonn, Germany

During recent years, breast MRI has emerged as a valuable adjunct to the conventional imaging modalities in the detection of primary and recurrent breast cancer (GILLES et al. 1993, 1994; HARMS et al. 1993; HEYWANG et al. 1990; HEYWANG 1994; KAISER and ZEITLER 1989; OREL et al. 1994; WEINREB and NEWSTEAD 1995). It is an extraordinarily sensitive imaging modality based on the characteristic contrast enhancement of malignant lesions due to their angiogenetic activity. There is broad agreement among authors that sensitivity of breast MRI approaches 100% for invasive malignant lesions and further improves the sensitivity of X-ray mammography for the detection of in situ cancers.

So far, breast MRI is mainly used in cases difficult to evaluate conventionally. This includes, e.g., cases of scarring after tumorectomy and radiation therapy or cases of reconstructive surgery with or without implants; high-risk patients and BRCA gene carriers with dense breasts; and cases where a firm diagnosis is not obtainable using conventional modalities or where there are discordant clinical or conventional imaging findings. Moreover, a growing field of breast MRI application is in the case of the pre-operative patient with known or suspected breast cancer, in whom multicentric disease has to be excluded before a breast-conserving therapy is initiated. In these patients, breast MRI detects conventionally invisible breast cancers in 34% (OREL et al. 1995); therapeutically relevant multicentric or contralateral disease is found in 20% of cases (FISCHER et al. 1994a).

Thus, in all these applications, but particularly in the pre-operative patient, it is a quite common diagnostic dilemma that breast MRI – owing to its unsurpassed sensitivity – reveals a suspicious lesion without imaging correlate on conventional mammography or breast ultrasound. In this situation, clarification of the lesion is not easy to obtain, e.g., because of the change from prone patient position during MR imaging to a supine position in the operating room – this will regularly cause major shifts within the parenchymal volume even between different quadrants, thus precluding an accurate and safe excision.

Image-guided localizations and fine-needle or core biopsies of non-palpable lesions are established techniques in X-ray mammography and breast ultrasound, accepted both by referring surgeons and patients (Elvecrog et al. 1993; Gisvold and Martin 1984; Gisvold et al. 1994; Goldberg et al. 1983; Kopans et al. 1984; Liberman et al. 1995; Parker et al. 1994; Rissanen et al. 1994; Silverstein et al. 1989). They allow a definite and tissue-sparing clarification of suspicious lesions that are clinically occult. As it is the declared goal to identify breast cancers at even earlier stages, the need to localize non-palpable lesions is ever increasing.

The necessity to also allow the pre-operative marking of MR-suspicious lesions has grown in parallel with the increasing availability of breast MRI and the increasing demand for pre-operative MR imaging. In this chapter, we will provide an overview of the different state-of-the-art solutions for MR-guided breast interventions and discuss the diagnostic and interventional accuracy achievable with the technique.

16.2 Stereotactic Devices

The stereotactic MR guidance of breast interventions requires:

- Sufficient fixation (usually compression) of the breast
- Preserved accessibility of the entire parenchyma including both retro-areolar and pre-pectoral locations
- Inclusion or addition of an imaging coil
- An accurate stereotaxy system that guarantees correct placement of the needle in the desired position

In principle, three different types of dedicated stereotactic devices for MR guidance of breast lesion imaging have been introduced so far, with differing patient position and coil design.

Heywang-Köbrunner and coworkers were among the first to report MR-guided interventions (wire localizations) with a prototype biopsy coil used with the patient in the prone position (Heywang-Köbrunner et al. 1994). It is a dedicated single-breast coil with built-in stereotaxy system designed in cooperation with Siemens (Erlangen, Germany). The breast is compressed by two plates that have MR-visible markers (fiducials) serving as reference coordinates for calculating lesion location. The plates are perforated to let the needle pass; sterile bushings are used to protect the needle. Orel and coworkers presented a home-built dedicated biopsy coil with comparable features (Orel et al. 1994a).

Fischer and coworkers developed a home-built stereotaxy system for use with the patient in the supine position (Fischer et al. 1994b, 1995a, 1995b). Here, the stereotaxy device is used in conjunction with a regular, rigid, circular surface coil ("eye-and-ear coil"). It consists of an arched frame that is used to support the surface coil and the stereotaxy system clamped into it (Fig. 16.1). The stereotaxy system consists of two semicircular perforated plates with a hinge in between to allow a ridgelike angulation of the plates against each other, thus producing gentle breast compression.

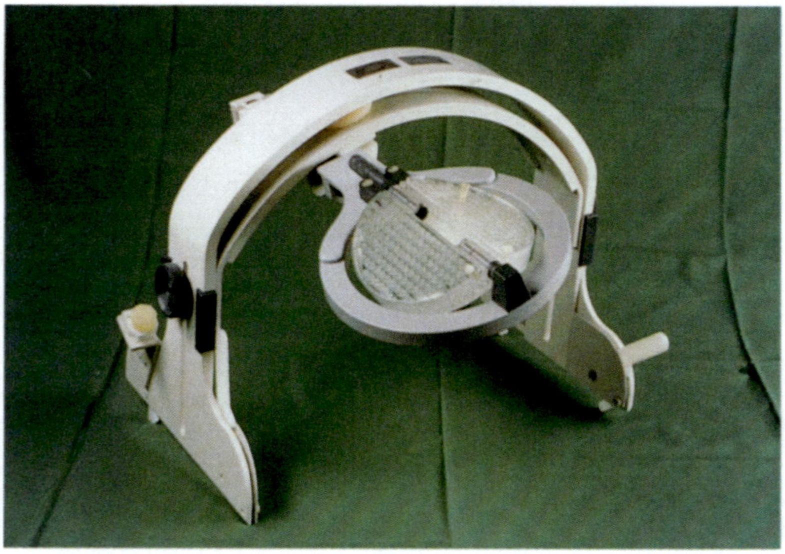

Fig. 16.1. Stereotactic localization and biopsy device for use with patients in the supine position, designed by Fischer and coworkers (Fischer et al. 1994b). Note the arched frame with the compression plates clamped into a regular, rigid, circular surface coil

Our group introduced a stereotactic device designed in cooperation with Philips Medical Systems (ELEVELT et al. 1995; KUHL et al. 1997b). It is used with the patient in a semi-prone position, tilted by about 20° away from the puncture side (Fig. 16.2a). Two compression plates with built-in stereotaxy system are used to immobilize the breast. There is no built-in coil; instead, a regular, flexible, circular surface coil is placed between patient support and chest wall, around the breast. Thus, the breast is not hidden by the coil, but may be pulled and positioned between the compression paddles to allow optimum exposure and even compression of the respective region of interest.

Apart from the differences described above, the problems and special requirements associated with MR guidance of breast lesion imaging stipulate most of the detail of a stereotactic biopsy device. In all types, breast compression ensues via MR-compatible (usually Plexiglass) perforated plates with holes every 2 to 4 mm to let the needle pass. The spatial coordinates of the lesion under study are determined with reference to MR-visible fiducials, the "stereotaxy system" in the narrow sense, which is integrated in, or clamped onto the compression plates.

The true-prone patient position and the closed walls of the dedicated biopsy coil introduced by Heywang and coworkers explain some difficulties associated with its use (FISCHER et al. 1995b); due to the true-prone position and chest wall parallel needle pathways, lesions in the pre-pectoral location and in the axillary tail are virtually inaccessible. This is even more important because the breast, hidden by the closed coil walls, may not be pulled and positioned to help expose lateral or pre-pectoral parenchymal tissue. Owing to these difficulties, the biopsy coil has not been widely used, but it is being re-evaluated to improve its design.

By using regular surface coils instead of built-in coils, other stereotaxy systems (FISCHER et al. 1995b; KUHL et al. 1997b) are probably more cost effective. With the semi-prone position, the advantages of the true-prone and the supine position are combined in that the breast extends away from the chest wall as with prone imaging, while accessibility of the entire breast parenchymal volume is preserved as with the supine position (Fig. 16.2b).

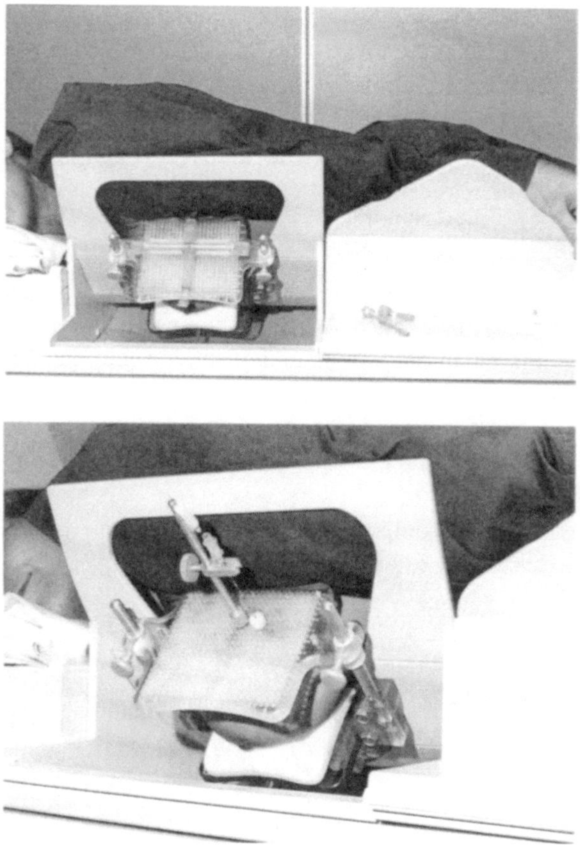

Fig. 16.2a,b. Stereotactic localization and biopsy device for use in the semi-prone position. a) View from the side. Note the tilted patient position and the compression plate with the stereotactic coordinate system clamped onto it. b) Detailed view of the compression plate with the external needle guide and the needle with a sterile bushing in the corresponding bore hole. Note the versatility of breast positioning and compression due to the broad access to the breast (KUHL et al. 1997b; ELEVELT et al. 1995)

16.3 Needles and Wires

For MR-guided breast interventions, preferably (but not inevitably) fully MR-compatible needles should be used. For MR-guided stereotactic hook wire localization, it is possible to use non-MR-compatible needles as long as the hook wires loaded within them fulfill MR-compatibility criteria. We have gained experience with use of the following needles and wires:

1. Hook wires
- Homer Mammalok [AD Krauth, Hamburg, Germany] (curved-end wire), 20G, 6.5–10cm (the wire is MR compatible; the needle is not) [Bjaerverskov, Denmark]

- Cook Kopans MReye MR compatible, 20G, 9cm (needle and wire are fully MR compatible)
- BIP/Bard Angiomed MR-compatible hook wire (needle and wire are fully MR compatible)
- E-Z-EM [Westbury, NY, USA] MR-compatible hook wire, 19.5G, 10cm (needle and wire are fully MR compatible)

2. Core biopsy systems

- Coaxial system by BIP/Bard [Tuerkenfeld, Germany] Angiomed. A 14G coaxial needle system is placed under MR guidance; after removing the trocar, a conventional 16G core biopsy needle system is loaded into the coaxial needle and used together with a conventional automatic core biopsy gun
- Full MR-compatible automatic 14G core biopsy system by E-Z-EM

16.4 Protocols

16.4.1 Planning the Intervention

Before MR-guided intervention of a lesion is recommended, we advise that any other options that may allow a conservative clarification of the lesion in question should be evaluated first. In particular, lesions visible by breast MRI alone that occur in premenopausal patients may correspond to areas of hormone-induced spontaneous enhancement [incidental lesion, "unknown breast object" (UBO)] (Kuhl et al. 1997a). These "lesions" may (and should) be clarified by follow-up imaging in a suitable phase of the menstrual cycle, i.e., during the 2nd week. The same holds true for post-menopausal women receiving hormonal replacement therapy. Apart from these patients, follow-up breast MRI is of course an option in other lesions rated "probably benign".

With the existing technology, breast MRI-guided interventions today follow a two-stage approach. After a suspicious lesion has been identified on a diagnostic breast MRI study, the following course of action has to be taken: in general, MR guidance should be reserved for lesions not visualized by other imaging modalities. First of all, therefore, every effort should be made to re-identify the lesion in retrospect on the conventional modalities (mammography, directed high-frequency breast ultrasound). If the lesion is clearly delineated on the conventional studies, then the intervention should be performed under mammographic or sonographic guidance. However, if the lesion is not unequivocally visualized by conventional images or if a conventionally visible, indeterminate lesion is not unequivocally attributable to the MR-suspicious lesion, the intervention under MR guidance is mandatory. As a rule of thumb, a non-palpable lesion should be localized or biopsied under guidance of the modality that first raised suspicion of it and first indicated biopsy.

MR-guided hook-wire lesion marking should be performed immediately preceding the excisional biopsy. Thus, the MR-guided intervention should be scheduled for the same day as the open biopsy; to prevent wire migration, we do not recommend lesion marking earlier than 4–6h prior to surgery. Obviously, this schedule requires good cooperation and communication between radiologists and surgeons. The only exception to this rationale is made in cases where there are bilateral findings. Here, two-stage lesion marking is necessary to allow adequate elimination of contrast material before the second contrast-enhanced study is obtained. We recommend marking of the first lesion on the preceding evening, while the contralateral lesion should be localized on the day of surgery. In these cases, an interesting approach is to insert an MR-compatible embolization coil (Cook, Bjaerverskov, Denmark) next to the lesion to enable a persistent lesion localization. (Müller-Schimpfle et al. 1977) Particularly in cases with a waiting time between intervention and surgery, precautions against guidewire migration (Owen and Kumar 1991) must be meticulously followed. The wire should be tightly fixed on the skin (we now prefer to suture it in place under local anesthesia with a purse string as for drainage tube fixation at surgery). The patient should be instructed to avoid moving the arm on the puncture side, particularly to avoid raising it above the level of the breast. If core biopsies are to be performed, communication with the pathologist is necessary to ensure a rapid and qualified processing of the specimen.

Before commencing, it is necessary to explain the whole procedure to the patient and to obtain her informed consent. Important points are:

- Complications associated with any needle localization or core biopsy procedures in general. Wire localization procedures can incur pain, bleeding, infection, and failure of directed surgery due to wire misplacement or wire migration. In cases scheduled for core biopsy add the possibility of hematoma; in non-parallel needle pathways, pneumothorax; the possibility of seed implanta-

tions along the needle tract is virtually excluded if the above-mentioned coaxial systems are used to minimize tissue traumatization and if the needle trajectory is excised during subsequent oncologic surgery in case a malignant lesion is found in the core. There is the possibility of false-negative core biopsies, thus the patient must undergo follow-up control imaging.
- Complications associated with MR guidance of MR-suspicious lesion imaging in particular: in pre-menopausal patients and in post-menopausal patients receiving hormone substitution therapy, the possibility should be mentioned that the lesion may have resolved and not be visible any more.

Table 16.1. Pulse sequence parameters for diagnostic and pre-interventional breast MRI

	Diagnostic MRI	Interventional MRI
Imaging coil	Double breast surface	Flexible circular surface
Type of pulse sequence	2D Gradient echo	2D Gradient echo
Orientation	Axial	Axial
TR/TE/flip angle	240/4.6/90°	240/4.6/90°
Thickness/gap	4 mm/no gap	4 mm/no gap
No. of sections	21	21
Field of view	280–330 mm	200–220 mm
No. of dynamic scans	10 (1 pre-contrast, 9 post-contrast)	4 (1 pre-contrast, 3 post-contrast; last scan delayed by 2 min)
Temporal resolution	42s/dynamic scan	42s/dynamic scan
Contrast agent	0.1 mmol/kg body weight Gd-DTPA	0.1 mmol/kg body weight Gd-DTPA
Post-processing	Subtraction	Subtraction

16.4.2 Interventional Protocol

16.4.2.1 Lesion Identification

During the intervention, the first step is to re-identify the suspected lesion. In most cases, it will be necessary to use contrast-enhanced studies to accurately demonstrate the lesion. This is almost always mandatory in case the lesion is surrounded by breast parenchyma. Lesions easily visualized in pre-contrast images are mostly those located within fatty tissue; however, as such, they should be easily visible with conventional methods and should therefore not be subjected to MRI.

We recommend using the same basic imaging sequence as used for diagnostic breast MRI study. However, since the pre-interventional dynamic study is used for lesion re-detection and not for lesion characterization, it is sensible to abridge the protocol in order to save time. For the diagnostic and pre-interventional dynamic studies, we use the protocol given in Table 16.1.

16.4.2.2 Determination of Stereotactic Coordinates

After re-identification of the lesion, its stereotactic coordinates are determined with reference to the MR-visible fiducials (Fig. 16.3). Details of this procedure will differ according to the varying design of the different stereotactic devices, so we will only discuss the common principles.

In-plane coordinates (on axial images and with medio-lateral compression, this is the lesion's antero-posterior and left-right offset) are easily calculated with the system's distance function (see Fig. 16.3d). To avoid calculation errors, it is important to draw the distance calculation lines strictly parallel or perpendicular to the potential needle pathways.

The third stereotactic coordinate is somewhat more difficult to obtain. Acquiring images in an additional orientation (e.g., sagittal) to determine it directly is problematic because lesion delineation will be poor on these late postcontrast images (see "vanishing target," Sect. 16.6). Other approaches, like multiplanar reformatting of early postcontrast subtracted images or use of fat-suppressed pulse sequences, harbor their own difficulties. The easiest and safest approach is to use the geometric information given by the offset of the section that best displays the lesion (on axial images, this is the section's cc-offset) and use this as the third dimension's coordinate.

The bore hole over the prospective lesion location is identified according to the stereotactic coordinates. We always insert a needle phantom into the bore hole and control its position to check for calculation errors before the actual puncture is performed. For this purpose, we repeat one scan of the two-dimensional (2D) gradient-echo series (imaging time is 42s).

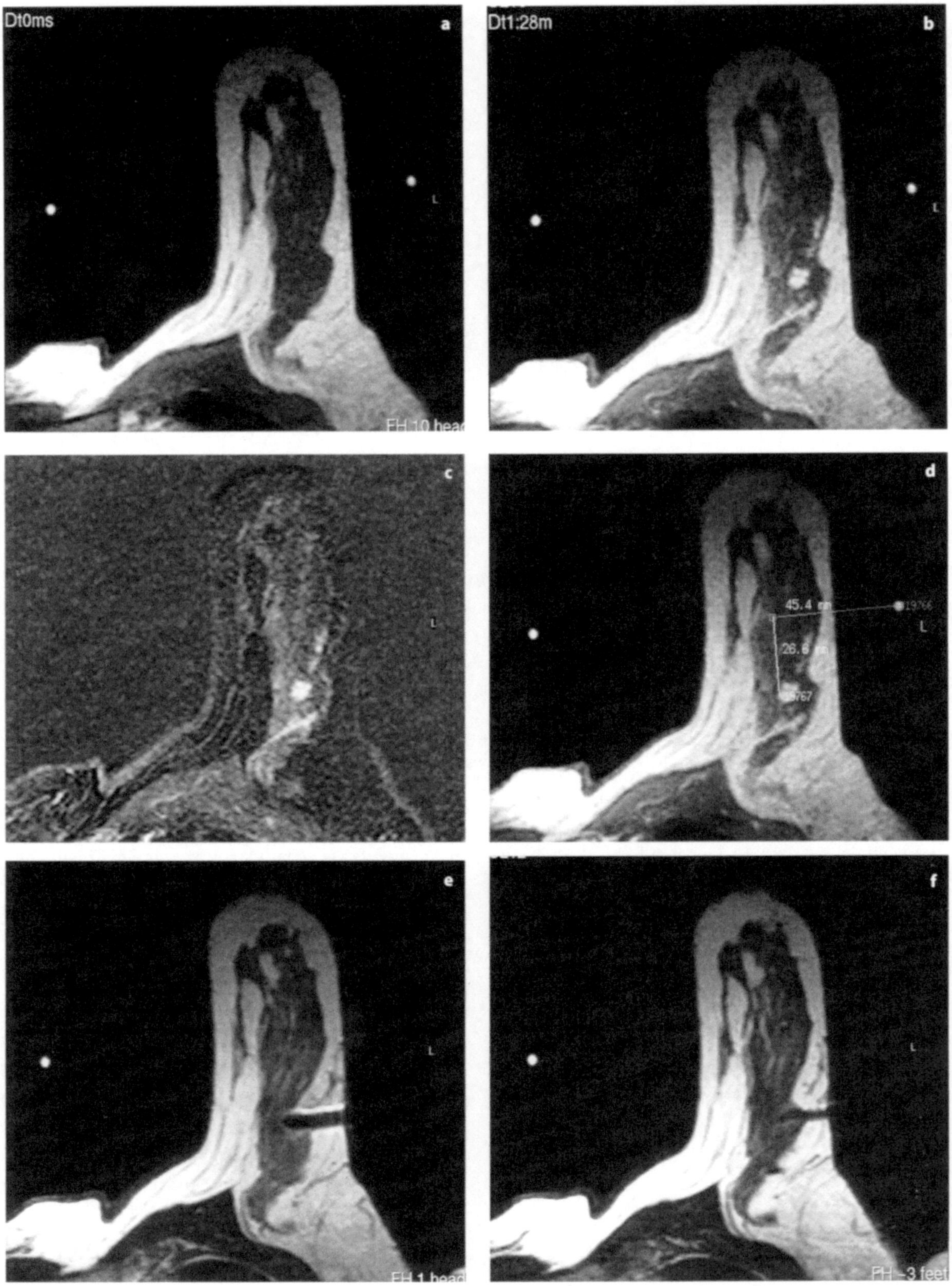

Fig. 16.3a-f. MR-guided 14G-core biopsy and lesion marking of a 7mm invasive ductal breast cancer in a 40-year-old high-risk patient. a)-c) Pre-interventional dynamic series: pre-contrast (a), early post-contrast (b), and subtracted image (c). Note the small, rapidly enhancing, irregular lesion. d)-f) Interventional study: calculation of lesion coordinates with reference to the MR-visible markers (d); a late post-contrast image with a 14G biopsy needle (E-Z-EM) in situ (e; core biopsy revealed invasive cancer); after additional insertion of a Kopan MR-compatible guidewire (Cook; f); subsequent excisional biopsy confirmed the diagnosis of early-stage breast cancer. Note the reduced lesion visibility due to the vanishing target phenomenon in e) and f)

16.4.2.3
Lesion Puncture

The puncture procedure corresponds to what is known from other image-guided interventions. The skin should be disinfected and local anesthesia should be applied. The latter is particularly important for stereotactic interventions because it is vital to prevent pain-related movement of the patient during the puncture. It should go without saying that it is necessary to talk to the patient and tell her every step in advance.

16.4.2.4
Position Control

For rapid orientation of the guidewire needle or coaxial needle position, we use T1-weighted Spin-echo (SE) images (TR 300/TE 11). Although reducing the number of sections of the control scans, as compared with the initial imaging scans, would save time, we do not change the image stack geometry in general or the number of sections in particular. The reason is that it is much easier to re-identify the calculated lesion location and to compare it with the actual needle position if these parameters are left unchanged. Rather, to save time we use a rectangular field of view of about 70% and reduce the image matrix.

If the needle position is satisfactory, the guidewire is released or the biopsy needle is advanced within it to take the cores. After releasing the wire, its position is controlled via the rapid 42s 2D gradient-echo scan mentioned above (Sect. 16.4.2.2). This scan is meant to serve two different purposes: first, it is used to give a rapid overview of the hook wire position; second, it is used to provide the surgeons with images that clearly show the wire (which produces a 4mm thick signal void on gradient-echo images). On the final SE scan (TR 300/TE 11) used for accurate delineation of the wire position, the wire is only visible as a very thin signal void which may be quite difficult to recognize for the non-radiologist.

16.5
Results

There are four teams with substantial experience of MR-guided breast interventions (Fischer et al. 1995b; Heywang-Köbrunner et al. 1994; Kuhl et al. 1997b; Orel et al. 1994a). The respective results are given in Tables 16.2 and 16.3. The data document the high accuracy and reliability of the different stereotactic devices concerning guidewire localization procedures. Failures occurred with the prone dedicated biopsy coil (Fischer et al. 1995b; Heywang-Köbrunner et al. 1994) and were due to the pre-pectoral location of the lesions.

A point of major importance is the size of the lesions localized under MRI guidance (see Fig. 16.4). Both of the larger series of MR-guided breast interventions (Fischer et al. 1995a; Kuhl et al. 1997b) agree in that the resected malignant lesions corresponded to pT1 tumor stages only. In our series, the mean size of malignant lesions was 8.7mm. This underlines the high sensitivity and accuracy of the technique. There is extensive evidence that nodal state, prevalence of metastatic seed and overall survival are closely related to the size of the breast cancer at the time of diagnosis. Thus, breast MRI in conjunction with MR-guided pre-operative lesion marking may have the potential to further improve the prognosis of breast cancer patients.

In contrast to MR-guided lesion marking, at this stage we would not recommend MR-guided core biopsy as a routine clinical modality for the confirmation of MR-suspicious lesions. The reason is that the requirements for spatial accuracy and consistency of position are much higher for core biopsies than for wire placements, while at the same time errors due to needle misplacement are much more severe and may be disastrous. This has led to the strategy of using MR-guided core biopsy only in lesions with a low probability of breast cancer (which explains the large fraction of benign lesions among the core biopsy specimens). However, to exc lude any false-negative diagnoses due to needle misplacement, histopathologic core diagnoses of mastopathic changes, including hyperplasia or epitheliosis, may *not* be regarded as definitive diagnosis, because these are non-specific findings that may as well correspond to the tissue next to the lesion that was intended to be biopsied. Only cores positive for either breast cancer, fibroadenoma, or other distinct pathologic entities, known to be associated with contrast enhancement, permit a firm diagnosis.

Until its diagnostic accuracy is established, we suggest that MR-guided core biopsy be regarded as a method under investigation. We recommend use of MR-guided core biopsies only in lesions larger than about 10mm; in smaller lesions, guidewire placement is mandatory. Moreover, we would recommend the accuracy of a device be first evaluated in a series

Table 16.2. Literature review and recent data on MR-guided interventions in the breast

Reference[a]	Total number of lesions localized and/or biopsied	MR-guided Interventions							
		Needle localization				Biopsy			
		Total	Success	Benign	Malignant	Total	Benign	Malignant	IM[c]
Heywang-Köbrunner et al.	11[b]	11	10	3	7	–	–	–	–
Recent data	n.p.	27	n.p.	15 (56%)	12 (44%)	31 (FNA, Core	23 (74%)	4 (13%)	4 (13%)
Orel et al. 1994[a], 1994[b]	11[b]	11	11	7	4	–	–	–	–
Recent data	n.p.	78	78	49 (63%)	29 (37%)	8 (FNA, Core	3	2	3
Fischer et al. 1995[b]	34	28	26	16	12	23 (FNA)	12	7	4
Recent data	112	112	112	58 (52%)	54 (48%)	28 (FNA)	16 (57%)	8 (29%)	4 (14%)
Kuhl et al. 1997[b]	97	97	97	44	53	5 (Core)	1	3	1
Recent data	104	104	104	47 (45%)	57 (55%)	7 (Core)	1	4	2

[a] Recent data correspond to personal communications of unpublished material as of April 1997
[b] Half of these lesions localized under MRI guidance were also visible by conventional imaging modalities
[c] IM means insufficient FNA or core biopsy material
FNA, Fine needle aspiration; n.p., data not provided; Core, core biopsy

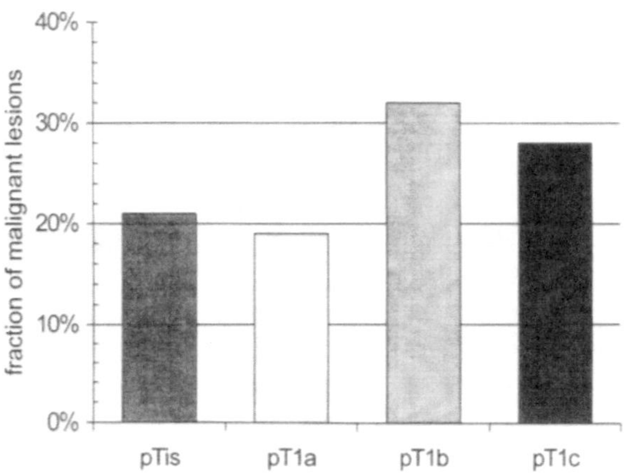

Fig 16.4. Distribution of tumor stages (pTNM classification) of breast cancers resected after MRI guidance

of MR-guided core biopsies, with subsequent insertion of guidewires and open biopsy. The results of the core biopsies may then be verified by the findings at excisional biopsy. Only after this, may the results of MR-guided core biopsies be allowed to have an impact on clinical patient management.

16.6 Troubleshooting: The Lacking, the Vanishing, and the Missed Target

There are specific difficulties associated with MR-guided interventions in the breast. We encountered three main problems: in chronological order (a) the "lacking" target, (b) the "vanishing" target and (c) "missed" target.

The lacking target: This was a reduced lesion enhancement or even an absence of lesion enhancement in the dynamic series of the interventional study, leaving us unable to re-identify the suspicious lesion on post-contrast subtracted images. In our series, three cases of invasive breast cancer, with typical, rapid, and strong enhancement in the preceding diagnostic breast MRI study, did not exhibit any enhancement in the corresponding interventional dynamic series. The lacking target was encountered particularly in patients in whom strong breast compression was applied to ensure optimal breast immobilization in the stereotactic device. We speculate that excessive breast compression may interfere with lesion enhancement. Accordingly, we modified the protocol so that the compression pressure was reduced to a level just sufficient to immobilize the breast. Since then, lesion enhancement has been almost comparable with that seen in the non-compressed, diagnostic study, and there have been no further cases of non-enhancing breast cancers.

It is essential to distinguish the lacking target from a reversible lesion that has actually resolved between the diagnostic and the interventional study (in case of a UBO in pre-menopausal patients). In the pre-menopausal patient, we therefore recommend the interventional study be scheduled for no later than 1 week after the diagnostic study. Moreover, if lesion re-identification, and thus the intervention, proves impossible, diagnostic breast MRI should be repeated the next day to rule out a lacking target phenomenon.

The vanishing target (Fig. 16.5): lesion visibility decreases progressively over time during the intervention, owing to wash-out of contrast agent from

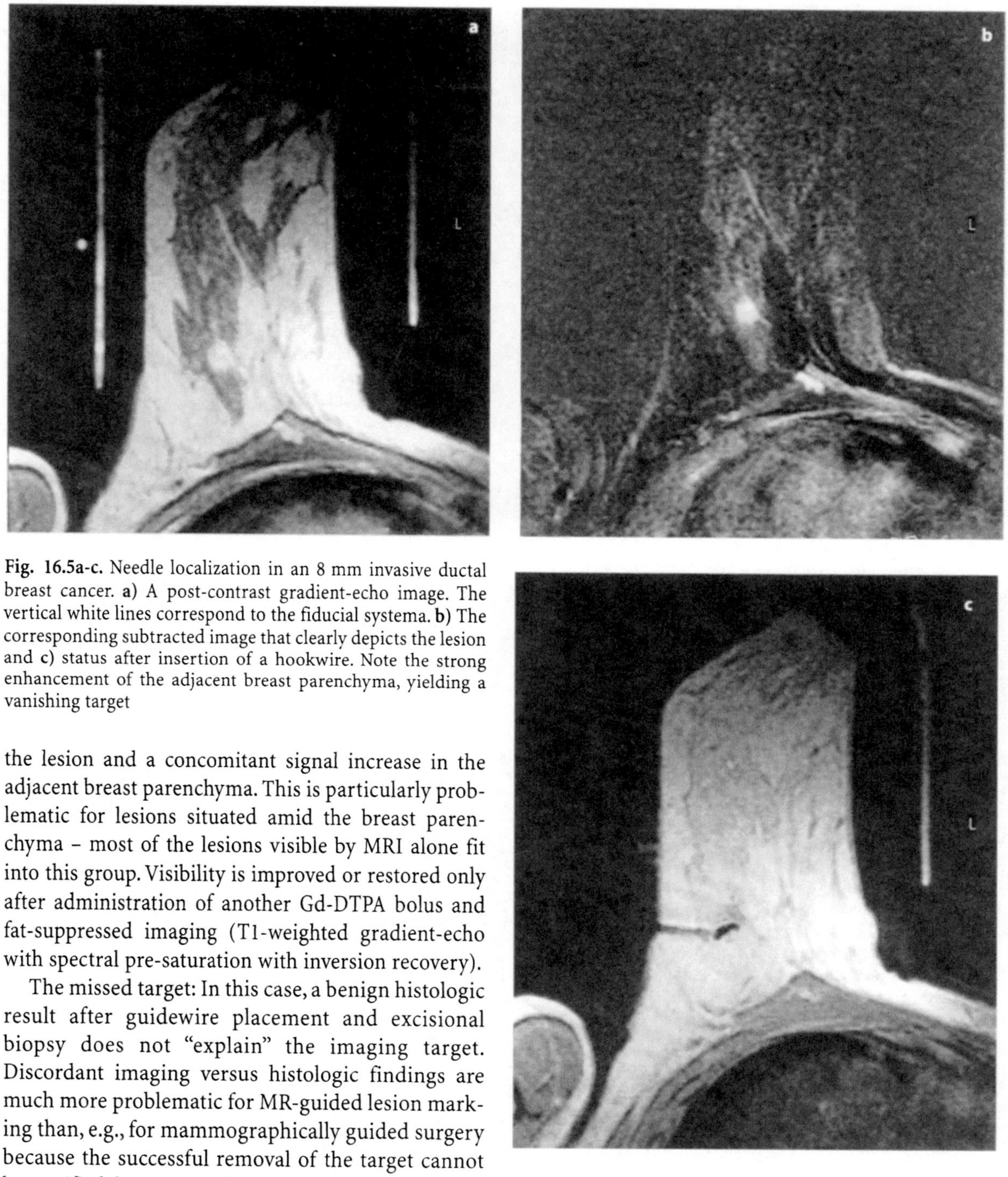

Fig. 16.5a-c. Needle localization in an 8 mm invasive ductal breast cancer. a) A post-contrast gradient-echo image. The vertical white lines correspond to the fiducial systema. b) The corresponding subtracted image that clearly depicts the lesion and c) status after insertion of a hookwire. Note the strong enhancement of the adjacent breast parenchyma, yielding a vanishing target

the lesion and a concomitant signal increase in the adjacent breast parenchyma. This is particularly problematic for lesions situated amid the breast parenchyma – most of the lesions visible by MRI alone fit into this group. Visibility is improved or restored only after administration of another Gd-DTPA bolus and fat-suppressed imaging (T1-weighted gradient-echo with spectral pre-saturation with inversion recovery).

The missed target: In this case, a benign histologic result after guidewire placement and excisional biopsy does not "explain" the imaging target. Discordant imaging versus histologic findings are much more problematic for MR-guided lesion marking than, e.g., for mammographically guided surgery because the successful removal of the target cannot be verified by specimen imaging. To control adequate excision of the suspected lesion, the findings should be discussed directly with the pathologist. Size and configuration of the imaging and the histologic lesions should be compared; moreover, it is important to carefully check for histologic lesion features that are known to be associated with contrast enhancement in breast MRI (e.g., hypervascularity, epithelial proliferation). If any doubt persists, we would recommend regular early post-operative control breast MR imaging within the first 24–72h. Out of the 15 early post-operative breast MRI studies of our series, the lesion was still present in 5, 3 of which eventually proved malignant.

In summary, during MRI-guided breast interventions, familiarity with the lacking, the vanishing, or the missed target is important to avoid false-negative results. We advise cautious application of breast compression. Lesion visibility in the late post-contrast interventional period is almost always reduced; it may be restored by a repeat injection of contrast agent plus fat-suppressed imaging. Early post-operative control of lesion removal is mandatory in patients with discordant histologic findings.

References

American Cancer Society (1996) Cancer facts and figures. American Cancer Society, Atlanta, Ga.

Elevelt A, Kuhl CK, Selder B, Gieseke J (1995) A new breast biopsy and localizer device designed for MR-guided interventional procedures. (abstract) Proceedings of Third Annual Meeting of the Society of Magnetic Resonance, p 146

Elvecrog EL, Lechner MC, Nelson MT (1993) Nonpalpable breast lesions: correlation of stereotaxic large core needle biopsy and surgical biopsy results. Radiology 188:453-455

Fischer U, Vosshenrich R, Probst A, Burchhardt H, Grabbe E (1994a) Präoperative MR-Mammographie bei bekanntem Mammakarzinom. Sinnvolle Mehrinformation oder sinnloser Mehraufwand? Rofo Fortschr Geb Röntgenstr Neuen Bildgeb Verfahr 161:300-306

Fischer U, Vosshenrich R, Keating D, Bruhn H, Döler W, Oestmann JW, Grabbe E (1994b) MR-guided biopsy of suspect breast lesions with a stereotaxic add-on device for surface coils. Radiology 192:272-273

Fischer U, Vosshenrich R, Bruhn H, Keating D, Raab BW, Oestmann JW (1995a) MR-guided localization of suspected breast lesions detected exclusively by postcontrast MRI. J Comput Assist Tomogr 19:63-66

Fischer U, Vosshenrich R, Doler W, Hamadeh A, Oestmann JW, Grabbe E (1995b) MR imaging-guided breast intervention: experience with two systems. Radiology 195:533-538

Gilles R, Guinebretière JM, Shapeero LG, et al (1993) Assessment of breast cancer recurrence with contrast-enhanced subtraction MR imaging: preliminary results in 26 patients. Radiology 188:473-478

Gilles R, Guinebretière JM, Lucidarme O, et al (1994) Nonpalpable breast tumors: diagnosis with contrast-enhanced subtraction dynamic MRI. Radiology 191:625-631

Gisvold JJ, Martin JK Jr (1984) Prebiopsy localization of nonpalpable breast lesions. AJR Am J Roentgenol 143:477-481

Gisvold JJ, Goellner JR, Grant CS et al (1994) Breast biopsy: a comparative study of stereotaxically guided core and excisional techniques. AJR Am J Roentgenol 162:815-820

Goldberg RP, Hall FM, Simon M (1983) Preoperative localization of nonpalpable breast lesions using a wire marker and perforated mammographic grid. Radiology 146:833-835

Harms SE, Flamig DP, Hesley KL et al (1993) MR imaging of the breast with rotating delivery of excitation off resonance: clinical experience with pathologic correlation. Radiology 187:493-501

Heywang SH (1994) Contrast enhanced magnetic resonance imaging of the breast. Invest Radiol 29:94-104

Heywang SH, Hilbertz T, Beck R, Bauer WM, Eiermann W, Permanetter W (1990) Gd-DTPA enhanced MR imaging of the breast in patients with postoperative scarring and silicon implants. J Comput Assist Tomogr 14:348-349

Heywang-Köbrunner SH, Huynh AT, Viehweg P, Hanke W, Requardt H, Paprosch I (1994) Prototype breast coil for MR guided needle localization. J Comput Assist Tomogr 18:876-881

Hurley SF, Kaldor JM (1992) The benefits and risks of mammographic screening for breast cancer. Epidemiol Rev 14:101

Kaiser WA, Zeitler E (1989) MR imaging of the breast: fast imaging sequences with and without Gd-DTPA. Preliminary observations. Radiology 170:681-686

Kopans DB, Meyer JE, Lindfors KK, Bucchianeri SS (1984) Breast sonography to guide cyst aspiration and wire localization of occult solid lesions. AJR Am J Roentgenol 143:489-492

Kuhl CK, Bieling HB, Gieseke J, Kreft B, Sommer T, Lutterbey G, Schild HH (1997a) Healthy premenopausal breast parenchyma in dynamic contrast-enhanced MRI of the breast: normal values of contrast enhancement and cycle phase dependency. Radiology 203:137-144

Kuhl CK, Elevelt A, Leutner C, Gieseke J, Pakos E, Schild HH (1997b) Clinical use of a stereotactic localization and biopsy device for interventional breast MRI. Radiology 204: 667–676

Liberman L, Dershaw DD, Rosen PP, Cohen MA, Hann LE, Abramson AF (1995) Stereotaxic core biopsy of impalpable spiculated breast masses. AJR Am J Roentgenol 165:551-554

Müller-Schimpfle M, Stoll P, Stern W, Huppert PE, Claussen CD. Präzise MR-gestützte Coil-Markierung von Mamma-Läsionen unter Verwendung einer MR-Standard-Spule. RöFö Fortschr. Geb. Röntgenstr. Neuen Bildgeb. Verf. (1997) 166:576

Orel SG, Schnall MD, Newman RW, Powell CM, Torosian MH, Rosario EF (1994a) MR-imaging-guided localization and biopsy of breast lesions: initial experience. Radiology 193:97-102

Orel SG, Schnall MD, LiVolsi VA, Troupin RH (1994b) Suspicious breast lesions: MR imaging with radiologic-pathologic correlation. Radiology 190:485-493

Orel SG, Schnall MD, Powell CM et al (1995) Staging of suspected breast cancer: effect of MR imaging and MR-guided biopsy. Radiology 196:115-122

Owen AW, Kumar EN (1991) Migration of localizing wires used in guided biopsy of the breast. Clin Radiol 43:251

Parker SH, Burbank F, Jackman RJ et al (1994) Percutaneous large-core breast biopsy: a multi-institutional study. Radiology 193:359-364

Rissanen TJ, Makarainen HP, Kiviniemi HO, Suramo II (1994) Ultrasonographically guided wire localization of nonpalpable breast lesions. J Ultrasound Med 13:183-188

Silverstein MJ, Gamagami P, Colburn WJ et al (1989) Nonpalpable breast lesions: diagnosis with slightly overpenetrated screen-film mammography and hook wire-directed biopsy in 1,014 cases. Radiology 171:633-638

Tabar L, Faberg G, Duffy S et al (1989) The Swedish two-country trial of mammographic screening for breast cancer: recent results and calculation of benefit. J Epidemiol Community Health 43:107

Weinreb JC, Newstead G (1995) MR imaging of the breast. Radiology 196:593-610

17 MR-Guided Cholecystostomy in Pigs

J.F. DEBATIN and S. GÖHDE

CONTENTS

17.1 Introduction

The MR experiment is highly sensitive to materials characterized by long T2 relaxation times. Bile fluid is such a material. Bile-filled structures can hence be displayed on heavily T2-weighted MR sequences without the use of any contrast medium. Use of very long repetition (TR) and echo times (TE) results in a selective display of the biliary system referred to as MR cholangiography (KAUFMANN et al. 1989; SCHUSTER et al. 1995). The MR images are acquired non-invasively in any desired plane, providing a truly three-dimensional perspective of the biliary tree, including any pathologic findings (KAUFMANN et al. 1989; SCHUSTER et al. 1995).

With the availability of open-configuration MR systems, percutaneous biliary interventions under MR-based guidance and control have become possible (JOLESZ and BLUMENFELD 1994; SCHENK et al. 1995). Fundamental to the safe and expeditious percutaneous accessing of the biliary tree is the visualization of puncture and manipulative instruments relative to the biliary system. With electrically active techniques (DUMOULIN et al. 1993) localization of a device is made possible by incorporating a miniature radiofrequency (RF) receive-only coil in the tip of the instrument (LEUNG et al. 1995a). This provides real-time tracking of a needle tip in any number of desired scan planes simultaneously (LEUNG et al. 1995b).

J.F. DEBATIN, MD, Institute of Diagnostic Radiology, Zurich University Hospital, Rämistr. 100, CH-8091 Zurich, Switzerland
S. GÖHDE, MD, Institute of Diagnostic Radiology, Zurich University Hospital, Rämistr. 100, CH-8091 Zürich, Switzerland

17.2 Material and Methods

The 14-G prototype MR-tracking needle (Fig. 17.1) was manufactured by BIP (Munich, FRG). Both style and cannula are made of polyethyleneketone (PEEK), a polymer composite. Biocompatibility and durability of PEEK have been documented in conjunction with its use as an orthopedic implant material (JOKISCH et al. 1992; MAHARAJ et al. 1994; ALBERT et al. 1994).

In order to ensure reliable cutting, the "cutting" style tip is made of ceramic. A simple untuned copper loop RF coil with an out diameter of 1.2 mm is incorporated in the style immediately distal to the cutting tip. To improve tracking robustness, a small 0.002-ml container, filled with a Gd-DTPA (Magnevist, Schering, Berlin, Germany) solution (0.5 M), was placed in the center of the coil as an internal signal source. It provides a consistent tracking signal for the antenna, allowing for tissue-independent MR tracking. To maximize the signal amplitude from the internal signal source, the RF coil is arranged 30° oblique relative to the axis of the needle (Fig. 17.1). The RF coil is attached to a coaxial cable which is interfaced to the workstation via a plug at the needle

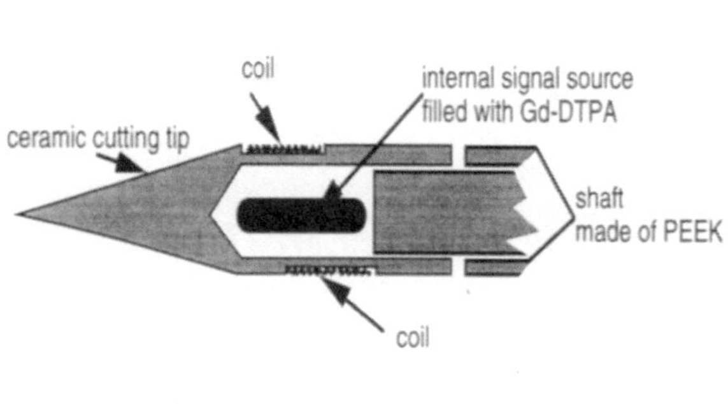

Fig. 17.1. Schematic diagram of the tracking needle tip containing the internal signal source (PEEK, polyethyleneketone)

base. Both RF coil and the coaxial cable are contained within the biocompatible needle material.

The experiments were performed in a superconducting, cryogen-free, 0.5-T open-configuration "interventional" MR scanner (Signa SP, GEMS, Milwaukee, Wis.). The tracking software was implemented on two Sparc workstations (Sun Microsystems, Mountain View, Calif.). Cholecystostomies were conducted on three fully anesthetized female pigs (body weight 40–45 kg). The animal experiments had been approved by the appropriate governmental regulatory committees.

The gallbladder and biliary system were displayed in all three orthogonal planes using a heavily T2-weighted fast spin-echo (FSE) sequence [echo train length 32, TR 200/TE 7000, number of excitations (NEX) 1, matrix 256×160, field of view (FOV) 32 cm]. Sections of 4-mm thickness were acquired in suspended respiration. Maximum pixel intensity projections of the biliary system were constructed. The gallbladder was targeted using two different approaches: along the axis of the magnet, as well as in a plane perpendicular to it. For planning purposes, the expected course of the needle was drawn on the "roadmap" images, which were displayed on liquid crystal display monitors placed in front of the interventionalist, positioned in the opening of the interventional magnet itself.

Based on these "cholangio-roadmaps" the coaxial MR-tracking needle was inserted percutaneously into the gallbladder under continuous MR guidance. Using the MR-tracking sequence (TR 30/TE 8 ms, 60° flip) the position of the coil was sampled using a Hadamard encoding strategy (Dumoulin et al. 1991) every 120 ms or 8 times/s. The position of the needle tip was displayed simultaneously on the two cholangio-roadmaps in real time (less than 10 ms delay from data acquisition; Leung et al. 1995b). Thus the biplanar positional information of the needle was advanced into the gallbladder (Fig. 17.2). The needle was manipulated solely under apnea conditions.

The success of the tracking process was confirmed in the second tracking mode by acquiring fast gradient-echo "update" images (TR 20/TE 4 ms, flip 20°, 10 mm sections, FOV 40 cm, matrix 256×128, 1 NEX) transsecting the tip of the puncture needle. The tracking information was used to ensure that each update image, regardless of the chosen imaging plane, was centered on the most recent coil position.

Once the needle was positioned inside the gallbladder, the bile was aspirated and MR cholangiography was repeated. Subsequently, a fast T1-weighted gradient-echo imaging series (TR 30/TE 14, flip 30°) was used to document the insufflation of the collapsed gallbladder by means of installation of undiluted paramagnetic contrast medium (Gd-DTPA, 0.5 M; Magnevist, Schering, Berlin, FRG; Fig. 17.3).

17.3 Results

Based on the heavily T2-weighted MR cholangio-roadmaps, the gallbladder was easily identified. The actual procedure time for the cholecystostomy was

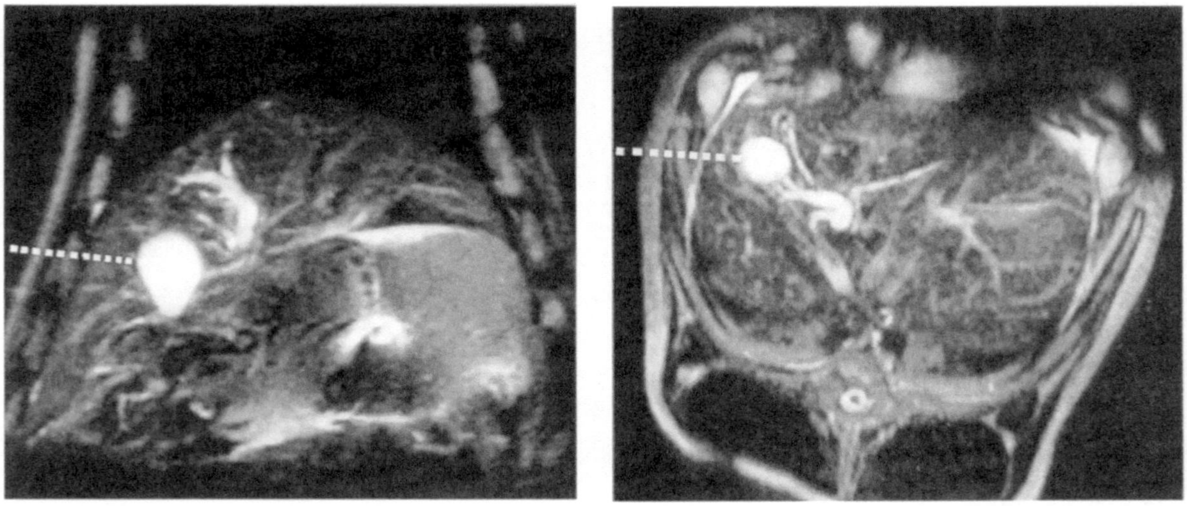

Fig. 17.2. Coronal *(left)* and axial *(right)* "cholangio-roadmaps" in a pig. On both orthogonal planes, the position of the needle tip is being projected in real time *(dotted line)* as it is advanced into the gallbladder. The gallbladder and portions of the bile ducts are identified as bright structures on these heavily T2-weighted images

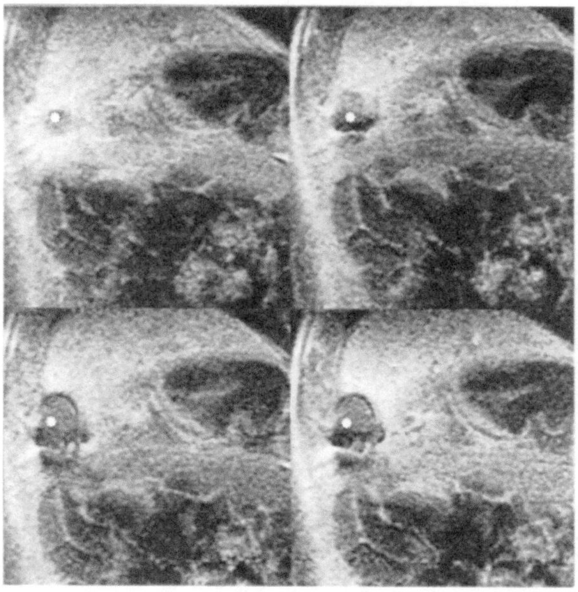

Fig. 17.3. Dynamically acquired gradient-echo images (one image update per s). The needle tip position is demonstrated by the white asterisk. Following aspiration of the bile from the gallbladder, paramagnetic contrast material (gadolinium-DTPA, 0,5 mmol) is instilled through the indwelling needle into the gallbladder. The lumen enlarges as the gallbladder is filled with paramagnetic contrast material, which is displayed as a relatively dark fluid inside the gallbladder

less than 5 min. Biplanar MR tracking was robust and remained totally unaffected by the surrounding tissues (tissue-independent tracking) throughout the interventions (Fig. 17.2). In all three animals cholecystostomies were successfully performed under MR guidance and control. The puncture needle was safely guided in real time using the MR-tracking algorithm, displaying the position of the needle simultaneously on two orthogonal cholangio-roadmaps. Aberrations from the pre-defined course could be corrected in real time by applying counter-pressure to the distal end of the needle. In addition, progress of the needle was documented by the interleaved acquisition of update images.

Following aspiration of bile from the gallbladder through the cannula of the coaxial MR-tracking needle system, MR cholangiograms confirmed a marked reduction in the size of the gallbladder. Fast T1-weighted gradient-echo imaging documented re-insufflation of the gallbladder achieved with installation of undiluted paramagnetic contrast medium through the needle into the collapsed gallbladder (Fig. 17.3). T2-shortening effects of the paramagnetic contrast agent rendered the growing outline of the gallbladder black.

17.4 Discussion

Cholecystostomies are possible under active biplanar MR-tracking guidance. This guidance and monitoring system combines real-time instrument visualization aspects of fluoroscopy, scan plane flexibility and ability to visualize the biliary system inherent to sonography with the spatial resolution of computed tomography. Based upon the non-invasive acquisition of MR cholangiograms, active biplanar MR tracking promises to provide a safe and efficient means of guiding devices into the biliary system for diagnostic as well as therapeutic purposes.

The cholecystostomy must be considered a first step with regard to using MR guidance for biliary interventions. The outlined biplanar target-directed active tracking approach appears sufficiently versatile to also permit accessing dilated biliary ducts for percutaneous biliary drainage procedures. By visualizing the needle tip in relation to the biliary tree at all times, the drainage cannula could be guided for optimal access. Procedure times could be reduced and exposure to ionizing radiation altogether eliminated. Insertion of coil-tipped MR-tracking guidewires and catheters (Wildermuth et al. 1995) into the biliary tree might enable the performance of more complex biliary interventions.

The presented device tracking technique is based on the separation of imaging data acquisition and the collection of the positional data of the device's tip. The device is not identified within the image, but instead its position is determined totally independent of the morphologic imaging process. The images based on which the intervention is guided and monitored can thus be acquired using the highest quality standards, including maximal lesion conspicuity. Images with different inherent contrast properties may be acquired of the same region: one image set will display the dilated biliary system, whereas a second set of images could be optimized to depict an obstructing tumor in relation to the surrounding vasculature.

Since the localization of the coil requires merely four MR experiments (Dumoulin et al. 1993; Leung et al. 1995a) with a TR of 15–30 ms, the spatial coordinates of the device can be updated 8–16 times per second: a temporal resolution far superior to most MR-imaging sequences. Fast data links and computing power enable display of the RF coil position with a delay of less than 10 ms. The biplanar implementation of the technique does not slow the tracking process. The coordinates of the coil are actively available in all three planes and can hence be projected onto any desired image, as long as it is collected in the same acquisition volume. The simultaneous tracking of the needle on two orthogonal images, both displaying the gallbladder, greatly facilitated guidance of the puncture needle. The real-time display permits the interventionalist to gauge adjustments to the course of the device in all three planes.

In case images do need to be updated, the positional information of the coil can be used to guide the imaging plane so that new images are acquired corresponding to the coil position. With the biplanar tracking option, updated images can even be acquired in two different planes, displaying the real-time position of the needle tip. The operator is free to choose whether to track the device on two previously acquired images or to have the scanner provide update images on one or both displays corresponding to the position of the RF coil.

Since the tracking algorithm finds the most intense point in the Fourier-transformed MR response signal, it will ideally track the signal source located in the center of the coil. The incorporation of an internal signal source in the center of the coil makes MR tracking of this particular needle tissue-independent. The design contributes to a robustness crucial for the successful performance of complex interventions. The tracking signal remains always present and of the same amplitude even if the coil is passing through air.

The results of these preliminary experiments demonstrate the feasibility of applying this active device tracking technique to biliary interventions. Fundamental to the functioning of this system is the use of PEEK for the construction of the MR biopsy needle. Two properties of the material make it suitable for this purpose. Firstly, it is rather inert in an MR environment. There is no torque on the needle when moved within the magnetic field. The associated susceptibility artifact is sufficiently limited so as not to dephase the tracking signal originating from the spins inside and outside the coil.

Furthermore, it should be noted that susceptibility artifacts and gradient non-linearities are prevented from affecting the tracked locations by the use of four-excitation Hadamard encoding scheme (Dumoulin et al. 1991). Secondly, PEEK provides the needle with sufficient stability to penetrate even firm tissues. To enhance the cutting ability, the cutting tip of the stylet is made of ceramic.

Clearly, the biplanar tracking concept will need to be proven in a clinical environment. The presented data suggests, however, a significant potential for the delivery of both diagnostic and therapeutic devices to the biliary system.

References

Albert K, Schledjewski R, Harbaugh M, Bleser S, Jamison R, Friedrich K (1994) Characterization of wear in composite material orthopedic implants. II. The implant/bone interface. Biomed Mater Eng 4:199-211

Dumoulin CL, Souza, SP, Darrow RD, Pelc NJ, Adams WJ, Ash SA (1991) Simultaneous acquisition of phase contrast angiograms and stationary tissue images with Hadamard encoding of flow-induced phase shifts. J Magn Reson Imaging 1:399-404

Dumoulin CL, Souza SP, Darrow RD (1993) Real-time position monitoring of invasive devices using magnetic resonance. Magn Reson Med 29:411-415

Jokish KA, Brown SA, Bauer TW, Merritt K (1992) Biological response to chopped-carbon-fiber-reinforced PEEK. J Biomed Mater Res 26:133-146

Jolesz FA, Blumenfeld SM (1994) Interventional use of magnetic resonance imaging. Magn Reson Q 10:85-96

Kaufmann L, Arakawa M, Hale J, et al (1989) Accessible magnetic resonance imaging. Magn Reson Q 5:283-297

Leung DA, Debatin JF, Wildermuth S, et al (1995a) Intravascular MR tracking catheter: preliminary experimental evaluation. AJR Am J Roentgenol 164:1265-1270

Leung DA, Debatin JF, Wildermuth S, et al (1995b) Real-time biplanar tracking for interventional MR- imaging procedures. Radiology 197:485-488

Maharaj G, Bleser S, Albert K, Lambert R, Jani S, Jamison R (1994) Characterization of wear in composite material orthopedic implants. I. The composite trunnion/ceramic interface. Biomed Mater Eng 4:193-198

Schenk JF, Jolesz FA, Roemer PB, et al (1995) Superconducting open configuration MR imaging system for image-guided therapy. Radiology 195:805-814

Schuster DM, Pedrosa MC, Robbins AH (1995) Magnetic resonance cholangiography. Abdom Imaging 20:353-356

Wildermuth S, Debatin JF, Leung DA, et al. (1995) MR-guided percutaneous intravascular interventions: in vivo assessment of potential applications. (abstract) Proceedings, Society of Magnetic Resonance, p 1161

18 Real-Time MR-Guided Neurosurgical Interventions

R. Bernays, S. Kollias, and B.J. Romanowski

CONTENTS

18.1 Introduction

The remote therapeutic manipulation of an invisible, intracranial target, monitored with real-time imaging, has long been a dream shared by generations of neurosurgeons. Several attempts toward this goal undertaken by neurosurgeons in the past were limited by the technical constraints of neuroimaging. The recent advent of open-configuration MRI systems seems to permit the implementation of strategies to overcome these limitations. The dream of remote therapeutic manipulation of intracranial lesions under real-time image guidance has come close to its realization.

18.2 Development of Stereotactic Procedures

The historical development of stereotactic procedures began with Zernov in 1889 (Kandel and Schavinsky 1972). He developed a guidance frame, which looked like a sieve, for advancing a probe into an abscess, directed by surface landmarks toward a clinically localized intracranial target. Horsley and Clarke (1908), in London, designed the first stereotactic frame for laboratory experiments. Each of these stereotactic procedures was based on superficial landmarks and were unsuccessful owing to the problem of anatomic variability, which had yet to be solved.

Spiegel and Wycis (1952), in Philadelphia, were the first to use the cerebral ventricles, visualized by ventriculography, as landmarks. These landmarks were related to deep brain structures with the help of an atlas. This important step toward image-guided therapy occurred just 49 years ago.

18.3 Indirect Neuronavigation

Today, several technologically advanced stereotactic systems are available. All of these systems rely on previously acquired images in the form of preoperative image data sets for navigation. These preoperative images are linked to the physical space by different types of referencing systems. Conventional stereotactic systems (Fig. 18.1) use a reference

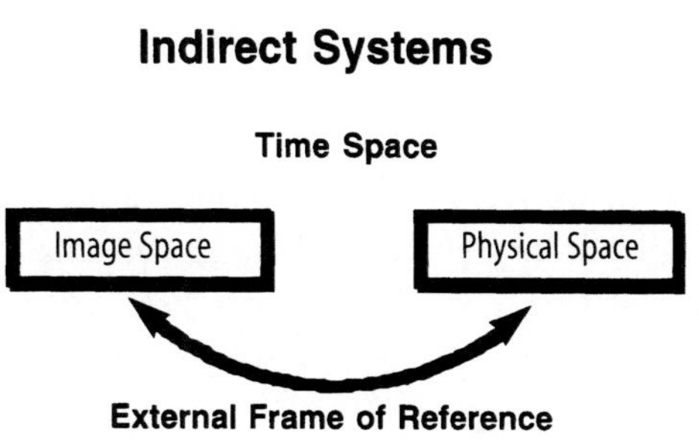

Fig. 18.1. An illustration of the conventional stereotactic approach based on preacquired images which are linked to the physical space by an external frame of reference. There is no compensatory mechanism for adjusting to changes in morphology during the procedure itself

R. Bernays, MD, Department of Neurosurgery, University Hospital Zurich, CH-8091 Zurich, Switzerland
S. Kollias, MD, Department of Neuroradiology, University Hospital Zurich, CH-8091 Zurich, Switzerland
B.J. Romanowski, RT, Research Coordinator, MRI Center, Institute of Diagnostic Radiology, University Hospital Zurich, Rämistrasse 100, CH-8091 Zurich, Switzerland

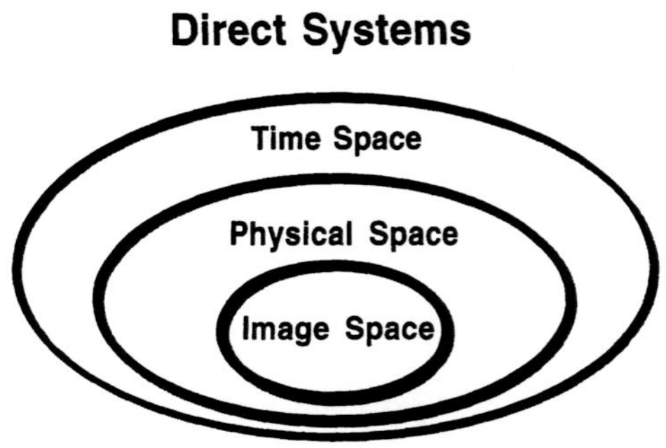

Fig. 18.2. Direct systems unify imaging, time and physical space. This reduces sources of navigational errors considerably, speeds up operating time and provides the neurosurgeon with real-time images displaying the position of the instruments relative to the surrounding morphology. Since images can be updated every 2 s, procedure-related changes in morphology are easily detected and can be incorporated into subsequent procedural planning

frame, while frameless systems incorporate an optical triangulation system to identify superficial reference points. The main drawback of these systems is that the preoperative images are rapidly outdated after the start of a surgical procedure because of tissue manipulation. The neuronavigational accuracy deteriorates because the surgical plan is based on pre-acquired images and the process of surgical intervention inevitably alters the target anatomy. These alterations cannot be compensated for.

18.4 Direct "Real-Time" Neuronavigation

Open-configuration interventional MRI in combination with external referencing systems unifies imaging, time and physical space (Fig 18.2). These basic conditions provide the surgeon with near-real-time imaging. The target lesion and the surgical instrument are presented on the same image. The flashpoint system (FPS; Image Guided Technologies) is a referencing device based on an optical triangulation system which projects the calculated position of an instrument and its virtual continuation on the near-real-time morphologic images. Near-real-time neuronavigation considerably increases positional accuracy while decreasing operating time.

18.5 Spectrum of Potential MR-Guided Neurosurgical Procedures

In order to develop neurosurgical concepts for procedures in open interventional MRI, it was necessary to evaluate which neurosurgical procedures benefit the most from the open environment and near-real-time neuronavigation. Clearly, the emphasis here lies on minimally invasive procedures. Such procedures include:

- Biopsies of intracranial lesions
- Puncture and evacuation of cysts and abscesses
- Ventriculotomies
- Endoscopic procedures
- Perforation and balloon dilatation of intraventricular septa
- Implantation of depth electrodes
- Laser induced thermal therapy (LITT)
- Photodynamic therapy (PDT)
- Focused ultrasound
- Micro-ultrasonic aspiration

Interventional MR is already in clinical use at several sites around the world, and many of these procedures have already been successfully performed. Beyond these limited procedures interventional MR holds considerable promise in the field of microneurosurgery. With further advances in image fusion, permitting the integration of functional MRI and positron emission tomography data into high resolution anatomical MR images, the vision of *functional and anatomical real-time neuronavigation* would become practicable. This would substantially increase surgical safety and virtually revolutionize neurosurgical practice. The potential yield of this development would translate into radical tumor removal with the preservation of functional cerebral integrity.

To date, many of these features are not yet fully developed. The current focus of the microneurosurgical work with interventional MR systems remains concentrated on pituitary and tumor surgery. The impact of the open interventional MR environment on tumor surgery to date has been a facilitation of radical, but nevertheless safe tumor removal. Preliminary studies, however, show that it is difficult to distinguish between tumor border and normal brain tissue in the wall of the cavity. Imaging in three-dimensional planes may be helpful for preserving important anatomic structures.

18.6 Neurosurgical Instrumentation for Open MR Procedures

Neurosurgical interventions of any kind require highly specialized instrumentation. The full range of microsurgical procedures in the brain within the MR environment cannot take place until MR-compatible instruments have reached a technical standard comparable to that of conventional microneurosurgical instrumentation. The availability of new, MR-compatible materials provides hope that this goal will indeed be achieved in the near future. Already today many such instruments, including an MR-compatible microscope, are available. A list of vendors is summarized in Chap. 36. In addition to commercially available instruments, such as the external referencing system (Flashpoint) Mayfield head frame, scalpels, scissors, clamps, high-speed drills and punches, many of the more specialized MR-compatible neurosurgical instruments still have to be developed.

For safety reasons, all instruments used in the MR environment need to be fully non-ferromagnetic. The further choice of materials for the different instruments is predicated upon their function. Instruments that manipulate a target structure under real-time imaging must be artifact-free. The most important region during a stereotactic procedure is the region adjacent to the instrument, e.g., the biopsy cannula. The use of nonmetallic MR-compatible materials for such instruments is advantageous, since most metals produce an artifactual shift of the displayed instrument position, in addition to a considerable susceptibility artifact (Ladd et al. 1996). Hence, the signal void produced by the instrument can appear to be at a different location from the actual instrument. Composite-based instruments proved to be artifact free and electrically nonconductive, but extremely difficult and expensive to produce (Figs. 18.3, 18.4, 18.5). They are visualized by a combination of passive signal void and active stereotactic triangulation. A "snapper-stereoguide" (Bernays 1997) was developed as a fixation device. It is positioned firmly in the burr hole and carries an instrument guide with a movement range of 30° that can be fixed at any angle and adapted to the FPS.

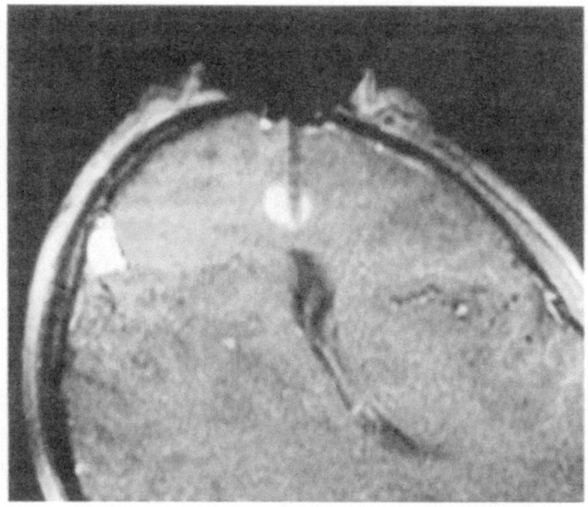

Fig. 18.3. An inserted composite-based cannula for stereotactic biopsy diagnostic in a high-grade tumor: the biopsy cannula is visualized by a signal void

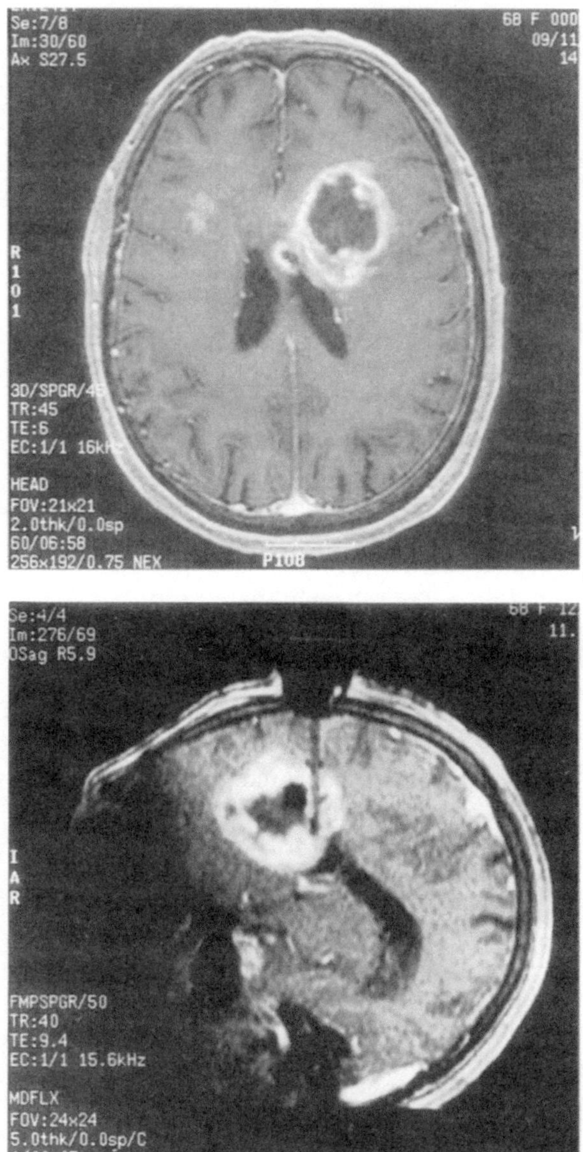

a

b

Fig. 18.4. **a** An axial image of a contrast-enhancing mass lesion acquired just prior to the procedure. **b** A near-real-time image acquired during the procedure depicts the composite biopsy needle as a signal void in excellent position for biopsy. Subsequent histopathological analysis revealed glioblastoma multiforme

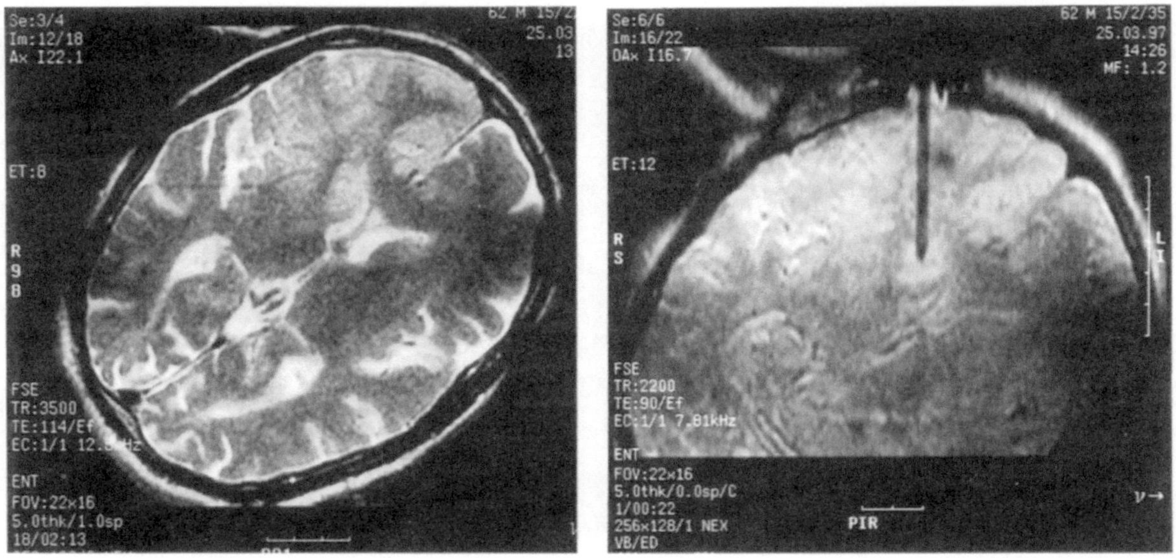

a b

Fig. 18.5 a A T2-weighted image of a mass lesion acquired just prior to the procedure. **b** A T2-weighted near-real-time image acquired during the procedure (acquisition time 22 s) depicts the composite biopsy needle as a signal void in excellent position for biopsy. Subsequent histopathological analysis revealed a grade II astrocytoma

Another area that will need refinement is the development of dedicated MR coils for specific anatomic neurosurgical regions, such as the pituitary gland. This will potentially increase image quality and provide anatomic detail that will be of great value to assist in surgical procedures.

18.7 Steps for Real-Time MR-Guided Neurosurgical Procedures

The steps of a surgical procedure in the open MR intervention include:

1. Preoperative imaging (image segmentation, functional MR, perfusion MR, virtual trajectory planning)
2. Positioning of the patient, positioning of the MR coils
3. Transfer of the patient into the scanner
4. Skin preparation and draping
5. Trajectory planning
6. Burr hole
7. Dural detachment, dural incision
8. Insertion of the snapper-stereoguide
9. Fixation of the FPS to the instrument guide
10. Trajectory tuning, verification
11. Insertion of biopsy cannula, endoscope, balloon, perforator or electrode
12. Fixation of instrument guide
13. Performance of biopsy or other definitive procedure
14. Removal of instrument, detachment of FPS, removal of snapper-stereoguide
15. Postprocedure imaging

18.8 Preliminary Experience with MR-Guided Neurosurgical Interventions

The first 20 stereotactic operations in our institution included 16 biopsies of supratentorial tumors, 3 abscess evacuations and 1 ventriculotomy. There were no perioperative complications. All biopsies were diagnostic, and the accuracy of the FPS adapted to the snapper-stereoguide was within 1–2 mm (annotation/cannula).

The snapper-stereoguide in conjunction with the FPS proved a useful tool for doing stereotactic procedures in open MRI. The near-real-time visualization of the biopsy procedure is an obvious advantage of the open compared with conventional MRI systems. Compared with conventional brain biopsies in an operating theater, the operative times could be significantly reduced when the procedures were performed in the interventional magnet system. Interventional MRI sets a new standard for neurosurgical stereotactic procedures against which all current neuronavigation systems must be measured.

References

Bernays R et al. (1997) a new guidance device for frameless, stereotactical near-real-time neurosurgical procedures in the open interventional MR (submitted for publication)

Horsley V, Clarke RH (1908) The structure and functions of the cerebellum examined by a new method. Brain 31:45-125

Kandel EI, Schavinsky YV (1972) Stereotaxic apparatus and operations in Russia in the 19th century. J Neurosurg 37:407-411

Ladd ME, Erhart P, Debatin JF, Romanowski BJ, Boesiger, McKinnon GC (1996) Biopsy needle artifacts. Magn Reson Med 36:646-651

Spiegel EA, Wycis HAT (1952) Stereoencephalotomy (thalotomy and related procedures). 1. Methods and stereotaxic atlas of the human brain. Grune and Stratton, New York

19 Neuronavigation of Cerebral Lesions

U. Spetzger

CONTENTS

19.1 Introduction

The central nervous system has no, or only limited, potential for regeneration, and surgically damaged nervous tissue remains permanently dysfunctional. Therefore, cranial neurosurgery differs from other surgical procedures in many respects. Even the access to the lesion can be a major problem in cerebral operations because surgical damage to physiological cerebral tissue around the lesion bears the risk of severe postoperative neurological deficits. This particular situation demands detailed preoperative planning of the surgical approach and the microsurgical strategy. A fundamental prerequisite for minimally invasive neurosurgical management is the exact knowledge of the location of the target area within the brain. Nowadays, the exact localization of the lesion with respect to the surrounding anatomy can be determined by sophisticated neuroradiological imaging techniques, but the transfer of this indispensable knowledge into surgical practice still remains difficult. Navigation systems have realized this transfer by the virtual linkage of digitized neuroradiological data with real anatomical structures.

Neuronavigation is an evolving field and is becoming an important component of the modern neurosurgical armamentarium.

U. Spetzger, MD, Department of Neurosurgery, University of Technology Aachen, Pauwelsstrasse 30, D-52057 Aachen, Germany

19.2 Concept of Neuronavigation

The basic principle of neuronavigation is the coupling of the spatial coordinates of radiological images with the real spatial coordinates of the patient. This registration procedure allows excellent three-dimensional (3D) orientation through real-time graphical-anatomical interaction. The accuracy of the primary data depends on the quality of the neuroradiological investigation and the exactness of the patient-image registration via external fiducials. The precise localization of the lesion by navigated neurosurgical techniques will minimize the invasiveness of operative procedures and improve the surgical results.

19.2.1 Navigation System

The navigation system (EasyGuide Neuro, Philips Medical Systems, Best, The Netherlands) is comprised of the following basic elements: (1) a workstation with positioning computer (Unix 4.0) with the implemented stereotactic software and a high resolution monitor integrated in a mobile trolley; (2) an optical localizing system with two infrared-sensitive cameras positioned on a single camera stand which can easily be secured to the operating table; (3) multiple, differently shaped pointers (straight and bayonet) or probes with infrared light-emitting diodes connected via a cable to the navigation unit (Fig. 19.1).

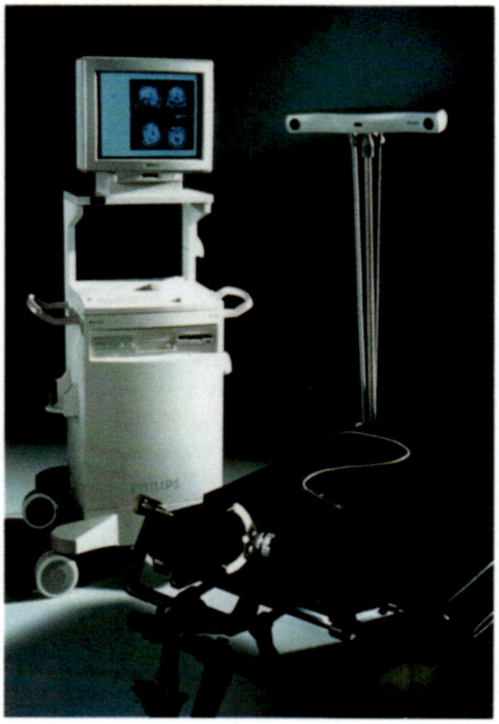

Fig. 19.1. The navigation system EasyGuide Neuro used in this series consists of the unix 4.0 workstation with the implemented software, a high-resolution monitor, infrared camera system and a wire-connected infrared light-emitting probe

19.2.2
Additional Equipment

Several devices have been developed as additional equipment to facilitate the intraoperative application of the navigation system. Instead of the pointer, an infrared light-emitting bipolar forceps can be used during surgery. Also, an articulated arm as a multifunctional instrument holder has been designed to support frameless stereotactic procedures. The arm consists of four segments which are connected by three joints and contains a lockable ball with the option to hold different navigated instruments (e.g., biopsy needles, catheters, endoscopes, etc.).

19.2.3
MR Data Acquisition

After the attachment of ten hydrogel multimodality skin markers (external fiducials) to the scalp, the patient is examined by MRI (Gyroscan ACS NT, 1.5 T, Philips Medical Systems, Best, The Netherlands). Routinely, the gadolinium-enhanced MR examination is performed using the following standardized protocol: 3D scan mode, fast field echo with TE 4.5/TR 30 ms, field of view 230–240 mm, matrix 256MaL256 and slice thickness 3 mm. At present, the data transfer from the MR image to the navigation system is performed via optical disk.

After data transfer of the radiological images to the graphical workstation (EasyGuide Neuro), an individual 3D voxel model of the patient's head and brain is reconstructed. The coordinate system of the resultant 3D model is then correlated with the actual position of the patient's head by touching the skin fiducials with the probe. The coordinates of the skin markers are thereby adjusted to the neuroradiological coordinates, establishing the correlation of the patient's head relative to the 3D digitizer. This so-called patient-image registration procedure optically links the tip of the pointer with its presentation on the screen, and the displayed image dynamically shows an exact localization in three perpendicular sectional two-dimensional views.

19.3
Application

Neuronavigation is used for trephination planning and intraoperative orientation, determination of the optimal approach and localization of small and, especially, deep-seated lesions not visible at the surface of the cerebral cortex, for targeted puncture of various lesions, as well as for frameless stereotactic operations.

19.3.1
Surgical Planning

The lesion is dynamically displayed on the monitor screen in three perpendicular images permitting exact surgical planning. A computer simulation of surgical procedures is also made possible and, furthermore, the local anatomy can be studied in detail.

19.3.2
Image-Guided Neurosurgery

Positioning of the patient's head and fixation of the infrared camera system to the operating table are carried out first. By touching the skin markers with the pointer, the image coordinates and spatial coordinates are matched by the navigation system (patient-image registration). The whole setup takes about 10 min and after this procedure the system is usable.

The neuronavigation system is an excellent tool for neurosurgical training. The dynamic 3D representation allows the exact target area and the neighboring anatomical structures to be studied in detail. Consequently, all surgical steps can be simulated and the appropriate approach determined. Neuronavigation offers the surgeon a repeated "virtual walk" through the region of interest, providing an excellent visualization of the individual anatomy. The computer-based preoperative planning and graphical-interactive learning procedure is a benefit in modern neurosurgical training.

The system offers the possibility of a virtual pointer elongation. This option enables virtual intracerebral navigation and planning of the surgical access or can be used to measure the depth of a biopsy needle in a virtual "unbloody" procedure (see Fig. 19.4).

19.4 Experiences

The wide range of 74 neurosurgical procedures (including 62 microsurgical operations and 12 navigated punctures and biopsies) performed between January 1996 and February 1997 using the navigation system EasyGuide Neuro is demonstrated in Table 19.1. The intraoperatively proven localization accuracy ranged from 1.5 to 6.9 mm. There are several technical reasons for reduced accuracy, especially incorrect patient-image registration. Major craniotomy and extensive dural openings with massive release of cerebrospinal fluid definitively change the relative position of the cerebral structures. The avoidance of such extended dural and arachnoidal opening at the beginning of surgery can retard this so-called brain-shift. However, anatomical relationships also change due to continuous tumor debulking or the evacuation of cystic lesions. The en bloc resection of lesions has therefore been proposed to avoid this problem (Barnett et al. 1993; Kelly 1992a,b).

Table 19.1. Application of the navigation system in 74 neurosurgical operations for the treatment of different intracranial lesions

Surgical application	*n*
Navigated microneurosurgery	***62***
Deep-seated intracerebral lesion	39
Miscellaneous	16
Transnasal approach	7
Biopsy and puncture	***7***
Ventricle catheter insertion	3
Cerebral abscess	2
Intracranial cyst	1
Malignant glioma	1
Frameless stereotaxy	***5***
Cerebral abscess	2
Intracerebral hematoma	2
Metastasis	1

19.4.1 Neuronavigation in Different Cranial Neurosurgical Operations

19.4.1.1 Navigated Microneurosurgery

Surgery is performed with the patient under general anesthesia positioned on the operating table, and the skull is fixed with a three-point fixation clamp. The size of the craniotomy flap is traced with the probe and the skin incision is centered over the tailored approach. After guided trephination and opening of the dura, the cortical approach is defined. Especially in the case of deep-seated tumors with an overlaying intact cerebral surface, the fissure or sulcus allowing for optimal access to the lesion can be easily determined (Fig. 19.2). If necessary, navigation can be additionally controlled and supported by the use of intraoperative ultrasound which provides online images (Mayfrank et al. 1994). After microsurgical preparation of the approach and detection of the lesion, the resection is performed. The navigation system proved a valuable tool for intraoperative localization and orientation, and enabled a lesion-directed and minimally traumatic surgical approach to the target in all of our 62 cases (Fig. 19.3).

19.4.1.2 Navigated Biopsies and Punctures

These surgical procedures are also performed under general anesthesia with rigid fixation of the patient's head in a clamp. An articulated arm is used as the instrument holder to facilitate the procedure. The skull is opened via a small burrhole and the canula for the biopsy forceps is introduced under continuous control of the navigation system. Tumor biopsies and drainages of intracerebral abscesses were successfully performed. In three selected patients with narrow ventricular chambers requiring ventricular shunting the catheter was inserted under control of the navigation system (Fig. 19.4).

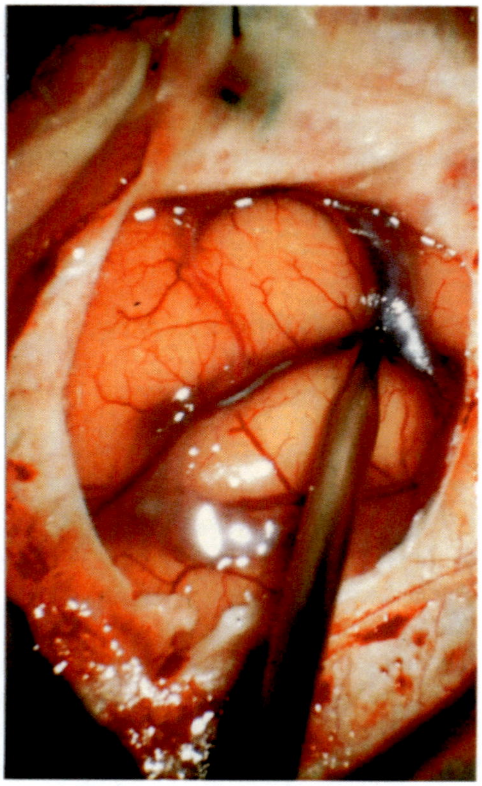

Fig. 19.2. A guided 3 cm × 3 cm craniotomy with a U-shaped opening of the dura was performed. The intraoperative photography demonstrates the planning of the microsurgical approach to a subcortical tumor. The probe is pointing to a bifurcation of a cortical vein used as a natural anatomical landmark at the completely intact superficial cerebral cortex. In this patient a transsulcal approach was used to resect the deep-seated lesion

19.4.1.3
Frameless Stereotactic Procedures

All surgical procedures are performed under local anesthesia and the patient's head is fixed with adhesive tape. The skin markers are left uncovered allowing re-registration. The clinically proven accuracy was slightly reduced (range 4.7–6.9 mm) owing to the non-rigid, frameless fixation of the patient's head as compared with navigated microsurgery. However, in the cases we selected for navigated frameless stereotaxy, pinpoint accuracy was not mandatory because the mean diameter of the five lesions was 2.1 cm. The fast and simple handling is an advantage over the more time-consuming and complex frame-based stereotactic procedure.

19.4.2
Challenges

Neuronavigation is a helpful tool in current neurosurgery. Exact preoperative planning and improved intraoperative orientation reduce surgical trauma and improve the postoperative results. However, the major problem of all neuronavigational systems is the lack of on-line information, resulting in progressive inaccuracy during intracranial surgery because the devices cannot accommodate to the continuously changing anatomical situation (Reinhardt et al. 1996; Spetzger et al. 1995). At present, the so-called brain-shift is still an unsolved problem (Sipos et al. 1996; Spetzger et al. 1997a,

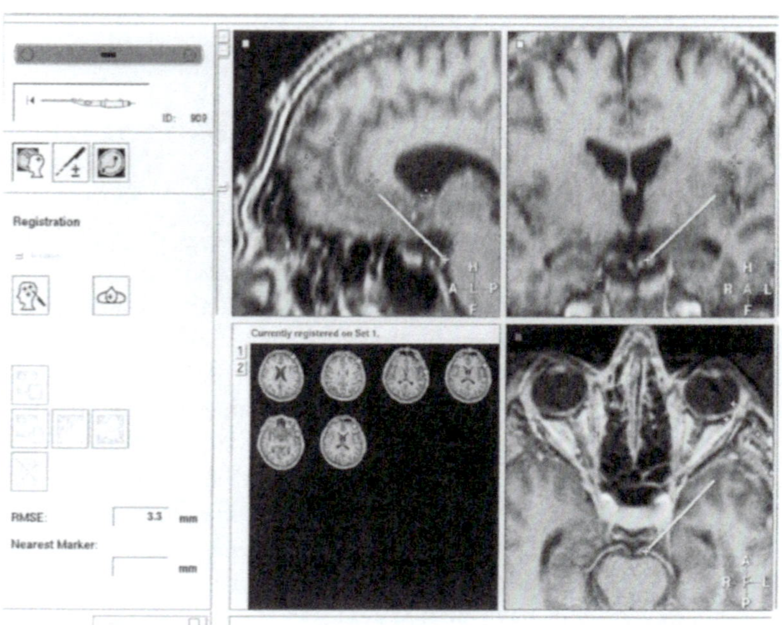

Fig. 19.3. Monitor screen display during microsurgical selective amygdalo-hippocampectomy in a patient with drug-resistant temporal lobe epilepsy. The position of the probe is dynamically indicated in three perpendicular MR images allowing an exact graphic-interactive orientation and intraoperative localization during surgery. The tip of the probe is directed via a transsylvian approach to the left posterior cerebral artery

1997b). Initial expectations to control the degree of intracerebral tumor resection using neuronavigational systems have not been met because debulking of the lesion changes the relationship to the surrounding tissue (KATO et al. 1991; KELLY 1992a, 1992b). Since the navigation system proceeds with preoperative neuroradiological images that no longer correspond to the true surgical anatomy, the progressive loss of accuracy is inevitable (ADAMS et al. 1990; GUTHRIE and ADLER 1992, KELLY 1992a, 1992b; LABORDE et al. 1992; SPETZGER et al. 1997a, 1997b; WATANABE et al. 1987, 1991; ZAMORANO et al. 1992).

19.5 Perspectives and Future Developments

Permanent on-line data refreshment during ongoing surgery could solve the problem of brain-shift. In the near future, this readaptation could be achieved by repeated intraoperative neuroradiological investigations (SPETZGER et al. 1995). A combination of neuronavigation with functional modalities such as electrophysiological brain mapping (BUCHNER et al. 1994) is desirable.

References

Adams L, Krybus W, Meyer-Ebrecht D, Rügger R, Gilsbach J, et al (1990) Computer assisted surgery. Comput Graph Appl 10:43-50 Barnett GH, Kormos DW, Steiner CP, Weisenberger J (1993) Use of a frameless, armless stereotactic wand for brain tumor localization with two-dimensional and three-dimensional neuroimaging. Neurosurgery 33:674-678

Buchner H, Adams L, Knäpper A, Rügger R, Laborde G, Gilsbach JM, et al (1994) Preoperative localization of the central sulcus by dipole source analysis of early somatosensory evoked potentials and three-dimensional magnetic resonance imaging. J Neurosurg 80:849-856

Guthrie BL, Adler JR Jr (1992) Computer-assisted preoperative planning, interactive surgery, and frameless stereotaxy. Clin Neurosurg 38:112-131

Kato A, Yoshimine T, Hayawaka T, Tomita Y, et al (1991) A frameless, armless navigational system for computer-assisted surgery. J Neurosurg 74:845-849

Kelly PJ (1992a) Computer interactive volumetric stereotactic resection of brain mass lesions. In: Kall BA (eds) Computers in stereotactic neurosurgery. Blackwell, Boston pp 295-312

Kelly PJ (1992b) Stereotactic resection and ist limitations in glial neoplasms. Stereotact Funct Neurosurg 59:84-91

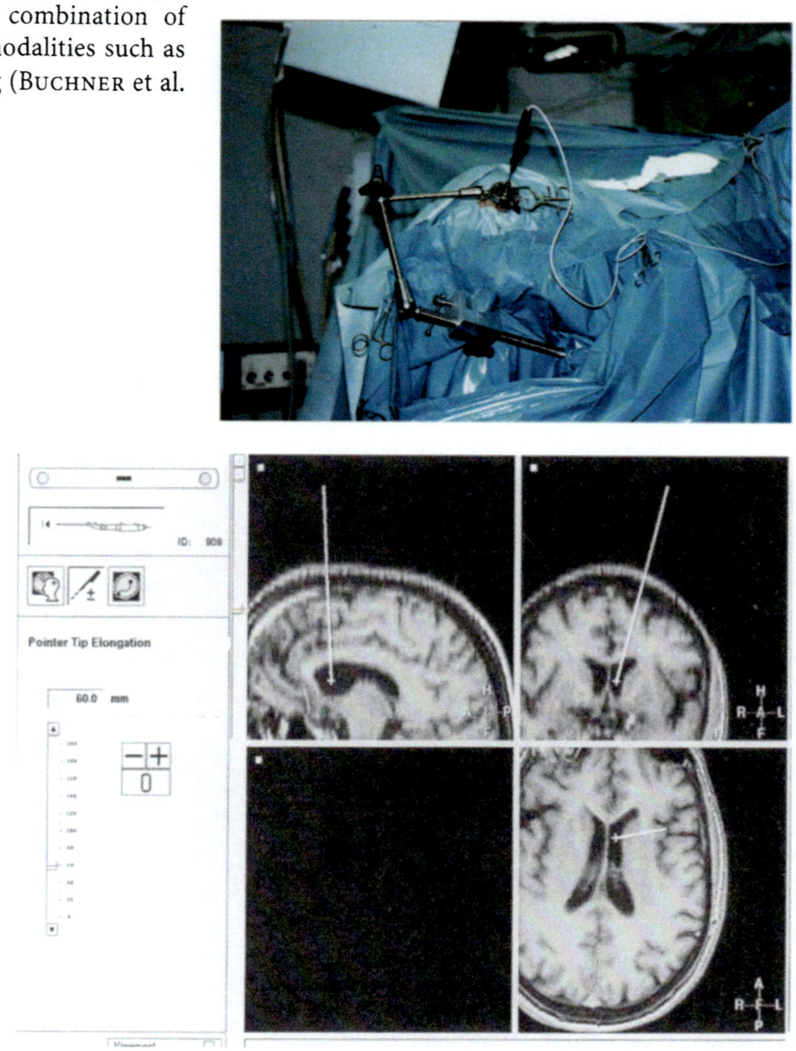

Fig. 19.4. a Intraoperative application of the articulated arm during the planning of a navigated ventricular puncture. The pointer is fixed, the cerebral access is planned and the length of the catheter can be measured by means of the virtual pointer elongation. **b** Monitor screen display showing the virtually elongated pointer (60.0 mm) within the frontal horn of the ventricular system

Laborde G, Gilsbach J, Harders A, Klimek L, Mösges R, Krybus W (1992) Computer assisted localizer for planning of surgery and intraoperative orientation. Cta Neurochir (Wien) 119:166-170

Mayfrank L, Bertalanffy H, Spetzger U, Klein HM, Gilsbach JM (1994) Ultrasound-guided craniotomy for minimal invasive exposure of cerebral convexity lesions. Acta Neurochir (Wien) 131:270-273

Reinhardt HF, Trippel M, Westermann B, Horstmann GA, Gratzl O (1996) Computer assisted brain surgery for small lesions in the central sensorimotor region. Acta Neurochir (Wien) 138:200-205

Sipos EP, Tebo SA, Zinreich SJ, Long DM, Brem H (1996) In vivo accuracy testing and clinical experience with the ISG viewing wand. Neurosurgery 39:194-204

Spetzger U, Laborde G, Gilsbach JM (1995) Frameless neuronavigation in modern neurosurgery. Minimal Invas Neurosurg 38:326-330

Spetzger U, Gilsbach JM, Mösges R, Schlöndorff G, Laborde G (1997a) The computer-assisted-localizer, a navigation help in microneurosurgery. Eur Surg Res 29(6):

Spetzger U, Reinges MH, Krombach GA, Rohde V, et al (1997b) Experiences with the neuronavigation system EasyGuide Neuro. MIN III Springer, Berlin Heidelberg New York (in press)

Watanabe E, Watanabe T, Manaka S, et al (1987) Three-dimensional digitizer (neuronavigator): a new equipment for computed-tomography guided stereotaxic surgery. Surg Neurol 27:543-547

Watanabe E, Mayanagi Y, Yosugi Y, Manaka S, Takakura K (1991) Open surgery assisted by the neuronavigator, a stereotactic, articulated, sensitive arm. Neurosurgery 28:792-799

Zamorano L, Kadi M, Dong A (1992) Computer-assisted neurosurgery. Simulation and automation. Stereotact Funct Neurosurg 59:115-122

20 MR-Guided Biopsies of the Head and Neck

G.M. Kacl[1] and G. K. von Schulthess[2]

CONTENTS

20.1 Introduction

Reflecting the unsurpassed soft tissue contrast inherent to the MR experiment, MR imaging (MRI) has emerged as a major diagnostic tool in the assessment of various pathologies affecting the head and neck region. Most soft tissue pathologies of the head and neck are well depicted on fast-spin-echo (SE) images with fat suppression. Without the use of contrast medium, vascular morphology can be easily delineated on gradient-echo (GRE) sequences (Vogl et al. 1994a). Although computed tomography (CT) is superior in the assessment of osseous and air-filled structures, contrast-enhanced MRI is of major value in delineating tumors within the soft tissues and vessels (Vogl et al. 1993, 1994b).

Optimal image quality with high spatial resolution for delineation of small structures has been achieved at 1.5 T field strength. In comparison, MR images of the head and neck region acquired with low- and mid-field systems exhibit merely intermediate image quality. This drawback is offset by the "open" design of several of these scanners, allowing direct access to the patient during examination. In view of the high density of "vital" structures in the head and neck region, the concept of interactive MRI with integrated biopsy devices appears particularly attractive (Schenck et al. 1995; Silverman et al. 1995).

The use of MRI to guide biopsies in the head and neck is similar to its use in other organs as discussed in previous chapters. Susceptibility artifacts play a greater role due to the proximity of air-filled and osseous structures as well as dental work. In addition, the abundance of often rather small vital structures, such as vessels and nerves, further complicates MR-guided biopsies in this region.

MR-guided needle targeting in the head and neck is not only useful for biopsy of suspicious lesions, but may furthermore be used as a means to introduce tools for subsequent, minimally thermosensitive therapies such as laser or radio-frequency treatments. Once the non-ferromagnetic needle has been positioned within the lesion, aspiration biopsy, application of energy, or instillation of local drugs becomes possible.

This chapter will describe and illustrate different applications of head and neck biopsies using an open-configuration 0.5-T superconducting MR system. Imaging and biopsies of the thyroid and the parathyroid glands as well as the maxilla and skull base will be discussed.

20.2 Background

Image-guided biopsies in the head and neck region have been performed for several years using different imaging modalities. Fluoroscopes have proved helpful in guiding biopsy needles into bone lesions. Ultrasound-guided fine needle biopsies have become commonplace in the clinical work-up of head and neck lesions (Boland et al. 1993). The inability of sound waves to penetrate air-filled and osseous or cartilaginous structures, however, limits the use of ultrasound. Thus, CT has evolved into the modality of choice for most image-guided biopsies of the head and neck.

[1]G.M. Kacl, MD, Institute of Diagnostic Radiology, Zurich University Hospital, Rämistrasse 100, CH-8091 Zurich, Switzerland
[2]G.K. von Schulthess, MD, PhD, Division of Nuclear Medicine, Zurich University Hospital, Rämistrasse 100, CH-8091 Zurich, Switzerland

MRI established its leading role in imaging of the brain and soft tissue structures of the head in the 1980s. In particular, the high soft tissue contrast is responsible for the success of MRI in the head and neck region (Castelijns and van den Brekel 1993; Kraus et al. 1992). Delineation of head and neck tumors, including lymphomas as well as benign and malignant processes of the thyroid and parathyroid glands, is best with MRI. Most imaging protocols consist of multiplanar fast-spin-echo as well as contrast-enhanced gradient-echo acquisitions (Lufkin et al. 1993). With the help of fat suppression techniques, MRI has been shown to be superior to both ultrasound and CT in imaging of the head and neck (Vogl et al. 1994a).

Since MRI is rapidly replacing CT for the evaluation of head and neck pathologies, the need for MR-guided biopsies quickly arose. Correspondingly, a suitable MR-compatible needle system had to be developed. Lufkin et al. (1988a) were among the first to introduce and evaluate different techniques. Mueller et al (1986) introduced a non-ferromagnetic needle for liver biopsies which can be used in the head and neck regions as well. Further applications led to the introduction of nickel alloy (alloy c-276) needles in 1987 and 1988 (Lufkin et al. 1987, 1988a). Reduced susceptibility artifacts and image distortions associated with this new nickel-based needle greatly increased the application of MR-guided biopsies. With the development of other needle systems, Duckwiler and Lufkin introduced MR-guided biopsies of head and neck lesions based on thin section MRI-using a 0.3-T open-configuration magnet system (Duckwiler et al. 1989). In their study, ten patients underwent MR-guided fine needle aspiration biopsies of the head and neck with a 22-gauge bevel-edged needle from alloy c-276 by E-Z-Em, Westbury, N.Y. Apart from the high soft tissue contrast, MRI was found to be useful as it permitted the use of an angulated approach to the complex morphology of the head and neck. Various malignant and inflammatory lesions were biopsied using a submastoid, subzygomatic, retromandibular, infraorbital approach. The infraorbital approach could be documented using sagittal planes to avoid vital structures in the orbit (Lufkin et al. 1988a; Duckwiler et al. 1989). In order to avoid motion artifacts of the needle and allow proper placement of the biopsy device, a special stereotactic device had to be applied (Lufkin et al. 1988b).

In 1991, Han and coworkers reported MR-guided aspiration and drainage of a nasopharyngeal mucus retention cyst in a 40-year-old patient. A 22-gauge MR-compatible needle was introduced via a subzygomatic approach. Following insertion of the needle tip into the pharyngeal lesion, mucoid fluid could be aspirated, thereby avoiding cost-intensive surgical management (Han et al. 1991).

In early implementations, the MR-guided biopsy technique was performed in analogy to CT in a largely blinded fashion. Instead of actively tracking the motion of the needle, as is possible with fluoroscopy or ultrasound, the needle position was imaged only periodically.

Newly developed low- and mid-field MR systems permitting substantially improved patient access are now available. In addition, various instrument-tracking techniques capable of monitoring the motion of instruments have become available. In our experience, the frameless interactive guidance system (Flashpoint 5000, Image Guided Technologies, Boulder, Colo., USA) is well suited for this purpose. Installed in an "open-configuration" 0.5-T MR system (Signa SP, GE Medical Systems, Milwaukee, Wis., USA), it allows an image update every 1.5 s.

With the use of this stereotactic instrument, every conceivable imaging plane relative to the needle course or patient position can be interactively chosen, aiding the exact localization of the non-ferromagnetic needle and reducing the risk of complications.

20.3 Biopsies of the Thyroid and Parathyroid Glands

The utility of MRI in the assessment of thyroid and parathyroid disease has been explored by several authors. For optimal image quality, use of a surface coil is mandatory. Rather than replacing ultrasound and scintigraphy, MRI has evolved into a complementary imaging modality. Thus, MRI was found to be particularly helpful in staging malignant thyroid disease. Local tumor infiltration, extension into the mediastinum of skull base, and lymph node involvement are well depicted on MR images (Bagley et al. 1996). Furthermore, MRI has been shown to be useful in the assessment of local tumor recurrence following thyroidectomy (Freitas and Freitas 1994). The value of MRI in the assessment of benign thyroid disease remains limited at this time (Bagley et al. 1996). The emergence of "open-configuration" MR units in conjunction with the successful integration of laser treatments into an MR environment might be used in the future as an imaging framework for applying and monitoring energy to benign thyroid nodules, when elective surgery is not necessarily indicated. Since both benign and malignant thyroid lesions can be visualized, they can be targeted under MR guidance. In our laboratory, 15 patients with sonographically suspected thyroid nodules or complicated cysts were biopsied in an open 0.5-T MR system. The lesion size varied from 1 to 5 cm. While solid lesions were merely biopsied, cysts were aspirated.

Figure 20.1a–d depicts a cyst before and after aspiration on T2-weighted fast-spin-echo (FSE) images.

Using the frameless stereotactic imaging system (Flashpoint 5000), the interventional radiologist is able to choose between different planes while advancing the needle (Fig. 20.2a–d). The computed needle path coincides with the needle-induced susceptibility artifact. Cytology revealed the lesion to be benign.

In the study presented here, the size limit below which lesion targeting was not reliable was 1.5 cm. All other lesions were successfully targeted. The biopsy time with MRI (mean 20 min) exceeded that with ultrasound (mean 10 min). Thus, it is unlikely that MRI will replace ultrasound as the primary tool for guiding biopsies of the thyroid gland. It may, however, eventually serve as an imaging framework in future thermotherapy. The utility of such an application remains to be demonstrated at present.

MRI is valuable in the assessment of patients with hyperparathyroidism. Particularly in complex cases, including patients with recurrent disease or postoperative scarring, the utility of MRI has been proven (VON SCHULTHESS et al. 1988; NUMEROW et al. 1995; LEE et al. 1996; GIRON et al. 1996). Integrated imaging using scintigraphy, high-resolution ultrasound, and MRI has reached considerable sensitivity and specificity of 70%–90% according to recent articles (LEE et al. 1996). The appearance of parathyroid adenomas and hyperplasia in primary or secondary hyperparathyroidism varies in SE sequences. T2-weighted SE images with spectrospatial fat suppression have been found to be especially helpful in the delination of parathyroid adenomas and hyperplasia.

The example of a 40-year-old woman with an episode of urolithiasis beautifully demonstrates the diagnostic value of MRI in assessing the parathyroid glands. An oval lesion measuring 1.6 cm in diameter was seen to equal advantage of high-resolution ultrasound and coronal T2-weighted fast-spin-echo images (Fig. 20.3a).

Dynamic contrast-enhanced coronal GRE images revealed only minor contrast uptake. For targeting of the lesion, the interactive guidance system was used. The resolution of the T1-weighted GRE update images (Fig. 20.3b) was, however, not sufficient to assure accurate targeting. No representative material could be retrieved, and the patient underwent open surgery, revealing a single parathyroid adenoma located at the left lower thyroid pole.

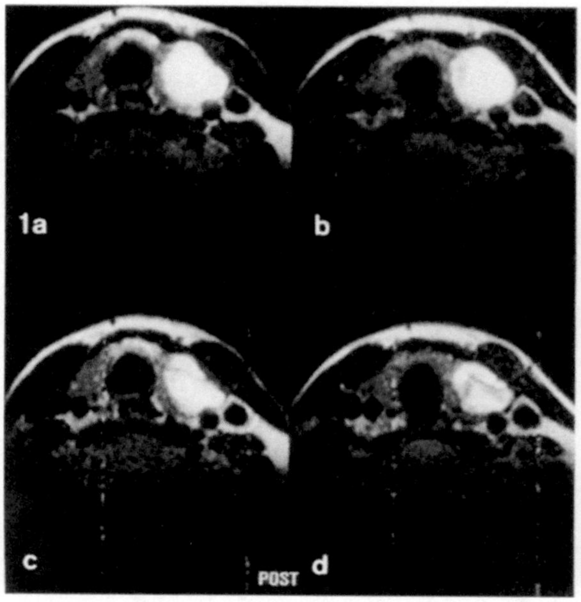

Fig. 20.1a-d. T2-weighted FSE images acquired before and after aspiration of a thyroid cyst

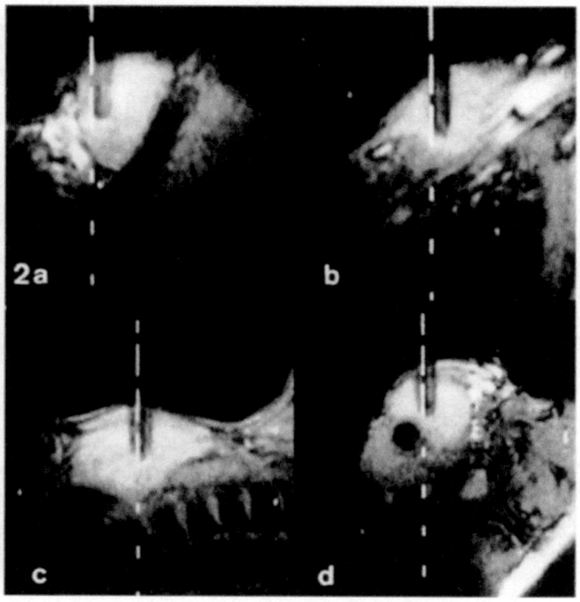

Fig. 20.2a-d. GRE image demonstrating different planes of the interactive guidance system in targeting a thyroid lesion

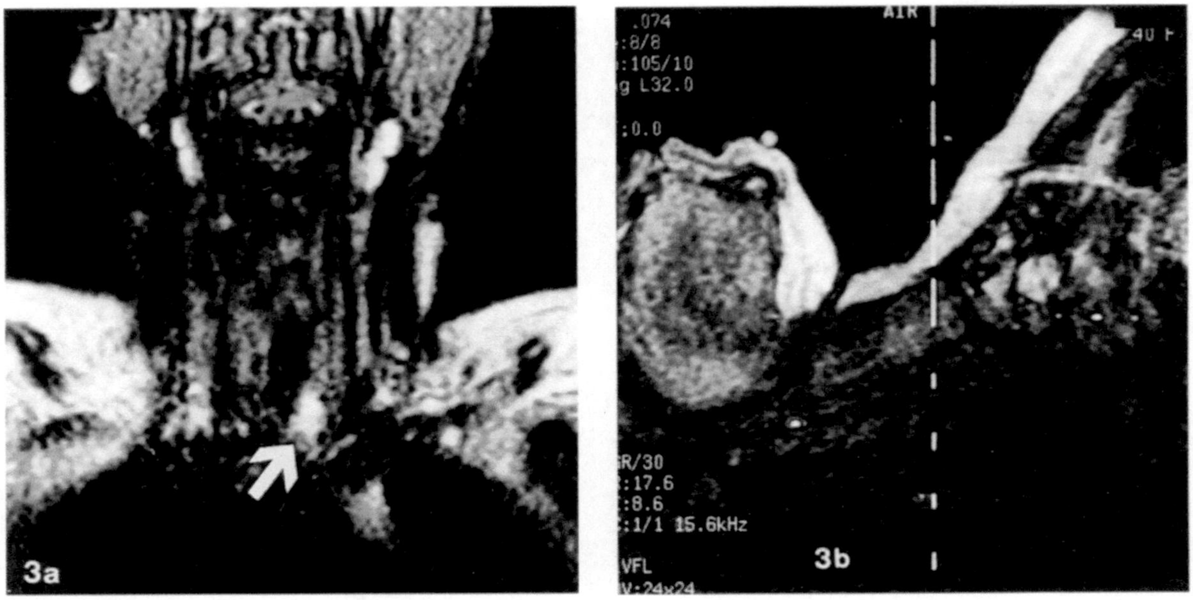

Fig. 20.3.a Coronal T2-weighted SE image demonstrated a parathyroid adenoma adjacent to the left lower thyroid pole (*arrow*). **b** The parathyroid tumor is not seen on the update GRE image

20.4 Biopsies of the Maxilla

MRI of the splanchnocranium is of high value to the oral surgeon. Multiplanar image acquisition and superior soft tissue contrast make MRI an important tool in preoperative tumor staging of lesions affecting the maxilla or skull base (Belkin et al. 1988). Pathohistological analysis remains the basis of any treatment consideration.

To date, CT- and MR-guided biopsy techniques have lacked interactive capabilities for fast and secure positioning of the biopsy needle. This has resulted in a reliance on open biopsy techniques for many tumors of the skull base and maxilla. With the introduction of open-configuration MR imagers in conjunction with interactive instrument-guidance systems, safe and accurate targeting of lesions in this area of complex morphology has become possible.

Using the "open-configuration" magnet with an integrated frameless stereotactical guidance system (Flashpoint), seven patients underwent MR-guided fine needle biopsy of solid and cystic tumors of the maxillary bone and the tooth-bearing parts. Three solid and four cystic lesions were targeted. In the case of several lesions, access required pursuance of an enoral exploratory approach. This was accomplished without problems in the open-configuration MR system. The interactive guidance system serves as a "third eye" to spare vital structures such as the carotid space and major cranial nerves.

All seven lesions were successfully targeted without complications. In all cases, diagnosis could be made on the basis of cytology alone. Surgical biopsy was not necessary in any patient. Histology of two of the solid tumors located in the upper jaw revealed the diagnosis of ameloblastomas. These rare lesions are benign tumors that appear solid or partially cystic (Jackson et al. 1996). If not diagnosed and resected properly, their tendency to recur is extremely high (Hotzinger et al. 1983). Recurrent ameloblastomas require skillful surgical therapy often associated with microsurgical and prosthetic reconstructions of the skull base and facial bones (Hell et al. 1994).

The third solid tumor turned out to be a non-Hodgkin's lymphoma (B cell type) affecting the maxillary sinus (Fig. 20.4). CT showed an infiltrating mass originating in the right maxillary sinus. MRI demonstrated infiltration of the skin and skull base. During the targeting process, the sagittal projection (Fig. 20.4) was particularly helpful.

Four of the lesions turned out to be benign cysts. An example is illustrated in Fig. 20.5. A 31-year-old patient complained of recurrent pain in the left maxillary bone. CT and MRI both depicted a cystic mass originating from the tooth-bearing part of the maxillary bone. The GRE image demonstrates the needle tip positioned in the cystic lesion (Fig. 20.5). Cytological material from the dorsal and rostral wall of the cyst could be selectively retrieved. The cytological material contained only benign epithelial cells consistent with a radicular cyst.

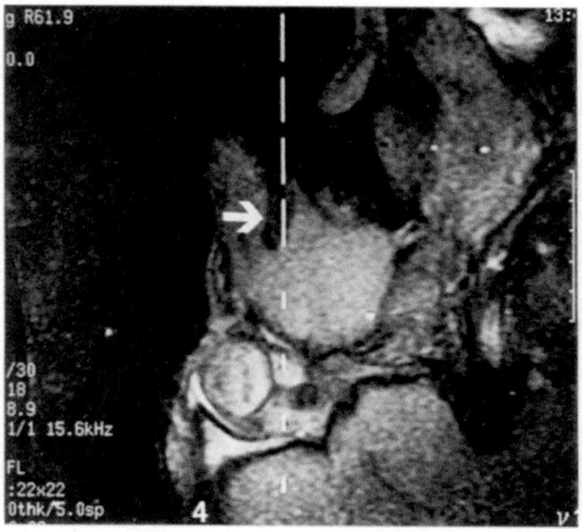

Fig. 20.4. Sagittal GRE image showing infiltrating non-Hodgkin's lymphoma of the right maxillary sinus. Note the susceptibility artifact emanating from the 22-gauge needle (*arrow*).

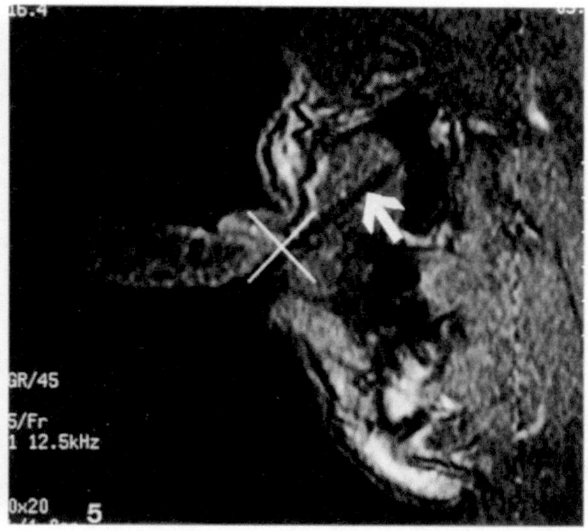

Fig. 20.5. Sagittal GRE image illustrates a radicular odontogenic cyst in the left maxillary sinus with the susceptibility artifact of a 22-gauge needle (*arrow*). The cross marks the entry point of the guidance system in the alveolar process

20.5 Biopsies of the Skull Base

MRI of the skull base is of great value in the preoperative planning of orofacial surgery. The preoperative work-up of lesions affecting the skull base frequently still requires open surgical biopsy. Access is often difficult, and an enoral transpharyngeal approach is often chosen to reach pathologies in the skull base.

Biopsy with the interactive MR guidance system now offers a valuable alternative to the open surgical approach. This technique allows visualization of the lesion in relation to the needle as well as to major vessels and nerves.

The following example illustrates the MR-guided biopsy of a lesion at the skull base of a 45-year-old man who had previously been operated upon for ameloblastoma. The lesion is characterized by increased signal on T2-weighted SE images (Fig. 20.6a). In order to differentiate recurrent tumor from granulation tissue, a biopsy using an enoral approach to the pharyngeal lesion was planned (Fig. 20.6b). The lesion was successfully targeted without complications following local anesthesia. The patient tolerated the procedure well. The presence of typical

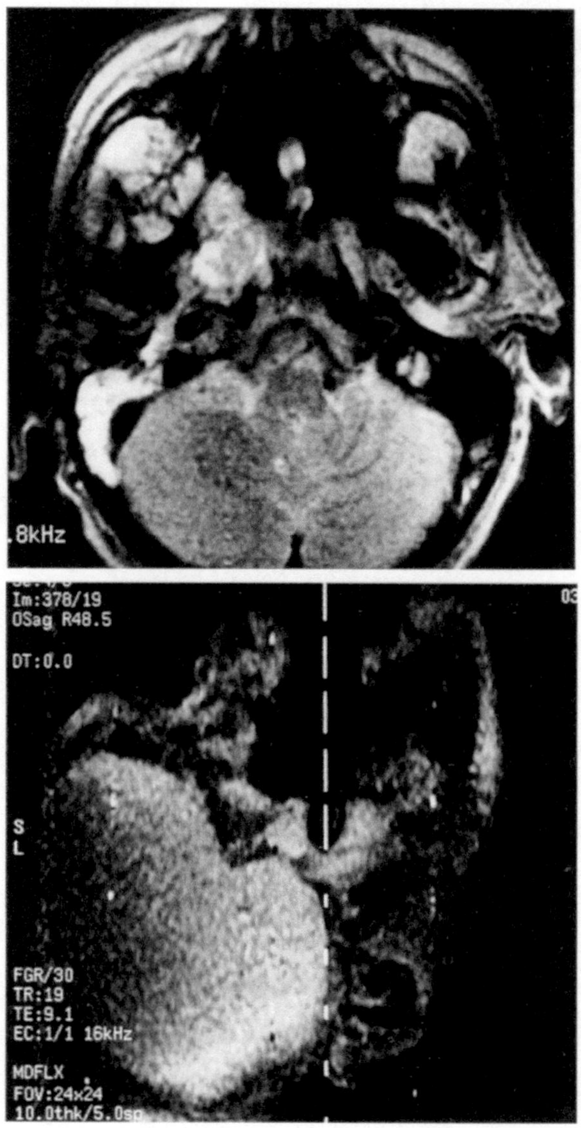

Fig. 20.6.a Ameloblastoma of the skull base: axial image demonstrating tumorous infiltration of the right skull base and extension to the carotid artery. **b** The following biopsy of the recurrent retropharyngeal ameloblastoma is demonstrated in axial view

basaloid cells consistent with ameloblastoma confirmed the diagnosis of recurrence. A more invasive and costly open surgical biopsy could thus be avoided.

20.6 Conclusions

Interactively MR-guided biopsies represent a welcome addition to the arsenal of diagnostic tools for the work-up of lesions in the head and neck region. Reflecting the unsurpassed soft tissue contrast inherent to the MR experiment, lesions are readily identified and can be delineated from vital structures including vessels and nerves. Interactive visualization of the instrument in relation to the lesion and surrounding structures permits safe targeting of lesions even in poorly accessible areas. The preliminary experience described in this chapter suggests that MR-guided biopsies obviate costly open surgical biopsy in many instances, particularly in the maxillary and skull base regions.

References

Bagley JS, Ewen SW, Smith FW, Krukowski ZH (1996) Magnetic resonance imaging of thyroid swellings. Br J Surg 83:828-829

Belkin BA, Papageorge MB, Fakitsas J, Bankoff MS (1988) A comparative study of magnetic resonance imaging versus computed tomography for the evaluation of maxillary and mandibular tumors. J Oral Maxillofac Surg 46:1039-1047

Boland GW, Lee MJ, Mueller PR, et al (1993) Efficacy of sonographically guided biopsy of thyroid masses and cervical lymph nodes. AJR Am J Roentgenol 161:1053-1056

Castelijns JA, van den Brekel MW (1993) Magnetic resonance imaging evaluation of extracranial head and neck tumors. Magn Reson Q 9:113-128

Duckwiler G, Lufkin RB, Teresi L, et al (1989) Head and neck lesions: MR-guided aspiration biopsy. Radiology 170:519-522

Freitas JE, Freitas AE (1994) Thyroid and parathyroid imaging. Semin Nucl Med 24:234-245

Giron J, Ouhayoun E, Dahan M, et al (1996) Imaging of hyperparathyroidism: US, CT, MRI and MIBI scintigraphy. Eur J Radiol 21:167-173

Han MH, Jabour B, Andrews J, et al (1991) MR-guided aspiration and drainage of a nasopharyngeal mucus retention cyst. Am J Neuroradiol 12:1185-1186

Hell B, Heissler E, Gazounis G, Menneking H, Bier J (1994) Microsurgical and prosthetic reconstruction of patient with recurrent ameloblastoma extending into the skull base. Int J Oral Maxillofac Surg 23:90-92

Hotzinger H, Barth HH, Ries G (1983) Recurrent ameloblastoma of the upper jaw — diagnosis. Morphol Med 3:89-96

Jackson IT, Callan PP, Forté RA (1996) An anatomical classification of maxillary ameloblastoma as an aid to surgical treatment. J Oral Maxillofac Surg 24:230-236

Jolesz F, Silverman SG (1995) Interventional magnetic resonance therapy. Semin Interventional Radiol 12:20-27

Kraus DH, Lanzieri CF, Wanmaker JR, et al (1992) Complementary use of computed tomography and magnetic resonance imaging in assessing skull base lesions. Laryngoscope 102:623-629

Lee VS, Spritzer CE, Coleman RE, et al (1996) The complementary roles of fast spin-echo MR imaging and double-phase 99m Tc-sestamibi scintigraphy for localization of hyperfunctioning parathyroid glands. AJR AM J Roentgenol 167:1555-1561

Lufkin RB, Teresi L, Hanafee W (1987) New needle for MR-guided aspiration cytology of the head and neck. AJR AM J Roentgenol 149:380-382

Lufkin RB, Teresi L, Chiu L, Hanafee W (1988a) A technique for MR-guided needle placement. AJR Am J Roentgenol 151:193-196

Lufkin RB, Duckwiler G, Spickler E, et al (1988b) MR body stereotaxis: an aid for MR-guided biopsies. J Comput Assist Tomogr 12:1088-1089

Lufkin RB, Robinson JD, Castro DJ, et al (1990) Interventional magnetic resonance imaging in the head and neck. Top Magn Reson Imaging 2:76-80

Lufkin RB, Davis WL, Osborn AG (1993) Overview of MR imaging modalities. J Comput Assist Tomogr Suppl 17:24-29

Moon Hee Nan, Kee Hyun Chang, In One Kim, et al (1993) Non-Hodgkin lymphoma of the central skull base: MR manifestations. J Comput Assist Tomogr 17:567-571

Mueller PR, Stark DD, Simeone JF, et al (1986) MR-guided aspiration biopsy: needle design and clinical trials. Radiology 161:605-609

Numerow LM, Morita ET, Clark OH, Higgins CB (1995) Persistent/recurrent hyperparathyroidism: a comparison of sestamibi scintigraphy, MRI and ultrasonography. JMRI 5:702-708

Schenck JF, Jolesz FA, Roemer PB, et al (1995) Superconducting open-configuration MR imaging system for image-guided therapy. Radiology 195:805-814

Silverman SG, Collick BD, Figueira MR, et al (1995) Interactive MR-guided biopsy in an open-configuration MR imaging system. Radiology 197:175-181

Vogl TJ, Dresel S, Juergens M, Assal J, Lissner J (1993) MR imaging with Gd-DTPA in lesions of the head and neck. J Otolaryngol 22:220-230

Vogl TJ, Mack MG, Juergens M, et al (1994a) Fat suppression in contrast-enhanced MRT of the skull base and of the head and neck area: its clinical value. RoFo Fortschr Geb Rontgenstr Neuen Bildgeb Verfahr 160:417-424

Vogl TJ, Mack MG, Juergens M, et al (1994b) MR diagnosis of head and neck tumors: comparison of contrast enhancement with triple-dose gadodiamide and standard-dose gadopentetate dimeglumine in the same patients. AJR Am J Roentgenol 163:425-432

Vogl TJ, Mack MG, Mueller P, et al (1995a) Recurrent nasopharyngeal tumors: preliminary clinical results with interventional MR imaging – controlled laser-induced thermotherapy. Radiology 196:725-733

Vogl TJ, Mack MG, Muller P, et al (1995b) MR-guided laser-induced thermotherapy in tumors of the head and neck region: initial clinical results. RoFo Fortschr Geb Rontgenstr Neuen Bildgeb Verfahr 163:505-514

von Schulthess GK, Weder W, Goebel N, et al (1988) 1.5 T MRI, CT, ultrasonography and scintigraphy in hyperparathyroidism. Eur J Radiol 8:157-164

Principles of MR-Guided Interstitial Therapy

21 Temperature-Sensitive MR Sequences

R. Botnar

CONTENTS

21.1 Introduction

Minimally invasive surgical interventions such as interstitial laser thermotherapy (LITT) or radio-frequency (RF) thermotherapy allow treatment of deep-seated tumors in the human body. Compared to conventional surgical interventions, these techniques may help to reduce health care costs and shorten patient recovery times. In order to guarantee safe treatment, temperature dissipation must be monitored in the target tissue. MR thermometry allows noninvasive monitoring of interventional thermal procedures inside the human body with high spatial and temporal resolution. Several temperature-dependent MR parameters such as the spin-lattice relaxation time T_1 (Parker et al. 1983; Jolesz et al. 1988; Cline et al. 1994), the molecular diffusion coefficient (LeBihan et al. 1989; Bleier et al. 1991), or the proton frequency shift (Hall et al. 1985; de Poorter et al. 1995; Ishihara et al. 1995) can be exploited for the purpose of temperature mapping.

Fast T_1-weighted sequences were used to monitor the local heating of various human tissues (Darkazanli 1993; Cline et al. 1994; Matsumoto et al. 1994). However, T_1 temperature dependency varies in different tissues and is influenced by thermoregulative processes and metabolic tissue changes.

Diffusion-weighted imaging is based on the thermal Brownian motion which can be described by the diffusion coefficient. The drawback of this method lies in the long scan time. If applied in vivo, it suffers from thermoregulative diffusion changes and from tissue motion.

Compared to the two aforementioned methods, the proton frequency shift technique has several advantages. It exploits the phase of the MR signal instead of the signal amplitude. (Hall et al. 1985; de Poorter et al. 1995; Ishihara et al. 1995). Temperature sensitivity is related to changes of the molecular screening constant. A disadvantage of this technique is the high sensitivity to frequency drifts due to system instabilities. These can, however, be reduced to a great extent by using suitable correct schemes.

In the following sections, the various sequences are discussed in greater detail. The last section describes the implementation of quantitative temperature mapping on an open-configuration 0.5-T MR scanner.

21.2 Temperature Effects in Tissue

21.2.1 Signal Intensity Change Due to T1-Effects

The signal intensity S of a spoiled gradient echo sequence (SPGR, FLASH) depends on several sequence parameters such as the echo time TE, the repetition time TR, the flip angle α and on the tissue and temperature dependent relaxation time T1.

$$S = M_0 * \frac{\sin\alpha\,(1 - E1)e^{-\frac{TE}{T2}}}{1 - E1\cos\alpha} \qquad [1]$$

$$E1 = e^{-\frac{TR}{T1}}$$

R. Botnar, PhD, MR Center, Institute of Diagnostic Radiology, Zurich University Hospital, Rämistrasse 100, 8091 Zurich, Switzerland

Signal intensity locally decreases if the temperature T of the imaged tissue increases $\Delta T = T - T_0$. This effect is based on temperature dependent alterations of the spin-lattice relaxation time T1 and the equilibrium magnetization M_0. T1 is linearly dependent on temperature changes ΔT whereby the slope m in Eq. 2 can be interpreted as temperature sensitivity of T1, which is tissue dependent (PARKER et al. 1983, DICKINSON et al. 1986, CLINE et al. 1994):

$$T1 = T1_0 + m\Delta T \quad [2]$$

$T1_0$ stands for the spin lattice relaxation time at the ambient temperature T_0. According to the Curie law temperature sensitivity of the equilibrium magnetization is proportional to the inverse of the ambient temperature $1/T_0$. Temperature dependence of the imaging sequence can be expressed by differentiation of Eq. 1 with respect to the temperature T (CLINE et al. 1994).

$$\frac{dS}{SdT} = -\frac{mTR\,E1\,(1 - \cos\alpha)}{(1 - E1)\,(1 - \cos\alpha\,E1)\,T1^2} - \frac{1}{T_0} \quad [3]$$

The first term describes the signal change due to temperature-dependent T1 variations, and the second describes the temperature dependency of the equilibrium magnetization. For bovine muscle, temperature sensitivity was determined as 1.0%±0.1% signal change per degree Celsius (TE/TR/α = 6.8 ms/13.9 ms/60°; CLINE et al. 1996).

If the T1-weighted method is used for temperature monitoring, it must be considered that the rate of signal change depends on the sequence parameters TE, TR, and α as well as on the tissue parameter T1. Therefore this technique is suited only for qualitative temperature visualization and not for quantitative temperature monitoring.

21.2.2 Signal Intensity Change Due to Diffusion

MR imaging is sensitive to the thermal Brownian motion described by the diffusion coefficient D(x,y). Temperature sensitivity is based on the exponential relationship between diffusion coefficient and the temperature T:

$$D \propto e^{-\frac{E_a}{kT}} \quad [4]$$

E_a describes the activation energy of the translation molecular motion, and k is Boltzmann's constant. E_a was determined by LeBihan as 0.18 eV (LEBIHAN et al. 1989). Differentiation of Eq. 4 with respect to temperature yields the relative change of the diffusion coefficient per degree Celsius (LEBIHAN et al. 1989).

$$\frac{dD}{DdT} = \frac{E_a}{kT^2} \quad [5]$$

Compared to T1-based signal changes, temperature sensitivity of the diffusion coefficient is high (2.4%/°C, E_a = 0.18 eV). From integration of Eq. 5 the non-linear relationship between temperature change and the diffusion coefficient can be derived:

$$T(x,y) = \frac{1}{\frac{1}{T_0} - \frac{k}{E_a}\ln\frac{D(x,y)}{D_0(x,y)}} \quad [6]$$

The diffusion coefficient D(x,y) can be derived if two diffusion-sensitive experiments have sequences with different b-factors (LEBIHAN et al. 1986):

$$D(x,y) = \ln\left(\frac{S_2(x,y)}{S_1(x,y)}\right) / (b_1 - b_2) \quad [7]$$

$$b = -\gamma^2 G^2 \delta^2 (\Delta - \frac{\delta}{3})$$

The b factor describes the exponential attenuation e^{-bD} of the transversal magnetization due to diffusion.

S_1 and S_2 are the signal intensities of the two experiments, G the strength, and δ the length of the flat portion of the diffusion gradients. Δ is the spacing between the leading edges of the two diffusion gradients. According to Eq. 6, temperature changes can be derived determining the diffusion coefficient D(x,y) at different temperatures. An advantage of diffusion-based temperature mapping is the relatively high temperature sensitivity. However, diffusion caused by thermoregulative microcirculation of the blood may affect the accuracy of this method. Further restrictions of real-time temperature mapping are the relatively long scan time compared to the T1-weighted or PFS-based techniques as well as the high sensitivity to motion. These factors limit the technique's application to a meaningful clinical environment.

21.2.3 Signal Phase Change Due to Proton Frequency Shift

The proton frequency shift (PFS) technique is known as an accurate method for quantitative two-dimensional temperature mapping. The resonance frequency of the spins is determined by the local magnetic field $\vec{B}_{loc}(\vec{r})$ at the proton (Yamada et al. 1990):

$$\vec{B}_{loc}(\vec{r}) \cong \vec{B}_{mac}(\vec{r}) - \left(\frac{2\chi(T(\vec{r}))}{3} + \sigma(T(\vec{r}))\right)\vec{B}_0 \qquad [8]$$

The macroscopic magnetic flux $\vec{B}_{mac}(\vec{r})$ is determined by the susceptibility distribution of the objects brought into a main magnetic field $\vec{B}_0$. Since the macroscopic magnetic flux does not take into account microscopic molecular screening effects of the proton, these have to be added as a correction term. This term contains the volume susceptibility χ of the object and the molecular screening constant σ of the water molecules. Higher order terms of χ and σ were neglected.

Temperature-induced frequency shifts of pure water are mainly related to changes of the molecular screening constant of water molecules. The molecular screening constant of water is influenced by hydrogen bonds that distort the electronic screening of the proton. Heating decreases the number of hydrogen bonds. As the temperature increases, electronic screening increases and therefore the local magnetic field decreases. The rate of change α of the molecular screening constant σ was determined for pure water at 0.1017 ppm/°C (Hindman 1966). The dependence of the phase shift $\Delta\Phi$ on molecular screening can be expressed according to Eq. 8 (Ishihara et al. 1992):

$$dB_{loc} \propto \Delta\Phi(\Delta T) = 2\,\pi\,\Delta f\,TE = 2\pi\gamma B_0\,\Delta\sigma T_E \qquad [9]$$

$$\Delta\sigma = \alpha\,\Delta\,T \qquad [10]$$

At 0.5 T, the frequency shift is 0.23 Hz/°C. ΔT stands for temperature change, T_E for echo time, and γ is the gyromagnetic ratio of ^1H. The linear relationship between temperature and the molecular screening constant $\sigma(T)$ is described by the temperature coefficient α.

α of muscle tissue was determined by several au thors (0.007–0.009 ppm/°C according to Kuroda et al. 1993; 0.0097 ppm/°C according to de Poorter 1995; 0.008 ppm/°C according to Cline et al. 1996). At 1.5 T, a temperature uncertainty of ± 2.4°C ($T_E/T_R/\alpha$ = 6.8 ms/13.9 ms/60°) has been reported by Cline et al. (1996). The frequency shift of fat is mainly influenced by the susceptibility change (0.01 ppm/°C according to Stollberger et al. 1996).

MR temperature calibration measurements in 1.5% agarose gel and muscle tissue carried out in an open configuration 0.5-T MR scanner correlated well with fiber-optical temperature measurements (Luxtron). For a receiver bandwidth (BW) of 3.9 kHz and an echo time of 19.3 ms, temperature uncertainty was determined at ± –1.8°C (Botnar et al. 1997). Figure 21.1 shows the calibration curves during a cooling process in 1.5% agarose gel. The temperature varied over a range of 20°C from 60° to 40°C. Low bandwidths and long echo times provided the greatest temperature accuracy (Fig. 21.2) but have the disadvantage of prolonged scan times.

21.3 Subtraction Technique

MR temperature mapping is a relative and not an absolute temperature quantification method. Temperatures measured with MRI are always derived relative to a reference temperature. The reference-temperature image usually is acquired before the thermal treatment. All three temperature-sensitive MR sequences described here are based on a subtraction technique. Quantitative temperature maps are calculated by subtracting the images acquired during the thermal procedure from the previously acquired reference image. The subtraction technique is illustrated in Fig. 21.3. A common way to visualize temperature changes is to overlay a color-coded temperature map on an anatomical MR image.

21.4 Artifacts

21.4.1 Breathing Artifacts

Temperature maps are generally generated by subtracting a reference image from a continuously updated actual image. In the abdomen and chest, the problem inherent to this technique, therefore, lies in its sensitivity to respiratory motion. The influence of this motion can be reduced by either acquiring the data in apnea or applying navigator scans to synchronize image acquisition to the respiratory cycle.

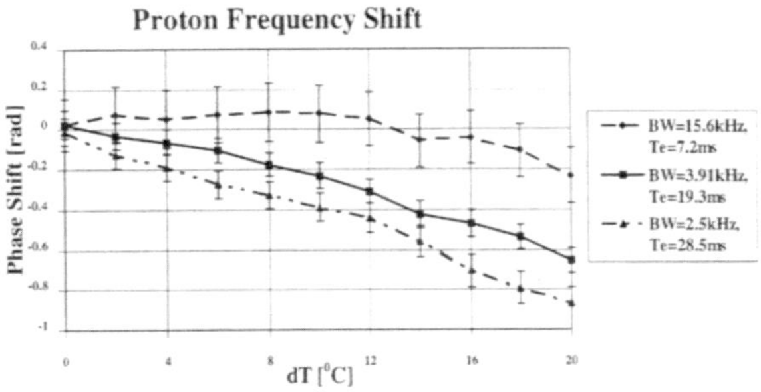

Fig. 21.1. Temperature-induced phase shift. Temperature sensitivity increases with prolonged echo times as predicted by equation 9 y-axis: phase shift in radians. x-axis: temperature change in degree Celsius

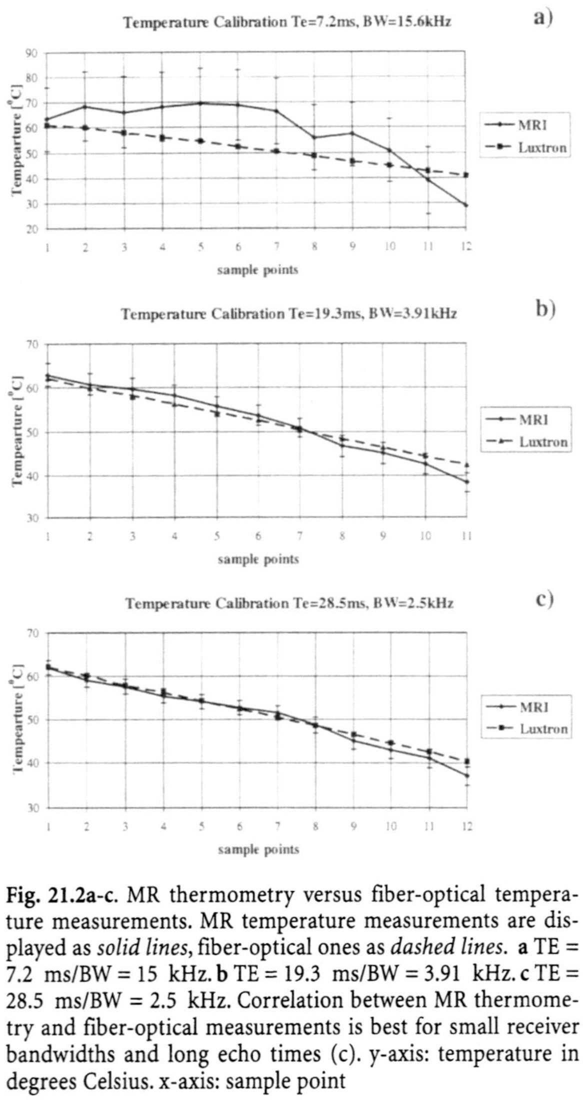

Fig. 21.2a-c. MR thermometry versus fiber-optical temperature measurements. MR temperature measurements are displayed as *solid lines*, fiber-optical ones as *dashed lines*. **a** TE = 7.2 ms/BW = 15 kHz. **b** TE = 19.3 ms/BW = 3.91 kHz. **c** TE = 28.5 ms/BW = 2.5 kHz. Correlation between MR thermometry and fiber-optical measurements is best for small receiver bandwidths and long echo times (c). y-axis: temperature in degrees Celsius. x-axis: sample point

21.4.2 Thermoregulative Blood Flow

T1 and diffusion-based temperature mapping have been reported to be difficult under in-vivo conditions because of signal changes caused by thermoregulative blood flow (Young et al. 1993).

Thermoregulative blood flow may also induce signal phase changes that affect the accuracy of PFS-based temperature maps. These changes are caused by susceptibility alterations arising from an altered oxygenation level of inflowing blood. During thermal treatment, local blood perfusion generally changes in the treated region. This may lead to an altered oxygen concentration in the treated tissue. Due to the changed susceptibility of blood, a phase shift is induced. Compared to the accuracy of this technique of 1°–2°C, the effect of thermoregulative blood flow appears to be quite negligible. Thus, experiments with a cuffed muscle (ischemic) revealed signal changes indicating an erroneous temperature decrease of 0.9°C when the cuff was inflated Young et al. 1996).

21.4.3 Aliasing Artifacts

Aliasing is a phenomenon known to affect phase-contrast blood flow measurements. Since the phase value corresponds to an angle, a phase value larger than π, e.g. a bright white pixel, is rotated by 2π, rendering the pixel black (aliasing). This effect may also appear if the PFS technique is applied to temperature mapping. Phase wraps can either be induced by the inhomogenity of the main magnetic field or by temperature changes causing a phase shift larger than π. Phase wraps caused by field inhomogenities, however, can be avoided if the phase difference image is calculated using complex images (Chung et al. 1996):

$$\Delta\Phi = \Phi_1 - \Phi_2 = \arctan\left\{\frac{Re2 * Im1 - Re1 * Im2}{Re1 * Re2 + Im1 * Im2}\right\} \quad [11]$$

Re and Im correspond to the real and the imaginary part of the complex MR image. The relationship between the anatomic image and its real and imaginary part is defined as follows:

$$\text{anatomic image} = \sqrt{Re^2 + Im^2} \quad [12]$$

21.5 "Real-Time" Temperature Monitoring

The availability of "open-configuration" MR magnets in conjunction with various tracking systems allows MR guidance of instruments as well as subsequent monitoring of thermal therapies in "real time".

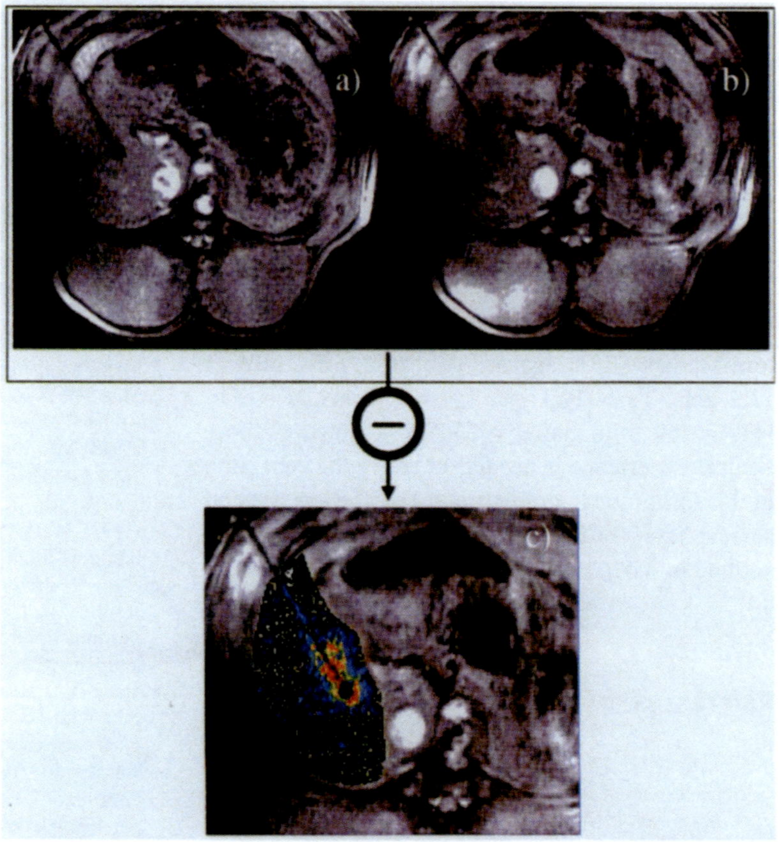

Fig. 21.3a-c. Subtraction scheme. **a** Magnitude image before thermal treatment (reference image). **b** Magnitude image during thermal treatment (actual image) **c** Anatomical background image overlayed with color-coded temperature map (difference image: a-b). Temperature increases from *blue* to *red*

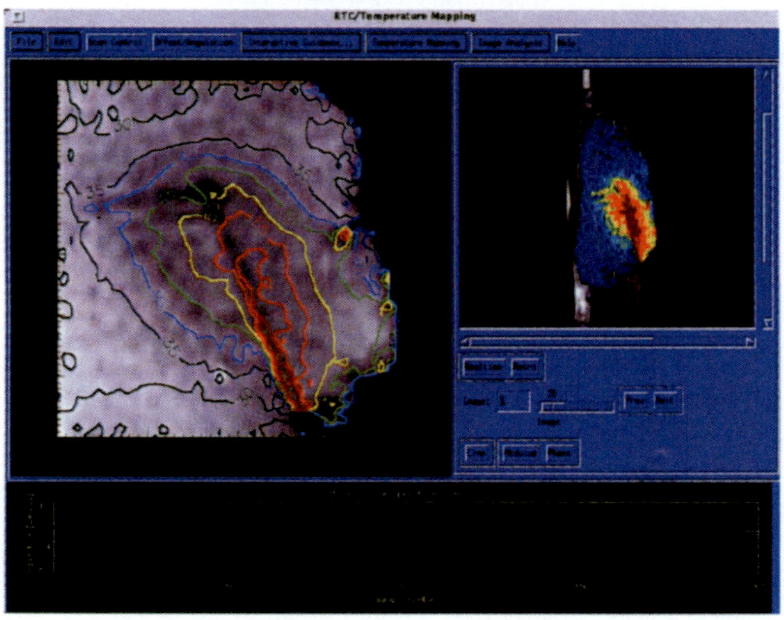

Fig. 21.4. "Real-time" temperature visualization and quantification tool. Temperature maps are usually updated every 1–5 s. Temperature can be visualized either as color-coded image or quantified using isotherms overlayed on an anatomical image

A software tool for "real-time" temperature quantification has been developed for a 0.5-T open-configuration MR scanner (Singa SP, GEMS, Milwaukee, Wis.) and implemented on a separate workstation (Sparc20, Sun Microsystems, Mountain View, CA) which controls the "real-time" communication with the MR scanner (Botnor et al. 1997). All procedures based on interactive image guidance, such as repositioning of the laser fiber can be easily handled. T1-weighted images as well as phase images can be managed accordingly. For temperature quantification and visualization, either color-coded images or anatomical images overlayed with isotherms can be displayed (Fig. 21.4). The isotherms help to estimate the size of the induced lesion and ensure that maximum temperature is kept below the critical temperature for carbonization of the tissue.

The software is compatible with optical image guidance tools (Flashpoint) integrated into the Signa SP open-configuration MR scanner. This provides direct access to the actual images acquired at the laser fiber tip, typically leading to an image update rate of 0.2-1.0 Hz. A new temperature map is acquired and displayed every 1–5 s. Preliminary experience suggests temporal resolution to be sufficient for most laser ablation applications.

Temperature accuracy was determined in phantom studies (1.5% agarose gel) at ± 1.8°C (BW = -3.9 kHz, T_E = 19.3 ms, T_R = 39.6 ms, α = 45°, FOV = 280 mm, matrix = 256*128). However, more clinical experience is needed to verify the reliability of this technique in predicting correct lesion size and correct temperature when thermal procedures are applied in vivo.

References

Bleier AR, Jolesz FA, Cohen MS, et al (1991) Real-time magnetic resonance imaging of laser heat deposition in tissue. Magn Reson Med 21:132-137

Botnar R, Steiner P, Erhart P, Debatin JF, von Schulthess GK (1997) Absolute temperature quantification in near real-time with an open 0.5 Tesla interventional MR-scanner. In: Proceedings of the International Society of Magnetic Resonance in Medicine 1997. Society of Magnetic Resonance in Medicine, Berkeley, Calif.

Chung AH, Hynynen K, Colucci V, Oshio K, Cline HE, Jolesz FA (1996) Optimization of spoiled gradient-echo phase imaging for in vivo localization of a focused ultrasound beam. Magn Reson Med 36:745-752

Cline HE, Hynynen K, Hardy CJ, Watkins RD, Schenck JF, Jolesz FA (1994) MR temperature mapping of focused ultrasound surgery. Magn Reson Med 31:628-636

Cline HE, Hynynen K, Schneider E, Hardy CJ, Maier SE, Watkins RD, Jolesz FA (1996) Simultaneous magnetic resonance phase and magnitude temperature maps in muscle. Magn Reson Med 35:309-315

Darkazanli A, Hynynen K, Unger B, Schenk JF (1993) On-line monitoring of ultrasonic surgery with MR imaging. J Magn Reson Imaging 3:509-514

de Poorter J, de Wagter C, de Deene Y, Thomsen C, Ståhlberg F, Achten E (1995) Noninvasive MRI thermotherapy with the proton resonance frequency (PRF) method: in vivo results in human tissue. Magn Reson Med 33:74–81

Dickinson RJ, Hall AS, Hind AJ, Young IR (1986) Measurement of changes in tissue temperature using MR imaging. J Comput Assit Tomogr 10:468-472

Hall LD, Talagala SL (1985) Mapping of pH and temperature distribution using chemical shift resolved tomography. J Magn Reson 65:501-505

Hindman JC (1966) Proton resonance shift of water in the gas and liquid states. J Chem Phys 44:4582-4592

Ishihara Y, Calderon A, Watanabe H, Mori K, Okamoto K, Suzuki Y, Sato K (1992) A precise and fast temperature mapping using water proton chemical shift. In: Works in progress of the International Society of Magnetic Resonance in Medicine 1992. Society of Magnetic Resonance in Medicine, Berkeley, Calif.

Ishihara Y, Calderon A, Watanabe H, Okamoto K, Suzuki Y, Kuroda K, Suzuki Y (1995) A precise and fast temperature mapping using water proton chemical shift. Magn Reson Med 34:814-823

Jolesz FA, Bleire AR, Jakob P, Ruenzel PW, Huttl K, Jako GJ (1988) MR imaging of laser-tissue interactions. Radiology 168:249-253

Kuroda K, Abe K, Tsutsumi S, Ishihara Y, Suzuki Y, Sato K (1993) Water proton magnetic resonance spectroscopic imaging. Biomed Thermol 13:43-62

LeBihan D, Breton E, Lallemand D, Grenier P, Cabanis EA, Jeantet ML (1986) MR imaging of intravoxel incoherent motions application to diffusion and perfusion in neurologic disorders. Radiology 161:401-407

LeBihan D, Delannoy J, Lewin RL (1989) Temperature mapping with MR imaging of molecular diffusion: application to hyperthermia. Radiology 171:853-857

Matsumoto R, Mulkern RV, Hushek SG, Jolesz FA (1994) Tissue temperature monitoring for thermal interventional therapy: comparison of T1-weighted MR sequences. J Magn Reson Imaging 4:65-70

Parker DL, Smith V, Sheldon P, Crooks LE, Fussel L (1983) Temperature distribution measurements in two-dimensional NMR imaging. Med Phys 10:321-325

Silverman SG, Collick BD, Figueira MR, et al (1995) Interactive MR-guided biopsy in an open-configuration MR imaging system. Radiology 197(1):175-181

Stollberger R, Renhart W, Huber D, Glanzer H, Rehak P, Ebner F (1996) Möglichkeiten und Grenzen des MR-Temperaturimaging mittels Protonenresonanzverfahren. In: Boenick U (ed) Biomedizinische Technik, vol 41. Schiele und Schön, Berlin, pp 132-133 (Suppl 1)

Yamada N, Imakita S, Sakuma T, et al (1990) Evaluation of the susceptibility effect on the phase images of a simple gradient echo. Radiology 175:561-565

Young IR, Hand JF, Coutts GA, Oatridge A, Prior M (1993) Problems arising from perfusion changes affecting temperature calibrations derived from T1 and diffusion weighted MRI. In: Proceedings of the International Society of Magnetic Resonance in Medicine 1993. Society of Magnetic Resonance in Medicine, Berkeley, Calif.

Young IR, Hajnal JV, Oatridge A, Roberts I, Wilson JA, Saeed N, Bydder GM (1996) Demonstration of in-vivo susceptibility variations developing phase changes that mimic those due to temperature measured by the chemical shift method. In: Proceedings of the International Society of Magnetic Resonance in Medicine 1996. Society of Magnetic Resonance in Medicine, Berkeley, Calif.

22 MR-Guided Laser Therapy

P. STEINER

CONTENTS

22.1 Introduction

Laser-induced thermotherapy (LITT), which was first described by BOWN in 1983, destroys tissues with near-infrared, continuous-wave laser energy which is directed into a tissue volume through one or more interstitially implanted optical fibres. So far, LITT has been used to treat unresectable, localised human tumours in the brain (JOLESZ 1995), head and neck (OHYAMA et al. 1988), liver and breast (AMIN et al. 1993; HARRIES et al. 1994). The central problem of interstitial laser treatments is the inability to predict size and geometry of the thermal lesions due to inherent tissue heterogeneities enhanced by the variability of blood flow and tissue perfusion. Effective and reliable LITT does, however, mandate a means to assure laser coverage of the entire lesion without damage to healthy surrounding tissues. This requires on-line monitoring of laser-induced energy distribution during application. Ultrasound has shown some promise in this regard. Experiments in the liver and pancreas found it to be sensitive to acute tissue modifications induced by boiling tissue water and diffusion of microbubbles in tissue structure (DACHMAN et al. 1990). Mere tissue heating, however, could not be visualised.

The use of magnetic resonance (MR) imaging in the diagnosis of different diseases has steadily increased over the past decade. In addition to its unsurpassed soft tissue contrast, the MR experiment has been shown to be sensitive to changes in tissue temperature (NELSON and TUNG 1987). In fact, there are three tissue properties measurable with MR that cause a reduction in signal intensity when tissue temperature increases: proton diffusivity (DELANNOY et al. 1991), proton resonance frequency shifts (DE POORTER et al. 1995) and the longitudinal nuclear-spin relaxation time T1 (MATSUMOTO et al. 1992).

In this chapter, we will familiarise the reader with some of the fundamentals of biomedical laser applications. Various techniques of MR-guided tissue targeting will be covered in greater detail. Subsequently, the chapter will focus on ex-vivo and in-vivo laser investigations performed in the 'interventional MR laboratory' at the Zurich University Hospital using an open-access interventional midfield MR unit. Finally, established and emerging clinical applications of MR-guided laser treatment will be described. A thorough discussion of the status of MR-guided LITT within the therapeutic algorithms is contained in subsequent chapters of this book.

22.2 Effects of Laser Radiation on Biological Tissue

Energy release from laser applicators into substances such as haemoglobin, melanin pigments and water leads to molecular vibrations that cause a local temperature rise. Sufficient continued energy release and absorption can result in a local temperature rise sufficient to induce protein denaturation (41°–65°C), water evaporation and boiling (up to 300°C),

P. STEINER, MD, MR Center, Institute of Diagnostic Radiology, Zurich University Hospital, Rämistrasse 100, 8091 Zurich, Switzerland thermolysis of proteins, and even the generation of gaseous decomposition products and of carbonaceous residue or char (>300°C). The clinical effect of this chain of thermal events is tissue ablation.

Currently, there are four lasers in large-scale, routine clinical biomedical use. They are employed to ablate, dissect and coagulate soft tissues. Two of the lasers, the carbon dioxide (CO_2) and argon ion (Arion) types, are gas-filled. The other two employ solid-state lasing media. One is the neodymium-yttrium-aluminium-garnet (Nd:YAG) laser, which operates at 1064 nm. Most of the LITT experience available is based on this solid-state laser. The other is the gallium-aluminium arsenide (GaAIAs) semiconductor diode laser. Smaller-scale uses have been described for some other biomedical lasers currently being tested for various biomedical applications. One of these is the holmium:YAG (Ho:YAG) laser, which emits pulses of 2.1 μm wavelength and is used in soft tissue ablation in joint surgery and laser discectomy (Quigley et al. 1994).

22.3 Implementation of Laser Treatment in the MR Environment

In comparison to CT- or ultrasound-guided laser therapy, the implementation of a laser in the MR environment is a far more demanding task. In the following paragraphs, the major aspects affecting implementation, including the advantages of different 'open-configuration' MR scanner designs, will be discussed.

22.3.1 General Considerations

In order to avoid damage to the laser machine induced by the magnetic field as well as corruption of the MR signal by the presence of a large, electrically powered object in the MR room, the laser machine is best positioned outside the MR suite. The laser fibre has to be directed from the laser source to the MR scanner. To avoid damage to the fibre, one might consider constructing an underground delivery channel through which a permanent laser fibre is fed. In our laboratory, a 12-m long fibre is guided through the ground and bridges the distance between the generator and a special connector installed directly next to the MR scanner. The connector allows the fitting of different fibres. Due to the special design of the extension fibre and the connector box, the power loss between generator and applicator amounts to merely 10% (Coherent, Palo Alto, Calif./personal communication). The availability of the connector box allows the individualised use of different conventional end-use fibres without having to change the long underground extension cable.

To date, most attempts to monitor MR signal changes during LITT have exploited the high signal-to-noise ratio inherent to high-field (1.5 T and more) magnets (Jolesz et al. 1988; Pignoli et al. 1995). In these magnet systems, however, patient access has been limited. Simultaneous instrument manipulation and MR imaging are not possible. This limitation has motivated the design and manufacturing of 'open-configuration' magnets.

22.3.2 Open Magnet Design

Over recent years, various 'open configuration' magnet designs enabling better access of the patient during MR examination have become commercially available. Most of these systems, however, were not primarily designed for MR-guided interventions, but instead for increased patient comfort. Since the number and severity of technical challenges, as well as the cost associated with the construction of such 'open-configuration' systems, appear directly related to field strength, most 'open' systems operate at less than 0.5 T. Reductions in field strength, however, significantly decrease the achievable signal-to-noise ratio (SNR), thereby limiting the speed of image updates, as well as the quality of the MR images themselves.

As is the case for most other interventions, safe and effective monitoring and guidance of laser ablation also requires rapid and robust updates of high-quality images. The utility of any 'interventional' magnet design is thus determined by two conflicting desires: maximal access with maximal SNR. One scanner characterised by a balanced approach to these conflicting requirements has been introduced by General Electric Medical Systems. Direct patient access in the form of a 'double doughnut' is combined with 0.5-T (mid-field) field strength (Signa SP, GE Medical Systems, Milwaukee, Wis.); Schenck et al. 1995). The scanner design is based on a cryogen-free, super-conducting magnet. This MR system has been especially engineered to integrate diagnostic imaging, tumour localisation with stereotactic targeting (Silverman et al. 1995), and monitoring of tumour thermotherapy. It has been available at our laboratory since September 1995.

22.3.3 Application of Laser Fibres

A major issue affecting the outcome of MR-guided laser therapy is the correct and safe application of laser fibres. For LITT, fibres are usually introduced percutaneously. Depending on the type of laser fibre used fibre placement may vary. Some investigators have successfully gained experience with a combination of specially produced laser fibres with light applicators at the tip (Vogl et al. 1995a). For LITT these are positioned within a Teflon catheter to prevent the fibre from breaking within the treated issue during or after therapy (Vogl et al. 1995b). Other groups use so-called bare fibres consisting only of plastic-clad fiber-optic light guides, easily fitting through standard 18-gauge needles (Harries et al. 1994).

If imaging is performed in a conventionally designed closed magnet, lesion targeting and placement of the fibre cannot take place inside the magnet. Approaches vary from CT- to ultrasound-guided applications of the laser fibre and subsequent transfer of the patient into the MR scanner (Harries et al. 1994; Mumtaz et al. 1996). In some instances, lesion targeting is performed in the MR suite with the patient table outside the magnet. None of these applications are truly 'MR-guided', however. Instead of active guidance, MR imaging is merely employed to document the position of the fibres. Repositioning of the applicator requires the patient to be moved in and out of the scanner. This task is often complicated by motion of the patient in between applicator manipulations. For an efficient approach, it would be desirable if lesion detection and characterisation, targeting, and monitoring of laser therapy could be achieved without having to transport the patient.

22.3.3.1 Interactive-Stereotactic and Active Laser Fibre Positioning

There are two fundamentally new methods for positioning of minimally invasive therapy applicators such as laser fibres: the interactive, frameless stereotactic approach using an external reference system (Silverman et al. 1995) and an active approach (Dumoulin et al. 1993), where the position of the instrument is defined by an incorporated miniature radio-frequency (RF) coil. Both are an integrated part of the interventional MR setup of the 0.5-T superconducting MR unit (Signa SP, General Electric, Milwaukee, Wis.).

The interactive, frameless stereotactic technique is based on the positional definition of a handheld probe by computer calculation. A needle can be connected to this probe. Three infrared cameras integrated into the roof of the interventional MR unit received infrared signals from two diodes affixed to the back of the handheld probe. The position of the two diodes determines the positional coordinates of the probe in real time (10 updates per second). Based on the availability of these coordinates, the position of any needle of predefined length can be calculated. MR images in different planes can be obtained on the basis of this positional information (Chap. 19). The MR images are continuously updated with a maximum speed of one image every 2 s. Furthermore, the MR plane can interactively be changed during the procedure, as in ultrasound, without the handheld probe having to be moved. The plane of the reference images can be chosen relative to the course of the needle or the position of the patient. Once the needle artefact is seen to lie within the targeted region, the correct position can be verified by obtaining images orthogonal to the projected course of the needle, traversing its tip. When correct placement has been confirmed, the positional information is stored and subsequently used to acquire images for monitoring of treatment effects.

Device visualisation as well as determination of the appropriate imaging section can also be accomplished with an electrically active technique referred to as MR tracking (Dumoulin et al. 1993). Device localisation is made possible by incorporating a miniature RF receive-only coil into the instrument. The coil receives signal only from its immediate vicinity. Following non-selective RF excitation, the three-dimensional position of the coil is frequency encoded. The coil position can be rapidly updated for real-time tracking and is displayed as a graphic overlay on any previously acquired 'roadmap' MR image (Leung et al. 1995). By transforming the coil's position onto a second reference plane, biplanar MR tracking in real time is possible. Moreover, based upon the constant availability of the three-dimensional coordinates of the coil and thus of the instrument itself, an imaging mode can be chosen whereby the collected images always transect the tip of the instrument, hence tracking the motion of the instrument. Once the instrument has reached the desired position, the positional information of the instrument tip can be employed for visualising laser heat effects.

For real-time interactive lesion targeting and subsequent monitoring of laser effects, it is desirable for the interventionalist to have visual control of the procedure. To this purpose, specially designed monitors can be integrated into the MR unit. The images available at the workstations outside the MR room are simultaneously projected onto these screens. In our laboratory, the radiologist performing the procedure inside the magnet is, furthermore, connected to the team at the consoles outside via headphones (Steiner et al. 1996a).

22.3.4 Safety Aspects and Patient Monitoring

During lesion targeting and laser application, it is mandatory to observe the patient closely. Open-configuration magnets facilitate this task. The interventionalist has direct contact to the patient. Furthermore, some sort of objective patient monitoring should be performed. MR-compatible patient monitoring systems are available and deliver continuous updates of patient vital signs during the investigation, including heart rate, blood pressure, oxygen saturation etc.

22.4 Visualisation of Laser Effects

The MR experiment is temperature sensitive. Changes in temperature translate into altered signal intensities. For monitoring and guidance of LITT, it is desirable to map temperature distribution as close to real time as possible in the affected tissue volume. The light dose can be adjusted to assure total destruction of the lesion, whilst at the same time preventing damage to surrounding normal tissues. In the following sections, the MR sequences most relevant for temperature mapping will be discussed in the context of extensive ex-vivo and in-vivo experiences.

22.4.1 T1-Weighted MR Imaging

The longitudinal nuclear spin relaxation time, T1, is sensitive to changes in temperature. Recent hardware and software advances have enabled the fast and ultrafast acquisition of temperature-sensitive T1-weighted sequences (Matsumoto et al. 1994). Attempts to monitor laser effects with T1-weighted MR sequences were primarily triggered by the fact that these sequences were readily available on routine MR scanners (Jolesz et al. 1988), including most 'open-configuration' scanners. Studies assessing the temperature sensitivity of different T1-weighted sequences at 1.5 T performed in vitro (gel phantoms) as well as ex vivo (liver and muscle tissue) revealed an almost linear SI decrease of 0.5%–1.1% per degree Celsius (Matsumoto et al. 1992, 1994). The quantitative relationship between absolute temperature and SI change, however, was found to be dependent on the tissue treated as well as on the type of T1-weighted sequence used. Sequences considered ranged from fast-spin-echo to gradient-echo type sequences. In addition, the temperature sensitivity of each sequence type is dependent on the magnetic field strength, echo time (TE), repetition time (TR) and flip angle, to mention just a few parameters. This explains variations in the reported experience regarding accuracy and feasibility of temperature mapping with T1-weighted sequences.

22.4.1.1 Ex-Vivo Studies

Experiments were performed on the open-configuration 0.5-T scanner. To assure adequate temporal resolution, the two fastest GRE sequences available (TR/TE 18/10 ms, 40° flip, 12.6 kHz bandwidth, 18×18 cm field of view, 256×128 matrix, one signal average) were evaluated with regard to temperature sensitivity and measurement accuracy. Both sequences enabled an image update every 2 s. One sequence was spoiled, destroying residual transverse magnetisation after each RF excitation (spoiled GRE: FSPGR), while the other was not (FGRE).

Experiments were performed on a wooden phantom filled with minced pig liver, as well as in explanted pig liver. During the experiments, the actual temperatures were measured using a fluorooptic four-sensor-array probe (Luxtron, Santa Clara, Calif.). The probes were positioned in defined distances from the laser fibre (Fig. 22.1). Following warming of the liver tissue to room temperature (20° C), LITT was applied at 5 W. As shown in Fig. 22.2, significant SI changes were observed as early as 15 s after initiation of laser treatment. The percentage SI loss was significantly higher for the non-

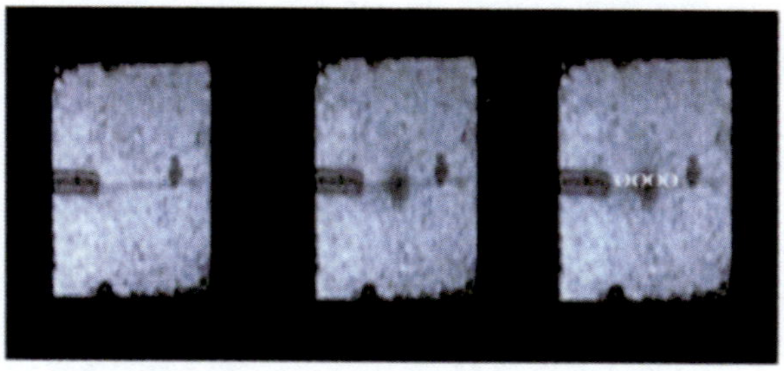

Fig. 22.1a-c. Laser-induced signal intensity change in minced porcine liver tissue (FGRE sequence). a,b Images demonstrate SI decrease around laser tip, which itself is not visible. c Circles representing regions of interest placed according to the positions of the four thermosensors

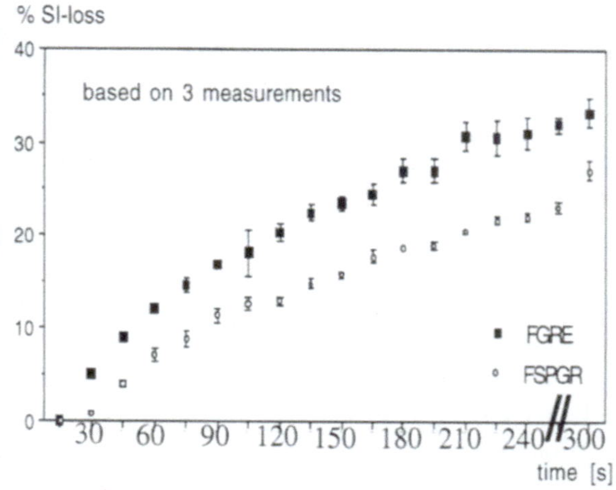

Fig. 22.2. Percent SI loss (± standard deviation) versus time of laser irradiation for the FGRE and FSPGR sequences

spoiled FGRE sequence. Comparison of fluoroptically measured temperature and SI change revealed good correlation for both sequences with the steeper slope (1.4 versus 1.0) again favouring the FGRE (Fig. 22.3).

Correlation between lesion size seen on MR images and macroscopic coagulation necrosis was good for both sequences (Fig. 22.4). Lesion size was slightly underestimated in the majority of cases. This observation confirmed previous results, documenting the value of non-spoiled T1-weighted GRE sequences for ex-vivo temperature mapping at 1.5 T (Cline et al. 1994). A possible explanation for the higher sensitivity of the non-spoiled GRE sequence in ex vivo experiments might be that the non-spoiled T2* effect synergistically contributes to the temperature-induced SI change. This emphasises the pitfalls associated with any direct transfer of SI changes seen on T1 images into absolute temperature determination. Studies attempting to correlate SI measurements with absolute temperatures in liver tissue revealed a 95% confidence interval of up to ±11°C (Pignoli et al. 1995). These errors associated with temperature measurements derived from T1-weighted MR imaging limit its potential use in mapping thermal distribution in clinical applications.

In order to further enhance the accuracy of imaging as well as the visual contrast between SI change and surrounding tissue, a colour-coded technique can be implemented. The continuously updated images obtained during laser therapy are subtracted from a baseline image obtained prior to laser application. The difference in SI between images is colour coded according to predefined colour scales (Steiner et al. 1996b). This bright signal is continuously updated and superimposed on the T1-weighted images. To further enable detection of tissue changes such as oedematous swelling, the con-

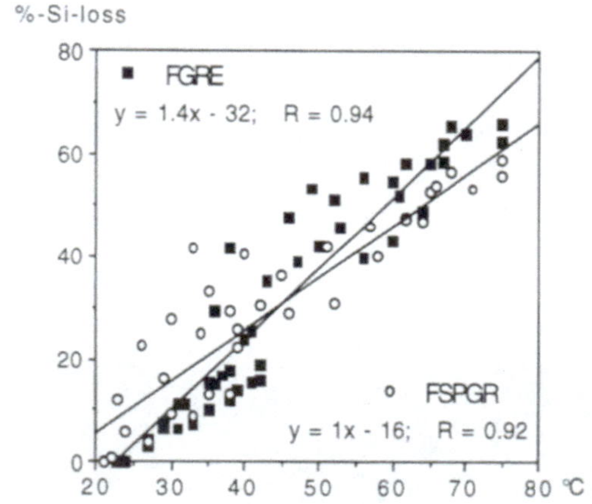

Fig. 22.3. Correlation between percent SI loss obtained by FGRE and FSPGR images and fluoroptically measured temperature

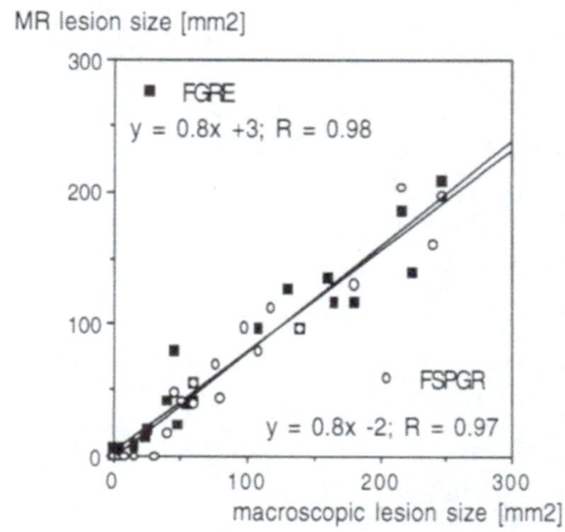

Fig. 22.4. Lesion size detected on MR imaging versus macroscopically verified lesion size. Data were obtained by FGRE and FSPGR sequences

tinuously updated T1-weighted source image is also displayed on the monitor of the workstation. In addition, the subtraction technique allows individualised definition of window level and width for displaying colours. Thus, temperature sensitivity can be restricted to the relevant change.

At our institution, the technique of transforming SI decrease into positive colour signals was also evaluated for percutaneous laser disc decompression, which is believed to be a useful treatment for herniated disc disease (Choy et al. 1992). Generally, Nd:YAG wavelengths are used to vaporise a small portion of the nucleus pulposus, thereby decompressing the disc. Tissue ablation is achievable within minutes. Application of laser energy is usually monitored endoscopically. This form of monitoring is limited to the visible surface. Thus, deep tissue penetration of laser energy cannot be assessed. In order to widen the application of percutaneous laser disc decompression, effective MR monitoring of laser effects is highly desirable. For an ex-vivo study, lumbar vertebral discs and vertebral bodies of cadavers were harvested. Using the stereotactic frameless MR-guiding system described above, a 16-French trocar was advanced from an anterior approach to the nucleus and then replaced by a bare-firing laser fibre. In all specimens, temperature distribution during lasing was visualised by a growing extension of the colour focus (Fig. 22.5). Following termination of lasing, the colour spread decreased in size. There was no direct correlation between laser energy deposition and tissue change based on either MR images or morphological tissue analysis. There was, however, good correlation of maximal size of MR signal changes and macroscopic extension of brittly altered, slightly discoloured tissue (Fig. 22.5). As a consequence of the high temperature sensitivity of the subtraction technique, monitored temperature spread surpassed macroscopically detectable lesions in the ex-vivo experiments. MR imaging, as we have shown, can depict temperature changes in a cross section through the whole intervertebral disc, thus minimising the risk of undetected energy deposition during percutaneous laser disc decompression. A study investigating the feasibility of MR-guided percutaneous laser disc decompression in humans is in progress at our institution.

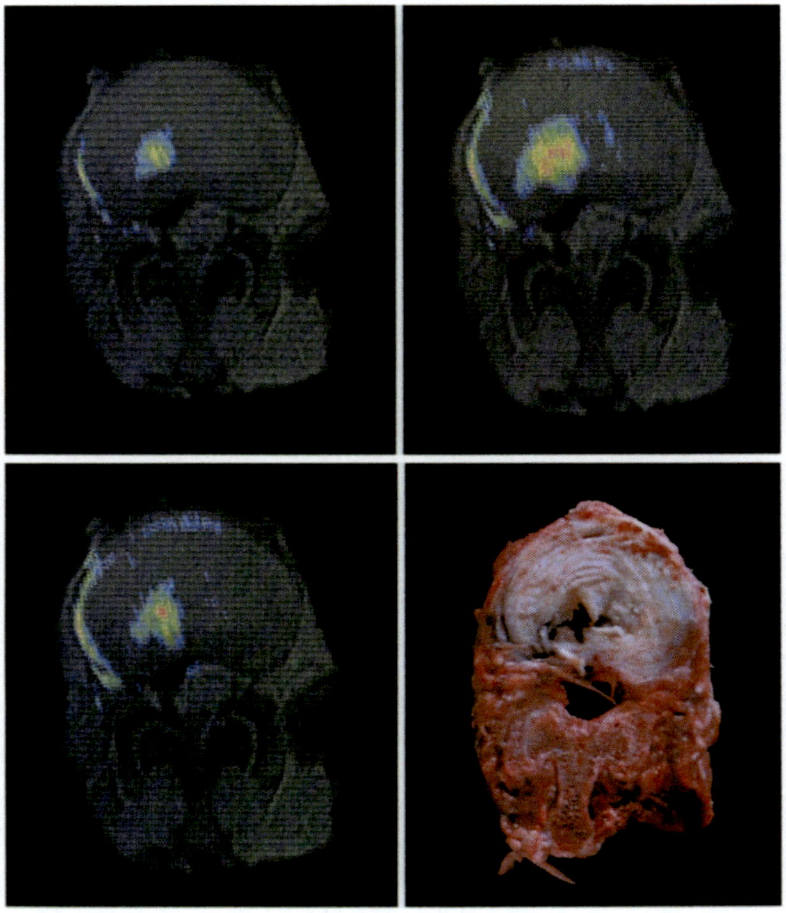

Fig. 22.5a-d. Real-time images and gross inspection of one laser-induced lesion in the ex-vivo assessment. This specimen was lased at a power setting of 25 W **a** Real-time MR image obtained 30 s after initiation of lasing shows main energy deposition in-plane to the track of the laser fibre. **b** Real-time MR image obtained 2 min after initiation and immediately before termination of lasing shows maximal extension of the main energy deposition. A small part of the energy found its way through the anulus and spread anteriorly along the disc. **c** Real-time MR image obtained 10 min after termination of lasing shows persisting colour changes. **d** Gross inspection of the specimen shows good correlation of brittly altered, slightly discoloured tissue and maximal extension on MR image. Charred tissue at gross inspection corresponds to persisting colour changes

22.4.1.2
In-Vivo Studies

In-vivo experience with T1-weighted temperature mapping for guidance of laser therapy has been gathered both in animal experiments and in patient studies. Analysis of the results reveals a strong dependence of the technique's success on the signal intensity of the underlying tissue under consideration. For tissues with an inherently high SI on T1-weighted images, such as liver tissue, a good correlation between the region of SI change and macroscopic coagulation necrosis was observed (Fig. 22.6). In tissues with lower SI, such as muscle or intervertebral discs, results were less promising. Here, adoption of the colour-coded subtraction technique resulted in some amelioration. Due to the physiologic changes occurring during heat application, especially in the periphery of the lesion (hyperaemia and others), SI change is not sufficiently predictable (Fried et al. 1996). This effect hampers the accuracy of temperature predictability on the basis of pure SI change on T1-weighted images. Based on data obtained from various animal studies, it is nowadays accepted that SI change can only be used to predict lesion size to a certain extent. Hope of also being able to quantify the local heat distribution has evaporated.

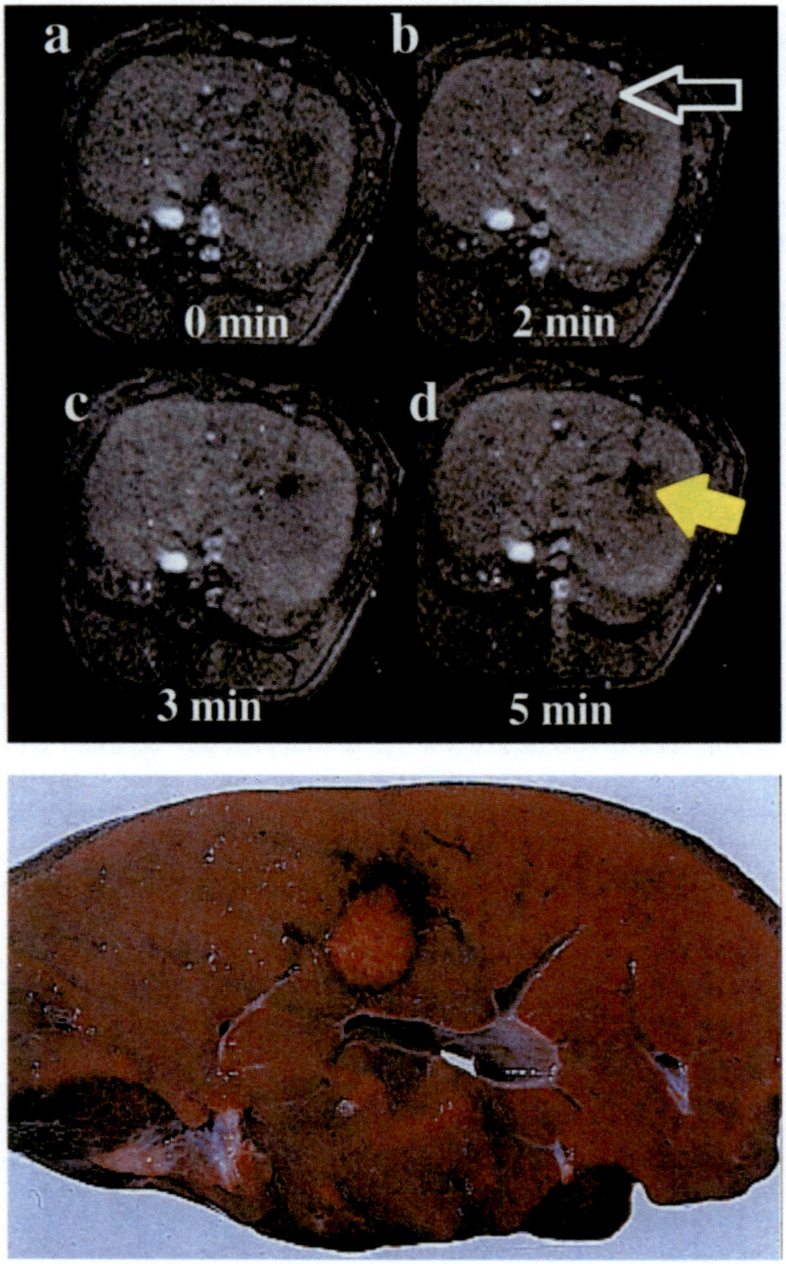

Fig. 22.6a-d. Laser-induced ablation in an in vivo porcine liver. **a-d** Images reveal SI decrease in left liver lobe during laser irradiation ranging from 0 to 5 min. Lesion (*arrow*) corresponds to macroscopic tissue change shown in **e**. *Open arrow* indicates laser fibre

In view of these limitations inherent to temperature mapping with T1-weighted imaging, it is interesting that for most clinical studies in which MR imaging were performed to monitor laser therapy, fast T1-weighted images were adopted (VOGL et al. 1995a,b; KAHN et al. 1996). In these studies, the laser-induced SI decrease correlated well with the size of coagulation necrosis. The colour-coded technique described previously was successfully adopted for guiding laser-induced brain tumour ablations (KAHN et al. 1996).

22.4.2 Proton-Frequency-Shift MR Imaging

As described in detail in Chap. 21, the proton frequency shift (PFS) is a temperature-dependent MR parameter influenced by the phase shift of proton frequency. Although the phase shift per degree Celsius is very small (0.64 Hz/°C for 1.5 T according to CHUNG et al. 1996; 0.23 Hz/°C for 0.5 T according to KURODA et al. 1993), it is theoretically favoured over T1 measurements because of its direct relationship to absolute temperature. Furthermore, PFS data can be obtained from GRE sequences, thus enabling image updates with time resolutions sufficient to monitor laser effects. The feasibility and accuracy of PFS have been evaluated both ex vivo (CLINE et al. 1996) and in vivo (CHUNG et al. 1996; DE POORTER et al. 1995), mostly in relation to the use of focused ultrasound. So far, no experience has been published concerning its value in monitoring laser irradiation in patients.

Experiments at 1.5 T have shown that the temperature accuracy of PFS based on GRE images acquired every 2 s is high. Temperature maps with 1-mm spatial resolution provide a 2°C temperature sensitivity in ex-vivo bovine muscle (CLINE et al. 1996). Similar results were achieved in vivo (skeletal muscle and kidney cortex). For best results, TE was optimised to correspond to the specific T2* value of the tissue under consideration, and the flip angle was chosen close to the Ernst angle (CHUNG et al. 1996). Together with the technique's sensitivity to motion artefacts, these requirements render the PFS approach difficult to implement.

In our laboratory, the PFS technique has been successfully implemented in the open 0.5-T environment (BOTNAR et al. 1997). The phase changes observed can be colour coded and displayed on simultaneously updated amplitude images (Fig. 22.7). For monitoring the progress of heat distribution during laser application, isotherms can also be displayed (Botnar, unpublished data).

22.4.3 Diffusion-Weighted MR Imaging

Diffusion-weighted MR imaging constitutes the third technique sensitive to thermal changes. Compared to T1-weighted temperature mapping, temperature sensitivity of the diffusion coefficient is high (2.4%/°C). However, besides other drawbacks, diffusion imaging requires relatively long scan times and is therefore highly sensitive to motion. These limitations make diffusion-weighted images unsuitable for rapid monitoring of heat distribution.

22.5 Requirements for 'Real-Time' Temperature Monitoring

MR imaging has been used to visualise therapy effects following laser treatment (MUMTAZ et al. 1996; HUCH-BÖNI et al. 1997). Reflecting the high soft tissue contrast inherent to the MR experiment, MR reveals tissue defects earlier than CT or ultrasound. This approach, however, cannot be considered 'MR-guided laser therapy'. To fully exploit the advantages of MR monitoring, temperature mapping should be performed during laser application.

To date, no consensus has been achieved regarding the temporal requirements of temperature mapping during LITT. Considering that the duration of most LITT lies in the range of minutes rather than seconds (VOGL et al. 1995b), an image update every 2–5 s does appear adequate. This resolution is achievable with most commercially available fast GRE sequences. The importance of short imaging times is underlined by the inability of seriously ill patients to hold their breath for a long time. Breathing or motion artefacts are obviously less of a concern in areas not subject to respiratory motion, such as the brain or joints (KAHN et al. 1996; HEINRICH et al. 1996).

While temporal resolution seems not to be of critical concern, the temperature accuracy, i.e. temperature resolution, is. As mentioned above, accurate quantification of temperature is not possible on the basis of T1-weighted sequences. The visualised SI decrease reflects a combination of various factors, including tissue destruction (vacuolisation, gas formation), heat distribution, diffusion mechanisms

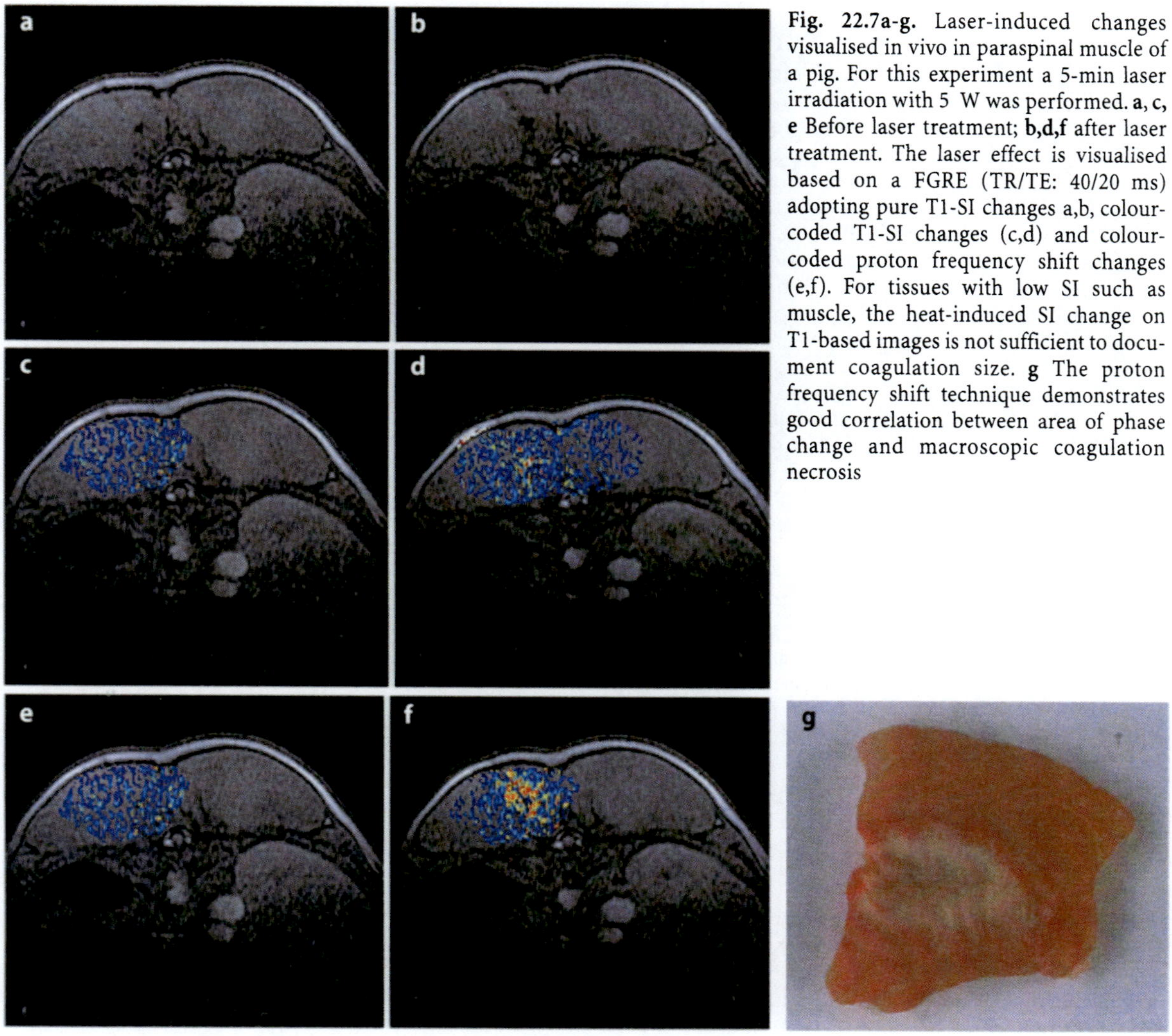

Fig. 22.7a-g. Laser-induced changes visualised in vivo in paraspinal muscle of a pig. For this experiment a 5-min laser irradiation with 5 W was performed. **a, c, e** Before laser treatment; **b,d,f** after laser treatment. The laser effect is visualised based on a FGRE (TR/TE: 40/20 ms) adopting pure T1-SI changes a,b, colour-coded T1-SI changes (c,d) and colour-coded proton frequency shift changes (e,f). For tissues with low SI such as muscle, the heat-induced SI change on T1-based images is not sufficient to document coagulation size. **g** The proton frequency shift technique demonstrates good correlation between area of phase change and macroscopic coagulation necrosis

etc. So far, the available clinical information is too limited to warrant a definitive statement with regard to the ability to predict SI coagulation size based on SI changes on T1-weighted images.

PFS enables tissue-independent temperate quantification. It is more difficult to implement than T1-weighted imaging, however. If acquisition parameters are optimised to achieve maximal temperature accuracy (±2°C), imaging time tends to become too long for a single breath hold (Chung et al. 1996). If these parameters are altered to enforce faster image updates, temperature accuracy deteriorates (Cline et al. 1996). As with temporal resolution, there is no agreement on minimum temperature accuracy. One would suppose that an accuracy of ±5–10°C should be appropriate for laser treatment. This theoretically should be obtainable with PFS based on fast GRE with image updates ranging between 2 and 5 s. However, as yet no clinical studies have been published that have tested this hypothesis in patients.

22.6 Clinical Applications of MR-Guided LITT

MR-guided LITT stands to gain clinical acceptance as a minimally invasive method if heat distribution can be monitored safely and accurately. The increasing availability of open-configuration magnets, interactive device-localisation methods and fast and accurate temperature-sensitive MR-imaging sequences appear promising in this respect. To date, experience in treating patients with MR-guided LITT remains limited. Nevertheless, a variety of lesions have been successfully treated. These include lesions in the brain (Kahn et al. 1996), the head and neck region and the liver (Vogl et al. 1995a,b). In addition, laser discectomies have been performed under MR guidance (Schoenenberger et al. 1997).

Before the true value of MR-guided laser therapies can be assessed, more clinical experience is needed.

References

Amin Z, Donald JJ, Masters A, Kant R, Steger AC, Bown SG, Lees WR (1993) Hepatic metastases: interstitial laser photocoagulation with real-time US monitoring and dynamic CT evaluation of treatment. Radiology 187:339-347

Botnar R, Steiner P, Erhart P, Debatin JF, von Schulthess GK (1977) Absolute temperature quantification in near real-time with an open 0.5 Tesla interventional MR-scanner. In: Proceedings of the International Society of Magnetic Resonance in Medicine 1997. Society of Magnetic Resonance in Medicine, Berkeley, Calif, p. 1957

Bown SG (1983) Phototherapy of tumors. World J Surg 7:700-709

Choy DSJ, Ascher PW, Ranu HS, et al (1992) Percutaneous laser disc decompression. A new therapeutic modality. Spine 17:949-956

Chung AH, Hynynen K, Colucci V, Oshio K, Cline HE, Jolesz FA (1996) Optimisation of spoiled gradient-echo phase imaging for in vivo localisation of a focused ultrasound beam. Magn Reson Med 36:745-752

Cline HE, Hynynen K, Hardy CJ, Watkins RD, Schenck JF, Jolesz FA (1994) MR temperature mapping of focused ultrasound surgery. Magn Reson Med 31:628-636

Cline HE, Hynynen K, Schneider E, Hardy CJ, Maier SE, Watkins RD, Jolesz FA (1996) Simultaneous magnetic resonance phase and magnitude temperature maps in muscle. Magn Reson Med 35:309-315

Dachman AH, McGehee JA, Beam TE, Burris JA, Powell DE (1990) US-guided percutaneous laser ablation of liver tissue in a chronic pig model. Radiology 176:129-133

Delannoy J, Chen CN, Turner R, Levin L, LeBihan D (1991) Noninvasive temperature imaging using diffusion MRI. Magn Reson Med 19:333-339

de Poorter J, de Wagter C, de Deene Y, Thomsen C, Ståhlberg F, Achten E (1995) Noninvasive MRI thermometry with the proton resonance frequency method: in vivo results in human muscle. Magn Reson Med 33:74-81

Dumoulin CL, Souza SP, Darrow RD (1993) Realtime position monitoring of invasive devices using magnetic resonance. Magn Reson Med 29:411-415

Fried MP, Morrison PR, Hushek SG, Kernahan GA, Jolesz FA (1996) Dynamic T1-weighted magnetic resonance imaging of interstitial laser photocoagulation in the liver: observation on in vivo temperature sensitivity. Lasers Surg Med 18:410-419

Harries SA, Amin Z, Smith MEF, et al (1994) Interstitial laser photocoagulation as a treatment for breast cancer. Br J Surg 81:1617-1619

Hendrich C, Jakob PM, Breitling T, Schäfer A, Berden A, Haase A, Siebert WE (1996) Kernspintomographische Messung der Temperaturverteilung in Knorpelgewebe nach Lasertherapie. Orthopäde 25:17-20

Huch-Böni RA, Sulser T, Jochum W, Romanowski B, Debatin JF, Krestin GP (1997) Laser ablation-induced changes in the prostate: findings at endorectal MR imaging with histologic correlation. Radiology 202:232-237

Jolesz FA (1995) MR-guided thermal ablation of brain tumors. Am J Neuroradiat 16:49-52

Jolesz FA, Bleier AR, Jakab P, Ruenzel PW, Huttl K, Jako GJ (1988) MR imaging of laser-tissue interactions. Radiology 168:249-253

Kahn T, Schwabe B, Bettag M, et al (1996) Mapping of the cortical motor hand area with functional MR imaging and MR imaging-guided laser-induced interstitial thermotherapy of brain tumors. Radiology 200:149-157

Kuroda K, Abe K, Tsutsumi S, Ishihara Y, Suzuki Y, Sato K (1993) Water proton magnetic resonance spectroscopic imaging. Biomed Thermol 13:43-62

Leung DA, Debatin JF, Wildermuth S, et al (1995) Real-time biplanar needle tracking for interventional MR imaging procedures. Radiology 197:485-488

Matsumoto R, Oshio K, Jolesz FA (1992) Monitoring of laser and freezing induced ablation in the liver with T1-weighted MR-imaging. J Magn Reson Imaging 2:555-562

Matsumoto R, Mulkern RV, Hushek SG, Jolesz FA (1994) Tissue temperature monitoring for thermal interventional therapy: comparison of T1-weighted MR sequences. J Magn Reson Imaging 4:65-70

Mumtaz H, Hall-Craggs MA, Wotherspoon A, et al (1996) Laser therapy for breast cancer: MR imaging and histopathologic correlation. Radiology 200:651-658

Nelson TR, Tung SM (1987) Temperature dependence of proton relaxation times in vitro. Magn Reson Imaging 5:189-199

Ohyama M, Nobori T, Moriyama I, Furuta S, Shima T (1988) Laserthermia on head and neck malignancies: experimental and clinical studies. Acta Otolaryngol Suppl (Stockh) 458:7-12

Pignoli E, Marchesini R, Curti L, Sichirollo AE, Tomatis S, Musumeci R (1995) Potential and limitations of magnetic resonance imaging for real-time monitoring of interstitial laser phototherapy. Acad Radiol 2:741-747

Quigley MR, Maroon JC, Shih T, Elrifai A, Lesiecki ML (1994) Laser discectomy. Comparison of systems. Spine 19:319-322

Schenck JF, Jolesz A, Roemer PB, et al (1995) Superconducting open-configuration MR imaging system for image-guided therapy. Radiology 195:805-814

Schoenenberger AW, Steiner P, Debatin JF, et al (1997) Real-time monitoring of laser discectomies with a super-conducting, open-configuration MR system. Am J Roentgenol (in press)

Silverman SG, Collick BD, Figueira MR, et al (1995) Interactive MR-guided biopsy in an open-configuration MR imaging system. Radiology 197:175-181

Steiner P, Schoenenberger AW, Penner EA, Erhart P, Debatin JF, von Schulthess GK, Kacl GM (1996a) Interaktive stereotaktische Interventionen im supraleitenden, offenen 0.5-Tesla-MR-Tomographen. RoFo Fortschr Geb Röntgenstr Neuen Bildgeb Verfahr 165:276-280

Steiner P, Schoenenberger AW, Erhart P, Penner EA, von Schulthess GK, Debatin JF (1996b) Optimization of MR sequences for detecting laser-induced tissue changes Radiology 201:389

Vogl TJ, Mack MG, Müller PK, et al (1995a) MR-guided laser-induced thermotherapy of tumors of the head and neck region: first clinical results. RoFo Fortschr Geb Röntgenstr Neuen Bildgeb Verfahr 163:505-514

Vogl TJ, Müller PK, Hammerstingl R, et al (1995b) Malignant liver tumors treated with MR imaging-guided laser-induced thermotherapy: technique and prospective results. Radiology 196:257-265

23 MR-Guided Focused Ultrasound Surgery

K. Hynynen

CONTENTS

23.1 Introduction

Ultrasound has several characteristics which make it well suited for MRI-guided noninvasive therapy. First, it is a mechanical wave with particle movements so small that the beam does not interfere with the process of MR data acquisition. Second, the frequency of the electrical signal driving the transducer is much lower than the Larmor frequency, making simultaneous sonication and imaging relatively easy to accomplish. Third, nonmagnetic applicators of practically any shape and size can be easily constructed with adequate power output to coagulate living tissues. Fourth, ultrasound penetrates soft tissues at frequencies where the wavelengths are in the order of a millimeter. The small wavelengths allow the beams to be focused and controlled, providing a completely noninvasive method for energy delivery deep into the body. Finally, the energy density at the focus can be increased to the point of tissue coagulation within a few seconds, resulting in perfusion-insensitive thermal exposures. Magnetic resonance imaging complements focused ultrasound by offering accurate information on the anatomy, for guiding the beam, and on temperature elevation, for verification of therapy location and quantification of the thermal exposure and biological effect.

K. Hynynen, PhD, Department of Radiology, Brigham and Women's Hospital and Harvard Medical School, 75 Francis Street, Boston, MA 02115, USA

23.2 Propagation Through Tissue

Ultrasound is a form of vibrational energy (at a frequency above the audible range) that is propagated as a mechanical wave by the motion of molecules within the medium. The wave causes compressions and rarefactions of the molecules. Thus, a pressure wave is propagated along with the mechanical movement. The characteristics of the wave are a function of both the source generating the motion and the acoustic properties of the medium through which it travels. The propagating wave is typically longitudinal with the molecules vibrating along in the direction of the propagation. (For the theory and references see Wells 1977.)

The ultrasound energy is attenuated according to an exponential law in tissue. The rate of energy flow through a unit area normal to the direction of the wave propagation is called the acoustic intensity (I). For a plane wave of a frequency f, the intensity $I(x)$ at the depth x is described by the following formula:

$$I(x) = I(0)\, e^{-2\alpha x f}$$

where $I(0)$ is the intensity at the surface and α is the amplitude attenuation coefficient per unit path length (an average value for soft tissues = 5 Npm^{-1} MHz^{-1}). Thus, at 1 MHz the ultrasound wave is attenuated approximately 50% while it propagates through 7 cm of tissue. At 2 MHz the wave is reduced to approximately 25% of its initial value by the same tissue. Ultrasound attenuation in tissues is a sum of the losses due to absorption and scattering. In the scattering process the elastic discontinuities within the tissue absorb the energy and then re-emit it away from its original direction of propagation.

In an ideal, pure elastic medium, the energy in an ultrasonic field is either in kinetic or potential form, and the pressure wave is in phase with the particle velocity. In a real medium there are also viscous forces between the moving particles, which cause a lag between the particle pressure and velocity. Therefore, an energy loss during each cycle will result. The absorption in a viscoelastic medium depends on the square of the frequency (f^2). This is true in many liquids but not in tissues, where the absorption has been shown to increase almost linearly as a function of frequency (Goss et al. 1979) due to multiple relaxation mechanisms that cause additional ultrasound absorption. During the compressive part of the pressure wave, energy is stored in the medium in a number of forms, such as lattice vibrational energy, molecular vibrational energy, translational energy etc. This stored energy is returned to the wave during the expansion phase. At the same time, the temperature of the medium returns to the original level. However, in tissue the increased kinetic energy of the molecules is not in balance with the environment, and the system tries to redistribute the energy. The transfer of energy takes time, and thus, during the decompression cycle, energy will return out of phase to the wave and absorption results. In addition, a portion of the stored energy remains in various forms within the medium. This mechanism of energy absorption is called relaxation. The ultrasound absorption mechanism in tissues has been reviewed in detail by Wells (1977), and the acoustic properties have been compiled elsewhere (Goss et al. 1978, 1980).

Ultrasound is effectively transmitted from one soft tissue layer to another with a small (few percent) amount of wave reflected back. At soft tissue-bone interfaces about one third of the incident energy is reflected back at normal incidence. In addition, the amplitude attenuation coefficient of ultrasound is about 10–20 times higher in bone than in soft tissue. This causes the transmitted beam to be absorbed rapidly, resulting in a hot spot on the bone surface (Hynynen and DeYoung 1988; Lehmann et al. 1967). At a soft tissue–gas interface all of the energy is reflected back.

23.3 Focused Beams

Due to the short wavelength (1.5 mm at 1 MHz) the ultrasound beams can be focused by using focused radiators, lenses or reflectors. Focusing can also be achieved by using transducer arrays that are driven with signals having the proper phase difference to obtain a common focal point (electrical focusing). The wavelength imposes a limitation on the size of the focal region. The sharpness of the focus is determined by the ratio between the aperture of the radiator to the wavelength. A focal diameter of 1 mm can be achieved in practice at 1.5 MHz. The length of the focus is typically 5–20 times larger than the diameter. Since the ultrasound beam is transmitted from an applicator that is several centimeters in diameter, the ultrasound intensity at the focal spot can be several hundred times higher than in the overlying tissues. Similarly, the ultrasound exposure drops off rapidly across the focus, thus limiting the ultrasound exposure to the focus.

23.4. Tissue effects

The ultrasound beam can interact with tissue at the target volume primarily via two different mechanisms. First, it can elevate the tissue temperature due to energy absorption from the wave, resulting in different degrees of thermal damage to the tissue depending on the temperature reached. The effect of elevated temperature on cells and tissues is characterized by a nonlinear function of both time and temperature (Landry and Marceau 1978; Sapareto and Dewey 1984; Crile 1963; Moritz and Henriques 1947). It has been shown that above 43°C an increase of 1°C in temperature reduces the required treatment time to half. This relationship has been verified up to 57°C (Borrelli et al. 1990; Landry and Marceau 1978). For exposures of a few seconds, temperatures of above approximately 60°C are needed to coagulate proteins, resulting in tissue necrosis. The elevated temperature also blocks micro vasculature and stops blood perfusion in the coagulated tissue volume. Occlusion of surgically exposed veins by thermal effects of ultrasound has also been demonstrated (Delon-Martin et al. 1995). When the temperatures reach 100°C, gas formation results. The gas blocks the propagation of the ultrasound beam and significantly modifies the energy deposition pattern.

The second mechanism, cavitation requires pressure amplitudes that are large enough to form gas bubbles within the tissue (ter Haar et al. 1982; Frizzell et al. 1983; Coakley 1971). The pressure wave causes the bubbles to expand and then collapse. The collapse of the bubbles causes high temperatures

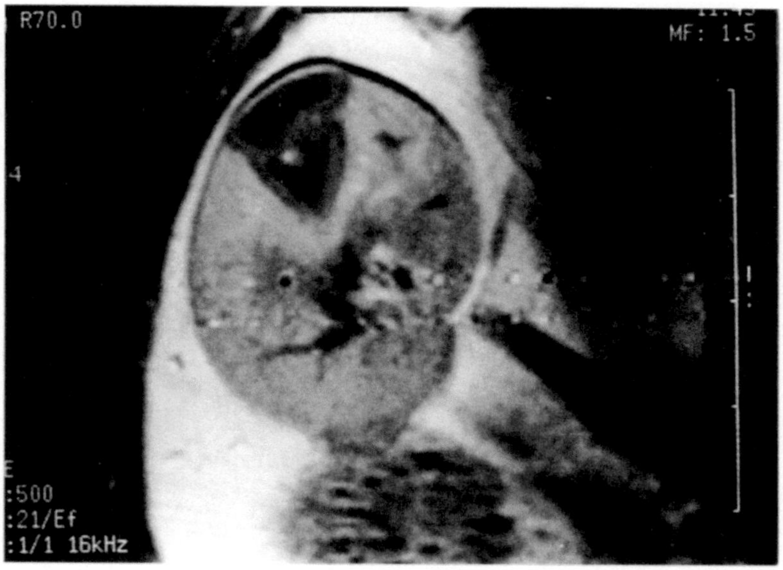

Fig. 1. Fast spin echo (FSE) T1-weighted contrast-enhanced image of a rabbit kidney after ultrasound was used to occlude a branch of an artery (HYNYNEN et al. 1996b).

and pressures that can cause direct mechanical damage to the tissue. This phenomenon is called transient or inertial cavitation. Histologic studies have shown that cavitation can offer different therapeutic options than thermal exposures. These are: breakage of the blood-brain barrier, selective vascular damage, and tissue necrosis (VYKHODTSEVA et al. 1995). NONINVASIVE occlusion of deep arteries (HYNYNEN et al. 1996b) (Fig. 1) has been demonstrated. In addition, animal tumor studies have shown that focused ultrasound-induced cavitation can activate certain chemicals (UMEMURA et al. 1989). The disruption of arteriosclerotic plaques and thrombi is also cavitation mediated (ROSENSCHEIN et al. 1990; SIEGEL et al. 1989). Finally, high-amplitude focused ultrasound beams can also be distorted to shock waves at the focus (CARSTENSEN et al. 1981) and thus potentially influence the cell membrane permeability in a similar way to the shock waves generated by pulsed laser exposures (DOUKAS and FLOTTE 1996). This may offer new therapeutic options.

23.5 Large target volume

The small size of the focal spot that is one of the main strengths of focused ultrasound is also its weakness when large tumors or target volumes are treated. The coagulated tissue volume depends on the transducer characteristics (frequency, diameter, and radius of curvature), sonication time and achieved temperature (DAMIANOU and HYNYNEN 1994), but is seldom great enough to cover a large lesion with a single sonication. Therefore, multiple exposures are required to coagulate a typical tumor. Unfortunately multiple exposures need to be separated by an interval sufficient to avoid temperature build-up in the more superficial tissue volumes that are exposed by multiple sonications due to the large beam diameter outside of the focal spot (FAN and HYNYNEN 1996; DAMIANOU and HYNYNEN 1993). Using sharply focused transducers, only small tumors (a few cubic centimeters in volume) can be treated in a reasonable amount of time. It has been shown theoretically that by increasing the focal spot size the total treatment time can be reduced to a practical level (FAN and HYNYNEN 1996). In principle, special lenses (LALONDE and HUNT 1995; LALONDE et al. 1990; TAKAYAMA and ITOH 1989), multiple overlapping beams (HYNYNEN et al. 1993) and phased arrays can be used to increase the focal spot size and reduce the treatment time. Phased arrays may control the ultrasound distribution within the focus and offer the highest flexibility.

23.6. Ultrasound Systems

Noninvasive surgery using focused, high-intensity ultrasound beams was first proposed in 1942 (LYNN et al. 1942). The technique was later modified and used in the destruction of central nervous system tissue for therapeutic purposes (FRY et al. 1955). Since then ultrasound has been extensively tested for trackless surgery of brain both in animals (LELE 1962; BASAURI and LELE 1962; FRY et al. 1955) and in humans (Heimburger 1985; Fry and Fry 1960). During the past few years new clinical trials using ultrasound for noninvasive surgery of the prostate, kidney, bladder (Vallancien et al. 1993; Madersbacher et al. 1995; Foster et al. 1993) and eye (Coleman et al. 1985) have shown promise. In principle all of the systems use spherically curved ultra-sound transducers that have a small, fixed focus. The location of the focus in tissue can be moved by mechanically moving the transducer. The sonication system is connected to an ultrasound imaging device to aim the therapeutic beam into the treatment area.

Small catheters capable of necrosing cardiac muscle tissue have also been developed (Hynynen et al. 1997a; Zimmer et al. 1995; He et al. 1994). These catheters are now under evaluation for ablation of abnormal electric pathways that are responsible for arrhythmias. Ultrasound can also be delivered interstitially either using cylindrical ultrasound sources (Hynynen and Davis 1993) or external sources with a small wave guide (Jarosz 1996).

23.7 The role of MR Guidance

Recently, the feasibility of performing ultrasound surgery in an MRI scanner utilizing imaging to guide and monitor the therapy has been demonstrated by several groups (Smith et al. 1995; Stepanow et al. 1995; Suzuki et al. 1995; Cline et al. 1993, 1995; Hynynen et al. 1993, 1994, 1995, 1996; Darkazanli et al. 1993). MRI offers several advantages over other imaging techniques for guiding and monitoring ultrasound exposures: First, MRI has good soft tissue contrast and resolution to allow the beam to be accurately aimed at the target volume. Second, several MRI sequences can be made sensitive to temperature changes. This allows the temperature elevation to be detected prior to the induction of any irreversible tissue damage (Hynynen et al. 1997b). Thus, the location of the focus can be detected at low powers to verify targeting accuracy. Third, temperature-sensitive sequences allow an estimation to be made on the achieved focal temperature and thus on the thermal exposure produced. This can be useful in ensuring that the target volume is adequately covered and surrounding normal structures and spared. Finally, the tissue changes induced by the sonications can be detected using MRI. Tissue damage results in signal changes on both T1- and T2-weighted images. Similarly, tissue perfusion can be assessed by utilizing contrast agent uptake (Hynynen et al. 1994).

Good temperature resolution has been obtained using the proton resonance frequency (PRF). Changes in the PRF induced by the temperature are linearly related to temperature and can be mapped by using changes in phase images. The disadvantage of the frequency shift technique is its insensitivity to temperature changes in fat. In in vitro studies by Kuroda et al. (1995) with different soft tissues, the maximum variations in the temperature dependency of the proton frequency from tissue to tissue were found to be small enough to localize the focus with low-power test exposures and to ensure that temperatures between 60 and 100°C are reached during the 10-s therapy exposures. The temperature history can be used to calculate the biological effect or thermal dose induced by thermal exposure (Chung et al. 1996b) (Fig. 2). In addition, the imaging can be used to monitor normal tissue temperatures for safety. The upper temperature limit of 100°C has been set to avoid boiling and the resulting formation of gas bubbles that could distort the ultrasound beam. Thus, the exposure limits are wide enough to accommodate some uncertainty in the temperature monitoring.

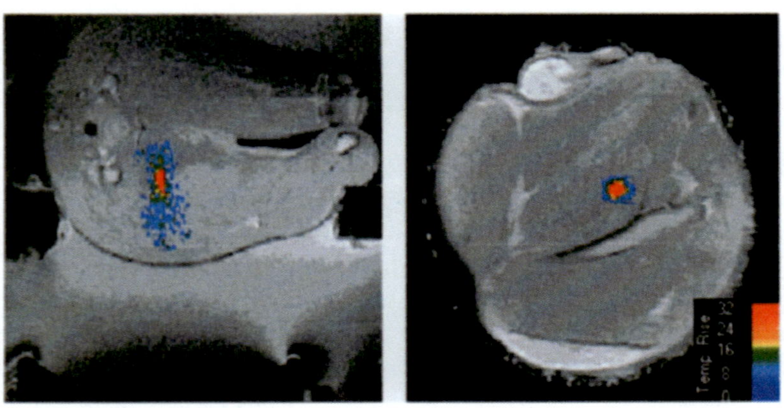

Fig. 2. FSE T2-weighted image of a rabbit thigh muscle with a superimposed temperature elevation map derived from phase-difference images. *Left*: along the axis of the ultrasound beam; *right*: across the focus of the beam (Chung et al. 1996a)

23.8
MR-Guided Ultrasound System for Clinical Tests

The first prototype ultrasound device was manufactured for the surgery of breast tumors, by General Electric Medical System in collaboration with the personnel from the Brigham and Women's Hospital (Fig. 3). The ultrasound fields were generated by a single, focused, air-backed transducer that was mounted in a standard MRI table. The transducer could be moved by a computer-controlled positioning device in the x, y, and z directions in the waterbath that acted as a coupling medium. A workstation that controlled the transducer motion was programmed to aim the ultrasound beam at a location defined on an MR image (HYNYNEN et al. 1996c; CLINE et al. 1995).

During a typical treatment execution the target volume is outlined on a series of MRI scans. A low-energy test pulse is aimed at the target volume. The workstation registers the target, aims the focus at that location, sonicates a low-power test pulse and transfers the temperature-sensitive image obtained during the sonication. If the location of the temperature elevation does not overlap the target volume a correction can be made and the test pulse resonicated to verify the alignment accuracy. Following the test pulses, the complete target volume is sonicated using multiple pulses placed so that the coagulated volumes overlap. Figure 4 illustrates this principle. The dimensions of the coagulated tissue volume for each sonication depend on the duration of the sonication and the applied power.

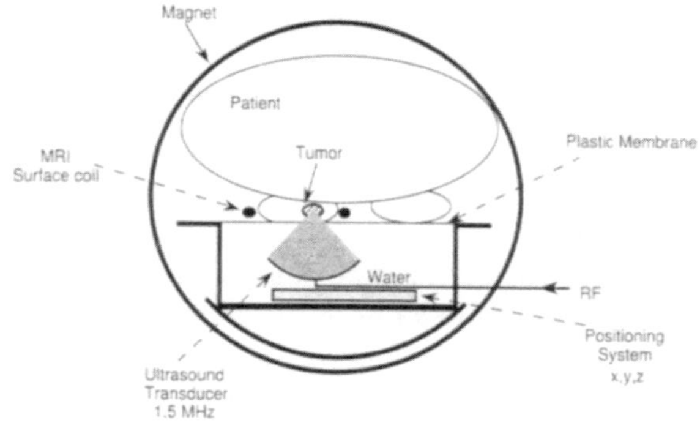

Fig. 3. Diagram of the clinical MR-guided focused ultrasound system (HYNYNEN et al. 1996c; CLINE et al. 1995).

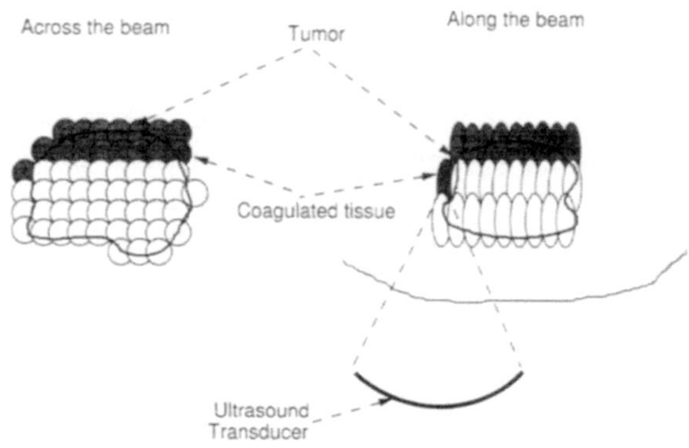

Fig. 4. Diagram of a multiple sonication treatment.

23.9
Clinical tests and potential

A clinical evaluation of this system is now in progress. Fibroadenomas of the breast are treated. An example of a contrast-enhanced MR image of a breast tumor treated a week earlier is shown in Fig. 5. The treated (lower) tumor shows no contrast up-

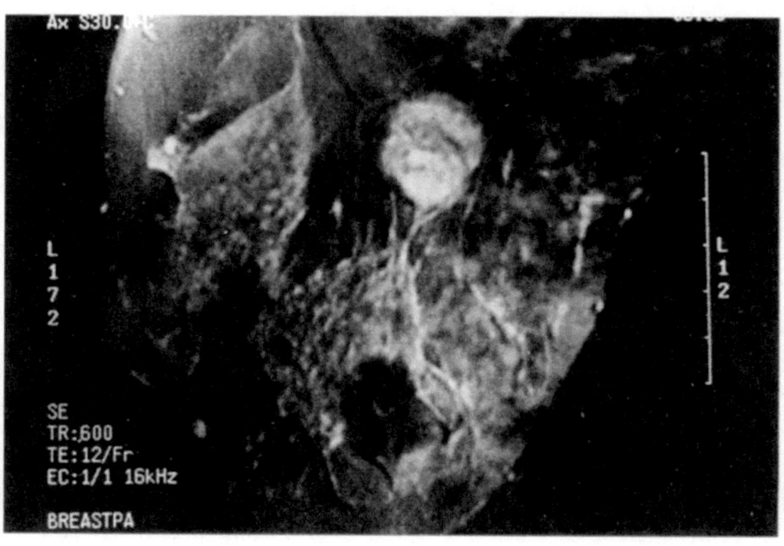

Fig. 5. Axial T1-weighted FSE image (TR 600 ms, TE = 12 ms, echo train length 4, one data acquisition, field of view 16 cm, slice thickness 5 mm) with contrast of the sonicated breast 7 days after the treatment (*below*, sonicated tumor; *above*, untreated tumor) (HYNYNEN et al. 1996c).

take, whereas the untreated (upper) tumor closer to the chest wall enhances. The two tumors had similar contrast uptake prior to treatment. While it is too early to make any conclusions on the clinical efficacy or toxicity of the treatment, initial results appear promising.

The proposed ultrasound surgery could be used to replace some present forms of tumor treatment. Potentially treatable lesions require a soft tissue window which allows passage of the ultrasound beam avoiding gas or bone. In addition to the breast, some liver tumors could be treated with MR-guided focused ultrasound. Secondary liver cancer is a common problem with a poor prognosis. However, the treatment of liver tumors is complicated by ribs and bowel gas that limit the available ultrasound window. In addition, movement of the liver caused by respiration has to be compensated for. Prostate cancer, benign prostatic hyperplasia, bladder cancer, as well as kidney tumors are also potential targets for MR-guided ultrasound treatments. Many prostate tumors could be reached through the ultrasound window created by a full bladder or specially developed rectal applicators. Both bladder and kidney tumors could be reached using external ultrasound applicators. As was shown in early clinical trials, deep target volumes in the brain can also be reached by ultrasound if a piece of skull is removed (Fig. 6). The development of large phased arrays may allow the ultrasound beam distortion caused by skull bone to be corrected and the energy focused adequately for trans-skull brain therapy (Thomas and Fink 1996; Smith et al. 1977). This would allow some brain tumors and functional disorders that can be visualized by MRI to be treated using focused ultrasound.

Blood vessel occlusion is useful for treating arteriovenous malformations (AVM) in different parts of the body and for treatment of some tumors with an identifiable blood supply. It may also be useful for controlling abdominal, peritoneal, and pelvic hemorrhage and in the treatment of some trauma victims.

23.10 Future technical development

It is expected that new site specific-devices will be developed for MR-guided ultrasound therapy. Eventually many of the systems will utilize phased arrays that offer several characteristics which are desirable for clinical treatments. First, an optimal focal size and ultrasound field distribution can be tailored for each target volume based on pretreatment planning. Second, the focal size can be controlled during a treatment requiring multiple sonications. Third, the effects of overlying tissues on the focal location can be compensated for by modifying the driving signals. Finally, phased arrays offer the flexibility of allowing the focal spot to be electrically moved without physically moving the transducer.

Several different array configurations have been tested for MR-guided focused ultrasound therapy (Hutchinson et al. 1996; Fjield and Hynynen 1997; Hynynen et al. 1996a). All of these experiments have shown that phase array applicators with adequate power output to coagulate tissue are feasible. Both the ability to move the focus electronically and to control the necrosed tissue volume has been demonstrated (Hynynen et al. 1996a). In addition, the phased arrays offer the potential for optimizing the energy deposition pattern (Fjield and Hynynen 1997). The feasibility of constructing MR-guided intracavitary ultrasound arrays has opened new potential for the treatment of targets located close to body cavities (for example the prostate).

23.11 Summary

Focused high-power ultrasound beams are well suited for noninvasive local coagulation of deep target volumes. The feasibility of guiding the ultrasound beam using MR has been shown both in ani-

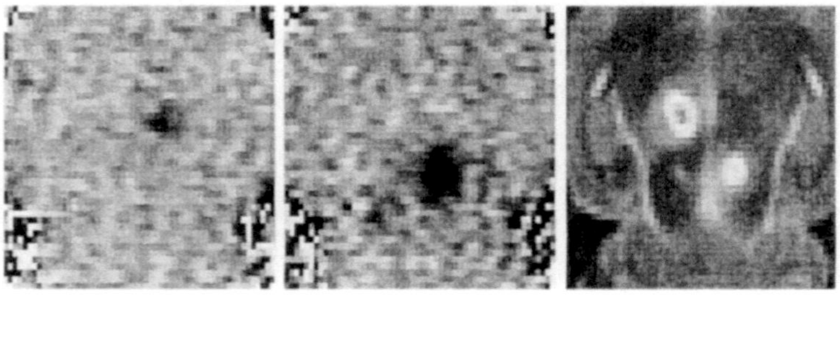

Fig. 6. Rabbit brain sonication: phase-difference images during the 10-s sonications. *Left*: 3.5-W sonication. *Middle*: 10.5-W sonication. *Right*: T2-weighted image after a total of four sonications. The location of the 3.5-W sonication does not show any signal intensity changes, while the 10.5-W sonication location shows a clear tissue effect. The two other locations visible in the T2-weighted image were sonicated at 7 W (*bottom left*) and 14 W (*top left*) (Hynynen et al. 1997b)

mals and in the clinical setting and shows promise. However, more clinical testing and device development is needed prior to its routine clinical use.

References

Basauri L, Lele PP (1962) A simple method for production of trackless focal lesions with focused ultrasound: statistical evaluation of the effects of irradiation on the central nervous system of the cat. J Physiol 160:513–534

Borrelli MJ, Thompson LL, Cain CA, Dewey WC (1990) Time-temperature analysis of cell killing of BHK cells heated at temperatures in the range of 43.5 °C to 57 °C. Int J Radiat Oncol Biol Phys 19 S:389–399

Carstensen EL, Becroft SA, Law WK, Barber DB (1981) Finite amplitude effects on thresholds for lesion production in tissues by unfocussed ultrasound. J Acoust Soc Am 70:302–309

Chung A, Hynynen K, Cline HE, Colucci V, Oshio K, Jolesz F (1996a) Optimization of spoiled gradient-echo phase imaging for in vivo localization of focused ultrasound beam. Magn Reson Med 36:745–752

Chung A, Hynynen K, Cline HE, Jolesz FA (1996b) Quantification of thermal exposure using proton resonance frequency shift. Proc SMR 4th Meeting ISSN 1065–9889, 3:1751 (Abstract)

Cline HE, Schenck JF, Watkins RD, Hynynen K and Jolesz FA (1993) Magnetic resonance guided thermal surgery. Mgn Reson Med 31:628–636

Cline HE, Hynynen K, Watkins RD et al. (1995) A focused ultrasound system for MRI guided ablation. Radiology 194:731–737

Coakley A (1971) Acoustical detection of single cavitation events in a focussed field in water at 1 MHz. J Acoust Soc Am 49:792–801

Coleman DJ, Lizzi FL, Driller J, Rosado AL, Chang S, Iwamoto T, Rosenthal D (1985) Therapeutic ultrasound in the treatment of glaucoma. Ophthalmology 92:339–346

Crile G (1963) The effect of heat and radiation on cancers implanted on the feet of mice. Cancer Res 23:372–380

Damianou C, Hynynen K (1993) Near-field heating during pulsed high temperature ultrasound hyperthermia treatment. Ultrasound Med Biol 19:777–787

Damianou C, Hynynen K (1994) The effect of various physical parameters on the size and shape of necrosed tissue volume during ultrasound surgery. J Acoust Soc Am 95: 1641–1649

Darkazanli A, Hynynen K, Unger E, Schenck JF (1993) On-line monitoring of ultrasound surgery with MRI. J Magn Reson Imaging 3:509–514

Delon-Martin C, Vogt C, Chigner E, Guers C, Chapelon JY, Cathignol D (1995) Venous thrombosis generation by means of high-intensity focused ultrasound. Ultrasound Med Biol 21:113–119

Doukas AG, Flotte TJ (1996) Physical characteristics and biological effects of laser-induced stress waves. Ultrasound Med Biol 22:151–164

Fan X, Hynynen K (1996) Ultrasound surgery using multiple sonications — treatment time considerations. Ultrasound Med Biol 22:471–482

Fjield T, Hynynen K (1997) The combined concentric-ring and sector-vortex phased array for MRI guided ultrasound surgery. IEEE Trans Ultrason Ferroelectr Freq Contr (in press)

Foster RS, Bihrle R, Sanghvi NT, Fry FJ, Donohue JP (1993) High-intensity focused ultrasound in the treatment of prostatic disease. Eur Urol 23:29–33

Frizzell LA, Lee CS, Aschenbach PD, Borrelli MJ, Morimoto RS, Dunn F (1983) Involvement of ultrasonically induced cavitation in the production of hind limb paralysis of the mouse neonate. J Acoust Soc Am 74:1062–1065

Fry WJ, Barnard JW, Fry FJ, Krumins RF, Brennan JF (1955) Ultrasonic lesions in the mammalian central nervous system. Science 122:517–518

Fry WJ, Fry FJ (1960) Fundamental neurological research and human neurosurgery using intense ultrasound. IRE Trans Med Electron 7:166–181

Goss SA, Johnson RL, Dunn F (1978) Comprehensive compilation of empirical ultrasonic properties of mammalian tissues. J Acoust Soc Am 64:423–457

Goss SA, Johnson RL, Dunn F (1980) Compliation of empirical ultrasonic properties of mammalian tissues. II. J Acoust Soc Am 68:93–108

Goss SA, Frizzell LA, Dunn F (1979) Ultrasonic absorption and attenuation in mammalian tissues. Ultrasound Med Biol 5:181–186

He DS, Zimmer JE, Hynynen K, Marcus FI, Caruso AC, Lampe LF, Aguine ML (1994) Preliminary results using ultrasound energy for ablation of the ventricular myocardium in dogs. Am J Cardiol 73:1029–1031

Heimburger RF (1985) Ultrasound augmentation of central nervous system tumor therapy. Indiana Med 78:469–476

Hutchinson EB, Dahleh M, Hynynen K (1996) MRI feedback control for phased array prostate hyperthermia. IEEE Ultrasonics Symp. Vol 2, pp 1285–1288

Hynynen K, Darkazanli A, Unger E, Schenck JF (1993) MRI-guided noninvasive ultrasound surgery. Med Phys 20: 107–115

Hynynen K, Darkazanli A, Damianou C, Unger E, Schenck JF (1994) The usefulness of contrast agent and GRASS imaging sequence for MRI guided noninvasive ultrasound surgery. Invest Radiol 29:897–903

Hynynen K, Damianou CA, Culucci V, Unger E, Cline HE, Jolesz FA (1995) MR monitoring of focused ultrasonic surgery of renal cortex: experimental and simulation studies. J Magn Reson Imaging 5:259–266

Hynynen K, Chung A, Fjield T et al. (1996a) Feasibility of using ultrasound phased arrays for MRI monitored noninvasive surgery. IEEE Trans Ultrason Ferroelectr Freq Contr 43:1043–1053

Hynynen K, Colucci V, Chung A, Jolesz FA (1996b) Noninvasive artery occlusion using MRI guided focused ultrasound. Ultrasound Med Biol 22:1071–1077

Hynynen K, Freund W, Cline HE, Chung A, Watkins R, Vetro J, Jolesz FA (1996c) A clinical noninvasive MRI monitored ultrasound surgery method. Radiographics 16:185–195

Hynynen K, Dennie J, Zimmer JE, Simmons WN, He DS, Marcus FI, Aguirre ML (1997a) Cyclindrical ultrasound transducers for cardiac catheter ablation. IEEE Trans Biomed Eng 44:144–151

Hynynen K, Vykhodtseva NI, Chung A, Sorrentino V, Colucci V, Jolesz FA (1997b) MRI detection of the thermal effects of focused ultrasound on the brain. Radiology (in press)

Hynynen K, Davis KL (1993) Small cylindrical ultrasound sources for induction of hyperthermia via body cavities or interstitial implants. Int J Hyperthermia 9:263–274

Hynynen K, DeYoung D (1988) Temperature elevation at muscle-bone interface during scanned, focussed ultrasound hyperthermia. Int J Hyperthermia 4:267–279

Kuroda K, Abe K, Tsutsumi S, Ishihara Y, Suzuki Y, Sato K (1995) Water proton magnetic resonance spectroscopic imaging. Biomed Thermol 13:43–62

Jarosz BJ (1996) Feasibility of ultrasound hyperthermia with waveguide interstitial applicator. IEEE Trans Biomed Eng 43:1106–1115

Lalonde R, Worthington A, Hunt JW (1990) Hyperthermia: Field conjugate acoustic lenses for deep heating. IEEE/EMBS Conference, Philadelphia, Pa, pp 235–236

Lalone R, Hunt JW (1995) Variable frequency field conjugate lenses for ultrasound hyperthermia. IEEE Trans Ultrason Ferroelectr Freq Contr 42:825–831

Landry J, Marceau N (1978) Rate-Limiting events in hyperthermic cell killing. Radiat Res 75:573–585

Lehmann JF, deLateur BJ, Warren CG, Stonebridge JS (1967) Heating produced by ultrasound in bone and osft tissue. Arch Phys Med Rehabil 48:397–401

Lele PP (1962) A simple method for production of trackless focal lesions with focused ultrasound: Physical factors. J Physiol 160:494–512

Lynn JG, Zwemer RL, Chick AJ, Miller AE (1942) A new method for the generation and use of focused ultrasound in experimental biology. J Gen Physiol 26:179–193

Madersbacher S, Pedevilla M, Vingers L, Susani M, Marberger M (1995) Effect of high-intensity focused ultrasound on human prostate cancer in vivo. Cancer Res 55:3346–3351

Moritz AR, Henriques FCJ (1947) Studies of thermal injury. II. The relative importance of time and surface temperature in the causation of cutaneous burns. Am J Pathol 23:695–720

Rosenschein U, Bernstein JJ, DiSegni E, Kaplinsky E, Bernheim J, Rozenzsajn LA (1990) Experimental ultrasonic angioplasty: disruption of atherosclerotic plaques and thrombi in vitro and arterial recanalization in vivo. IEEE Trans Ultrason Ferroelectr Freq Contr 43:1043–1053

Sapareto SA, Dewey WC (1984) Thermal dose determination in cancer therapy. Int J Radiat Oncol Biol Phys 10:787–800

Siegel RJ, Cumberland DC, Myler RK, DonMichael TA (1989) Percutaneous ultrasonic angioplasty: initial clinical experience. Lancet 2 (8666) 722–774

Smith NB, Webb AG, Ellis DS, Wilmes LJ, O'Brien WD (1995) Experimental verification of theoretical in vivo ultrasound heating using cobalt detected magnetic resonance. IEEE Trans. Ultrason Ferroelectr Freq Contr 42:489–491

Smith SW, Phillips DJ, von Ramm OT, Thurstone FL (1977) Some advances in acoustic imaging through skull. In: Hazzard DG, Litz ML (eds) Symposium on biological effects and characterizations of ultrasound sources. Food and Drug Administration, Department of Health, Education and Welfare, Rockville, MA, pp 37–52

Stepanow B, Huber P, Brix G, Debus J, Bader R, van Kaick G, Lorenz WJ (1995) Fast MRI temperature monitoring: application in focused ultrasound therapy of malignant tissue in vivo. Proc SMR 3rd Meeting, ISSN 1065–9889 2:1172

Suzuki T, Fujimoto K, Aida S et al. (1995) MRI monitoring during high-intensity focused ultrasound treatment Proc SMR 3rd Meeting, ISSN 1065–9889, 2:1177

Takayama N, Itoh T (1989) Investigation of ultrasonic heating with a non-axial symmetric acoustic lens. In: Sugahara T, Saito M (eds) Proceedings, 5th Int. Symp. Hyperthermic Oncology. Taylor & Francis, New York, pp 919–920

ter Haar GR, Daniels S, Eastaugh KC, Hill CR (1982) Ultrasonically induced cavitation in vivo. Br J Cancer 45: 151–155

Thomas J-L, Fink MA (1996) Ultrasonic beam focusing through tissue inhomogeneities with a time reversal mirror: application to transskull therapy. IEEE Trans Ultrason Ferroelectr Freq Contr 43:1122–1129

Umemura S, Yumita N, Nishigaki R, Umemura K (1989) Sonochemical activation of hematoporphyrin: a potential modality for cancer treatment. Proc IEEE Ultrasonics Symp 955–960

Vallancien G, Chartier-Kastler E, Bataille N, Chopin D, Harouni M, Bougaran J (1993) Focused extracorporeal pyrotherapy. Eur Urol 23:48–52

Vykhodtseva NI, Hynynen K, Damianou C (1995) Histologic effects of high intensity pulsed ultrasound exposure with subharmonic emission in rabbit brain in vivo. Ultrasound Med Biol 21:969–979

Wells PNT (1977) Biomedical ultrasound, Academic Press, Boston

Zimmer JE, Hynynen K, He DS, Marcus FI (1995) The feasibility of using ultrasound for cardiac ablation. IEEE Trans Biomed Eng 42:891–897

24 MR-Guided Cryotherapy

J. TACKE[1] and R. SPEETZEN[2]

CONTENTS

24.1 Introduction

Cryotherapy is a well-known method of tissue ablation in medicine. In general, the procedure is based on the contact or proximity of a cryoprobe to the target tissue. When a cooling agent or cryogen is circulated through the cryoprobe, the water content of the tissue within a certain distance of the probe begins to freeze. After a period of freezing, cryogen flow is stopped and the tissue is allowed to thaw. After removal of the probe, the previously frozen tissue is left in situ to be disposed of by an inflammatory scarring process. The origins of this kind of treatment go back to the mid-1850s, when iced saline solution was used to treat advanced breast and cervix carcinoma, which resulted in pain relief and tumor size reduction (BIRD 1949). Further advances in cryotherapy, however, did not take place until colder cryogens were developed. Between 1870 and 1900, when liquefaction of air became possible, the treatment of various skin diseases including skin cancer was reported. Much later, between 1950 and 1960, invasive cryotherapy techniques using cooled alcohol were developed to freeze cerebral tumors during craniotomy (ROWBOTHAM et al. 1959). Modern cryotherapy is based to a great extent on the development of automated cryosurgical instruments using liquid nitrogen (COOPER et al. 1963). At present, cryotherapy is a widely used ablation technique in superficial organs (ophthalmology, dermatology), in endoscopically accessible regions (pulmonology, gastroenterology) and during surgery (urology, hepatic surgery). The major advantages of this ablation technique are as follows: (1) The therapeutic effect is limited to ice formation in or near the target lesion, so there are no long-term side effects as with irradiation or chemotherapy. (2) One can regulate precisely the extent of the cytotoxic effect of cryotherapy. (3) No toxic or reactive by-products are created during freezing or thawing of the target lesion. (4) The bleeding risk in cryotherapy is low compared to other surgical or nonsurgical ablation techniques.

In several experimental studies (GILBERT et al. 1992; MATSUMOTO et al. 1992; RUBINSKI et al. 1993), MRI has been shown to be an excellent tool for imaging of iceball extension during freezing. Although still experimental, MRI of cryotherapy has some important advantages over ultrasound and CT. It has multiplanar imaging capabilities, allowing the operator to choose an anatomically optimal field of view of the treated area. It is less operator dependent than ultrasound and has superior soft tissue contrast, which provides better characterization of the target lesion during treatment and follow-up studies, MRI is highly sensitive to temperature and water content. In particular, MRI can accurately differentiate frozen from nonfrozen tissue. Due to an extremely short T2 relaxation time (MATSUMOTO et al. 1992), frozen tissues exhibit a signal void on MR images, whereas the adjacent tissue remains visible.

24.2 Mechanisms of Freezing Damage

The principle of cryotherapy is based upon tissue necrosis, which is induced by rapid freezing of a limited tissue volume. The exact mechanism(s) by which freezing causes damage are still being dis-

J. TACKE, MD, Department of Diagnostic Radiology, Aachen University of Technology, Pauwelsstrasse 30, 52057 Aachen, Germany
R. SPEETZEN, BEng, Helmholtz Institute for Biomedical Engineering, Aachen University of Technology, Pauwelsstrasse 20, 52057 Aachen, Germany

cussed (Rubinsky et al. 1987, 1990). If there is a high cooling rate (i.e., a rapid temperature decrease), intracellular ice causes damage to the intracellular structures directly. At lower cooling rates, extracellular ice causes dehydration of the surrounding cells. Due to the resultant osmotic shift, small vessels may expand to twice their normal diameter. This destroys the structural integrity of the vascular system and deprives those cells which have escaped direct cryotherapy damage of their blood supply. In addition, cryotherapy-induced thrombosis of smaller vessels further augments this ischemic damage mechanism. A final postulated mechanism is direct mechanical disintegration of tissue structure. Important factors controlling the extent of tissue damage are the cooling rate and the lowest temperature. The cooling rate is limited by the cryogen and the design of the apparatus. Thus, only empirical data exist for the optimum cooling rate which is estimated to be 100°C/min (Gage et al. 1982). In experiments in vitro, the lethal temperature for liver tissue (i.e., the temperature at which 100% of the frozen cells are damaged) has been found to be -50°C (Gage et al. 1985). The histological outcome of freezing damage is coagulation necrosis. In the liver, after an inflammatory phase of approximately 7 days the total extent of the lesion is visible and the scarring process begins. Dermatological and ophthalmological cryotherapy results have shown that the scarring process following freezing damage is very moderate and cosmetically benign.

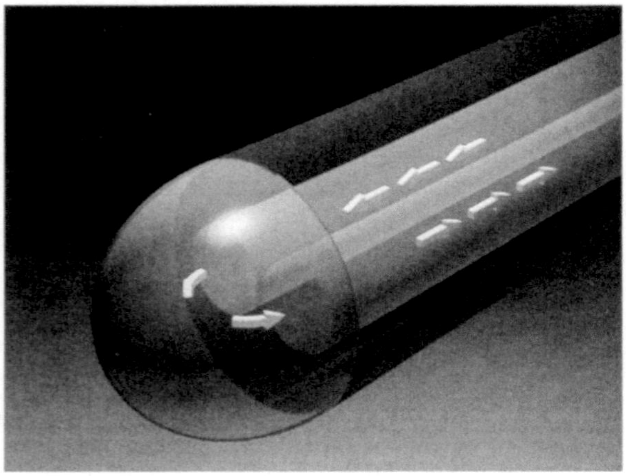

Fig. 24.1. Schematic model of the tip of the liquid nitrogen-cooled, MR-compatible glass probe. *Arrows* indicate the flow direction of the cryogen within the inner lumens towards and from the noninsulated tip. The outer lumen provides vacuum insulation

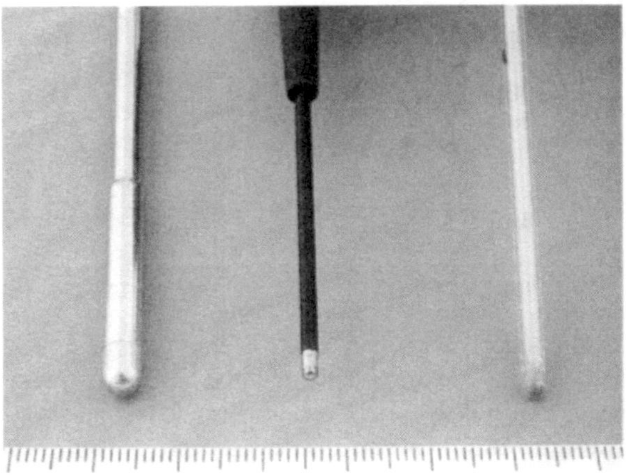

Fig. 24.2. Different probes for interstitial cryotherapy. *Left*: Nitrogen-cooled, vacuum-insulated stainless steel cryoprobe with a brass tip (diameter of the tip 5 mm, SMT, Praha, Czech Republic). *Middle*: Nitrous oxygen-cooled probe with a stainless steel tip. No vacuum isolation. (Diameter of the tip 2 mm, Erbe, Tübingen, Germany). *Right*: Nitrogen-cooled, vacuum-isolated glass probe. (Overall diameter 3 mm, designed by the Helmholtz Institute for Biomedical Engineering, Aachen University of Technology, Aachen, Germany). This probe is an updated model of the probe that was used in the study. The study probe had a slightly conical shape and the diameter at the tip was 3.5 mm

24.3 Experimental MR-Guided Cryotherapy of the Liver

24.3.1 Materials and Methods

MR-Compatible Cryoprobe. In order to combine minimally invasive cryotherapy with the imaging capabilities of MRI, a percutaneously insertable, MR-compatible and nitrogen-cooled cryoprobe was developed (Speetzen et al. 1997; Tacke et al. 1997). The cryoprobe was built of glass and contains three lumens (Figs. 24.1, 24.2): Inflow and outflow of liquid nitrogen were performed using the inner two lumens. The outer lumen, which encased the probe except for its tip, provided vacuum isolation. The probe length was 70 mm and the diameter at the noninsulated tip 3.5 mm. The liquid nitrogen lumens were connected via thermally insulated PTFE (polytetrafluoroethylene) tubes to a commercially available liquid nitrogen source and to an open collecting receptacle. In order to shorten the cooling time of the tube system, a bypass valve was placed between the supply tube and the exhaust tube 50 cm in front of the probe. The system pressure, which was kept below a maximum value of 5 bar, was regulated manually by a second valve in the supply tube. The cooling capacity of the cryoprobe was measured to be 12 (±1) W in water at a temperature of 37°C. The cryoprobe system was fixed to the table by a custom-made apparatus which was freely adjustable and thus allowed fixation of the probe in any position within the magnet.

In-Vivo Study. In order to test the feasibility of this new probe, a study was carried out in ten female chinchillas. General anesthesia was used for all procedures. All interventions and examinations were performed using a 1.5-T Gyroscan ACS-NT system (Philips, Best, The Netherlands), and a receive-only surface coil with a diameter of 13 cm. The system has an additional console on the magnet itself, which allows the operator to start a preloaded sequence at the magnet. In-room monitors permit the operator to observe MR images at the magnet. Planning of the approach to the liver, percutaneous insertion of the probe, and image control during freezing and thawing were performed using a gradient echo sequence (TR/TE/FA = 15/5.4/25°, slice thickness 5 mm, FOV 195×195 mm, 141×256 matrix). During the freezing procedure, images were obtained every 3 s by manually starting each scan at the magnet. After cooling the supply tube, the bypass valve was closed and the liquid nitrogen was allowed to flow through the probe. Because maximum iceball size was achieved after 1 min of freezing, duration of the freezing procedure was limited to 3 min. The increase in size of the iceball and its subsequent decrease after shut off of the liquid nitrogen supply were monitored by the same gradient echo scans. The freeze/thaw cycle was repeated three times per animal without changing the probe position and with a 5-min delay between cycles. Follow-up examinations were performed 3 and 7 days after cryotherapy using axial T1 and T2-weighted spin echo (SE) sequences (T1: TR/TE/FOV = 550/20/175, slice thickness 2 mm; T2: 1800/100/170, slice thickness 3 mm, 410×512 matrix), respectively. T1-weighted SE imaging was repeated after a bolus injection of gadopentetate dimeglumine (Magnevist, Schering, Berlin, Germany) at a dosage of 0.1 mmol/kg body weight. Seven days after cryotherapy, all animals were killed and the livers resected, sectioned, and stained with hematoxylin eosin (HE) and trichrome (Goldner and Masson) stains. In each animal, the lesions were analyzed as to their gross pathological and histological appearance and correlated with the MR image data.

24.3.2 Results

MR-guided cryotherapy was performed successfully in all animals. No complications occurred during placement of the probe or during the freezing procedure. Neither the cryoprobe nor the fixation device caused artifacts on gradient echo imaging. The average precooling time of the liquid nitrogen supply tube was 1 min. The inactive probe appeared hypointense (Fig. 24.3A, B). After a freezing time of approximately 1 min, maximum iceball size was between 9 and 12 mm in diameter (mean 11.8 mm; Fig. 24.3C, D). There was no MR- or histologically visible ice formation along the insulated probe shaft. In follow-up scans 3 days after freezing, the liver lesions appeared hyperintense on T2-weighted SE images, which has been found to represent an edematous reaction of liver tissue after freezing (Matsumoto et al. 1993). On plain T1-weighted SE images, the lesions were nearly invisible or, at most, slightly hyperintense. After injection of Gd-DTPA, the rim of the lesions showed a slight signal increase. Seven days after freezing, the lesions appeared only slightly hyperintense on the T2-weighted SE sequences as the edema dissipated. The signal on the plain T1-weighted SE images was also decreased. After contrast administration, the rim of the lesions showed a strong signal increase that enabled precise delineation between the lesion and normal liver (Fig. 24.4). The lesion center showed no contrast enhancement. Histologically, the lesions had the appearance of areas of coagulation necrosis with preserved, but nonvital (i.e., without intact nuclei) cellular architecture. All blood vessels less than 0.5 mm in diameter with perivascular connective tissue were not damaged. At the rim of the lesions, a thin wall of granulation tissue with neovascularity and regenerating bile ducts was found.

This granulation tissue correlated exactly with the contrast-enhancing tissue layer on the contrast-enhanced T1-weighted SE images. The parenchymal cells, intracellular architecture, and blood vessels in the surrounding liver were not affected. Maximum iceball diameter and the size of the lesions 3 and 7 days after freezing as seen on MR scans agreed very well with the extent of histological necrosis. No statistically significant differences (Wilcoxon test for unpaired samples) were seen between the size of the iceballs, the size of the lesions on MR images and the size of the lesions on histological examination.

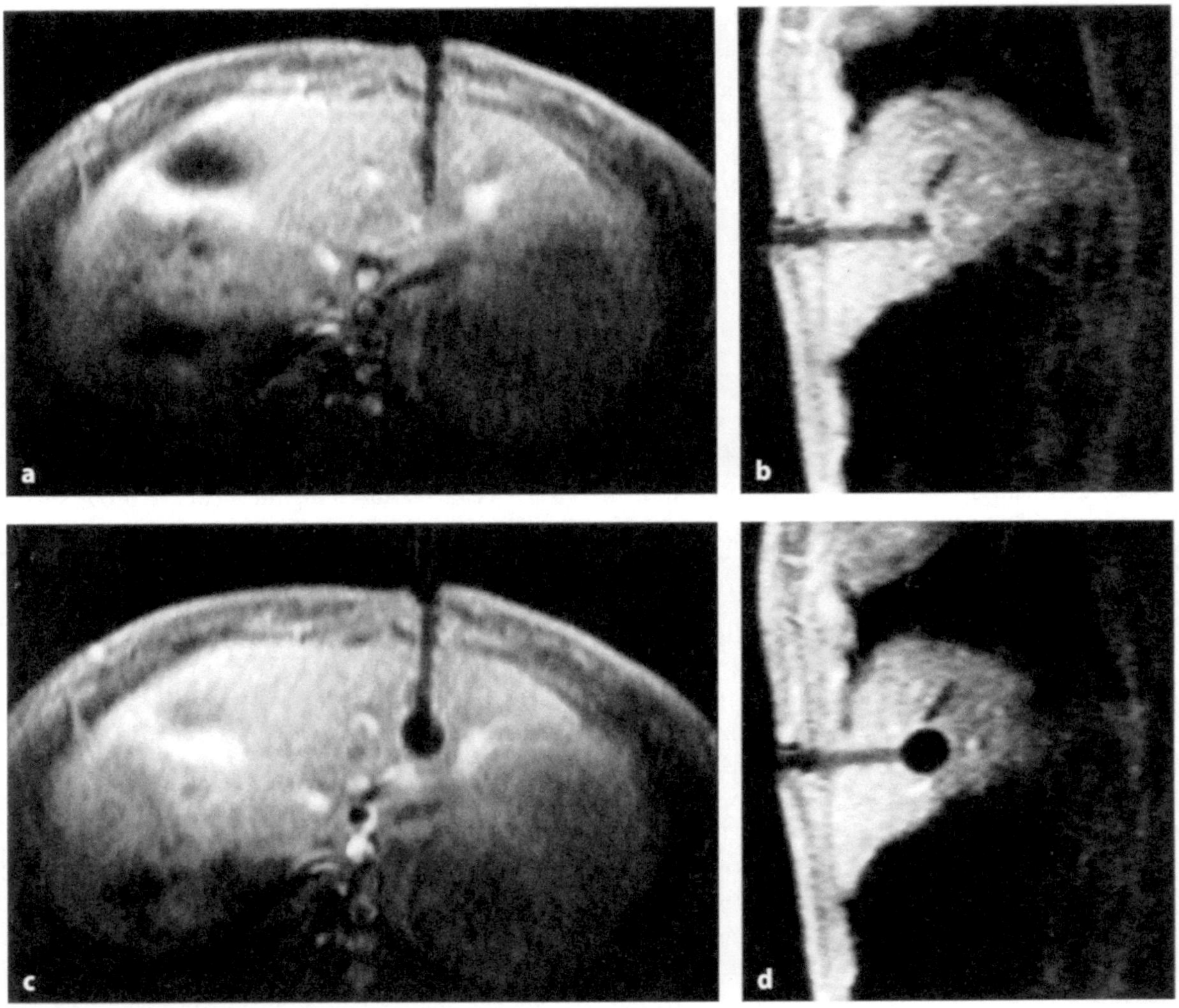

Fig. 24.3. a, b. Inactive probe within liver tissue. Gradient echo sequence (TR/TE/FA/FOV = 15/5.4/24°/195, slice thickness 5 mm). **a** Axial, **b** sagittal cross section with the cryoprobe in situ. **c, d** Cryoprobe and hypointense ice ball (diameter 9.1 mm) after 1 min of freezing. Gradient echo sequence (TR/TE/FA/FOV = 15/5.4/25°/195, slice thickness 5 mm). **C** Axial, **D** sagittal cross section with the cryoprobe in situ

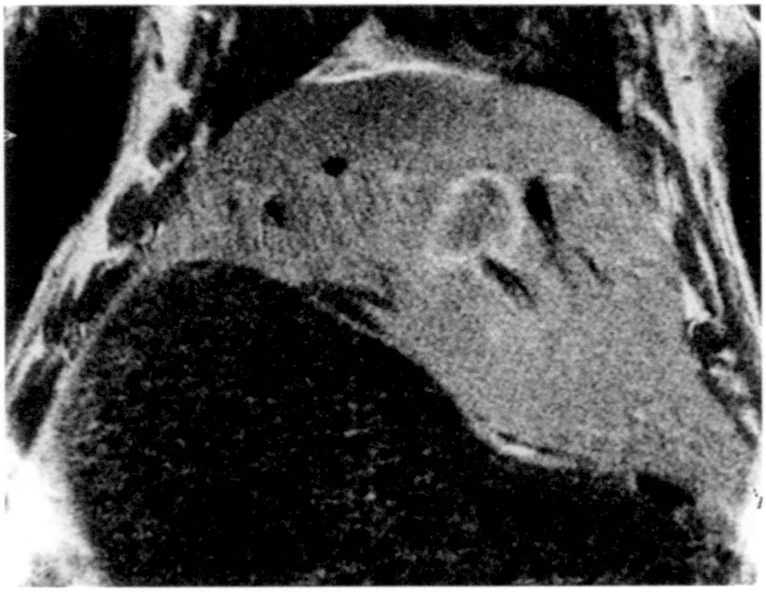

Fig. 24.4. Follow-up 7 days after the freezing procedure. T1-weighted spin echo sequence (TR/TE/FOV = 550/20/175) after bolus injection of gadopentetate dimeglumine (0.1 mmol/kg body weight). A strong signal increase is seen at the rim of the lesion, whereas the center is hypointense compared to the normal enhanced liver tissue. Histologically, the rim corresponds to a thin granulation tissue layer between coagulation necrosis and adjacent vital liver tissue

24.3.3 Discussion

24.3.3.1 Imaging of Cryotherapy

Ultrasound. The most common method of imaging interstitial cryotherapy is ultrasound. Originally described by Onik et al. in 1986, the method is based on the altered echogenicity of frozen tissue. During freezing, the growth of the iceball appears sonographically as a hyperechoic rim with posterior acoustic shadowing. This is due to the complete reflection of the ultrasound waves at the interface of nonfrozen tissue and the iceball. Thus, the tissues and the part of the iceball posterior to the "leading edge" of the iceball remain invisible. Depending on the tissue type and the location of the target lesion, it may be necessary to scan the ice formation from several different projections. Numerous reports about ultrasound as a monitoring system for cryotherapy in the liver (Gilbert et al. 1985; Ravikumar et al. 1987; Onik et al. 1991) and the prostate (Onik et al. 1993; Miller et al. 1994) have confirmed the clinical value of this method. The main advantage of ultrasound as an imaging tool for cryotherapy is its high temporal resolution which permits instantaneous redirection of the freezing procedure as needed. The primary disadvantages are low spatial resolution for deeper structures and non-visualization of tissue posterior to the iceball. These disadvantages are less significant during intraoperative cryotherapy, where the target lesion is less distant and the difficult of changing scan direction around the organ surface is minimized. They may however prevent a percutaneous approach.

Computed Tomography. Another possibility of imaging interstitial cryotherapy is computed tomography. As originally described by Reiser et al. in 1983, the phase shift of water from liquid to solid state appears on CT as a decrease in density. In experimental studies of the brain, the difference in density between frozen and unfrozen tissue was approximately 80 Hounsfield units (Moser et al. 1987). In a clinical case report about percutaneous cryotherapy of a pelvic tumor (Saliken et al. 1996), the attenuation value for the frozen tissue was approximately 30 Hounsfield units. However, the delineation of the interface between ice and adjacent tissue seems less precise on CT scans than with ultrasound. Moreover, CT image quality during cryotherapy is diminished by the artifacts caused by metal probes. As a result, CT has played a minor role as a monitoring modality for cryotherapy.

MRI. The technique of MR monitoring was originally described in 1989 by Isoda, who monitored the freezing of the thighs of rats with a liquid nitrogen-drenched gauze pad. Probably because this contribution was in Japanese, greater attention was paid to the reports of Gilbert et al. (1992), Matsumoto et al. (1992), and Rubinsky et al. (1993). Gilbert and coworkers performed cryotherapy of rabbit brains using an experimental cryoprobe under MR control. They used conical Pyrex centrifuge tubes with two lumens for inflow and outflow of the cryogen that were placed on the surface of the brain after surgical exposure. The probe used by Matsumoto and coworkers was made of a polystyrene cup in which there was a small aluminum foil "window" that was placed in contact with the surface of the surgically exposed rabbit livers. Both systems allowed artifact-free MRI of the freezing process but were limited to a superficial approach to the organs. Both groups reported well-delineated, signal-free ice formation on T1-weighted spin echo sequences, gradient echo sequences, and T1-weighted RARE sequences. The histological analysis of the frozen brain and liver showed well-delineated coagulation necrosis which corresponded nicely to the frozen region on MRI. Rubinsky et al. (1993) performed cryotherapy of a dog's prostate percutaneously using a three-lumen, liquid nitrogen-cooled brass probe. Although the probe caused susceptibility artifacts on MR scans, the signal-free ice formation within the prostate was larger in size than the artifact. In order to predict the outcome of cryotherapy more precisely, the group of Hong et al. reported in 1994 on a quantitative MRI technique that calculated and displayed the temperature distribution in the frozen region, which is homogeneously signal-free on standard MR images.

24.3.3.2 Applications of Interstitial Cryotherapy

Liver. Cryotherapy of the liver has been shown to be a useful and potentially complete ablative technique for liver metastases and primary liver tumors. In studies of more than 100 patients with primary unresectable hepatic carcinomas, the safety and efficacy of cryotherapy were clearly demonstrated (Ravikumar et al. 1987, Zhou et al. 1989). Depending on the location of the tumor, the cryoprobe is put on the organ surface adjacent to the tumor or, in less superficial cases, placed into the center of the tumor via a trocar technique. Placement of the probe and monitoring of the freezing procedure were first performed under sonographic control by ONIK et al. in 1986. Until recently, hepatic cryotherapy has been performed during laparotomy due to the lack of cryoprobes with a high cooling capacity and a sufficiently small diameter. In this context, the term "interstitial" is misleading, because it implies a minimally invasive approach. To the best of our knowledge, no percutaneous hepatic cryotherapy in humans has been reported to date.

Prostate. Cryotherapy of the prostate is a well-established ablation technique for prostate cancer. It is usually performed by a percutaneous, perineal or transurethral approach under endorectal sonographic guidance (ONIK et al. 1993). Reports about percutaneous cryotherapy of prostate cancer include series of 210 patients and more (MILLER et al. 1994; BAHN et al. 1995). The primary advantage of this minimally invasive technique is the low rate of complications and side effects compared to radical prostatectomy.

Brain. Except for some isolated reports (TSYMBALIUK 1995), cryotherapy of the has been an uncommon ablation technique in modern neurosurgery. This is presumably not a result of lesser efficacy for cryotherapy, but rather a consequence of substantial improvement in modern microsurgical techniques. Experimental studies have shown that interstitial cryotherapy of the brain results in a sharply demarcated region of coagulation necrosis which corresponds to the iceball size seen either with ultrasound (QUIGLEY et al. 1992) or CT (MOSER et al. 1987).

24.4 Conclusion

At present, MR-guided interstitial cryotherapy remains experimental. It has been shown that minimally invasive cryotherapy and MR monitoring can be successfully combined. Moreover, because of the close correlation between iceball extension as seen on MRI and cryonecrosis and the potential for quantitative predictability of the extent of tissue necrosis, this combination holds great promise. If major problems of temperature-resistant materials and probe design are solved, this technique has the potential for clinical introduction in the near future. In the liver, the most likely indication would be for percutaneous therapy of liver metastases or primary liver neoplasms, when surgical management is refused or impossible. Another target organ could be the brain. Based on the experience with stereotactic interventions, MR-guided cryotherapy could make a significant contribution to the field of minimally invasive neurosurgery of cerebral neoplasms. However, the next step in the evolution of MR-guided therapy must be the development of safe, biocompatible probes with increased cooling capacity.

References

Bahn DK, Lee F, Solomon MH, Gontina H, Klionsky DL, Lee FT (1995) Prostate cancer: US-guided percutaneous cryoablation. Radiology 194:551–556

Bird HM (1949) James Arnott, M.D. (Aberdeen) 1797–1883: A pioneer in refrigeration analgesia. Anaesthesia 4:10–17

Boethius J, Greitz T, Kyulenstierna R, et al (1984) Stereotactic cryosurgery in a CT scanner. Acta Neurochir Suppl (Wien) 33:553–557

Charnley RM, Doran J, Morris DL (1989) Cryotherapy for liver metastasis: a new approach. Br J Surg 76:1040–1041

Cooper IS (1963) Cryogenic surgery: a new method of destruction or extirpation of benign or malignant tissues. N Engl J Med 268:743–749

Fraunfelder F, Zacarian S, Wingfield D, Limmer B (1984) Results of cryotherapy for eyelid malignancies. Am J Ophthalmol 97:184–188

Gage AA, Montes M (1982) Destruction of hepatic and splenic tissue by freezing and heating. Cryobiology 19:172–179

Gage AA, Guest K, Montes M, Caruana JA, Whalen DA (1985) Effect of varying freezing and thawing rates in experimental cryosurgery. Cryobiology 22:175–182

Gilbert JC, Onik GM, Hoddick WK, Rubinsky B (1985) Real time ultrasonic monitoring of hepatic cryosurgery. Cryobiology 22:319–330

Gilbert JC, Roos MS, Wong STS, Brennan KM, Rubinsky B (1992) NMR monitored cryosurgery in the rabbit brain. In: Proceedings of The Society for Magnetic Resonance in Medicine, Berlin, p 1010

Gilbert JC, Rubinsky B, Roos MS, Wong STS, Brennan KM (1993) MRI-monitored cryosurgery in the rabbit brain. Magn Reson Imaging 11:1155–1164

Heberer G, Denecke H, Demmel N, Wirsching R (1987) Local procedures in the management of rectal cancer. World J Surg 11:499–503

Homasson J, Renault P, Angebault M, et al. (1986) Bronchoscopic cryotherapy for airway strictures caused by tumors. Chest 90:159–163

Homasson JP, Thiery JP, Angebault M, Ovtracht O, Maiwand O (1994) The operation and efficacy of cryosurgical, nitrous oxide-driven cryoprobe. Cryobiology 31:290–304

Hong JS, Wong S, Pease G, Rubinsky BV (1994) MR imaging assisted temperature calculations during cryosurgery. Magn Reson Imaging 12:1021–1031

Isoda H (1989) Sequential MRI and CT monitoring in cryosurgery – an experimental study in rats. Nippon Igaku Hoshasen Gakkai Zasshi 49:1499–1508 (in Japanese)

Kuflik EG, Gage AA (1990) Cryosurgical treatment for skin cancer. Igaku-Shoin, New York, pp 243–248

Matsumoto R, Oshio K, Jolesz FA (1992) Monitoring of laser and freezing-induced ablation in the liver with T1-weighted MR imaging. J Magn Reson Imaging 2:55–562

Matsumoto R, Selig AM, Colucci VM, Jolesz FA (1993) MR monitoring during cryotherapy in the liver: predictability of histologic outcome. J Magn Reson Imaging 3:770–776

Miller RJ, Cohen JK, Merlotti LA (1994) Percutaneous transperineal cryosurgical ablation of the prostate for the primary treatment of clinical stage C adenocarcinoma of the prostate. Urology 44:170–174

Moser RP, Abbott IR, Stephens CL, Lee YY (1987) Computerized tomographic imaging of cryosurgical iceball formation in brain. Cryobiology 24:368–375

Onik G, Kane R, Steele G, et al. (1986) Monitoring hepatic cryosurgery with sonography. AJR Am J Roentgenol 14:665–669

Onik G, Rubinsky B, Zemel R, Weaver L, Diamond D, Cobb C, Porterfield B (1991) Ultrasound-guided hepatic cryosurgery in the treatment of metastatic colon carcinoma. Cancer 67:901–907

Onik G, Cohen JK, Reyes GD, Rubinsky B, Chang ZH, Baust J (1993) Transrectal ultrasound-guided percutaneous radical cryosurgical ablation of the prostate. Cancer 7:1291–1299

Quigley MR, Lesch DV, Shih T, Marquardt M, Lupetin A, Maroon JC (1992) Intracranial cryosurgery in a canine model: a pilot study. Surg Neurol 38:101–105

Ravikumar TS, Kane R, Cady B, et al. (1987) Hepatic cryosurgery with intraoperative ultrasound monitoring for metastatic colon carcinoma. Arch Surg 122:403–409

Ravikumar TS, Steele G, Kane R, King V (1991) Experimental and clinical observations on hepatic cryosurgery for colorectal metastases. Cancer Res 51:6323–6327

Reiser M, Drukier AK, Ulzsch B, et al (1983) The use of CT in monitoring cryosurgery. Eur J Radiol 3:123–128

Rowbotham GF, Haigh AL, Leslie WG (1959) Cooling canula for use in the treatment of cerebral neoplasms. Lancet 1:12–15

Rubinsky B, Lee CY, Bastacky J, Hayes TL (1987) The mechanism of freezing in biological tissue: the liver. Cryo Letters 8379–8381

Rubinsky B, Lee CY, Bastacky J, Onik G (1990) The process of freezing and the mechanism of damage during hepatic cryosurgery. Cryobiology 27:85–97

Rubinsky B, Gilbert JC, Onik G, Roos MS, Wong STS, Brennan KM (1993) Monitoring cryosurgery in the brain and in the prostate with proton NMR. Cryobiology 30:191–199

Saliken JC, McKinnon JG, Gray R (1996) CT for monitoring cryotherapy. AJR Am J Roentgenol 166:853–855

Shields J, Parsons H, Shields C, Giblin M (1989) The role of cryotherapy in the management of retinoblastoma. Am J Ophthalmol 108:260–264

Speetzen R, Heschel I, Fischer A, et al. (1997) Interstitielle Kryotherapie im Kernspintomographen. Ki Luft Kältetechnik 2:71–73

Tacke J, Adam G, Speetzen R, et al. (1997) MR-guided interstitial cryotherapy of the liver with a novel, nitrogen cooled cryoprobe. Magn Reson Med (in press)

Tsymbaliuk VI (1995) Cryotherapy in neurosurgical practice. Oral presentation at World Congress Cryosurgery, 31 May–3 June 1995, Paris. CAP92 Sarl, Ville D'Avray, France

Zacarian S (1983) Cryosurgery for cutaneous carcinomas. An 18-year study of 3022 patients with 4228 carcinomas. J Am Acad Dermatol 9:947–956

Zhou XD, Tang ZY, Yu YQ, Ma ZC (1989) Clinical evaluation of cryosurgery in the treatment of primary liver cancer. Cancer 61:1889–1892

25 MR-Guided RF Treatment

J.S. Lewin and T.L. Boaz

CONTENTS

25.1 Introduction

Advances in imaging and interventional technology have profoundly impacted medical diagnosis over the past decade. Interventional imaging-based procedures have included percutaneous and stereotactic biopsy that have decreased the need for open surgical procedures and have resulted in a great reduction in patient morbidity, mortality and expense (Gazelle and Haaga 1989). MR has many advantages over the current standard guidance techniques. Lack of ionizing radiation exposure for both patient and operator, multiplanar imaging capability, and exquisite tissue contrast make MR an attractive alternative for procedure guidance. Until recently MR was not a feasible option owing to long imaging times and the difficulty in accessing the patient within a cylindrical imaging system. This has been overcome in the past several years with the advent of system hardware and pulse-sequence improvements that have allowed the development of rapid imaging on open-imaging systems (Jolesz and Blumenfield 1994; Schenck et al. 1995; Silverman et al. 1995; Kaufman et al. 1989; Grönemeyer et al. 1989, Duerk et al. 1996). The feasibility of MR as a guidance modality has depended upon the development of needles and probes that are undeflected by the magnetic field and that create little or no field distortions or image degradation (Lufkin et al. 1987, 1988; Wenokur et al. 1992). Other innovations that have made MR an attractive guidance alternative include the in-room liquid crystal display (LCD) monitor and frameless stereotactic localization systems which allow interactive scan-plane manipulation analogous to real-time ultrasound imaging (Lewin et al. 1996b). These advances have stimulated the development of MR-guided interventional techniques.

25.2. Interventional MR

To date, clinical applications of MR-guided interventional techniques have been divided into diagnostic and therapeutic procedures. Diagnostic procedures have included biopsy, aspiration, and joint injection prior to MR arthrography (Lewin 1996a; Duckwiler et al. 1989; Silverman et al. 1995; Lufkin et al. 1987; Petersilge et al. 1996). Therapeutic procedures have been more varied. Much of the effort in the development of MR-guided therapy has concentrated on local cancer treatment through percutaneous MR-guided thermal or chemical tumor ablation. These techniques have significant potential to produce complete destruction of local tumor. Other centers have concentrated on the use of MR imaging in an operating room environment to guide surgery. In addition to the excellent soft tissue contrast and multiplanar capabilities of MR, the vascular conspicuity afforded by gradient-echo MR techniques also offers an advantage in many of these applications.

J.S. Lewin, MD, Department of Radiology, Case Western Reserve University, University Hospitals of Cleveland, 11100 Euclid Avenue, Cleveland, OH 44106, USA
T.L. Boaz, MD, Department of Radiology, Case Western Reserve University, University Hospitals of Cleveland, 11100 Euclid Avenue, Cleveland, OH 44106, USA

The diagnostic utility of MR is well documented. The exquisite detail, tissue contrast, and pathologic tissue conspicuity of MR is unrivaled. These strengths in conjunction with the development of open-imaging systems and MR-compatible needles have allowed interventional radiologists to perform many diagnostic procedures that would have been previously difficult if not impossible. Independence from the need for iodinated contrast agents is yet another advantage of MR-guided intervention. This allows accurate needle guidance while providing information regarding tissue vascularity and avoiding vessels.

The main focus of therapeutic interventional MR has been in the minimally invasive treatment of cancer and cancer metastases. Regional metastasis may be the only life-threatening component of disease in many patients. For example, of the 160 000 patients newly diagnosed with colorectal carcinoma each year, approximately 24 000 have metastatic disease at the time of diagnosis, another 30 000–50 000 will subsequently develop metastases, and at least half of these patients ultimately die of their metastatic disease (NIEDERHUBER and ENSMINGER 1993; ALEXANDER et al. 1996). For many, progressive involvement of the liver will be a major or sole determinant of their survival (NIH Consensus Conference 1990; WOOD et al. 1976). For patients who are surgical candidates, resection of hepatic metastases has been shown to alter the natural history of the disease, increasing survival from a median of 6 months to a median of 20–30 months, with up to a 40% 5-year survival (NIEDERHUBER and ENSMINGER 1993; AUGUST et al. 1985). By demonstrating that effective local therapy can significantly improve the outcome in this group of patients, this provides a major motivation and working model supporting the development of methods for local therapy.

With growing experience in interventional MR, investigators have turned to MR as an effective means of guidance for the percutaneous destruction of neoplastic tissue. To date the use of chemotherapeutic or chemoablative substances and thermal energy tissue destruction have been investigated. Chemoactive agents include absolute alcohol and various chemotherapy drugs (LEWIN et al. 1996a). More recently, attention has focused on the delivery of thermal energy creating thermoablative lesions. Current thermoablative modalities include laser interstitial therapy, radiofrequency (RF) thermal ablation, focused ultrasound, and cryotherapy (ANZAI et al. 1991; GOLDBERG et al. 1995; CLINE et al. 1995; MATSUMOTO et al. 1993). This second subset of therapeutic options is perhaps the most exciting owing to the inherent capability of MR to monitor temperature fluctuations in addition to MR-apparent changes in tissue characteristics (HALL et al. 1990; LE BIHAN et al. 1989). Through the combination of MR-image monitoring of tumor destruction with minimally invasive methods for tumor destruction, such as laser interstitial thermal ablation, RF thermal ablation, focused ultrasound, alcohol injection, or cryotherapy, these new techniques have the potential to interactively visualize and direct the ablative procedure in order to ensure complete tumor destruction with an adequate margin. This is a major difference to other ablative techniques and could markedly alter the options available to patients who are not currently surgical candidates.

The addition of MR temperature monitoring and necrosis confirmation to interstitial thermal ablation was initially made in brain tumors, using both laser and RF generators as sources of heat (TOMLINSON et al. 1991; ANZAI et al. 1995). Preliminary clinical data have thus far been very encouraging. Temperature-sensitive MR sequences have also been developed to enable accurate on-line monitoring of heat deposition (VOGL et al. 1995). The relationship of MR signal intensity change to tissue temperature is a complex phenomenon, and precise MR measurement of temperature is difficult. However, the phase transition from viable to necrotic tissue can also be imaged using changes in the tissue relaxation parameters, T1 and T2, that occur in the process of necrosis (MATSUMOTO et al. 1992; BLEIER et al. 1991). The accuracy of MR findings in defining thermal lesion size has been repeatedly demonstrated using several different energy sources (ANZAI et al. 1992; MATSUMOTO et al. 1993; TRACZ et al. 1993).

25.3 RF Thermotherapy

Interstitial RF thermal ablation depends upon the transfer of electrical energy to tissue with the deposition of heat secondary to the increased resistivity of the intervening tissue substrate to the passage of rapidly alternating current (ARONOW 1960). This is achieved by passing RF energy from an RF generator through a shielded electrode with an exposed tip of variable length which has been placed within a focus of abnormal tissue. Tissue heated to 60 °C or above undergoes coagulative necrosis and can be considered adequately treated in thermal ablative techniques such as interstitial RF thermotherapy. RF therapy is not a new therapeutic modality, and it has been used with great success for over three decades within the neurosurgical community (ANZAI et al. 1995). The placement of RF electrodes in pathological tissue has typically been performed under direct visualization of stereotactic guidance based on preoperative CT data. Indications for this form of therapy have historically included cordotomy, pallidotomy, leukotomy, and thalamotomy for the treatment of intractable pain and involuntary movement disorders (SWEET et al. 1960; TEW and KELLER 1977; HITCHCOCK and TEIXEIRA 1981; BROGGI et al. 1985; LAITINEN et al. 1992; ROSOMOFF et al. 1965; NASHOLD and OSTDAHL 1979). More recently, investigators have used RF ablative therapy in the abdomen using ultrasound to direct therapy in the treatment of primary and secondary hepatic tumors (ROSSI et al. 1996; MCGAHAN et al. 1990, 1993). However, assessment of success or failure of treatment in this setting has been dependent on follow-up imaging, typically performed with contrast-enhanced CT.

Interstitial RF thermotherapy is an attractive treatment option for several reasons. As described above, this modality has a long history of use, and complications resulting from RF ablation are uncommon, with the coagulation effect of the heating process contributing to a very low incidence of hemorrhage in the central nervous system (ZERVAS and KUWAYAMA 1972; FARAHANI et al. 1995) and abdomen, based on our preliminary data and that of others (ROSSI et al. 1996; LEWIN 1997). The generating equipment necessary to create RF lesions is typically readily accessible, as it is well established within the neurosurgical community and is relatively inexpensive in comparison to laser light sources. Reproducible tissue destruction has been observed in a variety of tissues. Furthermore, studies in both humans and animals have shown that thermal lesion shape and size can be controlled through electrode design and the duration and magnitude of the energy delivered (ARONOW 1960; ZERVAS 1965; ZERVAS and KUWAYAMA 1972; FARAHANI et al. 1995; CHUNG et al. 1996). Energy deposition is easy to control with RF ablation and allows gradual heating (ZERVAS and KUWAYAMA 1972). The presence of a thermistor in the electrode tip gives continuous temperature feedback, while impedance measurements provide another parameter related to tissue changes at the ablation site. These features are of particular importance when destroying tumors adjacent to neurovascular structures. Unlike radiation therapy, interstitial RF thermal ablation, like other thermal ablative therapies, can be repeated over and over without concern for cumulative dose.

25.4 Interstitial RF Thermotherapy with MR Guidance

The use of interstitial RF thermotherapy under MR guidance is based on the direct destruction of tissue through the application of RF energy. The methodology differs significantly from the empirical approach typically used in neurosurgical applications of RF ablation technology, for which variations in lesion size and shape due to unanticipated thermal conduction during treatment cannot be predicted and are not usually recognized until follow-up imaging studies are performed. The major contribution of MR imaging is its outstanding ability to monitor the zone of thermal tissue destruction during the procedure and therefore to provide real-time guidance for deposition of the RF energy. Through MR monitoring, thermal lesion size and configuration can be directly controlled by the operator and adjusted during the procedure to compensate for deviations from preoperative predictions. MR is exceptionally well suited for this purpose due to its lack of ionizing radiation, excellent soft tissue discrimination, spatial resolution, and its sensitivity to temperature and blood flow (SCHENCK et al. 1995; CLINE et al. 1993, 1995). This not only permits accurate destruction of the tumor, including margins, but also extends the application of RF ablation to the safe destruction of tumor within visceral organs and adjacent to vital neurovascular structures. Furthermore, MR is not hampered by difficulties due to changes in tissue imaging charcteristics brought about by RF ablation as has been described by some authors using ultrasound guidance (ROSSI et al. 1996).

Until recently, MR-guided RF therapy has been limited by the inability to actively monitor the lesion as it is created. This is secondary to the inherent imaging interference caused by the RF source. New software and hardware modifications have recently been developed that allow RF energy to be deposited during imaging between the brief sampling periods of temperature-sensitive sequences, thereby maintaining tissue temperature while making interference-free, real-time monitoring possible (J.L. DUERK, personal communication 1997).

Other recent improvements include the development of a water-cooled RF electrode designed by GAZELLE and colleagues, in which the electrode is cooled by constant infusion of iced saline (GOLDBERG et al. 1996). While lesion length is dependent upon exposed tip length, lesion diameter was previously limited to approximately 2 cm (McGahan et al. 1993). This was thought to be due to charring at the electrode/tissue interface, which in turn impaired energy transfer. With the new water-cooled electrode, charring at the interface is prevented, allowing energy to be transmitted farther. With this form of energy deposition, a second application of RF energy may be necessary without cooling once the desired margins are achieved in order to destroy the area adjacent to the cooled electrode. Lesions can be created with this electrode design that would have required multiple ablations with intervening electrode repositioning with a standard RF electrode.

25.5 Technical Considerations

Interstitial RF thermotherapy monitored by MR has been performed in patients in two ways to date, either with RF electrode placement outside of the scanner in a neurosurgical stereotactic frame or with the RF electrode interactively placed under MR guidance in an open interventional system (Anzai et al. 1995; Lewin 1997). Technical requirements differ primarily with regard to the MR imager and interventional accessories, as detailed below. Once the electrode is placed, energy deposition and treatment monitoring are performed in a similar manner.

25.5.1 Interstitial RF Thermotherapy with Interactive Electrode Placement

The primary focus at our institution has been on minimally invasive interstitial RF thermotherapy of tumors of the liver and retroperitoneum with electrode placement performed under direct MR guidance within the MR imager. MR-guided electrode placement and monitoring of therapy is performed using a commercially available c-arm MR system (Magnetom Open, Siemens, Erlangen, Germany) supplemented with: (1) an in-room 1024 × 1280 LCD monitor; (2) in-room imager controls; (3) an optically linked frameless stereotaxy system (developed in collaboration with Radionics, Burlington, Mass. and Siemens Medical Systems, Erlangen, Germany) to interactively drive image acquisition; (4) a 50–100 W RF generator (Radionics, USA); and (5) an MR-compatible 17 cm × 2 mm shielded electrode with a 2- to 3-cm exposed tip with or without water cooling (Fig. 25.1).

Electrodes are placed in the liver or retroperitoneum under continuous imaging with automated acquisition, reconstruction, and display in 1 to 2 s/frame using short TR/short TE gradient-echo sequences. Either fast imaging with steady-state precession (FISP) or true-FISP sequence designs are applied, depending upon the tissue contrast necessary for tumor visualization. Using a standard non-perfused electrode, interstitial RF thermal ablation is performed at an electrode tip temperature of 85–90 °C for periods ranging from 6 to 20 min at each electrode location prior to repositioning for larger tumors. The ablation time at each location and electrode repositioning is based on MR imaging during the ablation session to achieve maximal ablation tissue necrosis for the MR-compatible electrode in use. Electrode repositioning is performed in the scanner in an interactive manner under continuous MR-image guidance similar to that used for initial electrode placement.

Multiplanar short inversion time inversion recovery (STIR) and T2-weighted imaging are performed prior to the procedure. These sequences are repeated intermittently during the ablation session to monitor thermal lesion size and configuration. Following ablation, they are repeated with the addition of gadopentetate dimeglumine-enhanced T1-weighted images to confirm the final zone of tissue destruction.

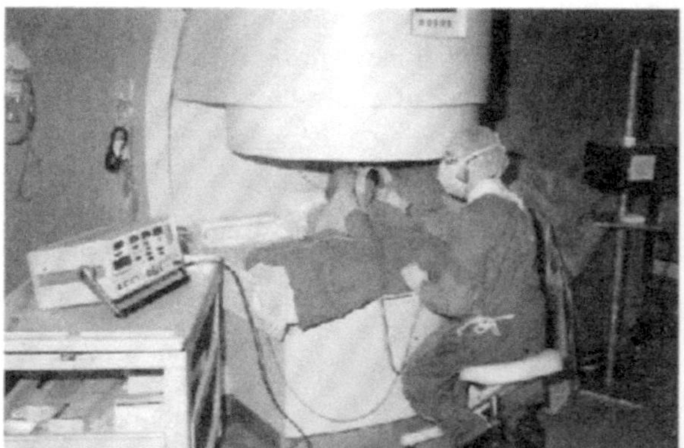

Fig. 25.1. Interventional MR suite. C-arm open imager allows access for radiofrequency (RF) electrode placement and manipulation while ablation is performed with the RF generator sitting adjacent to the MR imaging system. Anesthesia gases, surgical lighting, and an in-room LCD monitor facilitate electrode placement and thermal lesion generation

25.5.2 Interstitial RF Thermotherapy with Stereotactic Electrode Placement

The first reported use of RF thermotherapy monitored by MR imaging was at University of California at Los Angeles (UCLA) for the treatment of brain tumors. The initial series reported was performed on a standard "closed" superconducting imaging system with electrode placement being performed outside the gantry. Electrode placement was guided using an MR-compatible, stereotactic localizing device. The stereotactic coordinates were calculated using data from prior MR studies. After placement of the electrode, the patient was placed in the imager and RF lesions were created while the patient was awake in order to monitor for unwanted neurological changes. RF energy was applied heating brain tissue to approximately 80 °C for 1 min under MR observation. This was repeated until the desired lesion size was achieved. This technique has been used in the treatment of both primary and metastatic tumors (Anzai et al. 1995).

25.6 Current Experience

25.6.1 Animal Models

25.6.1.1 RF Thermal Brain Lesions

At UCLA, Farahani et al. (1995) monitored RF-induced thermal lesions in five rabbit brains with fast spin-echo T2-weighted images every 30 s for a period of 30 min. Analysis showed that MR accurately demonstrated temporal tissue changes induced by thermal ablation, with excellent histological correlation.

25.6.1.2 RF Thermal Hepatic Lesions

Experiments at our institution were performed to evaluate the detection and temporal evolution of heat deposition and in vivo tissue destruction during RF ablation under direct MR monitoring. Liver RF ablation thermal lesions were produced with a custom-designed MR-compatible electrode on a clinical 0.2-T scanner in a rabbit model under direct MR guidance. Heat deposition and thermal lesion extent were monitored with MR imaging during the procedure and for 20–40 min after treatment using phase-maps, T2-weighted (T2WI), and contrast-enhanced T1-weighted (T1WI) images (Fig. 25.2). Animals were sacrificed immediately following thermal lesion creation and pathological correlation was performed. Hepatic thermal lesions approaching 2 by 2–4 cm were produced, and it was possible to tailor thermal lesion size and shape under MR guidance. Tissue necrosis was marked by a ring of hyperintensity surrounding central hypointensity on T2WI and post-contrast T1W1, similar to the findings reported in the brain by Farahani et al. (1995). Correlation of MRI findings of tissue destruction with gross and histological analysis suggested that MR accurately guided electrode placement and predicted the size and shape of the region of tissue necrosis (Fig. 25.3; Boaz et al. 1996, 1997).

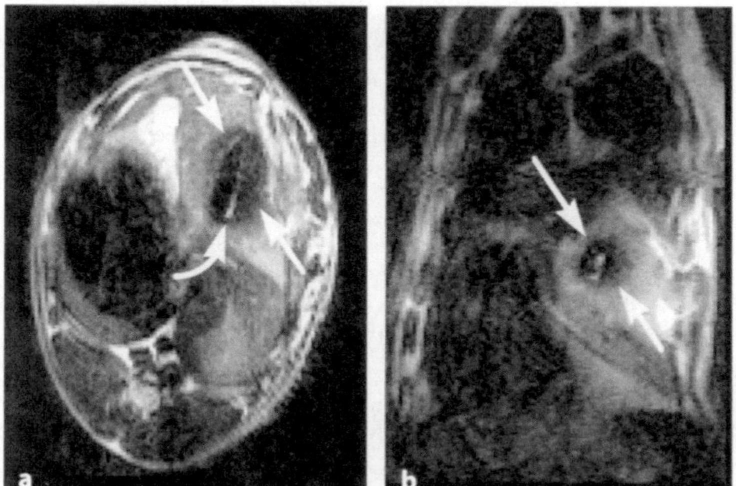

Fig. 25.2a,b. Rabbit model of hepatic ablation. **a** A T2-weighted axial image through the upper abdomen of a rabbit following hepatic RF thermal ablation. The thermal lesion demonstrates decreased signal intensity on this T2-weighted image, with its margins clearly demarcated (*straight arrows*). The 2-mm diameter RF electrode is identified within the central portion of the lesion (*curved arrow*). This is clearly separate from the remainder of the lesion. The electrode has minimal associated signal distortion and need not be removed to ascertain lesion size. **b** A T2-weighted coronal image through the upper abdomen of a rabbit following hepatic RF thermal ablation. The RF electrode is again identified centrally. A sharp lesion margin is present (*arrows*).

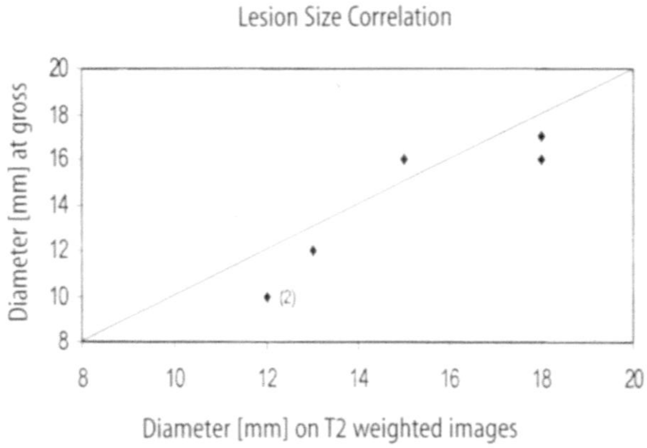

Fig. 25.3. A comparative plot of lesion size (in mm) as determined at gross evaluation and during procedure using T2-weighted images. As displayed, imaging diameter correlated well with actual diameter determined at gross. Estimated size was always within 2 mm. Imaging tends to slightly overestimate actual lesion size (modified with permission from BOAZ et al. 1997)

25.6.2 Clinical Experience

25.6.2.1 Abdomen and Pelvis

At our institution, eight tumors in six patients were treated during eight ablation sessions using this technique during 1996 as part of a phase I clinical trial. Five of the eight tumors treated were renal cell carcinoma metastases or local recurrence, two were metastic leiomyosarcoma, and one was an adenocarcinoma of unknown primary. Treated sites include the liver (n = 4), retroperitoneum (n = 2), diaphragmatic crus/abdominal wall (n = 1), and pelvis (n = 1). There were no technical failures or patient complications. Four tumors were considered >90% ablated at the time of the procedure; however, the length of follow-up is insufficient to confirm successful local control with reasonable confidence. In each tumor the region of tissue destruction could be accurately guided through sequential rapid T2WI and STIR images obtained during the ablation session and could be confirmed as an avascular zone or contrast-enhanced MR images obtained at the conclusion of the ablation session (Fig. 25.4; LEWIN 1996b; BOAZ et al. 1996). The maximal ablation size was an oblage spheroid of approximately 2.4 cm length and 2 cm diameter.

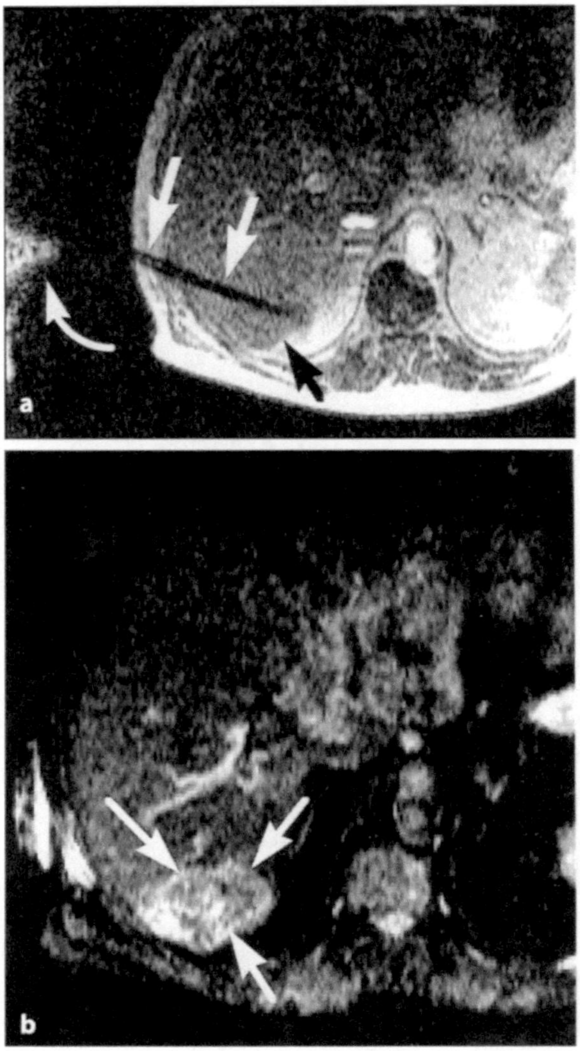

Fig. 25.4a,b. A 73-year-old patient with colon carcinoma metastatic to the liver. **a** Fast imaging in steady state procession (FISP; TR 17/TE 8, flip angle 90°) sequence used during interactive RF electrode insertion and manipulation. A single image from a series of images obtained during breath-hold at a frame rate of 2 s per image demonstrates the MR-compatible electrode (*straight white arrows*) being inserted into an exophytic mass in the posterior aspect of the right lobe of the liver (*black arrow*). The radiologist's hand can be seen advancing the electrode at the edge of the image (*curved arrow*). Delineation of the lesion was performed with T2-weighted images prior to RF electrode insertion. Currently, a true FISP sequence with T2 weighting is used for electrode insertion, with a frame rate of 1.5 s per frame for equivalent 128×256 resolution. The frame rate is often increased by using a rectangular field of view. **b** A short T1 inversion recovery axial image through the liver (TR 4470/TE 48, TI 110) demonstrates a central area of thermally induced necrosis which is decreased in signal intensity (*arrows*) and which is surrounded by increased signal consistent with edema. This pattern of signal changes correlates well with the experimental data in normal rabbit liver. Note is also made of a periportal metastasis on this image which was not treated during this RF thermal ablation session

Two weeks following the ablation session, tumors with greater than 50% volume ablation demonstrated a slight enlargement of the region of edema surrounding the central core of tissue necrosis, with subsequent reduction in tumor volume. In the patient with the longest follow-up thus far (9 months) there has been complete disappearance of the tumor on CT scan, with only minimal soft tissue distortion at the site of electrode placement on MR images. The remaining four tumors were incompletely ablated due to marked hypervascularity, size, or insufficient time to complete the procedure (LEWIN 1997).

No morbidity or toxicity has been encountered to date, although MR images obtained immediately following ablation have demonstrated a small amount of fluid adjacent to the liver in two patients following liver ablation, without associated symptoms, change in vital signs, or significant drop in hematocrit.

25.6.2.2
Brain

At UCLA, a total of 14 lesions in 12 patients were treated. Twelve of the tumors were metastases (adenocarcinoma $n = 6$, melanoma $n = 5$, and osteosarcoma $n = 1$), one was a glioblastoma multiforme, and one was an oligodendroglioma. Tumors ranged in size from 0.8 to 2.8 cm with an average of 1.3 cm. The tumors were treated for an average of 8.5 min with a range of 1–45 min. Five of the patients received adjuvant therapy (radiation $n = 3$, surgery $n = 1$, and chemotherapy $n = 1$). Reported follow-up ranged from 0.5 months to 10 months, with 4.1 months being average. In the brief follow-up no patients exhibited progression of the treated tumor; two did, however, develop new metastatic lesions elsewhere. Broca's aphasia complicated two treatments, one resolved completely, while the other patient had persistent speech difficulties (ANZAI et al. 1995).

25.6.3
Ultrasound-Guided RF Experience

As the follow-up period for MR-guided RF therapy is relatively short, comparison is made to the more established regimen of ultrasound-guided RF therapy. In a study using a very similar protocol of RF interstitial thermal ablation as performed at our institution, ROSSI et al. (1996) treated 50 patients with 41 hepatocellular carcinoma nodules and 13 metastatic hepatic nodules, with a mean follow-up of 22 months. Only 2 of the 50 patients treated demonstrated local recurrence at the treated site, although additional tumor nodules developed in other patients. The treatment appeared very well tolerated, without significant morbidity (ROSSI et al. 1996).

25.7
Conclusion

Radiofrequency therapy specifically has many intrinsic benefits, including ease of use, availability, low complication rate, and the ability to create thermal lesions of variable morphology (CHUNG et al. 1996). Recent advances in MR and RF technology are beginning to overcome previous shortcomings in this therapy/monitoring combination. Preliminary results suggest that this emerging modality has a promising future, with initial trials suggesting utility in the treatment of both intracranial and abdominal tumors. With the ability to immediately assess the results of treatment and to use this information to interactively vary the thermal lesion size and shape, the addition of MR monitoring to the technique of interstitial RF thermotherapy has significant potential to provide a much-needed therapeutic modality for the treatment of regional neoplastic disease.

References

Alexander HR, Bartlett DL, Fraker DL, Libutti SK (1996) Regional treatment strategies for unresectable primary or metastatic cancer confined to the liver. PPO Update 10(8):1–19

Anzai Y, Lufkin RB, Castro DJ, et al (1991) MR imaging-guided interstitial Nd:YAG laser phototherapy: dosimetry study of acute tissue damage in an in vivo model. J Magn Reson Imaging 1:553–559

Anzai Y, Lufkin RB, Hirschowitz S, et al (1992) MR-imaging histopathologic correlation of thermal injuries induced with interstitial Nd:YAG laser irradiation in the chronic model. J Magn Reson Imaging 2:671–678

Anzai Y, Lufkin RB, DeSalles A, et al (1995) Preliminary experience with MR-guided thermal ablation of brain tumors. AJNR Am J Neuroradio 16:39–48

Aronow S (1960) The use of radio-frequency power in making lesions in the brain. J Neurosurg 17:431–438

August DA, Sugarbaker PH, Ottow RT (1985) Hepatic resection of colorectal metastases. Ann Surg 201:210–218

Bleier Ar, Jolesz F, Cohen MS, et al (1991) Real-time magnetic resonance imaging of laser heat deposition in tissue. Magn Reson Med 21:132–137

Boaz TL, Lewin JS, Chung Y, et al (1996) Imaging of the temporal evolution of hepatic tissue destruction during MR-guided radiofrequency thermal ablation in a rabbit model (abstract). Radiology 201:389

Boaz TL, Lewin JS, Chung Y, et al (1997) A rabbit model for MR-monitoring of tissue destruction in MR-guided radiofrequency hepatic thermal ablation. Proceedings of the 5th Scientific Meeting and Exhibition of the International Society for Magnetic Resonance in Medicine, Vancouver

Broggi G, Franzini a, Giorgi C, et al (1985) Radiofrequency percutaneous trigeminal rhizotomy. Considerations in 1000 consecutive cases of essential trigeminal neuralgia. J Neurosurg Sci 29:165

Chung YC, Duerk JL, Lewin JS (1996) Generation and observation of radiofrequency thermal lesion ablation for interventional magnetic resonance imaging. Proceedings of the 4th Scientific Meeting and Exhibition of the International Society for Magnetic Resonance in Medicine, New York, p 1743

Cline HE, Schenck JF, Watkins RD, Jolesz FA (1993) Magnetic resonance-guided thermal surgery. Magn Reson Med 30:98–106

Cline HE, Hynynen K, Watkins RD, et al (1995) Focused US system for MR imaging-guided tumor ablation. Radiology 194:731–737

Duckwiler G, Lufkin RB, Teresi L, et al (1989) Head and neck lesions: MR-guided aspiration biopsy. Radiology 170: 519–522

Duerk JL, Lewin JS, Wu DH (1996) Application of keyhole imaging to interventional MRI: a simulation study to assess sequence requirements. J Magn Reson Imaging 6:918–924

Farahani K, Mischel PS, Black KL, et al (1995) Hyperacute thermal lesions: MR imaging evaluation of development in the brain. Radiology 1996:517–520

Gazelle GS, Haaga JR (1989) Guided percutaneous biopsy of intraabdominal lesions. AJR Am J Radiol 153:929–935

Goldberg SN, Gazelle GS, Dawson SL, et al (1995) Tissue ablation with radiofrequency: effect of probe size, gauge, duration, and temperature on lesion volume. Acad Radiol 2:399–404

Goldberg SN, Gazelle GS, Solbiati L, et al (1996) Radiofrequency tissue ablation: increased lesion diameter with a perfusion electrode. Acad Radiol 3:636–644

Grönemeyer DHW, Kaufman L, Rothschild P, Seibel RMM (1989) Neue Möglichkeiten und Gesichtspunkte der low-field-Kernspintomographie. Radiol Diagn 30:519–527

Hall AS, Prior MV, Hand JW, et al (1990) Observation by MR imaging of in vivo temperature changes induced by radio frequency hyperthermia. J Comput Assist Tomogr 14:430-436

Hitchcock ER, Teixeira MJ (1981) A comparison of results from center-median and basal thalamotomies for pain. Surg Neurol 15:341–351

Jolesz FA, Blumenfeld SM (1994) Interventional use of magnetic resonance imaging. Magn Reson Q 10:85–96

Kaufman L, Arakawa M, Hale J, et al (1989) Accessible magnetic resonance imaging. Magn Reson Q 5:283–297

Laitinen LV, Bergenheim At, Hariz MI (1992) Leksell's posteroventral pallidotomy in the treatment of Parkinson's disease. J Neurosurg 76:53–61

Le Bihan D, Belannoy J, Levin RL (1989) Temperature mapping with MR imaging of molecular diffusion: application to hyperthermia. Radiology 171:853–857

Lewin JS, Duerk JL, Varnes ME, et al (1996a) MR-monitoring of tissue necrosis following percutaneous ethanol injection in implanted rat hepatoma: evaluation of temporal signal changes at 0.2T. Proceedings of the 4th scientific meeting and exhibition of the International Society for Magnetic Resonance in Medicine 2, New York, p 895

Lewin JS, Duerk JL, Petersilge CA, et al (1996b) Interactive MRI of procedure guidance on a clinical C-arm system: a pilot biopsy study. Proceedings of the Third Meeting of the International Society for Magnetic Resonance in Medicine, New York, 27 April to 3 May

Lewin JS (1996c) Interactive MR-guided head and neck biopsy with a modified clinical C-arm system. (abstract) Proceedings of the 34th annual meeting of the American Society of Neuroradiology, Seattle, Washington, 21–27 June

Lewin JS (1996d) Magnetic resonance image guided therapy: clinical applications and future directions. Medical Physics 23:1146

Lewin JS (1997) Interactive MR-guided radiofrequency interstitial thermal ablation of abdominal tumors: a phase I clinical trial. (abstract) Proceedings of the 5th scientific meeting and exhibition of the International Society for Magnetic Resonance in Medicine, Vancouver

Lufkin R, Teresi L, Hanafee W (1987) New needle for MR-guided aspiration cytology of the head and neck. AJR Am J Radiol 149:380–382

Lufkin R, Teresi L, Chiu L, Hanafee W (1988) A technique for MR-guided needle placement. AJR Am J Radiol 151: 193–196

Matsumoto R, Oshio K, Jolesz FA (1992) Monitoring of laser and freezing-induced ablation in the liver with T1-weighted MR imaging. J Magn Reson Imaging 2:555–562

Matsumoto R, Selig AM, Colucci VM, Jolesz FA (1993) MR monitoring during cryotherapy in the liver: predictability of histologic outcome. J Magn Reson Imaging 73:770–776

McGahan MP, Browning PD, Brock JM, Tesluk H (1990) Hepatic ablation using radiofrequency electrocautery. Invest Radiol 25:267–270

McGahan JP, Schneider P, Brock JM, Tesluk H (1993) Treatment of liver tumors by percutaneous radiofrequency electrocautery. Semin Interv Radiol 10:143–149

Nashold BS, Ostdahl RH (1979) Dorsal root entry zone lesions for pain relief. J Neurosurg 51:59–69

Niederhuber JE, Ensminger WD (1993) Treatment of metastatic cancer to the liver. In: DeVita VT, Jr, Hellman S, Rosenberg SA (eds) Cancer: principles and practice of oncology, 4th edn, Lippincott, Philadelphia, pp 2201–2225

NIH Consensus Conference (1990) Adjuvant therapy for patients with colon and rectal cancer. JAMA 264:1444–1450

Petersilge CA, Lewin JS, Duerk JL, et al (1996) Imaging-guided MR arthrography of the shoulder (abstract). Radiology 201:156

Rosomoff HL, Carroll E, Brown J, Sheptak P (1965) Percutaneous radiofrequency cervical cordotomy, technique. J Neurosurg 23:639–644

Rossi S, di Stasi M, Buscarini E, et al (1996) Percutaneous RF interstitial thermal ablation in the treatment of liver cancer. AJR Am J Radiol 167:759–768

Schenck JF, Jolesz FA, Roemer PB, et al (1995) Superconducting open-configuration MR imaging system for image-guided therapy. Radiology 195:805–814

Siegfried J (1977) 500 percutaneous thermocoagulation of Gasserian ganglion for trigeminal pain. Surg Neurol: 126–131

Silverman SG, Collick BD, Figueira MR, et al (1995) Interactive MR-guided biopsy in an open-configuration MR imaging system. Radiology 197:175–181

Sweet WH, Mark VH, Hamlin H (1960) Radiofrequency lesions in the central nervous system of man and cat: including case reports of eight bulbar pain-tract interruptions. J Neurosurg 17:213–225

Tew JM, Keller JT (1977) The treatment of trigeminal neuralgia by percutaneous radiofrequency technique. In: Keener

EB (ed) Clinical neurosurgery. Williams and Wilkins, Baltimore, pp 557–578

Tomlinson FH, Jack CR, Kelly PJ (1991) Sequential magnetic resonance imaging following stereotactic radiofrequency ventralis lateralis thalamotomy. J Neurosurg 74:579–584

Tracz RA, Wyman DR, Little PB, et al (1993) Comparison of magnetic resonance images and the histopathological findings of lesions induced by interstitial laser photocoagulation in the brain. Lasers Surg Med 13:45–54

Vogl TJ, Muller PK, Hammerstingl R, et al (1995) Malignant liver tumors treated with MR imaging-guided laser-induced thermotherapy: technique and prospective results. Radiology 196:257–265

Wenokur R, Andrews JC, Abemayor E, et al (1992) Magnetic resonance imaging-guided fine needle aspiration for the diagnosis of skull base lesions. Skull Base Surg 2:167–170

Wood CB, Gillis CR, Blumgart LH (1976) A retrospective study of patients with liver metastases from colorectal cancer. Clin Oncol 2:285–288

Zervas NT (1965) Eccentric radio-frequency lesions. Confin Neurol 26:143–145

Zervas NT, Kuwayama A (1972) Pathological characteristics of experimental thermal lesions. Comparison of induction heating and radiofrequency electrocoagulation. J Neurosurg 37:418–422

Clinical Application of MR-Guided Interstitial Therapy

26 Interstitial Laser Therapy of Brain Lesions

T. KAHN, H.-J. SCHWARZMAIER, F. ULRICH

CONTENTS

26.1 Introduction

The goal of minimally invasive techniques is to reduce perioperative morbidity and mortality. These approaches are progressively gaining importance in all surgical fields, as well as in interventional radiology. In neurosurgery, tumors are often difficult to access and to distinguish from normal, functionally relevant brain tissue. Stereotactically guided resection of brain tumors using preoperatively obtained imaging data is an accepted therapeutic strategy. This method, however, does not allow real-time monitoring of the surgical procedure. Hence, our aim was to develop a therapeutic approach that can be controlled by online monitoring using an imaging modality.

Laser-induced interstitial thermotherapy (LITT) - a minimally invasive technique of local tumor destruction - fulfills this aim. It was first described by Bown in 1983. The laser energy is directed into the target volume through optical fibers implanted interstitially. Optical and thermal diffusion of the absorbed laser energy leads to damage of tissue following a distinct zonal architecture (SCHOBER et al. 1993; MASTERS and BOWN 1990). Several factors are involved in the initial laser light distribution, e.g., laser wavelength, fiber tip characteristics, wavelength-dependent absorption, and scattering properties of the tissue. The initial heat distribution is then modulated by heat conduction and convection by blood perfusion. Additionally, the optical parameters of tissue change during therapy and the optical properties of different tissues, especially tumors, vary significantly (CHEONG et al. 1990).

We used a special fiber-optic transmission system, the ITT light guide, which operates with reduced power density at the light guide tip compared with a bare fiber, minimizing the risk of carbonization (HESSEL and FRANK 1990). Temporal temperature profiles measured in vitro in pig brain and in vivo in rat brain revealed a steep decrease in temperature within several millimeters' distance from the ITT light guide (SCHOBER et al. 1993). The main advantages of LITT are precise delivery of energy to tissue and minimal damage to adjacent structures. Additionally, treatment of deep cerebral lesions usually inaccessible to surgical resection can be performed with preservation of superficial tissue.

The use of an imaging modality is a prerequisite for performing LITT in a clinical setting. Image guidance has to fulfill several aims: target definition, trajectory selection, laser light guide tracking, and monitoring the localization and volume of the induced lesion. Additionally, an overlay of the spatial temperature distribution on the anatomic data is desirable.

MRI is well suited to monitor LITT owing to its high soft tissue contrast and sensitivity to temperature changes (JOLECZ et al. 1988; TRACZ et al. 1992). Experimental studies in phantoms and animal models support the value of MRI in monitoring LITT (ANZAI et al. 1991; BLEIER et al. 1991; MATSUMOTO et al. 1992). There are three major temperature-sensitive MRI parameters: TI relaxation time, chemical shift, and diffusion constant (DEICHMANN and HAASE 1992; HARTH et al. 1995).

T. KAHN, MD, Institute for Diagnostic Radiology, Moorenstrasse 5, 40225 Düsseldorf, Germany
H.-J. SCHWARZMAIER, MD, Institute of Laser Medicine, Heinrich Heine University, Moorenstrasse 5, D-40225 Düsseldorf, Germany
F. ULRICH, MD, Department of Neurosurgery, Municipal Hospital of Krefeld, Lutherplatz 40, D-47805 Krefeld, Germany

26.2 MR Thermometry — In Vitro Results

The most promising approach to thermometry using MRI is based on the temperature-dependent chemical shift. The mean phase in a voxel built up during the specific echo time varies due to small temperature-related frequency shifts. These induced phase shifts can be measured with an appropriate gradient-echo sequence. Using an experimental setup with homogeneous heating of pig brain in vitro in a water bath, we could show a linear correlation between phase shift and temperature in a range of 20–60 °C using a 2D-FLASH sequence (TR 40/TE 14, flip angle 40°). Up to now, the phase method seems to demonstrate no tissue dependence - with the exception of fat - and offers a chance to accurately calculate actual temperature in vivo (Stollberger et al. 1993). Results with laser ablation of pig brain emphasize the capabilities of this method for monitoring LITT. Since 1996, we have been using this method for monitoring LITT. The complex raw data from the phase images are automatically transferred to a workstation, unwrapped and subtracted from a baseline phase image. The resulting temperature values are superimposed on an anatomical image. The temporal resolution is approximately 25 s. The program is integrated in a user surface that allows an arbitrary scaling of the upper and lower limits of the displayed temperature. Our preliminary experience with the application of the phase mapping method in vivo has indicated its feasibility. To avoid gross motion of the patient's head, tight fixation is required. However, tiny movements and intrinsic pulsations of the brain obviously do not affect the results to a significant extent.

On the other hand, MRI is capable of depicting irreversible lesions due to coagulation and vacuolization. In an experimental animal study, we found a typical zonal anatomy of a laser-induced lesion in rat brain with a central and a peripheral zone (Schober et al. 1993). In the central zone, the electron microscopic examination of the acute changes showed generalized damage of cellular and subcellular membranes surrounding the light guide track. Likewise, the intravascular red blood cells displayed membrane defects and appeared empty. On T1-weighted images this zone is displayed with high signal intensity and on T2-weighted images, with low signal intensity, presumably due to hemoglobin decomposition products.

The fine structural examination of the peripheral zone in experimental animals revealed no membrane disruptions but edema with generalized swelling and an empty appearance of nerve cell processes and astrocytic foot processes. The MR appearance with low signal intensity on T1-weighted images and high signal intensity on T2-weighted images is in good accordance with the histopathological findings.

26.3 Clinical Studies

26.3.1 Patient Population

After completing this detailed neuropathological study of laser–brain tissue interaction in an animal model, we started a clinical pilot study in 1992 in patients with brain tumors (Kahn et al. 1994, 1995). Thirty-one patients with brain tumors were enrolled in the study. All masses were located supratentorially and had an approximately spherical configuration with a diameter ranging from 18 to 35 mm (mean 27.9 mm) as determined by MRI. Neoplasms with intratumoral bleeding and mainly cystic components were excluded. All diagnoses were based on preceding stereotactic biopsy and histologic analysis.

There were 24 astrocytomas (WHO grade II), four anaplastic gliomas (WHO III–IV), two brain metastases of renal adenocarcinoma, and one malignant lymphoma. Eighteen neoplasms were located in or close to the sensorimotor cortical fields, one tumor was located in the hippocampus, one mass in the anterior corpus callosum, and one tumor in the thalamus.

26.3.2 Laser Equipment

An Nd:YAG laser (Medilas 4060N, 1 = 1064 nm, continuous wave; Dornier Medizintechnik, Germering, Germany) was used in combination with an ITT light guide (Dornier Medizintechnik). This device has a directed circumferential emission profile at the tip owing to a special fiber coupler. The length of the flexible light guide is 12 m. The laser unit was installed outside the magnet room. A built-in powermeter was used to control the power output. Additionally, before and after every laser therapy procedure, the system was calibrated with an external powermeter (Model 365 AT, detector head 38001, Scientech, Boulder, Colo.). Transmission loss varied between 10% and 15% of the given output power.

26.3.3 Patient Preparation

All patients underwent a detailed neurological and electroencephalographic examination. The patients with tumors in the sensorimotor cortical fields were additionally examined by neurophysiological methods (somatosensory evoked potentials, motor evoked potentials, and isometric precision force control). In seven patients, functional MR imaging using the "BOLD" method was performed in a single section technique with one acquisition using a 2D-FLASH sequence (TR 90/TE 60, flip angle 40°, matrix 128 × 128). Five images were acquired during rest and five images while the patient made repetitive finger flexion movements of the contralateral hand with respect to the side of the tumor. The procedure was repeated over six cycles resulting in a total of 60 measurements. The images were post-processed with a temporal correlation analysis and color coding of correlation coefficients (Fig. 26.1; Kahn et al. 1996). MR imaging was performed using a 1.5-T Magnetom (Siemens, Erlangen, Germany) with a circularly polarized head coil.

Immediately prior to LITT, a CT (Tomoscan 310 Philips, Best, The Netherlands) of the brain for guidance of stereotactic tumor biopsy was performed in each instance. The stereotactic coordinates were calculated with a Riechert-Mundinger stereotactic frame (Leibinger, Freiburg, Germany). Following the biopsy, a 7-F teflon sheath (Cordis, Erkrath, Germany) was implanted based on the stereotactic coordinates with the tip 5–10 mm proximal to the margin of the tumor. The sheath was later used to introduce the light guide. After fixing the sheath at the skull and removing the stereotactic frame, the patients were transferred to the MRI unit.

After placing the patients on the MR table, the sterile light guide was introduced via the sheath into the center of the tumor according to the stereotactic calculations. The light guide was fixed to the sheath and the MR table. The patients were awake and received no anesthesia. Patient contact was continuously maintained throughout the procedure.

26.3.4 MR Monitoring of LITT

For determining the position of the tip of the light guide and the sheath we used multiplanar reconstructions of a 3D-Turbo-FLASH sequence. Up until 1995, LITT monitoring was accomplished using a T1-weighted 2D-FLASH sequence with an acquisition time of 15 s. After calculation of the images, the sequence was started again and repeatedly applied during the course of the laser therapy. The temporal resolution of the 2D-FLASH studies, including reconstruction of the images, was approximately 20 s. The images were transferred automatically to a workstation, and subtraction of the baseline images acquired prior to LITT from the actual images was performed. We developed an evaluation program displaying the percentage of signal intensity changes with color coding. Images were analyzed according to size and intensity of signal changes. The LITT was terminated when the diameter of the laser-induced peripheral zone (decrease of signal intensity > 30%) was similar to the diameter of the tumor. In 15 of 16 patients the laser output was adjusted to 4 W; in one case, to 5 W. The time of irradiation varied from 10–20 min.

26.3.5 Results

During laser therapy typical changes of signal intensity were seen in all patients independent of tumor histology. A gradually increasing central zone of high signal intensity neighboring the tip of the light guide was surrounded by an increasing area of reduced signal intensity. The temporal and spatial development of these area was different. Our latest experience includes the use of phase-sensitive 2D-FLASH sequences. In accordance with experimental studies in vitro in pig brain, the irreversibly damaged zone is outlined by the 60–65° isotherm (Harth et al. 1997).

During follow-up, in all patients a central area of high signal intensity and a peripheral low signal intensity zone were displayed on T1-weighted images, corresponding to the 2D-FLASH scans during therapy. Moreover, in all cases a thin (1–3 mm) enhancing rim was evident on T1-weighted images after administration of Gd-DTPA, at the border of the peripheral zone. The diameter of these rims was considered the diameter of the total lesion. There was no apparent relation between lesion size

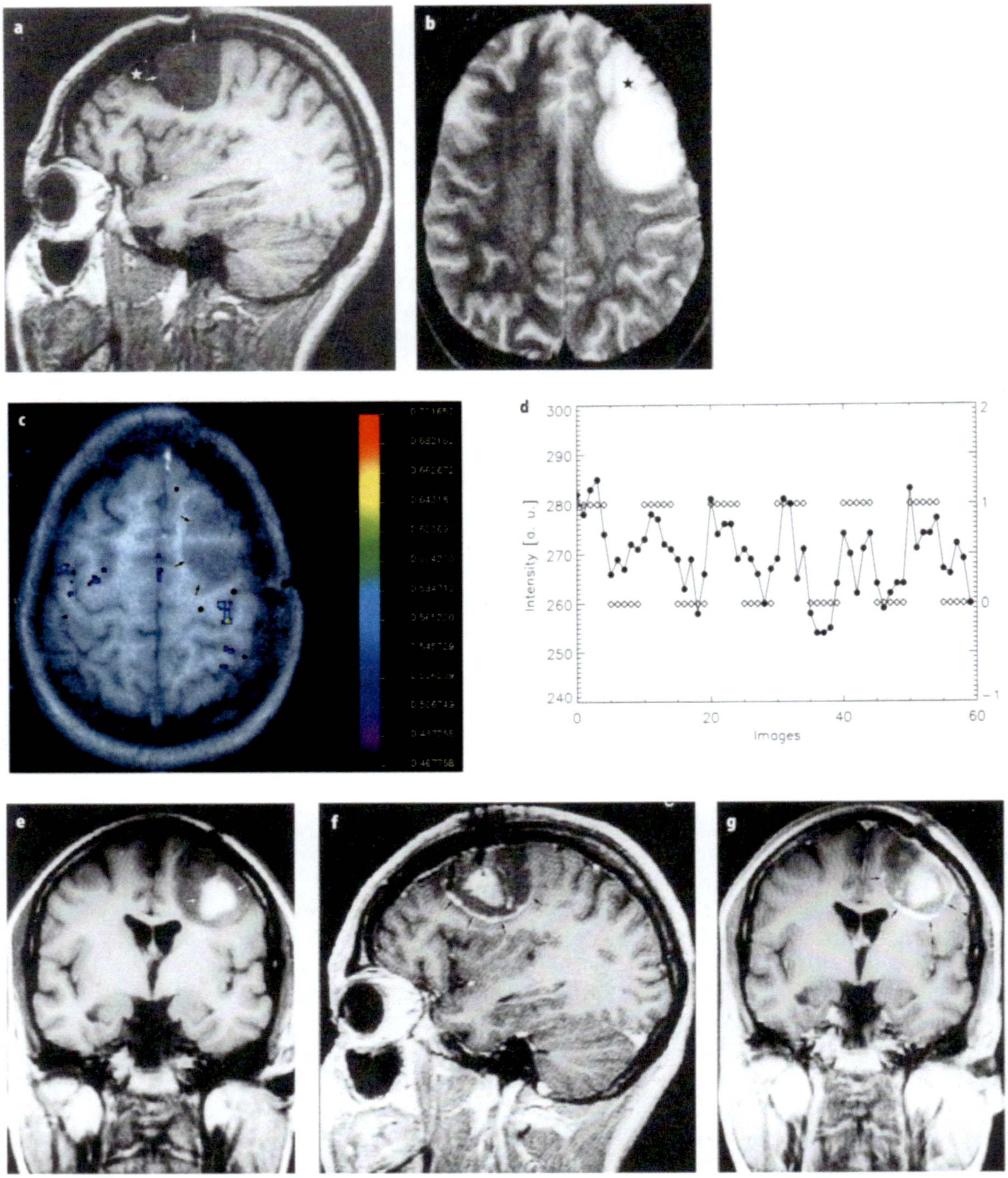

Fig. 26.1a-g. Images and data obtained in a patient with a recurrent left frontal-precentral astrocytoma (WHO grade II) who underwent surgery 22 months before laser-induced interstitial thermotherapy **a** Sagittal T1-weighted image (10/4) shows the recurrent tumor (*arrows*) that protrudes into the postoperative cavity (*). **b** T2-weighted image (2500/80) shows the mass with homogeneously high signal intensity. The cerebrospinal fluid within the postoperative cavity (*) also has high signal intensity. **c** Functional two-dimensional FLASH MR image (90/60) obtained during finger flexion of the right hand shows the results of the temporal correlation analysis with color coding of the pixels with correlation coefficients above the threshold. The mass (*arrows*) is adjacent to the partially infiltrated precentral gyrus (*). The spotlike cortical motor hand area is within the posterior bank of the precentral gyrus and is accompanied by some activity within the central sulcus. There is no activity within the mass. **d** Change in signal intensity over time in the center of the area within the posterior bank of the precentral gyrus. The anticipated slope of the signal intensity during rest and activation is indicated by ◊ (five-images acquired during rest and five images during activation per cycle) a.u., arbitrary units; **e** Coronal (614/14) T1-weighted obtained immediately after LITT shows a high signal intensity central zone (*arrows*). **f** Sagittal (10/4) and **g** coronal (614/14) T1-weighted images obtained after gadolinium administration show an enhancing rim (*arrows*) at the border of the laser-induced lesion. No neurologic deficits occurred during follow-up. (Reproduced with permission from Kahn et al. 1996)

and applied laser energy. The laser-induced lesion compromised 64–130% (mean 97%) of tumor size.

In those patients with a follow-up longer than 3 months the lesion size decreased by 13–87% (mean 48%).

The size of the central zone on T1-weighted images increased within 1–13 days by 7–180% (mean 42%). After the initial increase, the size and the signal intensity of the central zone decreased, resulting in a more homogeneous lesion without differentiation into two zones in further follow-up studies. In all patients the enhancing rim following Gd-DTPA administration was presenting in each follow-up study. However, the size, thickness, and the degree of enhancement decreased.

The T2-weighted images basically showed the reverse situation with regard to the signal intensities of the central and peripheral zones. The hyperintense channel of the light guide was surrounded by a central low signal intensity area and a peripheral high signal intensity zone. The follow-up studies revealed a demarcation of the peripheral zone from the surrounding brain by a thin hypointense rim. The diameter of total lesion size determined by T2-weighted images corresponded to the diameter on T1-weighted scans with Gd-DTPA.

In 28 or 31 patients the follow-up studies showed a slight to severe increase in perifocal edema on T2-weighted images that completely resolved within 2–5 weeks. There was neither an association between tumor grade and severity of edema nor between applied laser energy and severity of edema. None of the patients showed an increase in edema in immediate follow-up studies; 28 of 31 patients received steroids [dexamethasone (fortecortin, Merck) 12–32 mg/day] perioperatively.

During LITT there were two patients with neurological deterioration. In 29 patients, clinical and neurological conditions remained unchanged. In the postoperative period, 4 of 31 patients had transient deficits due to vasogenic edema after LITT. Persistent deficits were only observed in one patient. In this case, the laser-induced lesion exceeded the tumor margin.

Follow-up studies showed neurological improvement in 18 or 24 patients with astrocytoma WHO II, whereas 6 patients remained unchanged. The outcome of LITT in malignant gliomas was poor. All patients had tumor progression within 3–12 months.

26.4 Discussion

The results of our preliminary study show that MRI is well suited to monitor LITT. In all patients the evolving zonal architecture of the irreversible lesion was displayed during therapy. The central zone could readily be identified on the 2D-FLASH scans. The peripheral zone could be better discriminated on subtraction images, especially color-coded subtraction images. The central and peripheral zones together form the total lesion. This is supported by rim enhancement at the border of the peripheral zone after Gd-DTPA administration. Further follow-up studies with shrinkage of the lesion and accompanying diameter reduction of the enhancing rim after Gd-DTPA support the suggestion that the enhancing rim demarcates the outer border of the irreversibly damaged lesion. Tracz et al. (1993) found similar results in experimental animal studies in cat brain and a good correlation between final histological lesion size and diameter based on rim enhancement with Gd-DTPA.

The peripheral zone has to be distinguished from perifocal edema, which may show similar signal intensities. The peripheral zone has been labelled "necrotizing edema" or "delayed liquefaction necrosis", indicating the irreversible damage within this zone (Schober et al. 1993; Kiessling et al. 1990). In contrast, the surrounding vasogenic perifocal edema, which is not present immediately after therapy, is reversible within 15–40 days following LITT. A further improvement in monitoring LITT could be achieved by introducing phase-sensitive sequences displaying absolute temperature changes.

The time course for laser-induced expansion of the lesion following therapy is a controversial issue. Some authors report an increase in lesion size up to 100% (Eggert et al. 1985; Lindsberg et al. 1991). In our study there was an increase in size (mean 42%) based on diameter measurement of the enhancing rim after Gd-DTPA administration. With the light microscopic examination used in these studies it may be difficult to differentiate necrotizing edema of the peripheral zone from vasogenic perifocal edema. The sequential changes in the size of the central and peripheral zones after LITT support this hypothesis. In all patients the size of the central zone increased considerably after therapy, indicating an ongoing process of necrosis. Hence, in accordance with the experimental results of Anzai et al. (1991, 1992), MR imaging obviously is capable of demonstrating total lesion size accurately and may demonstrate irreversible effects, especially in the peripheral zone, earlier than these effects can be detected by light microscopy (Schober et al. 1993).

The advantage of therapeutic control by online monitoring of the conscious patient makes LITT particularly suitable in brain tumors that are located in areas of functional relevance. In our series, 18 patients had brain tumors located in or close to sensorimotor cortex fields (Bettag et al. 1995). As the majority of these tumors were benign or semibenign, usually slowly growing astrocytomas WHO II, it was particularly critical to avoid posttherapeutic neurological deficits. Using functional MRI in seven patients, we were able to determine the localization of the cortical motor hand area. This is important because it may vary, especially in the presence of space-occupying lesions close to or within the cortical motor hand area owing to dislocation or reorganization. In these patients, especially the border of the evolving, irreversible lesion facing the motor hand area was monitored, and LITT was terminated when the distance was less than 4–5 mm.

Currently available light guides for LITT are limited with respect to maximum lesion size. Newer developments are aimed at increasing inducible lesion size. Besides enlarging the fiber tip, this can be achieved by cooling the tissue area surrounding the optical fiber tips. This additional cooling offers also, in principle, the induction of asymmetrical tissue lesions (Schwarzmaier et al. 1994, 1995).

However, the role of LITT as a therapeutic alternative for brain tumors still has to be defined. There are only a few preliminary reports concerning the clinical applications of LITT in brain tumors (Roux et al. 1992; Ascher 1990; Bettag et al. 1992a, 1992b; Sakai et al. 1992). In our series, LITT was of low intraoperative morbidity and no mortality. There was only 1 out of 31 patients who suffered a persistent deficit. In this case, the laser-induced lesion exceeded the tumor margin. Transient neurological deficits occurred in the early postoperative period due to vasogenic perifocal edema. In all patients, recovery was obtained within 3–5 weeks. These results indicate that LITT is a safe therapy if the laser-induced lesion is confined to the tumor margins. In all patients, a marked tumor reduction was obtained; 18 of 24 patients with low-grade gliomas (astrocytoma WHO II) showed a neurological improvement, with decrease in severity and frequency of their seizures. Although definitive conclusions regarding the value of LITT cannot be drawn on the basis of our study, it seems that LITT can be of benefit in patients with low-grade gliomas. On the other hand, laser therapy in malignant gliomas – used as a monotherapeutic approach – was unsuccessful. Considering experimental results, a multitherapeutic approach of LITT in combination with radiotherapy and/or chemotherapy will probably improve the results in malignant brain tumors (Salcman and Ebert 1991; Salcman and Samaras 1981).

References

Anzai Y, Lufkin RB, Castro DJ, et al (1991) MR imaging guided interstitial Nd:YAG laser phototherapy: dosimetry study of acute tissue damage in an in vivo model. J Magn Reson Imaging 1:553–559

Anzai Y, Lufkin RB, Hirschowitz S, Farahani K, Castro DJ (1992) MR imaging – histopathologic correlation of thermal injuries induced with interstitial Nd:YAG laser irradiation in the chronic model. J Magn Reson Imaging 2:671–678

Ascher PW (1990) Interstitial thermal therapy of brain tumors with Nd:YAG laser under real time MRI control SPIE 12000:242–245

Bettag M, Ulrich F, Schober R, Sabel M, Kahn T, Bock WJ (1992a) Laser-induced interstitial thermotherapy in malignant gliomas. Adv Neurosurg 22:253–257

Bettag M, Ulrich F, Bock WJ, Kahn T, Schwarzmaier HJ, Hessel S (1992b) MR-guided laser interventions. SPIE 1643:242–245

Bettag M, Kunesch E, Kahn T, Ulrich F, Schmitz F, Bock WJ (1995) Neurological and functional changes after laser-induced interstitial thermotherapy (LITT) of brain tumors. In: Müller G, Roggan A, (eds) Laser-induced interstitial thermotherapy, vol PM25. SPIE Press, 382–392

Bleier AR, Jolecz FA, Cohen MS, Weisskopf RM, Dalcanton JJ, Higuchi N, Feinberg DA, Rosen BR, McKinstry RC, Hushek SG (1991) Real time magnetic resonance imaging of laser heat deposition in tissue. Magn Resol Med 21:132–137

Bown SG (1983) Phototherapy of tumours. World J Surg 7:700–709

Cheong WF, Prahl SA, Welch AJ (1990) A review of the optical properties of biological tissues. IEEE J Quantum Electron 26:2166–2185

Deichmann R, Haase A (1992) Quantification of T1-values by snapshot-FLASH NMR-imaging. J Magn Reson 96:608–612

Eggert HR, Kiessling M, Kleihues P (1985) Time course and spatial distribution of Neodymium: Ytriium-Aluminum-Garnet (Nd:YAG) laser-induced lesions in the rat brain. Neurosurgery 16:443–448

Harth T, Kahn T, Rassek M, Schwabe B (1995) Temperature monitoring using fast T1-measurement. (abstract) Proceedings of the 3rd Annual Meeting of the Society for Magnetic Resonance, p 1170

Harth T, Schulze PC, Kahn T, Schober R (1997) Correlation of MRI-monitored LITT and histological changes in pig brain (abstract) Proceedings of the International Society for Magnetic Resonance in Medicine, Vancouver 264

Hessel S, Frank F (1990) Technical prerequisites for the interstitial thermotherapy using the Nd:YAG laser. Proc SPIE 1201:233–238

Jolecz FA, Bleier AR, Jakab P, Ruenzel PW, Huttl K, Jako GJ (1988) MR imaging of laser-tissue interactions. Radiology 168:249–253

Kahn T, Bettag M, Ulrich F, Schwarzmaier H-J, Schober R, Fürst G, Mödder U (1994) MRI-guided laser-induced interstitial thermotherapy of cerebral neoplasms. J Comput Assist Tomogr 18:519–532

Kahn T, Bettag M, Ulrich F, Schwarzmaier HJ, Harth T, Mödder U (1995) MRI-guidance of laser-induced interstitial thermotherapy of brain tumors – three-year experience. In: Müller G, Roggan A (eds) Laser-induced interstitial thermotherapy, vol PM25. SPIE Press, Bellingham, Wash, pp 325–339

Kahn T, Schwabe B, Harth T, Bettag M, Ulrich F, Rassek M, Schwarzmaier H-J, Mödder U (1996) Mapping of the cortical motor hand area with functional MR imaging and MR imaging-guided laser-induced interstitial thermotherapy of brain tumors. Radiology 200:149–157

Kiessling M, Herchenhan E, Eggert HR (1990) Cerebrovascular and metabolic effects on the rat brain of focal Nd:YAG laser irradiation. J Neurosurg 73:909–907

Lindsberg PJ, Frerichs KU, Burris JA, Hallenbeck JM, Feuerstein G (1991) Cortical microcirculation in a new model of focal laser-induced secondary brain damage. J Cereb Blood Flow Metab 11:88–89

Masters A, Bown SG (1990) Interstitial laser hyperthermia in the treatment of tumors. Lasers Med Sci 5:129–135

Matsumoto R, Oshio K, Jolecz FA (1992) Monitoring of laser and freezing-induced ablation in the liver with T1-weighted MR imaging. J Magn Reson Imaging 2:555–562

Roux FX, Merienne L, Leriche B, Lucerna S, Turak B, Devaux BC, Chokiewicz JP (1992) Laser interstitial thermotherapy in stereotactical neurosurgery. Lasers Med Sci 7:121–126

Sakai T, Fujishima I, Sugiyama K, Ryu H, Uemura K (1992) Interstitial laserthermia in neurosurgery. J Clin Laser Med Surg 1:37–40

Salcman M, Samaras GM (1981) Hyperthermia for brain tumors: biophysical rationale. Neurosurgery 9:327–335

Salcman M, Ebert PS (1991) In vitro response of human glioblastoma and canine glioma cells to hyperthermia, radiation, and chemotherapy. Neurosurgery 29:526–531

Schober R, Bettag M, Sabel M, Ulrich F, Hessel S (1993) Fine structure of zonal changes in experimental Nd:YAG laser-induced interstitial hyperthermia. Lasers Surg Med 13: 234–241

Schwarzmaier HJ, Goldbach T, Ulrich F, Schober R, Kahn T, Kaufmann R, Wolbarsht ML (1994) Improved laser applicators for interstitial thermotherapy of brain structure. SPIE 2132:4–12

Schwarzmaier HJ, Kaufmann R, Kahn T, Ulrich F (1995) Applicators for the laser-induced thermotherapy – basic considerations and new developments. In: Müller G, Roggan A, (eds) Laser-induced interstitial thermotherapy, vol PM25. SPIE Press, pp 249–264

Stollberger F, Ebner F, Ascher PW (1993) Real time temperature imaging of interstitial laser thermotherapy using the water proton chemical shift. (abstract) Proceedings of the 2nd Annual Meeting of the Society for Magnetic Resonance, p 1584

Tracz RA, Wyman DR, Little PB, Towner RA, Stewart WA, Schatz SW, Pennock PW, Wilson BC (1992) Magnetic resonance imaging of interstitial laser photo coagulation. Lasers Surg Med 12:165–173

Tracz RA, Wyman DR, Little PB, Towner RA, Stewart WA, Schatz SW, Wilson BC, Pennock PW, Janzen EG (1993) Comparison of magnetic resonance images and histopathological findings of lesions induced by interstitial laser photocoagulation in the brain. Lasers Surg Med 13: 45–54

27 Interstitial Laser Therapy of Head and Neck Lesions

M.G. Mack, T. J. Vogl

CONTENTS

27.1 Introduction

The head and neck area contains a multitude of small, complexly arranged anatomic structures; intimate knowledge of normal spatial relationships and variations is necessary in planning and implementing appropriate therapy. Lesions often lie near vital structures, complicating diagnostic and therapeutic procedures. Improved visualization during such procedures can therefore provide the physician with critical information, enhancing safety and improving outcomes (Duckwiler et al. 1989; Fried and Jolesz 1993; Yousem 1992).

Palliative treatment options for recurrent head and neck cancer are limited by the proximity of vital vascular and neural structures and the aggressive nature of most of these tumors. Laser-induced interstitial thermotherapy (LITT) is a recently developed minimally invasive treatment modality. It is used for local tumor destruction within solid organs (Vogl et al. 1995b).

Experimental work has shown that a well-defined area of coagulative necrosis is obtained around the fiber tip, with minimal damage to surrounding structures.

MR-guided laser-induced thermotherapy offers a number of potential treatment benefits (Amin et al. 1993; Anzai et al. 1992; Bihan et al. 1989; Blackwell et al. 1993; Castro et al. 1992a, 1992b; Cline et al. 1993; Paynch et al. 1992; Roggan et al. 1994; Schwarzmaier et al. 1994; Steger et al. 1992). First, MR imaging provides unparalleled topographic accuracy owing to its excellent soft tissue contrast and high spatial resolution. Second, the temperature sensitivity of specially designed MR sequences can be used to monitor the temperature elevation in the tumor and surrounding normal tissues (Dickinson et al. 1986; Higuchi et al. 1992; Jolesz et al. 1988; Kahn et al. 1994; Karlin et al. 1987; Matsumoto et al. 1994; Muschter et al. 1994; Welch 1994). This enables the exact visualization of the growing coagulative necrosis. On-line MR imaging during LITT is essential for avoiding local complications due to laser treatment. Third, recovery time, lengths of hospital stay, and the risk of infection and other complications can be reduced compared with conventional palliative surgery. Finally, successful implementation of such minimally invasive procedures would significantly reduce costs in comparison to surgical procedures. A further, indirect advantage is the psychological effect due to avoidance of cosmetic deformities that can result from major reconstructive surgery.

A number of studies have already been performed to evaluate the potential of laser treatment for the local treatment of liver metastases (Masters and Brown 1992; Masters al. 1992; Matsumoto et al. 1992; Robinson et al. 1993; Vogl et al. 1995a, 1996), as well as other tumors. Here we describe our experience in the use of LITT for the therapy of head and neck tumors.

M.G. Mack, MD, Department of Radiology, Virchow Hospital, Humboldt University, Augustenburger Platz 1, D-13353 Berlin, Germany
T. J. Vogl, MD, Department of Radiology, Virchow Hospital, Humboldt University, Augustenburger Platz 1, D-13353 Berlin, Germany

27.2 Material and Methods

27.2.1 Laser system and application set

Laser coagulation was performed using a Neodymium-YAG laser [Dornier (Germany) MediLas 5060, Martin (Tuttlingen, Germany) MY 30, Zeiss (Oberkochen, Germany) Opmilas] with a specially developed scattering dome light emitter. Furthermore, an application kit for percutaneous treatment was developed and optimized for our purposes.

Laser light with a wavelength of 1046 nm was transmitted to tissue with a diffusing applicator. Laser light of this wavelength penetrates deeply into biological tissue, where photon absorption and heat conduction lead to hyperthermic and coagulative effects. The tissue destruction may be immediate or delayed.

The laser application kit (Somatex, Berlin, Germany) consists of a cannulation needle with a tetragonally sharpened tip containing a guidewire, a sheath system with mandrin (15 cm, 7 Ch), and a special protective catheter (43 cm, 4 Ch) which is closed at the distal end. The protective catheter prevents direct contact of the laser applicator with the patient and enables complete removal of the applicator even in the unlikely event of damage to the laser fiber during treatment. This increases patient safety and simplifies the procedure. The catheter is transparent for laser radiation and resistant to heat (up to 400°C). Marks on the sheath and the protective catheter allow exact positioning of both in the lesion.

The system is fully compatible with MR imaging systems. Magnetite markers on the laser applicator allow for easy and accurate positioning. The laser itself is installed outside of the examination unit. The laser light is transmitted via a 10-m long optical fiber. The complete setup used for LITT is shown in Fig. 27.1.

27.2.2 Procedure monitoring and computer simulation

Critical in LITT is the on-line monitoring of the actual temperature distribution. First, a computer simulation is used to calculate the parameters for laser treatment, such as energy and total application time. The tissue damage state can be calculated numerically from the Arrhenius formula which

a

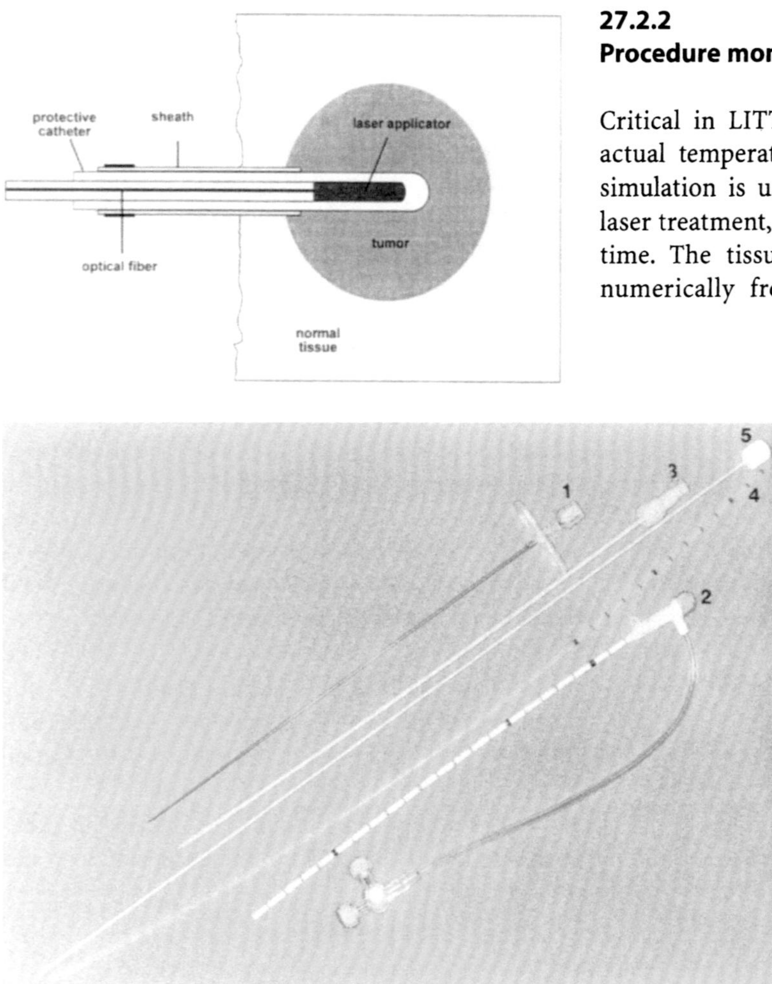

b

Fig. 27.1.a The drawing shows the laser-induced thermotherapy, (LITT) setup. **b** a laser application kit consisting of a cannulation needle (*1*) with a tetragonally sharpened tip, a sheath with an additional side-port (*2*), and the corresponding stylet (*3*). The protective catheter (*4*), which prevents the direct contact of the laser applicator with the patient, is closed at the distal end and also provided with a stylet (*5*) describes the process of coagulation as a rate equation:

$$\Omega(T,t) = A \int_{t_i}^{t_f} \exp\left(-\frac{E}{RT(t)}\right) dt$$

A and *E* are constants, depending on the specific tissue; R is the universal gas constant (8.31 J mol^{-1} K^{-1}); and *T* is the absolute temperature (K) at time *t*. Within the simulation the integral was solved numerically for each volume element. The damage integral describes the probability for protein denaturation, whereby 1 corresponds to a degree of denaturation of 63%. A value of 0.53 was used for irreversible tissue damage, corresponding to a change of the optical properties from the native to the coagulated values. For the constants *A* and *E*, only a few experimentally derived values are available. In our calculations, we used $A = 9.4 \times 10^{104}\ s^{-1}$ and $E = 6.68 \times 10^5\ Jmol^{-1}$.

27.2.3
Patients

Twelve patients (mean age 63.3 years) with recurrent head and neck tumors were treated using MR-controlled LITT. A total number of 13 lesions were treated. All patients had primary head and neck tumors (histologically undifferentiated squamous cell carcinoma, $n = 10$; pleomorphic adenoma, $n = 2$). The primary treatment modalities were surgical resection, postoperative radiation, radiochemotherapy, or a combination of these. Clinical examinations and MRI follow-up provided evidence for tumor recurrence 1–16 months following primary therapy. Nine patients presented with clinical signs of tumor recurrence, such as malfunction of the eustachian tube ($n = 6$), pain ($n = 7$), dysphagia ($n = 7$), hoarseness ($n = 3$), and symptoms of intracranial nerve involvement, e.g., diplopia.

27.2.4
Technique of MR-Guided LITT

Informed consent was obtained from all patients. Prior to LITT, all patients underwent CT and a contrast-enhanced MRI study at least 2 days prior to the intervention. After localization of the tumor with CT, 20 ml of 1% lidocaine was infiltrated in the surrounding tissues. If necessary patients were also sedated. The distance to the lesion and the puncture angle were calculated electronically. For targeting of both recurrent nasopharyngeal tumors and pleomorphic adenomas a subzygomatic approach to the lesion was chosen, which provided the best and safest access. Lesions of the larynx and the floor of the mouth were punctured directly. Following puncture of the lesion, a 7-F catheter was inserted via a percutaneous approach under CT guidance. Subsequently a special thermostable plastic catheter was introduced. After moving the patient from the CT to the MR table, the laser catheter was inserted into the guiding catheter. After the procedure, the cannulation channel was closed with fibrin glue (TISSUCOLL, Immuno, Heidelberg, Germany).

27.2.5
MR Thermometry

MR thermometry was performed with a TurboFLASH sequence (TR 7/TE 3/TI 400), as well as a Thermo-FLASH-2D sequence (TR 102/TE 8/flip angle 15°). The latter was found to be more sensitive to thermal changes.

Before and after LITT treatment T1-weighted [spin echo (SE and GE gradient echo), and T2-weighted (SE) images were obtained. Of particular significance is the acquisition of a dynamic TurboFLASH sequence which produces images both prior to and in short delays (6 s) following the intravenous administration of contrast medium over a period of 180 s. Follow-up studies including nonenhanced and contrast-enhanced sequences are performed 1, 4, 12, and 24 weeks following the laser therapy. Qualitative and quantitative parameters including size, morphology, and contrast enhancement pattern at early and late follow-up were evaluated.

27.3
Results

27.3.1
MR Thermometry

In vitro studies using muscle tissue demonstrated a reproducible loss of signal intensity corresponding to increasing tissue temperatures. Using an energy of 5 W and an application time of 12 min, the maximum diameter of the region with signal loss was 25 mm. This effect was best monitored using the Thermo-TurboFlash sequence at TR values of

300–400 ms, providing a nearly linear, inverse correlation between signal intensity and temperature. By comparison, this correlation was somewhat less linear using the FLASH-2D sequence; this sequence did, however, provide higher spatial resolution and clearer delineation of topographical structures.

27.3.2 In Vivo Study

Eleven patients tolerated the procedure well. One patient with a recurrent squamous cell carcinoma and infiltration of the sublingual gland developed pain 5 min after starting the laser treatment. No long-term side effects related to treatment were observed. The 2-year MR control study of the patients with the pleomorphic adenoma showed no recurrent tumor.

MR thermometry enabled on-line display of the hyperthermic effects, seen as progressively decreased signal from spaces surrounding the tumor. Criteria for evaluating success of treatment included clinical data such as pain or other local symptoms, as well as pre- and posttherapeutic changes in signal and tumor morphology. We were able to induce coagulative necrosis in all patients (Figs. 27.2, 27.3; volume range 3 cm^3 to 25 cm^3) and to reduce clinical symptoms in seven patients.

a

b

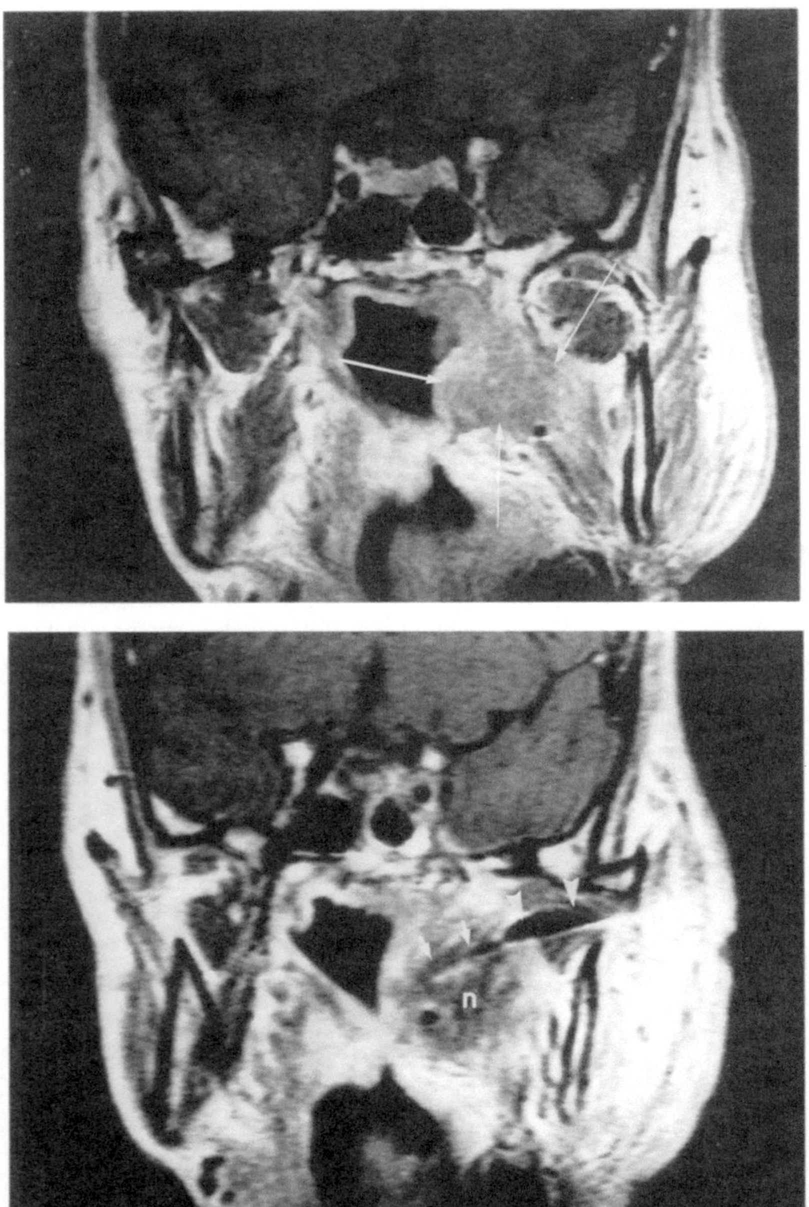

Fig. 27.2a, b. Recurrent nasopharyngeal carcinoma, 1 year postradiotherapy (70 Gy): a T1-weighted spin-echosequence in coronal slice orientation, TR 700/TE 14 before and after LITT. **a** A coronal T1-weighted image (TR 700/TE 15) acquired prior to laser treatment demonstrates the recurrent nasopharyngeal carcinoma (*arrows*) as a homogeneous mass involving skull base and parapharyngeal space. **b** This contrast-enhanced T1-weighted image, acquired following LITT (15 min, 4.5 W) reveals a significant amount of necrosis (*n*) in the middle and inferior compartments of the tumor. Note the magnetite marker (*arrowwheads*) and the active zone (*arrows*) of the laser applicator

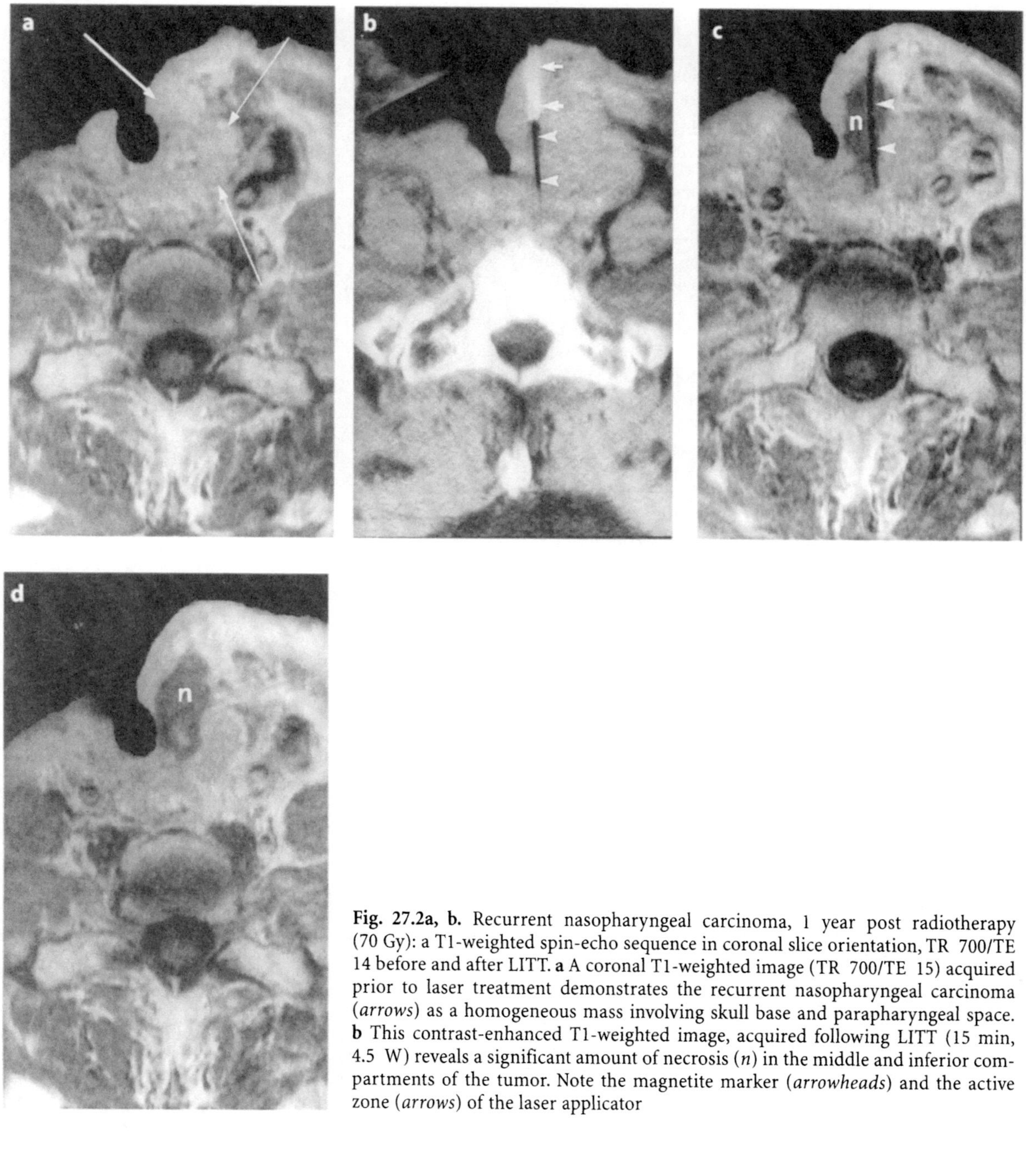

Fig. 27.2a, b. Recurrent nasopharyngeal carcinoma, 1 year post radiotherapy (70 Gy): a T1-weighted spin-echo sequence in coronal slice orientation, TR 700/TE 14 before and after LITT. **a** A coronal T1-weighted image (TR 700/TE 15) acquired prior to laser treatment demonstrates the recurrent nasopharyngeal carcinoma (*arrows*) as a homogeneous mass involving skull base and parapharyngeal space. **b** This contrast-enhanced T1-weighted image, acquired following LITT (15 min, 4.5 W) reveals a significant amount of necrosis (*n*) in the middle and inferior compartments of the tumor. Note the magnetite marker (*arrowheads*) and the active zone (*arrows*) of the laser applicator

In all patients the follow-up control studies showed an increase in the volume of coagulative necrosis between the 1- and 12-week control studies. The T1-weighted contrast-enhanced images revealed, up to 1 week following therapy, a central non-enhancing area of low signal intensity due to obtained coagulative necrosis in all patients. A rim of contrast enhancement surrounding the area of low signal intensity most likely represents reactive changes.

27.4 Conclusion

MR-guided LITT allows accurate on-line thermometry during the interventional procedure. Dynamic gadolinium-enhanced MRI is suitable for early and late follow-up studies for lesions treated with LITT. Follow up studies indicate that the laser-induced effects lead to reliable palliation in recurrent head and neck tumors.

References

Amin Z, Donald JJ, Masters A, Kant R, Steger AC, Bown SG, Lees WR (1993) Hepatic metastases: interstitial laser photocoagulation with real-time US monitoring and dynamic CT evaluation of treatment. Radiology 187:339–347

Anzai Y, Lufkin RB, Hirschowitz S, Farahani K, Castro DJ (1992) MR imaging-histopathologic correlation of thermal injuries induced with interstitial Nd:YAG laser irradiation in the chronic model. J Magn Reson Imaging 2:671–678

Bihan DL, Delannoy J, Levin RL (1989) Temperature mapping with MR imaging of molecular diffusion: application to hyperthermia. Radiology 171:853–857

Blackwell KE, Castro DJ, Saxton RE, et al (1993) Real time intraoperative ultrasonography as a monitoring technique for Nd:YAG-laser palliation of unresectable head and neck tumors: initial experience. Laryngoscope 103:559–564

Castro DJ, Lufkin RB, Saxton RE, Nyerges A, Soudant J, Layfield LJ, Jabour BA, Ward PH, Kangarloo H. (1992a) Metastatic head and neck malignancy treated using MRI guided interstitial laser phototherapy: an initial case report. Laryngoscope 102:26–32

Castro DJ, Saxton RE, Lufkin RB (1992b) Interstitial photoablative laser therapy guided by magnetic resonance imaging for the treatment of deep tumors. Semin Surg Oncol 8:233–241

Cline HE, Schenck JF, Watkins RD, Hynynen K, Jolesz FA (1993) Magnetic resonance-guided thermal surgery. Magn Reson Med 30:98–106

Dickinson RJ, Hall AS, Hind AJ, Young IR (1986) Measurements of changes in tissue temperature using MR imaging. J Comput Assist Tomogr 10:468–472

Duckwiler G, Lufkin RB, Teresi L, Spickler E, Dion J, Vinuela F, Bentson J, Hanafee W (1989) Head and neck lesions: MR-guided aspiration biopsy. Radiology 170:519–522

Fried MP, Jolesz FA (1993) Image-guided intervention for diagnosis and treatment of disorders of the head and neck. Laryngoscope 103:924–927

Higuchi N, Bleier AR, Jolesz FA, Colucci VM, Morris JH (1992) Magnetic resonance imaging of acute effects of interstitial neodymium:YAG laser irradiation on tissues. Invest Radiol 27:814–821

Jolesz FA, Bleier AR, Jokab P, et al (1988) MR imaging of laser tissue interactions. Radiology 168:629–631

Kahn T, Bettag M, Ulrich F, Schwarzmaier HJ, Schober R, Furst G, Modder U (1994) MRI-guided laser induced interstitial thermotherapy of cerebral neoplasms. J Comput Assist Tomogr 18:519–532

Karlin DA, Fisher RS, Krevsky B (1987) Prolonged survival and effective palliation in patients with squamous cell carcinoma of esophagus following endoscopic laser therapy. Cancer 59:1969–1972

Masters A, Bown SG (1992) Interstitial laser hyperthermia. Semin Surg Oncol 8:242–249

Masters A, Steger AC, Lees WR, Walmsley KM, Bown SG (1992) Interstitial laser hyperthermia: a new approach for treating liver metastases. Br J Cancer 66:518–522

Matsumoto R, Selig AM, Colucci VM, Jolesz FA (1992) Interstitial Nd:YAG laser ablation in normal rabbit liver: trial to maximize the size of laser-induced lesions. Lasers Surg Med 12:650–658

Matsumoto R, Mulkern RV, Hushek SG, Jolesz FA (1994) Tissue temperature monitoring for thermal interventional therapy: comparison of T1-weighted MR sequences. J Magn Reson Imaging 4:65–70

Muschter R, Hofstetter A, Hessel S (1994) Laser induced thermotherapy of benign prostatic hyperplasia. Min Invas Med 5:51–54

Panych LP, Hrovat MI, Bleier MI, Jolesz FA (1992) Effects related to temperature changes during MR imaging. J Magn Reson Imaging 2:69–74

Robinson PJ, Grant HR, Bown SG (1993) Nd:YAG laser treatment of a glomus tympanicum tumour. J Laryngol Otol 107:236–237

Roggan A, Handke A, Miller K, Müller G (1994) Laser induced interstitial thermotherapy of benign prostatic hyperplasia. Min Invas Med 5:55–63

Schwarzmaier HJ, Goldbach T, Kaufmann R, Ulrich F, Bettag M, Kahn T (1994) New applicators for the laser induced interstitial thermotherapy. Min Invas Med 5:32–35

Steger AC, Lees WR, Shorvon P, Walmsley K, Bown SG (1992) Multiple-fibre low-power intersitial hyperthermia: studies in the normal liver. Br J Surg. 79:139–145

Vogl TJ, Müller PK, Hammerstingl R, et al. (1995a) Malignant liver tumors treated with MR imaging-guided laser-induced thermotherapy: technique and prospective results. Radiology 196: 257–265

Vogl TJ, Mack MG, Müller P, et al. (1995b) Recurrent nasopharyngeal tumors: preliminary clinical results with interventional MR imaging-controlled laser induced thermotherapy. Radiology 196:725–733

Vogl TJ, Mack MG, Scholz WR, et al. (1996) MR imaging guided laser-induced thermotherapy. Min Invas Ther Allied Technol 5:243-248

Welch AJ (1994) The thermal response of laser irradiated tissue. IEEE J Quant Election 20:1471-1481.

Wyman DR, Whelan WM, Wilson BC (1992) Interstitial laser photocoagulation: Nd:YAG 1064 nm optical fiber source compared to point heat source. Lasers Surg Med 12:659-664

Yousem DM (1992) Dashed hopes for MR imaging of the head and neck: the power of the needle. Radiology 184:25-26

28 Interstitial Laser Therapy of Liver Lesions

T.J. Vogl and M.G. Mack

CONTENTS

28.1 Introduction

The liver is the most common site of metastatic tumor deposits, especially for colorectal cancer, which is the third leading cause of death in western communities, outnumbered only by lung and breast cancer. At the time of death, approximately two-thirds of the patients with colorectal cancer have liver metastases (Goslin et al. 1982; Jaffe et al. 1968; Petrelli et al. 1989; Weiss et al. 1986). Interstitial laser-induced thermotherapy (LTT) is a recently developed minimally invasive technique for local tumor destruction within solid organs (Amin et al. 1993b; Anzai et al. 1991; Dickinson et al. 1986; Vogl et al. 1995a, 1995b). Low-power laser application delivering light energy through thin optical fibers results in a well-defined area of coagulative necrosis. The focal nature of the tissue destruction by direct heating greatly limits damage to surrounding structures. Magnetic resonance imaging (MRI) has proved an ideal imaging tool for the exact positioning of the optical fibers in the target area. In addition, MRI is capable of providing real-time monitoring of the hyperthermic effects and the subsequent evaluation of the extent of coagulative necrosis (Castro et al. 1992; Cline et al. 1993; Matsumoto et al. 1992). In the following, an overview of the technical features and clinical results of MR-guided LTT of liver lesions will be presented based on the Berlin experience.

T.J. Vogl, MD, Department of Radiology, Virchow Hospital, Humboldt University, Augustenburger Platz 1, D-13353 Berlin, Germany
M.G. Mack, MD, Department of Radiology, Virchow Hospital, Humboldt University, Augustenburger Platz 1, D-13353 Berlin, Germany

28.2 Material and Methods

28.2.1 Laser System and Application Set

Laser coagulation was accomplished using a Neodymium-YAG laser [Dornier (Germany) MediLas 5060, Martin (Tuttlingen, Germany) MY 30] with a specially developed scattering dome light emitter. For an effective LTT procedure, a special diffusing applicator and an application kit for percutaneous treatment was developed and optimized.

Laser light with a wavelength of 1046 nm was transmitted to tissue with a diffusing applicator. A protective glass dome of 1.4-mm diameter was mounted on a 400-mm silica fiber core. The dome was frosted on its inner surface, which emitted laser light to an effective distance of 12–15 mm. Laser light of this wavelength penetrates deeply into biological tissue, where photon absorption and the conduction lead to coagulative and hyperthermic effects. The tissue destruction may be immediate or delayed.

The laser application kit (Somatex, Berlin, Germany) consists of a cannulation needle with a tetragonally sharpened tip, a guidewire, a sheath system containing a mandrin (15 cm, 7 Ch), and a special protective catheter (43 cm, 4 Ch) which is closed at the distal end. The protective catheter prevents direct contact of the laser applicator with the treated tissues and enables complete removal of the applicator even in the unlikely event of damage to the fiber during treatment. This increases patients' safety and simplifies the procedure. The catheter is transparent for laser radiation and resistant to heat of up to 400°C. Marks on the sheath and the protective catheter allow exact positioning of both in the liver lesion.

The system is fully compatible with MR imaging systems. Magnetite markers on the laser applicator facilitate visualization of the applicator in the MR image. This in turn enhances the positioning accuracy. The laser itself is installed outside the examination unit. The laser light is transmitted via a 10-m long optical fiber. The complete setup used for LTT is shown in Fig. 28.1.

28.2.2 Protocol During LTT

Informed consent was obtained from all patients enrolled in the study. The success of LTT depends on the accuracy of the optical fiber delivery to the target area, real-time monitoring of the treatment effects, and subsequent evaluation of the extent of thermal damage. The key to achieving these objectives lies in the imaging methods used.

Prior to LTT all patients underwent contrast-enhanced MRI studies. After localization of the tumor on CT images, pain control was achieved by infiltrating 20 ml 1% lidocaine locally and administering pethidine (20–50 mg) intravenously. A 7-F sheath was subsequently inserted via a percutaneous approach under CT guidance. Subsequently the special heat-resistant protective catheter was introduced. After re-positioning the patient on the MRI table, the laser catheter was inserted into the protective catheter.

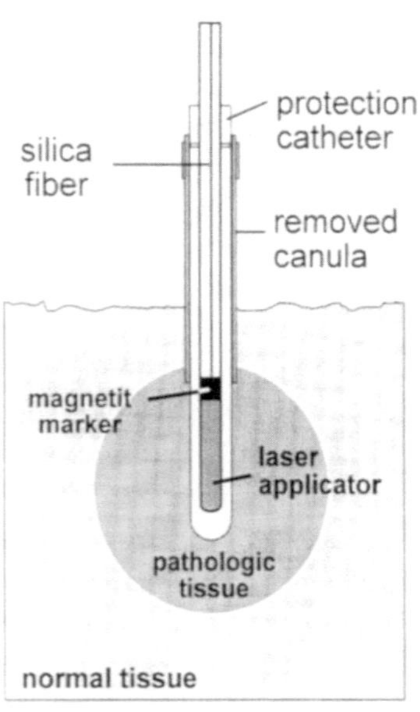

Fig. 28.1. Set-up of MR-guided laser induced thermotherapy

MR thermometry was performed using specially designed Turbo-FLASH (TR 7/TE 3/TI 400) and FLASH-2D (TR 102/TE 8 flip angle 15°) sequences, which had been optimized for the detection of thermal changes.

Before and after LTT T1-weighted [spin echo (SE) and gradient echo (GE)] and T2-weighted (SE) images were obtained. A conventional 1.5-T magnet system (Siemens SP 4000, Erlangen, Germany) was used for MR imaging. Follow-up examinations using native and contrast-enhanced (0.1 ml/kg body weight Gd-DTPA) sequences were carried out 2 days, 1 month, 3 months and every 6 months following the LTT procedure. Qualitative and quantitative parameters were evaluated, including size, morphology, and contrast enhancement pattern at early and late follow-up.

28.2.3 Definition of Patients for MR-Guided LTT of Hepatic Lesions

Patients chosen for LTT should have fewer than five lesions with none measuring more than 40 mm in diameter. They are generally non-surgical candidates owing to lesion distribution or localization, or refusal of operative resection. Patients with recurrent disease following partial resection of one hepatic lobe are also suitable for this therapy.

28.3 Results

To date 134 patients with a total 374 liver metastases of colorectal, esophageal, gastric, pharyngeal, testicular, or pulmonary origin were treated with LTT. A total of 1031 laser applications were performed.

The necrosis caused by the interstitial laser therapy was quantified by comparing the pre- and post-therapeutic plain and contrast-enhanced MR images. Various parameters including size, morphology, and contrast enhancement compared with pretherapeutic MR were helpful in deciding whether treatment could be terminated, or whether subsequent treatment sessions were required.

On the contrast-enhanced T1-weighted GE images necrosis is identified as a hypointense region that is well delineated from enhancing residual tumor tissue. A mean size of necrosis of 2 cm^3 of ellipsoid morphology can be achieved by LTT application lasting approximately 20 min at a power setting of 5–6 W using a single applicator system.

In our experience there are two methods to enlarge the area of necrosis. The choice of method depends on local conditions including tumor geometry or the presence of residual cancer in the vicinity of vital structures such as vessels. With the pull-back technique the region of necrosis can be enlarged longitudinally. The multi-applicator technique represents a more versatile alternative. The parallel positioning of two or three applicator systems can result in a necrosis size of up to 17 cm3 (Figs. 28.2, 28.3). The combination of both techniques enlarges the necrosis area by a factor of 2 or 3. Exploitation of these possibilities enhances the ability to achieve tumor control and patient survival (Fig. 28.4).

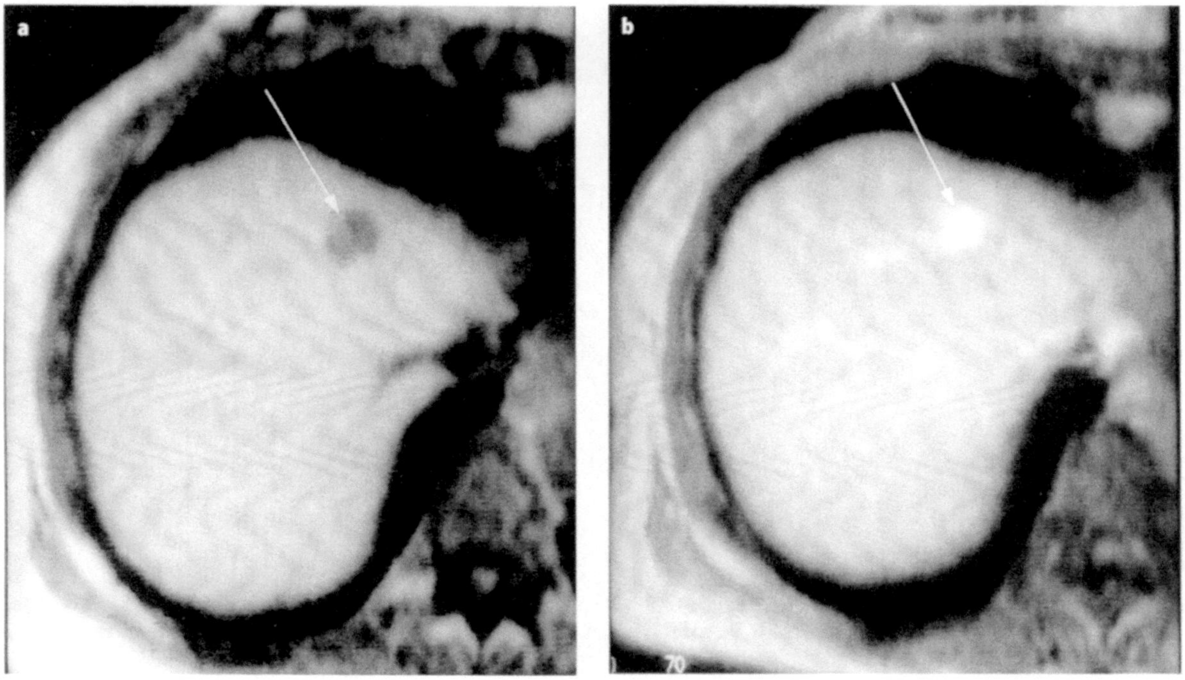

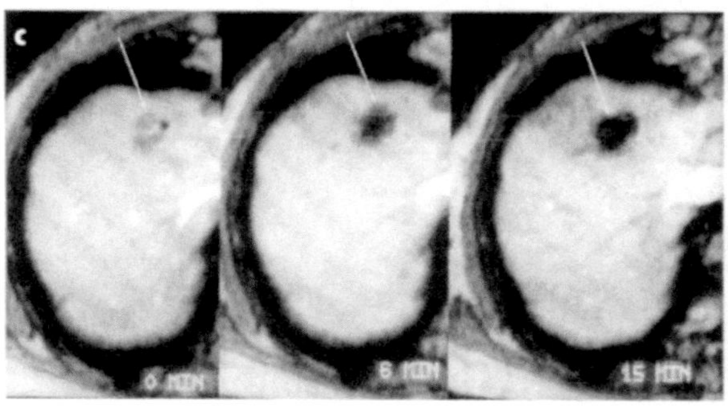

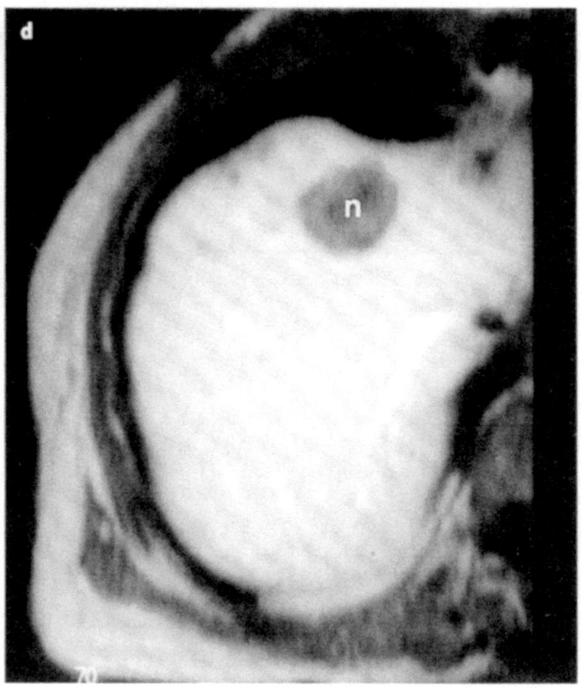

Fig. 28.2a-d. Liver metastases of a breast cancer. **a** An axial FLASH-2D image (TR 154/TE 6/flip angle 70°) reveals the size and location of the metastases in liver segment 8 (*arrow*) before LTT. **b** An axial contrast-enhanced FLASH-2D image (TR 154/TE 6/flip angle 70°) depicts the metastasis, before LTT, in liver segment 8 (*arrow*). The lesion is characterized by avid contrast-enhancement. **c** Thermosensitive FLASH-2D images (TR 102/TE 8/flip angle 15°) reveal a decrease of signal intensity during heating with the lesion (*arrows*). **d** An axial contrast-enhanced FLASH-2D image (TR 154/TE 6/flip angle 70°) obtained 2 days following LTT (15 min, 22.5 W) demonstrates the coagulative necrosis (*n*) suggesting total destruction of the metastasis.

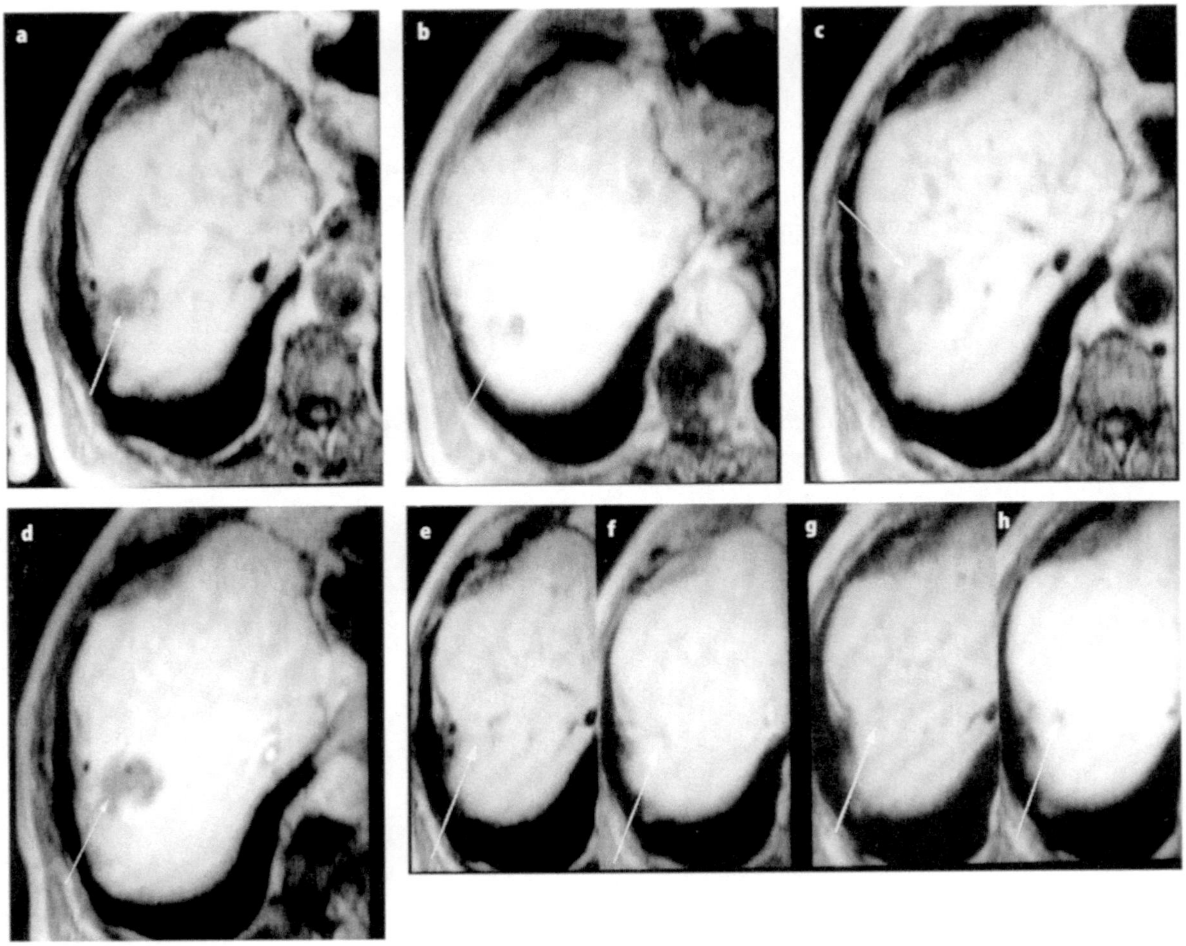

Figure 28.3a-h. Follow-up examination of a recurrent metastasis of a colorectal carcinoma following partial liver resection as the primary form of therapy. **a** A nonenhanced axial FLASH-2D image (TR 154/TE 6) prior to LTT delineates the hepatic metastases (*arrow*) of the colorectal carcinoma. **b** An axial contrast-enhanced FLASH-2D image following administration of 0.1 mmol/kg body weight Gd-DTPA demonstrates enhancement of the lesion (*arrow*) before LTT. **c** A nonenhanced FLASH-2D image acquired 2 days following LTT depicts the metastases with a slight central hemorrhage (*arrow*). **d** A contrast-enhanced FLASH-2D image obtained 2 days after the laser intervention (22 min., 5.8 W) shows the induced coagulative necrosis (*arrow*). Viable tumor is no longer documented. **e-h** Native (**e**) and contrast-enhanced (**f**) follow-up control studies obtained 3 months following LTT demonstrate an obvious decrease of lesion size (*arrow*). Similarly, the native (**g**) and contrast-enhanced (**h**) images obtained 1 year after LTT demonstrate no viable tumor. Only slight reactive changes are seen (*arrows*)

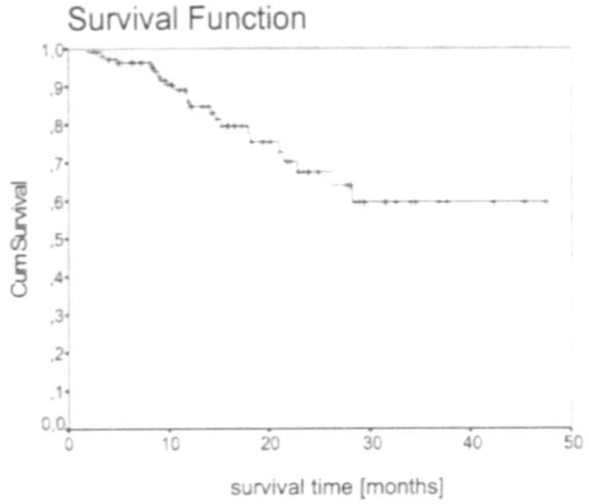

Fig. 28.4. Cumulative (*Cum*) survival rates of the consecutive patient series

28.4 Discussion

28.4.1 Benefits and Drawbacks of MR-Guided LTT Versus Conventional Therapy

Surgical resection of liver metastases is still considered the best option for a radical treatment of malignant tumors. However, only 20% of patients with hepatic metastasis are suitable candidates for surgical resection (Butler et al. 1986; Harned et al. 1994; Hughes et al. 1988; Scheele et al. 1991; Stangl et al. 1994; Steele 1994; Steele and Ravikumar 1989; Sugihara et al. 1993). The presence of lesions in both hepatic lobes or poor clinical condition of a patient exclude the possibility of surgical treatment. In addition, liver surgery is not without risk: it is associated with a mortality rate of approximately 5%. These facts have motivated the exploration of therapeutic alternatives in the treatment of liver metastases. These alternative strategies can be divided into oncologic therapies including systemic or locoregional chemotherapy, on the one hand, and interventional techniques including percutaneous alcohol injection (AMIN et al. 1993a), chemoembolization or percutaneous laser treatment on the other (GOLDENBERG 1994; LIURAGHI et al. 1995a, 1995b; PALMER et al. 1989). The clinical success of MR-guided LTT depends on three factors: the optimal localization of the applicator in the center of the lesion, optimal on-line monitoring of the temperature elevation in the tumor and surrounding tissue, and exact documentation of the local tumor destruction. On-line thermometry allows exact guidance of the interventional procedure. MRI provides unparalleled topographic accuracy owing to its excellent soft tissue contrast and high spatial resolution. Therefore, the early detection of local complications, like bleeding and hemorrhage, and treatment effects, like coagulative necrosis, is possible. Dynamic contrast-enhanced MR images represent the most important parameter for the evaluation of the treated lesions, especially the short-term evaluation.

The main benefits of this kind of treatment lie in the minimally invasive character of MR-guided LTT, the lack of short- or long-term side effects related to the treatment, and the patients' high tolerance of the procedure, combined with a short stay in hospital. The survival data (Fig. 28.4) compare most favorably with all other treatment alternatives in this non-surgical patient subset.

References

Amin Z, Bown SG, Lees WR (1993a) Local treatment of colorectal liver metastases: a comparison of interstitial laser photocoagulation (ILP) and percutaneous alcohol injection (PAI). Clin Radiol 48:166–171

Amin Z, Donald JJ, Masters A, et al (1993b) Hepatic metastases: interstitial laser photocoagulation with real-time US monitoring and dynamic CT evaluation of treatment. Radiology 187:339–347

Anzai Y, Lufkin RB, Castro DJ, et al (1991) MR imaging-guided interstitial Nd:YAG laser phototherapy: dosimetry study of acute tissue damage in an in vivo model. J Magn Reson Imaging 1:553–559

Butler J, Attiyeh FF, Daly JM (1986) Hepatic resection for metastases of the colon and rectum. Surg Gynecol Obstet 162:109–113

Castro DJ, Lufkin RB, Saxton RE, et al (1992) Metastatic head and neck malignancy treated using MRI guided interstitial laser phototherapy: an initial case report. Laryngoscope 102:26–32

Cline HE, Schenck JF, Watkins RD, Hynynen K, Jolesz FA (1993) Magnetic resonance-guided thermal surgery. Magn Reson Med 30:98–106

Dickinson RJ, Hall AS, Hind AJ, Young IR (1986) Measurement of changes in tissue temperature using MR imaging. J Comput Assist Tomogr 10:468–472

Goldenberg DM (1994) New developments in monoclonal antibodies for cancer detection and therapy. CA Cancer J Clin 44:43–64

Goslin R, Steele G Jr, Zamcheck N, Mayer R, MacIntyre J (1982) Factors influencing survival in patients with hepatic metastases from adenocarcinoma of the colon or rectum. Dis Colon Rectum 25:749–754

Harned RKN, Chezmar JL, Nelson RC (1994) Recurrent tumor after resection of hepatic metastases from colorectal carcinoma: location and time of discovery as determined by CT. AJR Am J Roentgenol 163:93–97

Hughes KS, Rosenstein RB, Songhorabodi S, et al (1988) Resection of the liver for colorectal carcinoma metastases. A multi-institutional study of long-term survivors. Dis Colon Rectum 31:1–4

Jaffe BM, Donegan WL, Watson F, Spratt JS Jr (1968) Factors influencing survival in patients with untreated hepatic metastases. Surg Gynecol Obstet 127:1–11

Livraghi T, Bolondi L, Buscarini L, et al (1995a) No treatment, resection and ethanol injection in hepatocellular carcinoma: a retrospective analysis of survival in 391 patients with cirrhosis. Italian Cooperative HCC Study Group. J Hepatol 22:522–526

Livraghi T, Giorgio A, Marin G, et al (1995b) Hepatocellular carcinoma and cirrhosis in 746 patients: long-term results of percutaneous ethanol injection. Radiology 197:101–108

Matsumoto R, Oshio K, Jolesz FA (1992) Monitoring of laser and freezing-induced ablation in the liver with T1-weighted MR imaging. J Magn Reson Imaging 2:555–562

Palmer M, Petrelli NJ, Herrera L (1989) No treatment option for liver metastases from colorectal adenocarcinoma. Dis Colon Rectum 32:698–701

Petrelli N, Douglass HO Jr, Herrera L, et al (1989) The modulation of fluorouracil with leucovorin in metastatic colorectal carcinoma: a prospective randomized phase III trial. Gastrointestinal Tumor Study Group. J Clin Oncol 1989; 7:1419–1426 (erratum 8:185)

Scheele J, Stangl R, Altendorf Hofmann A, Gall FP (1991) Indicators of prognosis after hepatic resection for colorectal secondaries. Surgery 110:13–29

Stangl R, Altendorf Hofmann A, Charnley RM, Scheele J (1994) Factors influencing the natural history of colorectal liver metastases. Lancet 343:1405–1410

Steele G, Jr (1994) Cryoablation in hepatic surgery. Semin Liver Dis 14:120–125

Steele G Jr, Ravikumar TS (1989) Resection of hepatic metastases from colorectal cancer. Biologic perspective. Ann Surg 210:127–138

Sugihara K, Hojo K, Moriya Y, Yamasaki S, Kosuge T, Takayama T (1993) Pattern of recurrence after hepatic resection for colorectal metastases. Br J Surg 80:1032–1035

Vogl TJ, Mack MG, Muller P, et al (1995a) Recurrent nasopharyngeal tumors: preliminary clinical results with interventional MR imaging – controlled laser-induced thermotherapy. Radiology 196:725–733

Vogl TJ, Muller PK, Hammerstingl R, et al (1995b) Malignant liver tumors treated with MR imaging-guided laser-induced thermotherapy: technique and prospective results. Radiology 196:257–265

Weiss L, Grundmann E, Torhorst J, et al (1986) Haematogenous metastatic patterns in colonic carcinoma: an analysis of 1541 necropsies. J Pathol 150:195–203

29 Interstitial Laser Therapy of Prostate Lesions

G.U. Müller-Lisse and A.F. Heuck

CONTENTS

29.1 Introduction

Increasing numbers of patients are diagnosed each year with prostate cancer (PC) or benign prostatic hyperplasia (BPH). Although both PC and BPH seldom occur in patients under the age of 50 years, they show a high and increasing prevalence in men over 60 years of age (Conrad et al. 1995). Throughout Europe and the USA, patients with PC usually undergo radical prostatectomy, radiation therapy, antiandrogenic therapy, or any combination of these modalities. In cases of infravesical (outlet) obstruction, transurethral electro-resection of the prostate (TUR-P) may precede radiation therapy or antiandrogenic treatment. However, despite early investigations in the field (Sander et al. 1982; Sander and Beisland 1984), neither laser therapy nor any other alternative surgical intervention plays an important role in PC therapy as yet. Cryosurgical ablation of the prostate in patients with PC has been reported as another alternative treatment with little associated morbidity (Onik et al. 1993), but the number of patients treated is relatively small and follow-up examinations with MRI could not reliably differentiate between therapy-induced changes and residual PC (Kalbhen et al. 1996).

In BPH, on the other hand, the increasing number of patients either unwilling to undergo or considered incapable of tolerating the "gold-standard" therapy of TUR-P has spurned the development of alternative therapies. Various therapies include application of laser energy to prostate tissue, and MRI has been used both to follow up and to monitor different types of laser therapy for BPH. This chapter introduces some of the alternative therapies for BPH and illustrates current applications of MRI in this field.

29.2 Therapies for Benign Prostatic Hyperplasia

The classical gold-standard therapy for BPH is transurethral electro-resection of the prostate. An electrical current is passed through a wire loop that is mounted on the shaft of a cystoscope. The cystoscope is inserted into the prostatic urethra and pieces of adenomyomatous prostate tissue are scraped out with the wire loop by passing the endoscope back and forth. Depending on the design of the wire loop, approximately 0.5–1.0 g of tissue are removed per minute. While the procedure is highly effective, its drawbacks lie in the blood loss (severe blood loss with subsequent blood transfusion in approximately 4% of patients; Conrad et al. 1995) and incorporation of irrigation fluids into the spongy adenomatous prostate tissue that is exposed once the urothelium has been scraped off the wall of the prostatic urethra. As a consequence of TUR-P, 50–68% of patients experience retrograde ejaculation, 4–15% complain of erectile dysfunction, 0.8–1.8% of incontinence, and 2.7–3.3% of urethral stricture (Hartung 1995).

An alternative for patients with large prostates or with frequently recurring BPH is suprapubic prostatectomy, an open surgical procedure whereby adenomatous tissue is digitally removed through the bladder. The procedure is associated with longer terms of hospitalization and a slightly higher mortality rate than TUR-P (Hinman 1994), while long-term morbidity is higher in TUR-P (Conrad et al. 1995).

G.U. Müller-Lisse, MD, Institute of Diagnostic Radiology, Ludwig Maximilians-Universität München, Klinikum Grosshadern, Marchioninistrasse 15, D-81377 Munich, Germany
A.F. Heuck, MD, Institute of Diagnostic Radiology, Ludwig Maximilians-Universität München, Klinikum Grosshadern, Marchioninistrasse 15, D-81377 Munich, Germany

Alternative therapies, including urethral stents (Gottfried et al. 1995) and thermal treatments with various energy sources, have been designed to decrease the risks, complications and side effects of the classical therapies. Medical lasers represent one such energy source. The term "laser" is an acronym for light amplification by stimulated emission of radiation. The optical waveguides utilized in laser prostatectomy devices are made of high-purity fused silica glass with minimal optical absorption and scattering. Less than 1% of the laser energy is actually lost during the series of reflections from one side wall to the opposite along the length of the fiber core of a typical optical fiber for medical applications. The active end of the fiber core is covered by a layer of lower refractive index glass or plastic termed "cladding" (Milam and Smith 1995). Depending on the design of the active fiber end, different laser instruments with different properties and modes of tissue interaction result. Presently, sidefire lasers are the class of instruments most frequently used for laser prostatectomy. The original (refractive) right-angle delivery system for coagulation prostatectomy was the transurethral ultrasonically guided laser-induced prostatectomy device (TULIP; IntraSonix, Burlington, Mass.) that diverts the laser beam 90° via a sapphire prism. Reflective sidefire systems utilize a gold-plated stainless steel reflector to deflect the laser beam laterally. Usually, the beam is not preserved but diverges to light a larger surface area, as in, for example, the Urolase device (Bard, Marietta, GA), with horizontal beam divergence of 25° and a sagittal divergence of 60°. Reflective systems absorb more energy than refractive systems (Milam and Smith 1995). Sidefire lasers are applied transurethrally in a non-contact mode, and laser energy is absorbed by prostatic tissue after passing through the urine or water contained in the prostatic urethra. Upon absorption, electromagnetic energy contained in the laser light waves is transformed into thermal energy which brings about tissue coagulation.

Clinical experience with the TULIP device has demonstrated that blood loss, incorporation of irrigation fluids, and the rate of postoperative retrograde ejaculation can be minimized, while peak urine flow and residual urine volume as well as prostate symptom scores improve considerably. The disadvantage of TULIP sidefire laser prostatectomy lies in the delayed relief of infravesical obstruction and a postoperative phase of bladder infection-like irritative symptoms (Schulze et al. 1995).

Randomized trials of visual laser-assisted prostatectomy (VLAP) with sidefire lasers versus TUR-P have shown that the clinical results (peak flow, residual urine) over 3–6 months after therapy are similar, while prostate symptom scores may be better with TUR-P (Conrad et al. 1995).

Sidefire VLAP and TUR-P are similar in that tissue is removed around the original prostatic urethra under visual control, which eventually creates a funnel-like crater depleted of urothelium with secondary reconstitution of the urothelial lining.

Interstitial laser-induced thermotherapy (LITT) takes a different approach. The cladded active end of an optical laser fiber is placed interstitially in the prostate (with immediate tissue contact) via a transperineal or transurethral approach (e.g., Dornier fibertom, Dornier Medical Systems, Germering, Germany). Laser light is evenly diffused by the cladding and produces ovoid or cylindrical coagulation lesions. LITT is highly effective in reducing both prostate and residual urine volumes and increasing peak urine flow as well as improving BPH symptoms (Muschter et al. 1993, 1995). While fiber end positions are controlled endoscopically or sonographically (in the transperineal approach), the process of interstitial coagulation itself cannot be monitored with these instruments. Another contact laser system consists of a 7-mm diameter round contact probe threaded onto a 600-mm optical fiber. The surface of the probe is covered with a black absorbent coating. The coating absorbs about 30% of the laser energy, causing intense probe heating. Contact between the hot probe and tissue produces tissue surface vaporization and subsurface coagulation (Contact Laser System, Surgical Laser Technologies, Oaks, CA). Contact laser systems utilize a conventional fiber-optic waveguide surrounded by a plastic cooling channel (Milam and Smith 1995).

Other sources of thermal energy include microwave generators, as in transurethral microwave thermotherapy (TUMT). A cooled microwave antenna is inserted into the prostatic urethra. Circular zones of coagulation develop in tissue around the urethra where temperatures exceed 45°C. Cooling of the antenna leads to preservation of 3–5 mm of tissue around the urethra. The clinical effectiveness of TUMT over up to 6 months has been demonstrated in studies comparing TUMT, TUR-P and sham treatment. However, while TUMT improves prostate symptom scores, it does not improve objective data like peak urine flow and residual urine volume. TUMT is considered to be a safe, minimally invasive treatment for patients with mild to moderate symptoms of BPH and only mild objective degrees of obstruction. It can be performed on an outpatient basis (Höfner et al. 1995).

Transrectal high-intensity focussed ultrasound (HIFU) has shown promising early clinical results, including improvement of peak urine flow and residual urine volume (MADERSBACHER et al. 1995).

Other, nonsurgical alternatives include pharmaceutical intervention with α_1-blockers (STOCKAMP 1995) or various phytotherapeutic drugs (DREIKORN and SCHÖNHÖFER 1995) whose value lies in the subjective relief of symptoms rather than in objective improvement of urine flow and residual urine. Hormone therapy with gonadotropin-relasing hormone agonists, cyproterone acetate and flutamide is effective, but rarely used in BPH owing to the side effects. New hormone derivatives with reduced side effects are currently under clinical investigation (HORNINGER and BARTSCH 1995).

29.3 Current Applications of MRI in the Monitoring of Interventions in Benign Prostatic Hyperplasia

Most examinations of the prostate with MRI are based on T2-weighted images since these allow differentiation of intraprostatic structures such as central (including transitional) and peripheral glandular tissue, the anterior fibromuscular band, the prostatic capsule, and, in cases of hyperplasia, the prostatic pseudocapsule that presents as a hypointense rim surrounding the hyperplastic adenomyomatous tissue in BPH (ALLEN et al. 1989; KAHN et al. 1989; MÜLLER-LISSE et al. 1996a, PHILLIPS et al. 1987; Fig. 29.1a). Unenhanced T1-weighted images outline the outer margins of the prostatic capsule

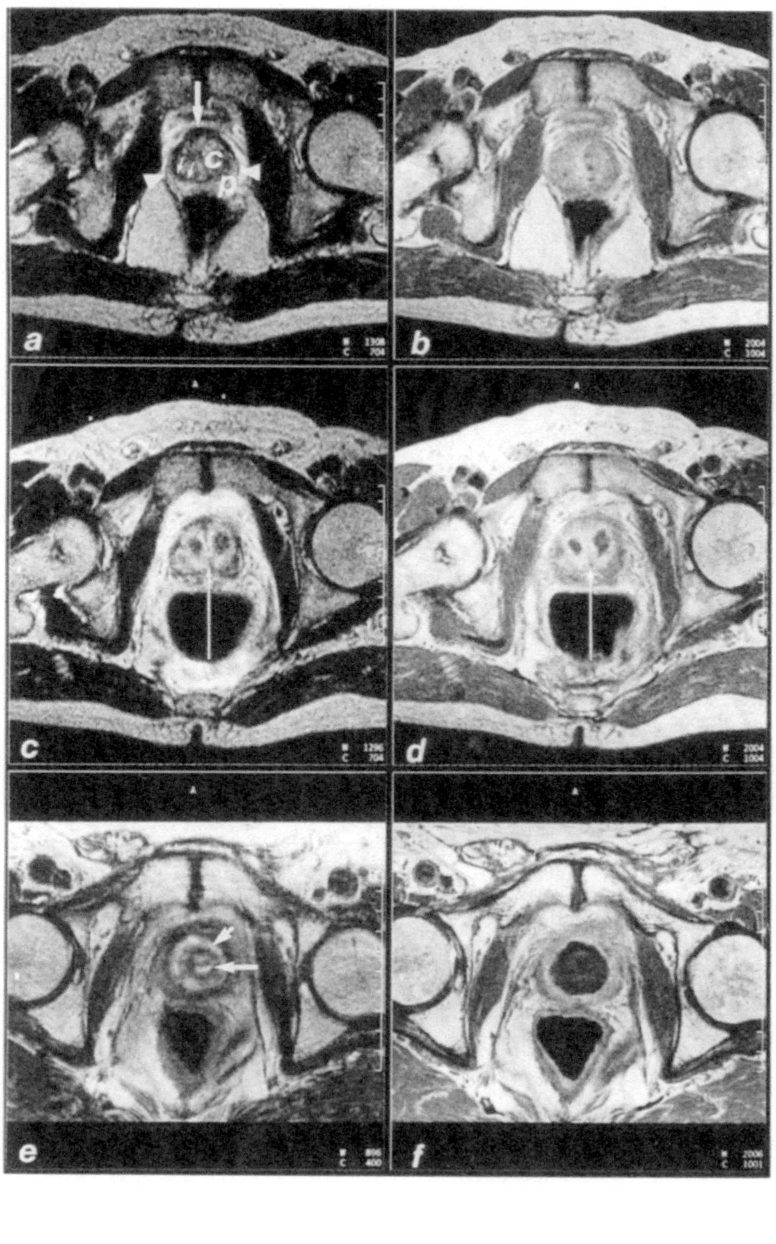

Fig. 29.1. Pretherapeutic appearance of the prostate in MR images **a,b,** post-therapeutic changes after visual laser ablation of the prostate (VLAP) **c,d** and interstitial laser-induced thermotherapy (LITT) **e,f** in patients with benign prostatic hyperplasia (BPH). Prior to therapy, T2-weighted images allow the differentiation of central (*c*) and peripheral (*p*) gland, prostatic capsule (*arrowheads*) and pseudocapsule (*small arrows*) and anterior fibromuscular band (*large arrow*) (**a**). On delayed contrast-enhanced T1-weighted images, the prostate appears more homogeneous (**b**). T2-weighted (**c**) and contrast-enhanced T1-weighted (**d**) images after LITT show low-signal-intensity cores of coagulated tissue surrounded by a 4–6 mm wide hyperintense enhancing rim of active inflammatory tissue that stands out against the peripheral zone of the prostate. The prostatic urethra lies in the central strand of preserved tissue (*arrow*). After VLAP, T2-weighted images (**e**) show a coagulated tissue remnant (*large arrow*) surrounded by urine (*small arrow*) in a smoothly outlined funnel that replaces the prostatic urethra and is distinguished from prostatic tissue by a hypointense rim of active scar tissue. Delayed contrast-enhanced T1-weighted images (**f**) show enhancing active scar tissue surrounding the urine-filled funnel with nonperfused remnants of coagulated tissue in its center.

against the periprostatic venous plexus and fibroadipose tissue, while differentiation of internal structures inside the prostate is impossible. Contrast-enhanced T1-weighted images, on the other hand, show homogeneous distribution of gadolinium-DTPA in the prostate on delayed scans (Fig. 19.1b). They permit delineation of necrotic regions based on their lack of enhancement (MUSCHTER et al. 1995; ROGGAN et al. 1994; MÜLLER-LISSE et al. 1996b).

Classical TUR-P does not necessitate MRI monitoring of intraoperative or postoperative results, since the resection is carried out under direct visual guidance through the endoscope. However, in an analysis with MRI of morphologic changes in hyperplastic prostate tissues following TUR-P, TAZAKI et al. (1995a) report reduction of hyperplastic tissue in the transitional zone, reepithelization of the prostatic urethra, and narrowing of the TUR-P-induced urethral channel within 8–12 weeks after the procedure as well as shrinking of the prostatic capsule and decrease in prostate size over 8–12 months after therapy. In their TUR-P patients, peak urine flow improved 78–81% within 8–12 weeks after the operation (TAZAKI et al. 1995a).

In patients undergoing TUMT, MRI shows no remarkable tissue reduction in the transitional zone shortly after treatment, but demonstrates areas of hemorrhagic necrosis beneath the epithelium of the prostatic urethra. Over 8–12 weeks, the hemorrhagic necrosis is replaced by scar tissue which leads to widening of the prostatic urethra. The urethral epithelium is left intact at all times, as proved by its more intense uptake of contrast media compared with the prostate (TAZAKI et al. 1995a).

The effects of VLAP also show a delayed course. While necrosis is visualized by contrast-enhanced MRI early after VLAP and reaches 0.7–1.0 cm deep into the periurethral prostatic tissue, the necrotic tissue is eventually sloughed off over 8–12 weeks (Fig. 29.1c, d), leaving a smoothly outlined cavity that reepithelializes secondarily (TAZAKI et al. 1995a, 1995b). DESOUZA et al. (1995), however, report different results in their MRI study of eight patients undergoing VLAP with a Urolase sidefire laser. They describe the formation of a poorly defined, low-signal-intensity region around the urethra on T2-weighted images immediately after therapy. This low-intensity region became less obvious after 1 week and was eventually replaced by a well-demarcated low-signal-intensity ring after 3 months on both T2-weighted and gradient-recalled echo images (DESOUZA et al. 1995).

LITT of the prostate, on the other hand, induces intraprostatic coagulation lesions. They are characterized by low-signal-intensity, surrounded by a high-signal-intensity rim of inflammatory tissue seen on both T2-weighted (MÜLLER-LISSE et al. 1996a) and contrast-enhanced T1-weighted images (MÜLLER-LISSE et al. 1996b; Fig. 29.1e, f). The lesions shrink to approximately 10% of their original size over a period of 6–12 months. This shrinkage is associated with a decrease of prostate volume averaging about 20% both for the central prostatic gland (including the hyperplastic transitional zone) and the total prostatic volume (Table 29.1). Correlation between the development of lesion volume and prostate volume amounts to 85–90% at various follow-up dates after LITT (Table 29.2). Since necrotic areas can be outlined on contrast-enhanced T1-weighted MR images immediately after LITT, the long-term volumetric outcome after LITT of the

Table 29.1. Development of total gland volume, central gland volume, and volume of laser-induced lesions over 6 to 12 months in relation to initial values in eight patients with LITT for BPH (mean %)

Volume	Pre –48–0 hours	Post 1 0–48 hours	Post 2 2–3 weeks	Post 3 6–8 weeks	Post 4 6–12 months
Total gland (%)	100	125	107	86	80
Central gland (%)	100	130	111	89	79
Lesion (%)		100	105	37	11

(modified from: MÜLLER-LISSE et al. 1996b)
BPH, benign prostatic hyperplasia; LITT, interstitial laser-induced thermotherapy

Table 29.2. Correlation of development of total gland volume and volume of laser-induced lesions after LITT in eight patients with BPH

Volume	Post 2 2–3 weeks	Post 3 6–8 weeks	Post 4 6–12 months
Total gland (ml)	+4.3	–8.7	–12.2
Lesion (ml)	+0.8	–8.3	–11.8
Correlation Coefficient	0.903	0.857	0.900
Significance (P)[a]	0.002	0.007	0.002

(modified from: MÜLLER-LISSE et al. 1996b)
[a]Pearson test

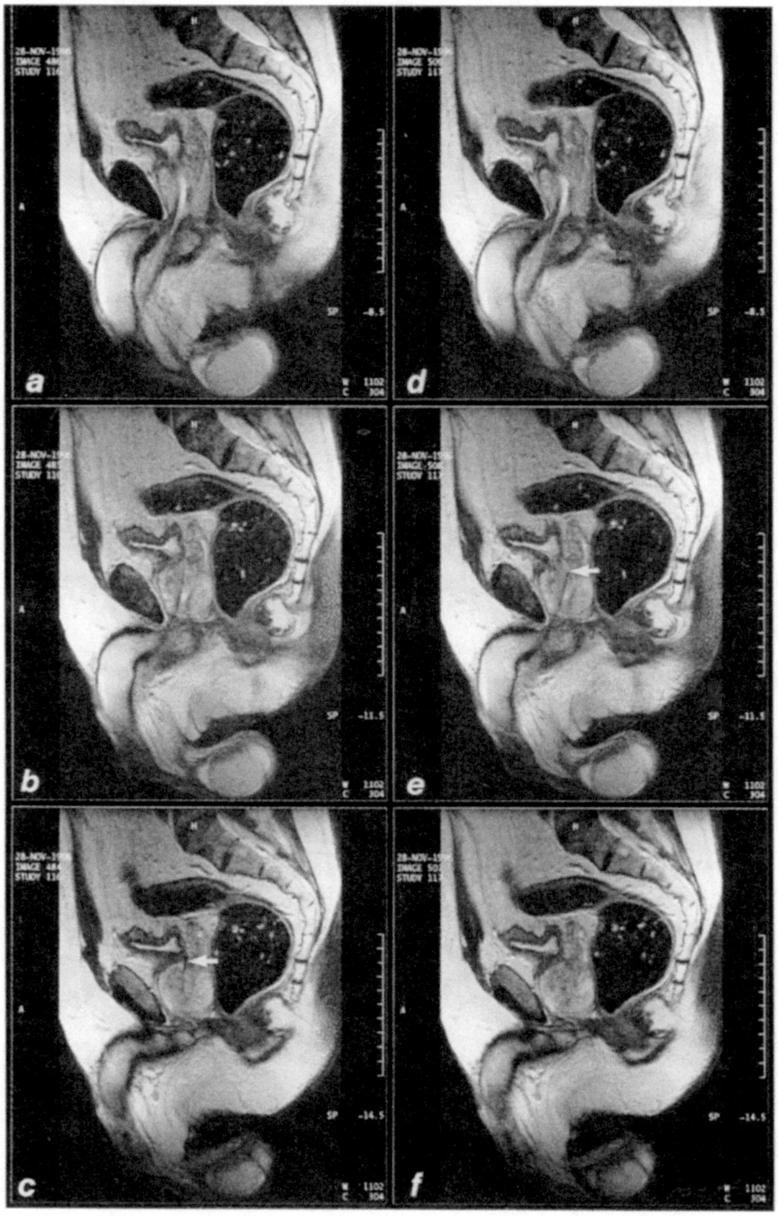

Fig. 29.2a-f. Correction of laser fiber position in MRI-guided LITT of BPH. The left column of adjacent T2-weighted MR images (**a-c**) shows the active end of the laser fiber to extend beyond the prostate, reaching the dorsal bladder wall (**c**, *arrow*). After pulling the fiber back by about 1 cm, the active end lies securely in the hyperplastic central gland (**e**, *arrow*)

prostate is predictable at therapy if carried out under MRI guidance (MÜLLER-LISSE et al. 1996b). Volumetric assessments based on MR images are accurate with intraobserver and interobserver reproducibility of measurements in the order of 5% (MÜLLER-LISSE et al. 1996a) and a correlation with prostate specimen volumes determined at pathology of around 93% (RAHMOUNI et al. 1992).

Online monitoring of thermal therapy of the prostate for BPH has been the subject of only two studies (DESOUZA et al. 1995; MÜLLER-LISSE et al. 1996b). The Urolase sidefire technique applied by DESOUZA et al. (1995) does not lend itself to continuous MRI monitoring during therapy, at least when conventional MR scanner designs are involved. Since sidefire VLAP requires that the operator observe the process of non-contact tissue coagulation continuously through the endoscope, deep tissue effects were intermittently monitored with MRI each time treatment of a quadrant of hyperplastic transitional tissue around the prostatic urethra had been completed. T1-weighted images obtained at intermissions showed decreased signal intensity in areas of the prostate that had just been treated with VLAP (DESOUZA et al. 1995).

LITT, however, does not require interactive visual guidance of the active end of the laser once this has been placed in the tissue. Therefore, the process of tissue coagulation can be monitored online even with conventionally designed tube-shaped MR scanners. Monitoring with T1-weighted sequences allows the recognition of the cladded active end of the laser

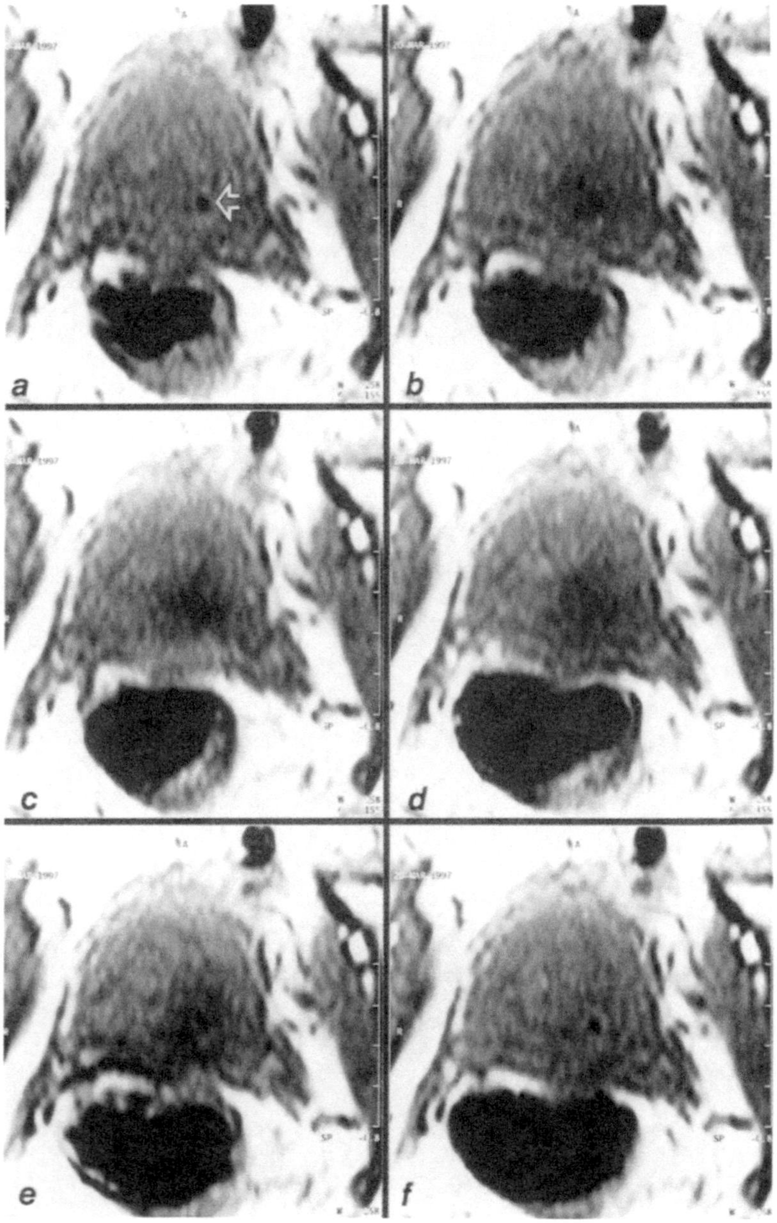

Fig. 29.3a-f. On-line monitoring with MRI of guided LITT of BPH. The active end of the laser fiber is well delineated on T1-weighted gradient-recalled echo images (**a-f**). Prostatic tissue appears more homogeneous prior to laser treatment (**a**, *open arrow*), while an area of decreased signal intensity spreads centrifugally from the fiber end during laser treatment (**b–e**, after 40, 80, 120, and 180 s of laser treatment) to disappear once the laser has been switched off (**f**)

fiber within the prostatic tissue and correction of fiber position (Fig. 29.2) as well as the development of a hypointense area around the laser fiber that spreads centrifugally with increasing duration of laser energy application, but completely disappears when the laser has been switched off and tissue temperature falls back to normal (Fig. 29.3). While in vitro studies in bovine prostate and seminal vesicles have shown high linear correlation of 88–98% between interstitial tissue temperature and signal intensity in T1-weighted gradient-recalled echo sequences in the temperature range of interest for coagulation thermotherapy, it remains impossible to exactly determine the margins of coagulation in prostatic tissue in vivo from these images (Müller-Lisse et al. 1996b).

29.4 Conclusions

Magnetic resonance imaging is developing a role in the monitoring of alternative therapies of the prostate. While there is some hesitance to apply alternative therapies such as visual laser ablation and interstitial laser-induced thermotherapy to prostate cancer, there is increasing interest in their application to relieve symptomatic BPH. Experience in the follow-up with MRI of patients who have undergone classical TUR-P, TUMT, visual laser ablation, and LITT has shown that MRI is capable of visualizing a variety of therapy-related intraprostatic changes and allows quantitative evaluation of their development.

One-stop therapy planning, therapy guidance and monitoring, and result control, including prediction of volumetric development of the prostate, are within reach in MRI-guided LITT. However, for online determination of the actual extent of the coagulated lesion, interstitial temperature mapping will be necessary. Color-coded temperature-related mapping of signal intensity development based on rapid T1-weighted MR images will be one option.

References

Allen KS, Kressel MY, Arger PH, Pollack HM (1989) Age-related changes of the prostate: evaluation by MR imaging. Am J Roentgenol 152:77–81

Conrad S, Gonnermann D, Heinzer H, Kabalin JN, Huland H (1995) Transurethrale Lasertherapie der benignen Prostatahyperplasie. Urologe A 34:25–34

deSouza NM, Flynn RJ, Coutts GA, et al. (1995) Endoscopic laser ablation of the prostate: MR appearances during and after treatment and their relation to clinical outcome. Am J Roentgenol 164:1429–1434

Dreikorn K, Schönhöfer PS (1995) Stellenwert von Phytotherapeutika bei der Behandlung der benignen Prostatahyperplasie (BPH). Urologe A 34:119–129

Gottfried HW, Schimers HP, Gschwend J, Brändle E, Hautmann R (1995) Erste Erfahrungen mit dem Memotherm,-Stent in der Behandlung der BPH (First experience with the Memotherm stent in the treatment of BPH). Urologe A 34:110–118

Hinman F (1994) Atlas urologischer Operationen. Rübben H and Altwein JE (eds. of German edition). Ferdinand Enke Verlag Stuttgart, 1124 pp

Hartung R (1995) Die BPH – ein altes Krankheitsbild – neu betrachtet. Urologe A 34:77–83

Höfner K, Krah H, Tan HK, Kuczyk M, Jonas U (1995) Thermotherapie der benignen Prostatahyperplasie (Thermotherapy in benign prostatic hyperplasia). Urologe A 34:16–24

Hofstetter A (1991) Interstitielle Thermokoagulation (ITK) von Prostatatumoren. Lasermedizin 7:179

Horninger W, Bartsch G (1995) Hormonelle Therapie der benignen Prostatahyperplasie (Hormone therapy for benign prostatic hyperplasia). Urologe A 34:9–15

Kahn T, Bürrig K, Schmitz-Dräger B, Lewin JS, Fürst G, Mödder U (1989) Prostatic carcinoma and benign prostatic hyperplasia: MR imaging with histopathologic correlation. Radiology 173:847–851

Kalbhen CL, Hricak H, Shinohara K, et al. (1996) Prostate carcinoma: MR imaging findings after cryosurgery. Radiology 198:807–811

Madersbacher S, Kratzik C, Susani M, Marberger M (1995) Minimal invasive Therapie der benignen Prostatahyperplasie mit fokussiertem Ultraschall (High-intensity focussed ultrasound as a minimally invasive treatment for benign prostatic hyperplasia). Urologe A 34:98–104

Milam DF, Smith JA (1995) Laser prostatectomy devices and their tissue effects. J Endourol 9:85–88

Müller-Lisse UG, Heuck AF, Schneede P, Muschter R, Scheidler J, Hofstetter AG, Reiser MF (1996a) Postoperative MRI in patients undergoing interstitial laser coagulation thermotherapy of benign prostatic hyperplasia. J Comput Assist Tomogr 20:273–278

Müller-Lisse GU, Heuck A, Stehling MK, et al. (1996b) MRT-Monitoring vor, während und nach der interstitiellen laserinduzierten Thermotherapie der benignen Prostatahyperplasie. Erste klinische Erfahrungen (MRI monitoring before, during, and after interstitial laser-induced thermotherapy of benign prostatic hyperplasia: first clinical experience). Radiologe 36:722–731

Muschter R, Hessel S, Hofstetter A, Keiditsch E, Rothenberger KH, Schneede P, Frank F (1993) Die interstitielle Laserkoagulation der benignen Prostatahyperplasie. Urologe A 32:273–281

Muschter R, Zellner M, Hessel S, Hofstetter A (1995) Die interstitielle laserinduzierte Koagulation (ILK) der Prostata zur Therapie der benignen Prostatahyperplasie (BPH) (Interstitial laser-induced coagulation of the prostate in the treatment of benign hyperplasia). Urologe A 39:90–97

Onik GM, Cohen JK, Reyes GD, Rubinsky B, Chang Z, Baust J (1993) Transrectal ultrasound-guided percutaneous radical cryosurgical ablation of the prostate. Cancer 72:1291–1299

Phillips ME, Kressel HY, Spritzer CE et al. (1987) Normal prostate and adjacent structures: MR imaging at 1.5 T. Radiology 164:381–385

Rahmouni A, Yang A, Tempany CMC, Frenkel T, Epstein J, Walsh P, Leichner PK, Ricci C, Zerhouni E (1992) Accuracy of in-vivo assessment of prostatic volume by MRI and transrectal ultrasonography. J Comput Assist Tomogr 16:935–940

Roggan A, Handke A, Miller K, Müller G (1994) Laser induced interstitial thermotherapy of benign prostatic hyperplasia – basic investigations and first clinical results. Min Invasive Med 5:55–63

Sander S, Beisland HO, Fossberg E (1982) Neodymium YAG laser in the treatment of prostatic cancer. Urol Res 10:85–86

Sander S, Beisland HO (1984) Laser in the treatment of localized prostatic carcinoma. J Urol 132:280–281

Schulze H, Martin W, Hoch P, Finke W, Senge T (1995) TULIP-Erfahrungen an über 80 Patienten (TULIP – experience in over 80 cases). Urologe A 34:84–89

Stockamp K (1995) Therapie der BPH mit α-Rezeptorenblockern (α-blockers in the treatment of benign prostatic hyperplasia). Urologe A 34:3–8

Tazaki H, Deguchi N, Baba S, Imai Y, Nakashima J (1995a) Magnetic resonance imaging following microwave thermotherapy, laser ablation and transurethral resection in patients with BPH. Urologe A 34:105–109

Tazaki H, Nakashima J, Nakagawa K (1995b) MRI evaluation of cavitation induced by laser prostatectomy. J Endourol 971–173

30 Interstitial Laser Therapy of Breast Lesions

M.A. Hall-Craggs

CONTENTS

30.1 Introduction

The concept of limited breast-conserving surgery (usually coupled with radiotherapy) in selected patients with breast cancer is now widely accepted, and several prospective randomised trials have shown that neither the disease-free interval nor overall survival are adversely affected in patients treated with breast-conservation surgery as compared with mastectomy (Veronesi et al. 1990; Fisher et al. 1989; Jacobson et al. 1995). However, it is not always associated with a good cosmetic result, and there may be post-therapeutic deformity and scarring. The known safety of breast conservation has prompted research into the application of minimally invasive therapies to breast cancers.

Another group of patients seeking an improved cosmetic result from the management of their breast disease consists of women with benign breast fibroadenomas. These masses, which are considered to be aberrations of normal breast tissue rather than truly neoplastic tumors, occur most commonly in young women in their early twenties and they are frequently multiple. To date these tumours have been managed either conservatively or by surgical excision. The main disadvantages of the conservative approach are that the patient has to live with a palpable lump(s) and, since the natural history of fibroadenomas is variable, the tumours may increase in size. On the other hand, surgery results in multiple scars in those patients requiring multiple excisions. In these women, percutaneous, minimally invasive therapies potentially offer a cosmetically superior result than surgical excision and a more predictable outcome than conservative management.

A number of minimally invasive therapies have been applied to the treatment of solid tumours and these can be loosely divided into thermal treatments [including interstitial laser photocoagulation (ILP), radiofrequency thermal ablation and high intensity focused ultrasound] and non-thermal techniques (photodynamic therapy and brachytherapy). Of these treatments, the method which has been developed most extensively in the breast is ILP, which in our own institution has been applied to the treatment of both benign and malignant tumours.

The ultimate aim of minimally invasive therapy to breast disease is to provide a one-stop, effective, safe and cosmetically acceptable treatment. With breast cancers, the aim is to completely destroy the cancer at a single outpatient treatment session, to modify and validate the extent of therapy at the time of the procedure and to obtain sufficient, clear margins akin to the 10-mm margins aimed at by surgeons. To do this, the biological effect of the therapy must be understood, the treatment must be controllable and reproducible. The treatment must be locally effective and at least equal to surgical excision (i.e. complete tumour resection with adequately clear resection margins). In the long term it must result in therapeutic benefit which equals or exceeds that presently available and must not confer adverse mortality or morbidity, such as an increase in local tumour recurrence, on the patient.

In order to be able to treat tumours effectively, there are a number of prerequisites for imaging the tumour and therapeutic effects. The tumour must be visualised and the locoregional extent of disease must be mapped accurately. It must be possible to

M.A. Hall-Craggs, MR-Unit, The Middlesex Hospital, University College London Hospitals, Mortimer Street, London W1N 8AA, UK measure the extent of the therapeutic effect after, or preferably during, treatment, and the extent of residual disease must be identified. It is to these issues that research efforts have been addressed.

30.2 Laser Properties

Interstitial laser photocoagulation (ILP) therapy is a technique which was first described in 1983 at our own institution (Bown 1983) as a minimally invasive method of causing localised tumour destruction in solid organs. Low-poor laser light energy is delivered directly to the target organ via optical fibres inserted into tissue, and tumours are destroyed by direct heating. ILP is now being used in routine clinical practice for some solid tumours, including liver metastases and head and neck tumours (see Chaps. 27 and 28).

Initial research into ILP showed that the shape and size of thermal lesions were difficult to predict and very variable owing to biological variability (Cheong et al. 1990), fibre-tip charring and changing optical and thermal conductivity properties of tissue during ILP (Svaasand et al. 1985). The use of ILP in primary breast cancer was first described by Stegar et al. (1989) in a patient with breast cancer who had rejected all conventional treatment. In this patient, treatment at three sites within the tumour by ILP produced a reduction in tumour volume as measured by ultrasound examination.

Using the semiconductor diode laser (Diomed-25, Diomed, Cambridge, UK), operating at 805 nm and coupled to 400-μm bare optic fibres, initial experiments made using laser parameters of 2–3 W for a duration of 500–750 s showed that the volume of the coagulative necrosis was variable (Harries et al. 1994). It was noticed in these early experiments that the diameter of the damaged tissue was greater if the fibre became charred during the procedure (median diameter 6 mm vs 13 mm for the clean and charred fibres, respectively). This led to further experiments comparing clean and pre-charred needles which showed that charring the fibre before the procedure consistently produced larger areas of necrosis (median diameter 9 mm vs 14 mm for clean and charred fibres, respectively) and that the burn was more consistent and less variable in size. Pre-charring can be performed in two ways; either a drop of the patient's blood can be placed on the optical fibre tip and the laser fired at a higher power (10 W for 20 s) or, if the fibre has already been placed within the breast, adequate charring can be obtained by a similar high-energy burst with the fibre tip in situ.

The use of diffuser tips was explored early in these studies as a method of increasing the volume of ILP-induced necrosis, but the bare pre-charred fibre tip was found to produce better results, possibly related to the thermal rather than optical effects of the therapy. A larger array of diffuser tips is now available but their efficacy in the breast is largely untested.

30.3 Treatment Technique

Laser technology has been developed sufficiently such that it is now reliable, portable, easy-to-use and deliverable in an MR environment. In our studies we have used the semiconductor diode laser (Diomed-25, Diomed, Cambridge, UK) which is compact, lightweight and does not require either sophisticated water cooling or a three-phase electrical supply. This laser operates at 805 nm, although a new generation of diode lasers are becoming available which can operate with variable wavelengths (Amin 1995). The laser light source is directly coupled to either a single optical fibre or, via a beam splitter, to several fibres. Each fibre is calibrated separately for output before treatment. By using long fibres (up to several metres long) the lasers can be used in an MR environment operating at high field strength as the source can remain within the scanner console room outside the 5 gauss line and the fibres passed through wave guides into the scanning room itself. The optical fibres themselves are 400 μm in diameter and thus pass easily through 18-G introducer needles. The fibres are freshly cleaved and sterilised before each treatment and before the pre-charring procedure.

The technique for treating tumours is simple although therapy has to be carried out in an isolated area with full laser safety precautions in place and with aseptic technique. As the laser damage is due to thermal heating, if unsedated, patients experience a feeling of heat and quite severe discomfort deep within the breast, as well as burning at the skin surface. Consequently all our patients receive intravenous sedation and analgesia before treatment. In our practice the tumour is usually localized using ultrasound and up to four 18-G needles (MR-compatible if the patient is to be studied in the MR scanner) are inserted into the tumour. The fibres, which measure 400 mm in diameter, are pre-charred, placed through the needles and positioned such that the tips lie a few millimetres distal to the needle tip. Treatments are made with 2–2.5 W per fibre delivered for 500 s (>1000 J per fibre).

As successful ILP potentially results in the destruction of all tumour tissue it is essential that the tumour type (benign or malignant, histological characteristics and grade) is characterised as completely as possible before treatment by adequate cytological and/or histopathological examination. For breast cancer, histology (and in some centres, cytology) is used for tumour grading, prognostic stratification and to determine the need for adjuvant treatment.

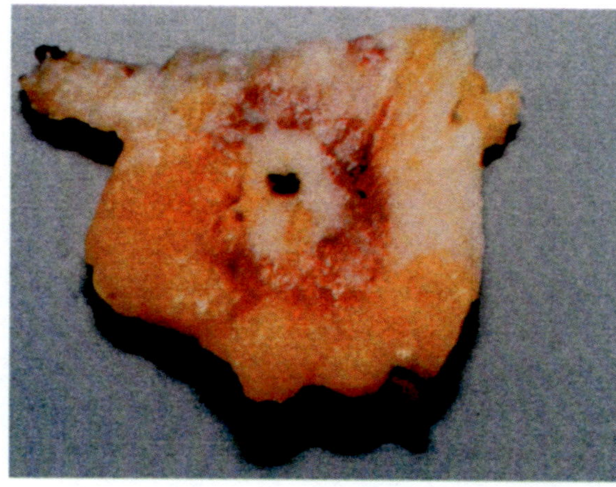

Fig. 30.1. Macroscopy of an interstitial laser photocoagulation (ILP) burn. The lesion made by ILP has a three-layered appearance macroscopically, with a central charred hole surrounded by a white zone of in situ fixation. Around this is a haemorrhagic region. All three layers are non-viable

30.4 Histopathology of ILP in the Breast

The macroscopic appearances of a laser burn show a three-zoned lesion which has a central charred hole due to a cavity left around the laser fibre. Surrounding this is a broad region of white tissue and peripheral to this there is a thinner haemorrhagic rim (Fig. 30.1). The histopathological features of the laser burn are consistent and confirm the three-zoned lesion (Fig. 30.1). The charred central cavity shows complete tissue destruction and tissue loss. The white tissue seen macroscopically is a zone of tissue which shows in situ fixation. This is characterized by cells which have smeared nuclei and a featureless, hyperchromatic appearance. The cell cytoplasm is hypereosinophilic, consistent with the presence of coagulated protein. The haemorrhagic rim contains cells which show structurally less damage. They contain unsmeared, slightly hyperchromatic nuclei which retain their chromatin pattern and nucleoli. These cells are surrounded by proliferating fibroblasts, blood vessels and extravasated red blood cells. The dimensions of the in situ fixation show inter-patient variability dependent upon the site of the laser fibre in the tumour and its relationship to normal breast tissue and fat. Fat has an insulating effect and lesions sited within it or bordering it are smaller. The histology of the haemorrhagic area varies in the intensity of the granulation tissue and fibroblastic response with respect to the time between the laser therapy and the surgical resection. All three zones have been shown to be non-viable by immunohistochemical analysis. Experience of the long-term appearances of healing of the lesion is limited to a single case in a patient who declined surgical excision of the tumour for 9 months after ILP. In this tumour the laser burn has healed by dense, hypocellular fibrosis.

30.5 ILP Treatment of Breast Cancers

To date most experience in the treatment of breast cancers has been with single fibres (Harries et al. 1994; Mumtaz et al. 1996a), but this results in a small volume of necrosis, insufficient to ablate anything other than the smallest tumours. The development of fibre splitters facilitated multifibre therapy, and work in hepatic metastases showed that larger volumes of necrosis could be produced with the use of multiple fibres – up to 16 fibres (Amin et al. 1993) – and by using a "pull back" technique. This involves the repositioning of fibre tips immediately after treatment by withdrawing the fibres 5–10 mm within the tumour and reapplying the ILP.

In the breast we have found that when a single pre-charred fibre is used, this reliably results in a burn with a median diameter of 11 mm (Mumtaz et al. 1996a). The effect can be increased by using two of four fibres simultaneously and by using the "pull back" (Fig. 30.2). These manoeuvres can result in burns with diameters of up to 40 mm, sufficient to ablate small cancers and treat tumour margins.

30.6 Imaging

As discussed above, imaging is critical to achieving successful tumour ablation for defining the tumour size and extent and for guiding and monitoring therapy. Finally, it is one of the tools that can be

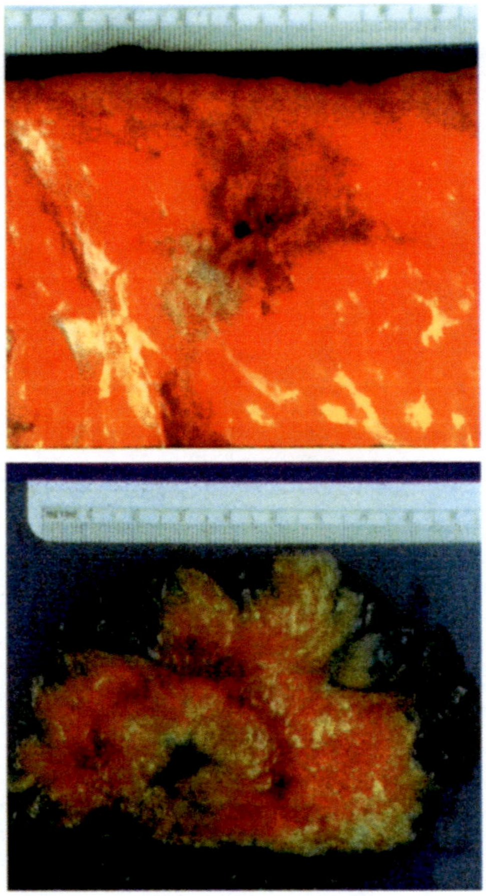

a

b

Fig. 30.2. Macroscopy of **a** a single-fibre burn vs **b** a multifibre burn. With a single fibre, the size of the necrotic lesion is on average about 11 mm for the standard parameters used in our laboratory. This can be increased up to 40 mm with the use of four-fibre treatment

applied to identifying the presence of residual tumour following treatment.

30.6.1 Tumour Localisation

Not all tumours are visible on ultrasound or X-ray mammography, and estimation of tumour size, margins and multifocality and multicentricity is not reliable using these techniques. The high sensitivity of contrast-enhanced MR to detect and show the locoregional extent of breast cancers is now well established (Orel et al. 1994, 1995; Boetes et al. 1995). Further, it is more sensitive than mammography for the detection of multifocal and multicentric disease, and measurements of tumour size on contrast-enhanced MR correlate closely with histological measures of tumour extent (Mumtaz et al. 1997). If ILP ever develops as a definitive treatment for breast cancer, accurate assessment of disease will be necessary to select those patients with multicentric disease or extensive in situ disease in whom more radical treatment is necessary. A further advantage of MR is the temperature dependence of T1 relaxation times, as this offers a method of monitoring the thermal effects of laser ablation during treatment. For these reasons MR has been used for the development of ILP to the breast as a means of localising tumours and guiding and monitoring therapy.

In our studies we have used a conventional 1-T magnet (42 SP Magnetom, Siemens, Erlangen, Germany) and a double breast, receive only coil has been used for diagnostic imaging and locoregional staging. The interventional therapeutic procedures have been performed using a side-access breast coil (MRI Devices, USA).

30.6.2 Image Guidance to Therapy

Initial experiments applying ILP to breast cancers were made using ultrasound and CT as methods of defining the tumour size and monitoring the effect of treatment. However, neither of these techniques could accurately map the tumour or the therapeutic effect. When ultrasound is used during treatment, a hyperechoic region gradually develops around the fibre tip, probably due to the formation of microbubbles, but the size of this region does not correlate with the size of the burn as measured histopathologically.

MR imaging offers several potential advantages to the monitoring of laser-tissue interactions. High soft tissue contrast can be generated with or without the use of contrast agents, and the dependence of some MR parameters on temperature can be exploited to monitor thermal effects of therapy. In addition, the optical fibres and laser light are not affected by the magnetic field, nor does the optical fibre disturb the MR signal (Jolesz and Blumenfeld 1994).

In our studies we have found that, when contrast-enhanced MR is performed 24–48 h after single fibre ILP treatment, it is possible to see the extent of laser damage as areas of non-enhancement appear in previously enhancing tumours and these correspond with areas of necrosis seen histopathologically (Fig. 30.3). The size of the non-enhancing area and the histological measurement of the area of necrosis correlate closely ($r^2 = 0.86$; Mumtaz et al. 1996a). In patients treated with a single fibre, residual enhanc-

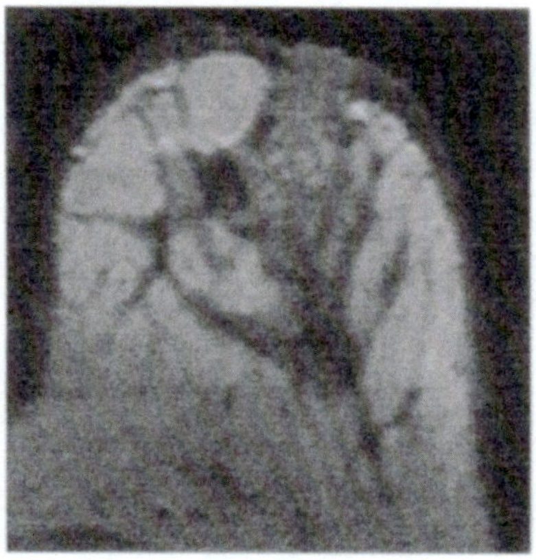

Fig. 30.3. Contrast-enhanced MRI of a single fibre burn. A 12-mm zone of non-enhancement can be seen in residual enhancing tumour in this patient with proven breast cancer treated with single-fibre ILP. This correlated accurately with the extent of necrosis measured histopathologically

ing material corresponds accurately with the extent of residual viable disease. If imaging is performed immediately or within a few hours of treatment, the results are unpredictable and in the majority of cases no treatment effect is visible.

With multifibre treatment, the situation is far less clear. With more aggressive therapy, significantly more surrounding inflammation occurs and this confuses the imaging appearances. Delayed imaging (by >1 week) or dynamic-enhancement imaging may be more helpful in defining the treatment effect and differentiating tumour from inflammation in these patients.

30.6.3 Dynamic MRI

To facilitate total tumour destruction, ideally the therapeutic effect requires monitoring during the treatment procedure. By doing this, therapy can be modified by repositioning of needles, changing laser parameters, etc., to ensure that the whole tumour and tumour margins are adequately covered. Peri-procedural imaging could also prevent the complications of ILP as changes leading to inadvertent damage of muscle and skin could be visualised during therapy, and fibres could be repositioned.

We have examined pre-procedural or "dynamic imaging" in 14 women with biopsy-proven unifocal, lateral quadrant breast cancers treated by ILP within a 1-T magnet (42 SP, Siemens, Erlangen, Germany; Hall-Craggs et al. 1996). Access to the patient is limited in this conventional bore system, but facilitated to a limited extent by the use of a side-access breast coil (MRI Devices). The needles can either be positioned through the coil side window with the patient lying in the breast coil or, as in most cases in our series, pre-positioned on a trolley under ultrasound guidance and then the patient transferred into the coil (with great care taken not to dislodge the needles). Once the needles are in place and the patient positioned in the coil, laser fibres can be introduced through the side port into the needles and positioned within the breast tumour. The needle position is then checked using MRI. In this study seven women were treated with single-fibre therapy (eight fibres in seven women), and seven women with multiple fibres (five with two fibres and two with four fibres). Pull-back techniques were used in three patients.

To monitor treatment we have exploited the thermal sensitivity of T1-weighted images to generate contrast between cool and heated tissue. Using two-dimensional (2D) FLASH imaging (TR 111/TE 10, flip angle 60°, slice thickness 10 mm, 3 slices) we have been able to acquire three slices every 30 s. With the present MR system, these images cannot be

a, b

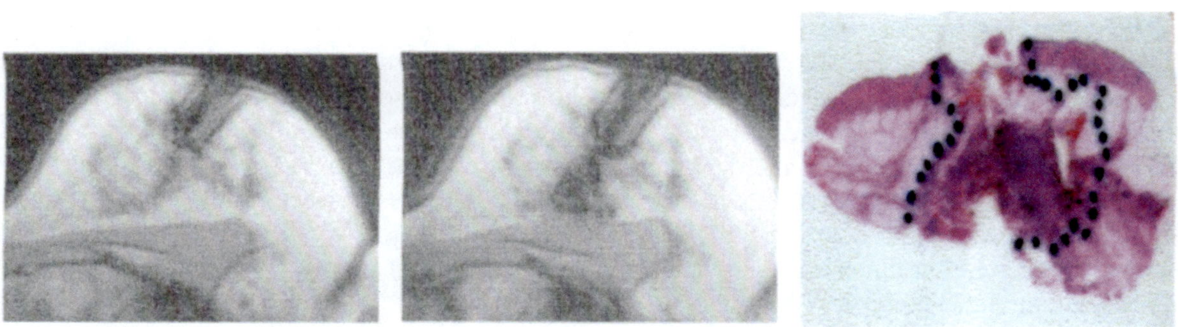

c

Fig. 30.4a-c. Dynamic monitoring of ILP using MR. **a, b** The MR scans show 2D FLASH images acquired before (a) and towards the end of a two-fibre ILP treatment (b). A region of low signal has appeared around the laser fibre tips. The fibres were withdrawn and the lesion treated more superficially (the "pull-back" technique). **c** The macroscopy of the tumour is shown with the extent of the necrosis marked by blue dots. The extent of necrosis found histopathologically correlated well with the size of the regions of low signal seen on the MRI scans.

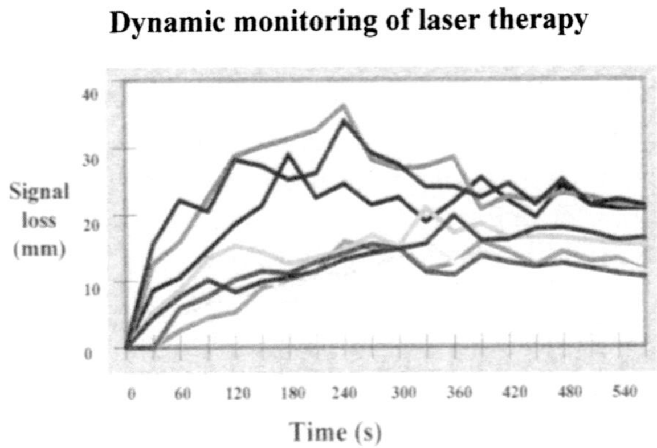

Fig. 30.5. Dynamic monitoring of ILP. The diameter of the low signal region appearing during ILP around the tip of the optical fibre (y axis) plotted against time for a group of patients treated with between one and four fibres. With single-fibre treatments, after achieving a maximum size the zone of low signal reaches a plateau. In contrast in the patients treated with multiple fibres a maximum is reached and then there is a very slight drift downwards as the zone decreases a little during the latter stages of the treatment

viewed until the end of the acquisition period for the entire scan series, but with more advanced scanners, this is clearly not a technical limitation. During the ILP an expanding zone of low signal appears around each optical fibre (Fig. 30.4), first seen after about 30 s and peaking at between 270–400 s (Fig. 30.5). In the patients treated with single fibres, the size of this zone reaches a plateau at the maximum level. In patients treated with multiple fibres following the maximum peak, the low signal zone reduces marginally in size and then either remains stable or drifts down slightly. The reason for the differences in the biological behaviour of the burns is unclear and may be due to differences in peripheral vasodilatation around the treated area with consequent differences in tissue cooling, or changes in thermal conductivity of the tissue.

In this study each patient underwent surgical resection of the breast cancer and the size of the low signal zone identified on the MR scanner was correlated with the histopathological dimensions of the laser burn. With single fibres the correlation was marginally better (median size 13 mm vs 11 mm for MR vs histology, respectively) than for multiple fibres (median size 26 mm vs 30 mm for MR vs histology, respectively) but the overall correlation coefficient for the entire group was satisfactory at 0.86.

A further observation of this study was that the contrast between the breast cancer and the laser effect could be improved by giving intravenous contrast medium immediately before treatment was started. The low signal "burn" can then be seen more clearly against the high signal enhancing tumour using the fairly heavily T1-weighted 2D FLASH sequence.

So to date we have shown that fairly large areas of laser necrosis can be generated, that these can be documented during treatment using fast imaging techniques and after treatment by follow up contrast-enhanced MR studies of the breast. However, there are a large number of technical and logistic difficulties that remain between these experiments and definitive therapy and these are discussed below.

30.7 ILP Treatment of Fibroadenomas

In most cases of fibroadenomas, a definite diagnosis of a benign mass can be made using conventional triple assessment (a combination of clinical assessment, mammographic and/or ultrasound appearances and cytology) and they do not require surgical excision for diagnostic purposes. ILP in these tumours seems to produce larger areas of necrosis than in breast cancers for the same treatment factors, presumably due to differences in optical and thermal conductivity of the tumours. A single two-fibre treatment can destroy tumours of 30–40 mm. Following treatment, most tumours swell slightly during the first week and then gradually decrease in size over the next few weeks. Although a residual mass is seen on ultrasound, the majority of tumours become impalpable. In our series we treated 15 women who had opted for surgical excision as their primary treatment and were awaiting surgery. Following ILP, ten of these patients were so satisfied with the therapeutic and cosmetic result of the ILP that they refused further surgery (Mumtaz et al. 1996b).

Some fibroadenomas appeared to respond better to ILP than others. It is likely that this was because some tumours were less completely treated. We are currently evaluating a variety of imaging techniques to see whether we can assess the adequacy of treatment at the time of the procedure in order to avoid under-treatment. More aggressive treatment with more fibres is also likely to achieve more complete tumour ablation.

30.8 Problems and Complications

At the present time, using conventional scanners, access to the patient is restricted and it is awkward to manoeuvre needles and fibres quickly and easily. These problems are likely to be partially assuaged by the use of the new generation of "open access" MR scanners and the development of MR fluoroscopy.

Localising the fibre tip position is difficult. Even MR-compatible needles cause sufficient susceptibility artefact at 1 T to obscure small targets, and at the present time the optical fibres are "MR invisible". Although fibres can be coated to make them visualisable, none of these methods has received Food and Drug Administration (FDA) approval and can only be used in experimental objects.

The only patient complications we have encountered in our studies have been from skin and pectoralis muscle burns from misplaced optical fibres, again largely because we cannot "see" the fibres. Real-time imaging during therapy would almost certainly avoid these as the laser effect is clearly seen in these tissues, as well as in the target tumour.

The validation of adequately treated margins remains an issue. At the present time a peripheral enhancing rim may be seen 2–3 days after treatment on contrast-enhancement MRI, due either to residual tumour or to an inflammatory response to treatment. Multiple biopsies of the periphery of the mass guided either by MR or ultrasound will probably be necessary to confidently ensure adequate treatment margins. Further work is also needed to develop "dynamic" monitoring of ILP, to refine the technique such that tumours are consistently completely necrosed with sufficiently treated margins.

30.9 Future Developments

To date the work with breast cancers has been developmental and there is a long way to go before it is proven to be a reliable method of treating breast tumours. Even if ILP can be shown to remove all tumours it seems likely that ILP will only be used to treat small cancers (<2 cm). However, owing to the success of the screening programmes, more of the smaller cancers are being detected. In the long term, outcome measures will be necessary to ensure that the long-term survival of these women is not prejudiced.

References

Amin Z (1995) Diode lasers. Experimental and clinical review. Laser Med Sci 10:157–163

Amin Z, Donald JJ, Masters A, et a (1993) Hepatic metastases: interstitial laser photocoagulation with real-time US monitoring and dynamic CT evaluation of treatment. Radiology 187:339–347

Boetes C, Mus RDM, Holland R, et al (1995) Breast tumours: comparative accuracy of MR imaging relative to mammography and US for demonstrating extent. Radiology 197: 743–747

Bown SG (1983) Phototherapy of tumours. World J Surg 7: 700–709

Cheong WF, Prahl S, Welch AJ (1990) A review of the optical properties of biological tissues. IEEE J Quantum Electron 26:2166–2185

Fisher B, Redmond C, Poisson R, et al (1989) Eight year result of a randomized clinical trial comparing total mastectomy and lumpectomy with or without radiation in the treatment of breast cancer. N Engl J Med 320:822–828

Hall-Craggs MA, Mumtaz H, Paley M, et al (1996) Dynamic guidance of laser therapy to breast cancer. Radiology 201:177

Harries SA, Amin Z, Smith ME, et al (1994) Interstitial laser photocoagulation as a treatment for breast cancer. Br J Surg 81:1617–1619

Jacobson JA, Danforth DN, Cowan KH, et al (1995) Ten-year results of a comparison of conservation with mastectomy in the treatment of stage I and II breast cancer. N Engl J Med 332:907–911

Jolesz FA, Blumenfeld SM (1994) Interventional use of magnetic resonance imaging. Magn Reson Q 10:85–96

Mumtaz H, Hall-Craggs MA, Wotherspoon A, et al (1996a) Laser therapy for breast cancer: Magnetic resonance imaging and histopathological correlation. Radiology 200:651–658

Mumtaz H, Hall-Craggs MA, Buonnacorssi G, et al (1996b) Image-guided interstitial laser photocoalgulation for fibroadenoma of the breast. Radiology 201:177

Mumtaz H, Hall-Craggs MA, Davidson T, et al (1997) Staging symptomatic primary breast cancer with MR imaging. AJR Am J Roentgenol (in press)

Orel SG, Schnall MD, LiVolsi VA, et al (1994) Suspicious breast lesions: MR imaging with radiologic-pathologic correlation. Radiology 190:485–493

Orel SG, Schnall MD, Powell CM, et al (1995) Staging of suspected breast cancer: effect of MR imaging and MR guided biopsy. Radiology 196:115–122

Stegar AC, Lees WR, Walmsley K, et al (1989) Interstitial laser hyperthermia: a new approach to local destruction of tumours. Br Med J 299:362–365

Svaasand LO, Boerslid T, Oeveraason M (1985) Thermal and optical properties of living tissue: application to laser-induced hyperthermia. Laser Surg Med 5:589–602

Veronesi U, Luini A, Beretta E, et al (1990) Conservative treatment of early breast cancer. Long-term results of 1232 cases treated with quadrantectomy, axillary dissection and radiotherapy. Ann Surg 211:250–259

Intraoperative MRI

31 Image-Guided Neurosurgery with Intraoperative MRI

F.A. Jolesz, J. Kettenbach, and R. Kikinis

CONTENTS

31.1 Introduction

Image-guided, computer-assisted neurosurgery has emerged as an alternative to frame-based stereotaxy and conventional neurosurgery. Image-based information can improve localization and targeting of the operational field and thereby reduce invasiveness. The use of interactive image plane selection-based surgical navigators (Shelden et al. 1980; Kelly 1986; Roberts et al. 1986; Watanabe et al. 1987, 1991; Kato et al. 1991; Barnett et al. 1993a, 1993b; Tan et al. 1993; Reinhardt et al. 1993; Golfinos et al. 1995; Grimson et al. 1995), three-dimensional (3D) models (Gleason et al. 1994; Kikinis et al. 1996; Nakajima et al. 1997a, 1997b; Kettenbach et al. 1997; Aoki et al. 1992; Schwartz et al. 1992; Castillo and Wilson 1994), and surgical simulations (Hu et al. 1990; Koyama et al. 1995; Tampiere et al. 1995; Hsiang et al. 1996; Gibson et al. 1997) have resulted in substantial changes in planning and performing neurosurgical procedures. Further change in neurosurgery is anticipated from the intraoperative use of complex surgical robots (Kelly et al. 1986, 1988; Kelly 1988; Hata et al. 1996; Pillay 1997), intraoperative computed tomography, (CT), fluoroscopy (Katada et al. 1996), and open-configuration magnetic resonance (MR) imaging systems (Jolesz and Blumenfeld 1994; Schenck et al. 1995; Silverman et al. 1995; Moriarty et al. 1996; Kaufman et al. 1989; Gronemeyer et al. 1989, 1991, 1995; Ortendahl and Kaufman 1995; Lu et al. 1997; Anzai et al. 1993). The realisation of these truly revolutionary visions is based on the availability of high performance computers, which are playing an increasing role in neurosurgery.

We have been conducting various forms of image-guided neurosurgery for several years. Our combined image-guided therapy program consists of surgical planning, intraoperative guidance using preoperative images, and, currently, intraoperative guidance using real-time MR images. We are convinced that modern image-guided neurosurgery requires the full integration of image processing, surgical planning, interactive image guidance (frameless stereotaxy) and real-time image-based intraoperative guidance. Our working hypothesis is that, for optimal image-based guidance, the integration of preoperative planning and simulation with registration techniques is necessary in order to utilize image data intraoperatively. In addition, these preoperative image-based techniques could be combined into a fully integrated intraoperative guidance system in which frequent image update can account for the unavoidable morphologic and physiologic changes induced by the surgical intervention itself.

31.2 Surgical Planning

In the surgical planning laboratory, 3D images are reconstructed based on image data from CT, MR imaging, and MR angiographs (MRA), as well as single photon emission tomography (SPECT). Registration between images from each modality is performed using the "maximization of mutual informa-

F.J. Jolesz, MD, Director of MR Division and Image Guided Therapy Program, Department of Radiology, Harvard Medical School and Brigham and Women's Hospital, 75 Francis Street, Boston, MA 02115, USA
J. Kettenbach, MD, Image Guided Therapy Program and Surgical Planning Laboratory, Department of Radiology, Harvard Medical School and Brigham and Women's Hospital, 75 Francis Street, Boston, MA 02115, USA
R. Kikinis, MD, Director of Surgical Planning Laboratory, Department of Radiology, Harvard Medical School and Brigham and Women's Hospital, 75 Francis Street, Boston, MA 02115, USA

tion" method. After the segmentation of each anatomical structure, such as the brain, a tumor, or vessels, a 3D model is constructed and displayed using surface rendering. We can rotate, translate, change color, and make translucent each structure on the computer display.

Preoperatively, the 3D models are used to optimize the trajectories of intervention and select the best surgical approach (Fig. 31.1). In the operating room, either the video registration method or laser registration with instrument tracking is used for navigation. The 3D model is superimposed onto the surgical field using a video mixer for the video registration system (Fig. 31.2). The surgical navigator can display the tip of the probe on the 3D model and original MR images (Fig. 31.3). The main active research and clinical projects in the laboratory include surgical planning and simulation (Gleason et al. 1994; Kikinis et al. 1996; Nakajima et al. 1997a, 1997b), intraoperative image-guidance, longitudinal study using computerized image processing for the analysis of multiple sclerosis (Guttmann et al. 1996), the study of morphologic abnormalities in schizophrenia (Shenton et al. 1992), virtual endoscopy (Jolesz et al. 1997), intracranial compartment volume analysis (Matsumae et al. 1996a, 1996b), and numerous other studies related to medical image processing. These research projects are supported by both commercial software and an extensive library of in-house software.

31.3 Intraoperative MRI

The intraoperative MRI project is integrated into a prototype MR imaging system which was developed in collaboration with GE Medical Systems (Milwaukee, Wis.) and was installed at the Department of Radiology, Brigham and Women's Hospital, in March 1994. This unit consists of two vertical components which provide 0.5 T magnetic field be-

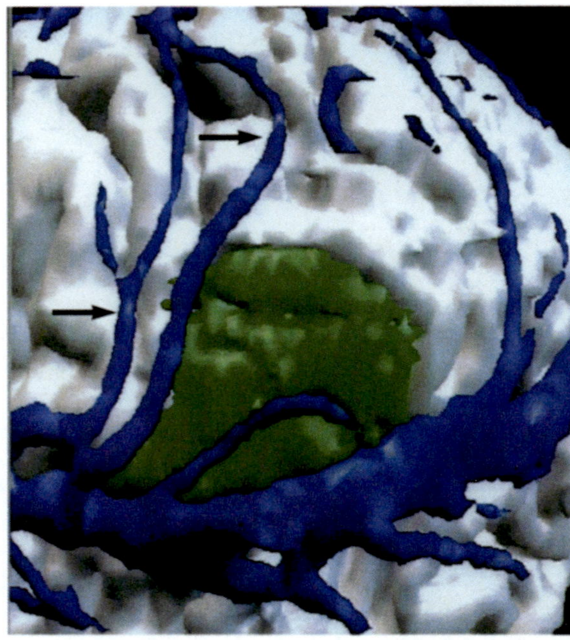

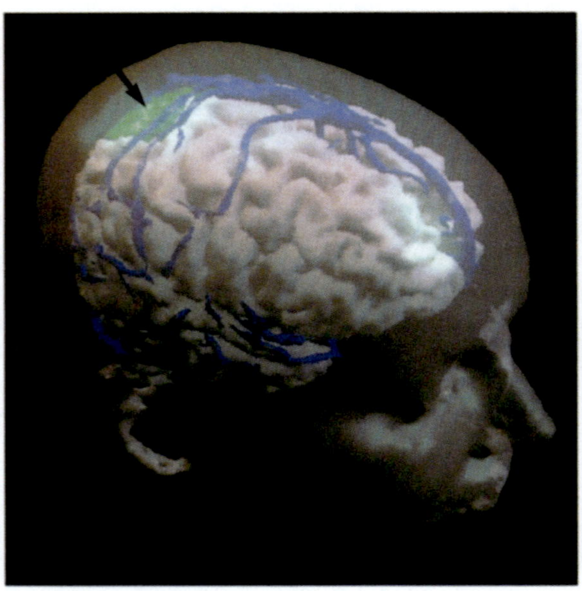

Fig. 31.1. For surgical planning a three-dimensional (3D) model was reconstructed from MR images and an MR angiogram. The tumor (*colored green*) is mainly in the right parietal lobe (*arrow*), surrounded by large cortical vessels

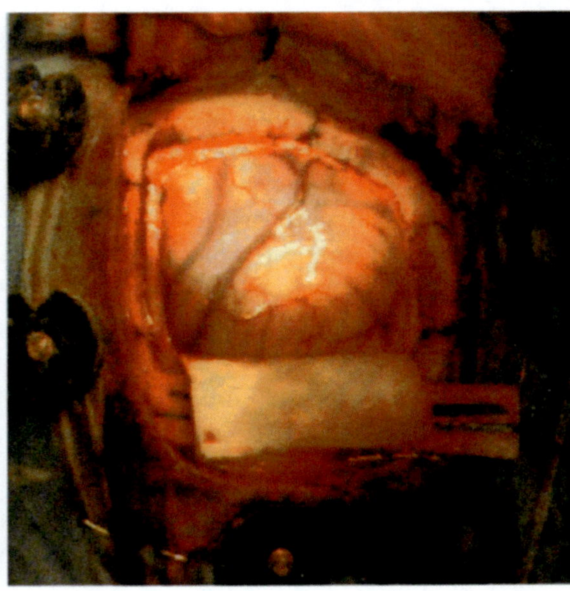

Fig. 31.2a,b. Vessel to vessel registration: The cortical vessels (*arrows*) were used for registering **a** the 3D model and **b** the patient's cortical surface

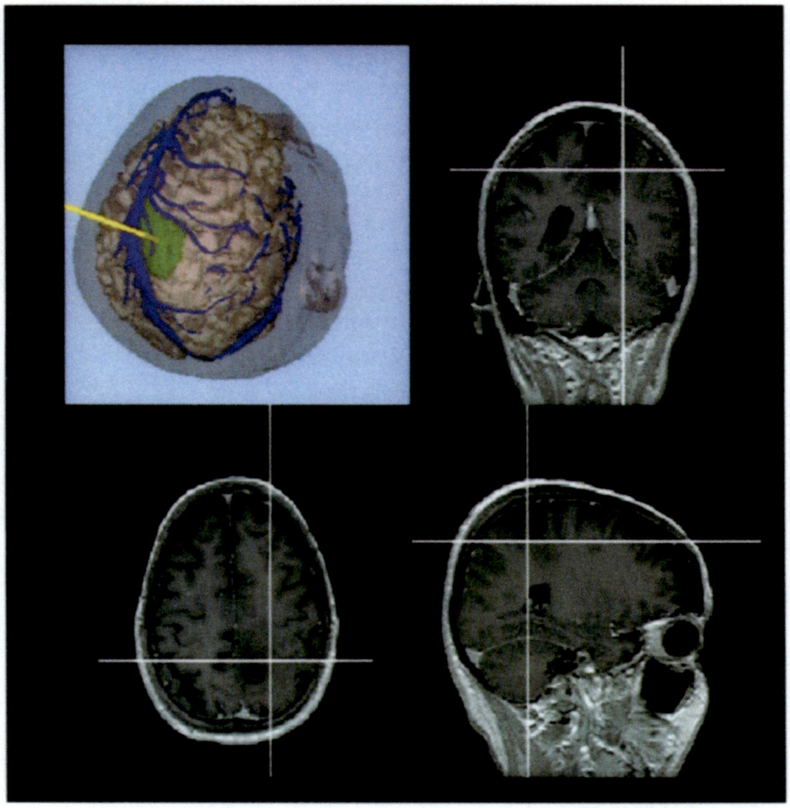

Fig. 31.3. The interface of the surgical navigator, showing the 3D model, as well as three orthogonal multiplanar MR images. The *yellow line* on the 3D model shows the position and direction of the probe pointing to the tumor margin. White crosses on the magnetic resonance images show the corresponding position of the probe's tip. (Courtesy of E. Grimson and M. Leventon)

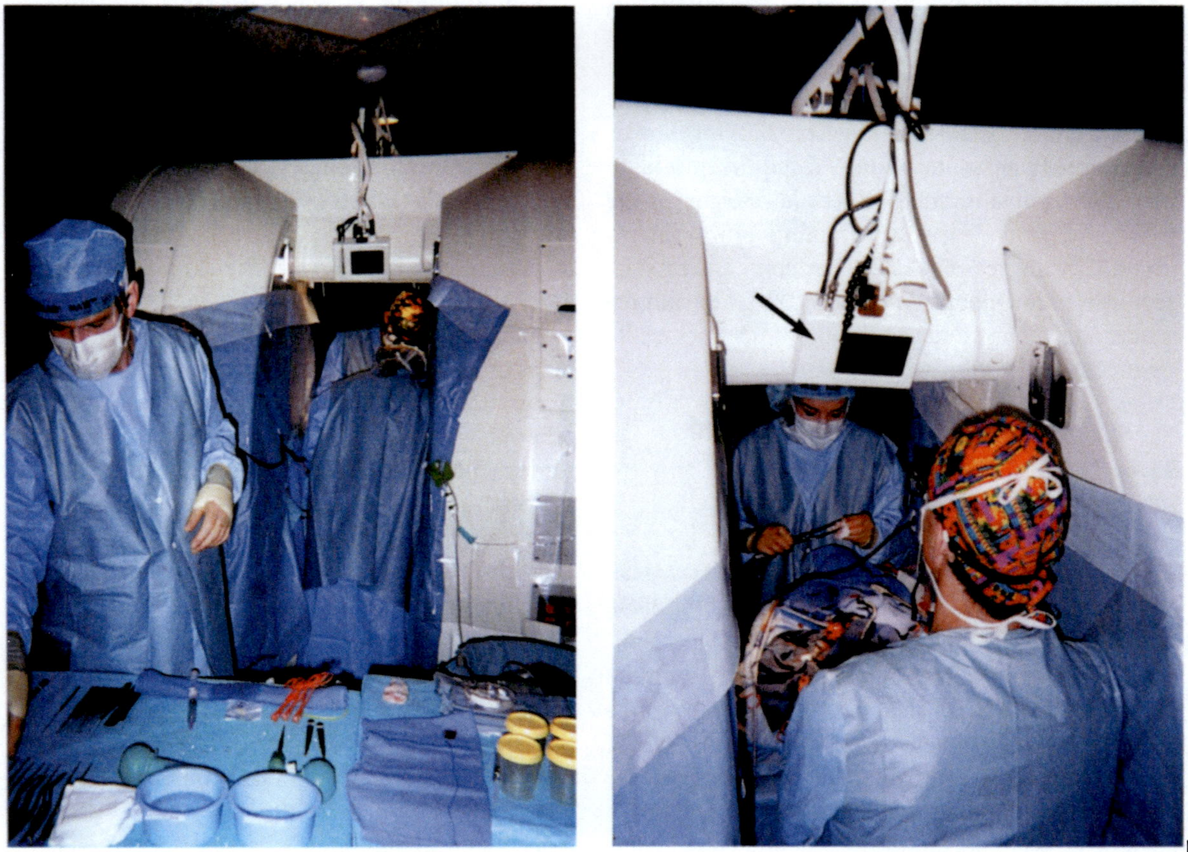

a **b**

Fig. 31.4 a The open-configuration MR imaging system during neurosurgery. **b** Surgeons can see the images using two liquid crystal display monitors (*arrow*) the procedure. All surgical and anesthesiological equipment is MR compatible tween them. The height of the coils is 184 cm and the space between these coils, where a physician has access to the patient, is 56 cm. There are two liquid crystal display monitors, so that surgeons can see the MR images during procedures (Jolesz and Blumenfeld 1994; Schenk et al. 1995; Silverman et al. 1995). Two surgeons can have simultaneous access to a patient during the MR scanning (Fig. 31.4). They can operate on the patient while monitoring the patient with the MR scanner. The first neurosurgical case, a brain biopsy, was performed within this unit in 1995. The intraoperative MRI suite is now used as one of the operating rooms and there are four to six open surgeries performed in the unit per week. Ongoing research involves the development and testing of new dynamic MR imaging sequences, MR-compatible surgical instruments, and several new procedures for minimally invasive treatment, including laser thermal ablations, cryosurgery, and MR-guided focused ultrasound surgery. Many MR sequences are available in this system, including T1-weighted spin-echo, T2-weighted spin-echo, and T1-weighted gradient-echo sequences. From the surgical viewpoint, there are two categories of scanning procedures. One is the "intraoperative" mode. This is the same scanning method as with an ordinary MR unit. It takes a few minutes to generate a series of 10–15 slices. For example, a neurosurgeon can obtain MR images after tumor removal by scanning the patient's brain. Usually, the relevant slice appears as an abnormal part of the brain. This mode is useful to check for residual tumor. The second category is the "real-time" mode. The scanner obtains a two-dimensional (2D) image every 1.5 s. Therefore, a neurosurgeon can follow the procedure in a 2D plane almost immediately. This mode is useful to track the needle tip during tumor biopsy.

31.4 Intraoperative Real-Time Guidance

The intraoperative, real-time mode allows surgical navigation. A 3D digitizer device (Flashpoint 5000, Image Guided Technologies, Boulder, Colo.) is installed in this system so the probe tip is displayed on the intraoperative MR images (Fig. 31.5). Since three cameras for infrared detection are fixed on the top of the unit and the real-time image is used, it is not necessary to register the MR image of the patient's head. The accuracy of the navigation system has been strictly calibrated and maintained within the working space. Interactive "near real-time" imaging is accomplished using a hand-held 3D optical tracking device mounted with three light-emitting diodes (LEDs), three high resolution video cameras located above the magnet's isocenter which detect the LED emissions and specialized image guidance software implemented on an interactive workstation (Sun Microsystems, Mountain View, Calif.). A series of images is obtained at specified distances from the edge of the localization device in order to determine an appropriate trajectory in three planes with a resolution of 1 mm. Once a track is chosen, a burr hole or craniotomy is drilled in the skull overlying the entry site.

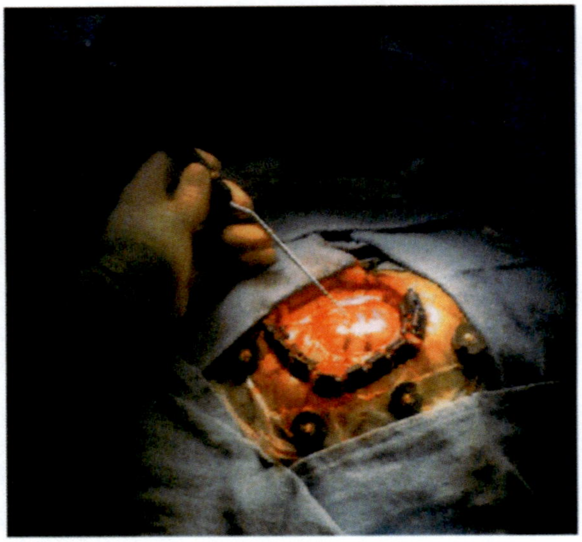

Fig. 31.5. The probe with two mounted light-emitting diodes for 3D registration. The probe specifies three imaging planes, two along the probe and one perpendicular to the probe

The open-configuration MR imaging system combines the surgical navigation with real-time imaging. Integration of cortical mapping, functional MRI and other imaging modalities (SPECT; positron emission tomography) will improve its effectiveness for intractable epilepsy cases or for tumor removal close the primary motor or language cortex.

With the 3D digitizer system and intraoperative MR images, the open-configuration MR imaging system is appropriate for surgery of deep lesions requiring biopsy, lesions requiring accurate stereotactic guidance, and lesion resection. In particular, this system is powerful for intraventricular tumor cases or tumors with a cystic component. During surgery, the lesion shifts after the fluid removal, but it is possible to monitor the tissue deformation in the open-configuration MR imaging system based on the real-time updates.

The ideal approach to each lesion is determined using a combination of the interactive hand-held tracking device and serial volume imaging. The operator can thus successfully avoid vital vascular structures and critical brain regions.

For biopsies, the MR-compatible biopsy needle and tracking device are fixed to the flexible arm of an MR-compatible Bookwalter metallic arm (Codman, Boston, Mass.), which allows precise control of the needle as it is manipulated using near real-time imaging. If preprocedure imaging reveals the brain lesion to enhance densely, imaging in the open magnet is performed following the injection of gadolinium DTPA with T1-weighted fast spin-echo (FSE) images acquired every 7–10 s. Biopsies and resections of nonenhancing lesions are performed using T2-weighted FSE images acquired every 14 s.

Continuous imaging during biopsy procedures allows the clinicians to be certain of the location of the biopsy needle when specimens are taken, thus obviating the need for multiple needle passes and frozen tissue sectioning. To date there have been no long-term complications noted in our patient population. In one patient undergoing biopsy, hemorrhage was noted in the operative site, which necessitated conversion to a craniotomy and resection of the clot; this case demonstrated the importance of immediate feedback of postprocedure complications, which would have been unavailable without the use of interactive MR imaging.

For resections, the approach to the lesion is easily determined using the interactive near real-time system. To determine the margins of the tumor and to define enhancing, cystic, or necrotic parts during surgery interactive imaging with a virtual pointer is employed. In smaller lesions (i.e., small tumors or cavernous hemangiomas) accurate localization and targeting is obtained using interactive imaging. Once resection has begun, serial volume imaging is performed using 3D fast spoiled gradient T1-weighted imaging or T2-weighted FSE images. The extent of resection can also be continuously evaluated; in many cases, tumor tissue invisible to direct viewing was seen on MR images and successfully removed under MR guidance (Fig. 31.6).

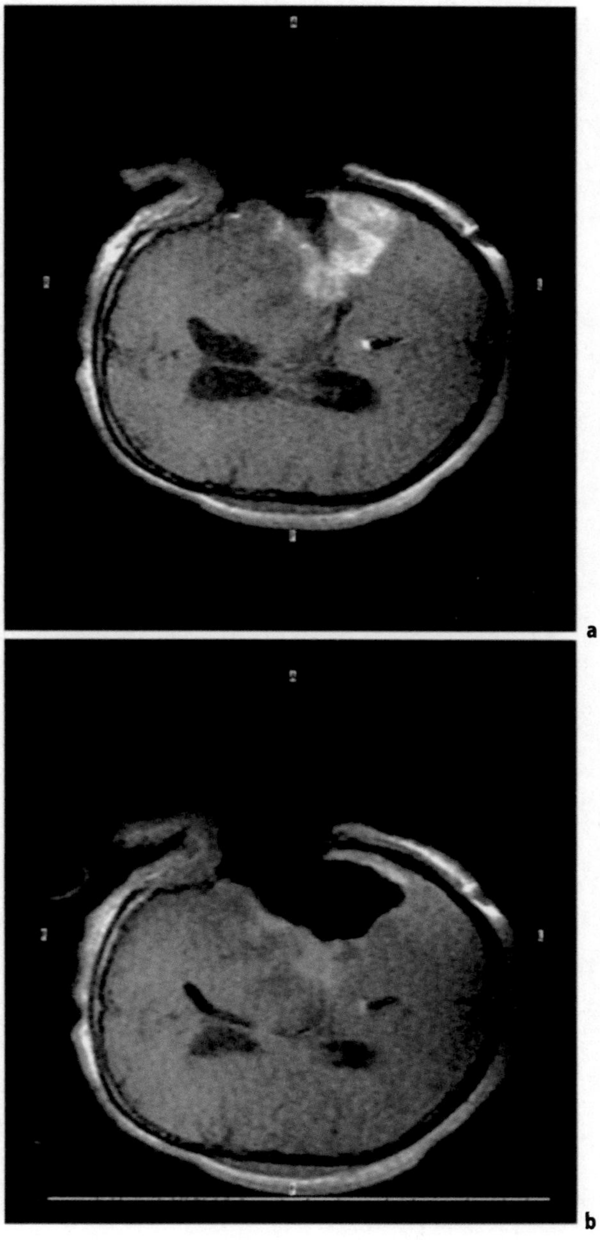

Fig. 31.6 a,b. Tumor resection using the open-configuration MR unit. **a** The intraoperative MR image shows residual tumor, so the surgeon continued removing the tumor after the scanning. **b** There is no residual tumor shown in the intraoperative MR image

In the case of intracranial cysts, isoosmotic gadolinium solution can be instilled into the cyst to determine if it communicates with the subarachnoid cerebrospinal fluid (CSF) space. Serial imaging was performed to elucidate the internal characteristics of the cyst and the rapidity with which CSF entered the subarachnoid cisterns. If the contents of the cyst were under pressure, a drain was placed within the cyst through the same approach used for the contrast agent injection. If free communication was demonstrated, no further intervention was performed. If no communication could be shown, the cyst was opened after craniotomy was performed. Gadolinium injection into extra-axial fluid collections differentiated free communication with the CSF space. The noncommunicating intracranial cyst and subdural collections were drained satisfactorily.

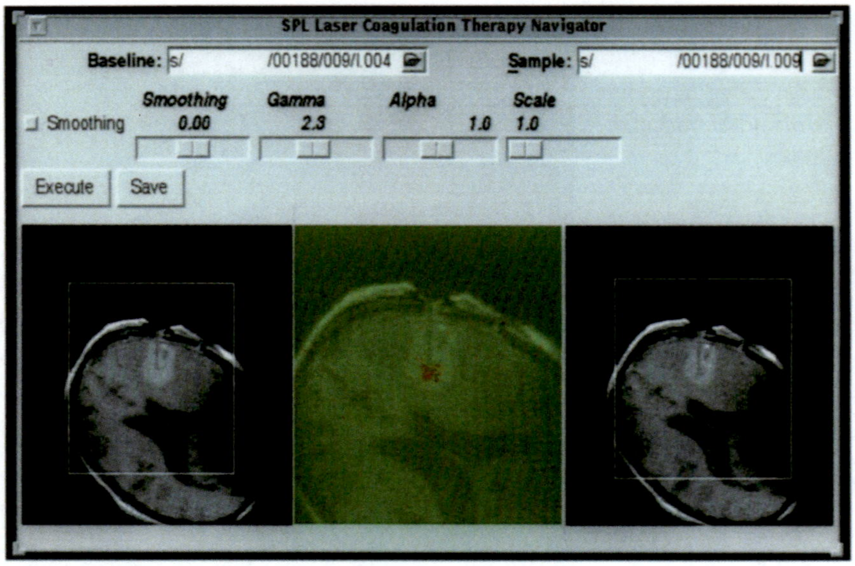

Fig. 31.7. Interstitial laser therapy of brain metastasis. T1-weighted fast spin-echo (FSE) images, obtained during laser therapy (*right*) in the open magnet, were subtracted from the baseline image (*left*) obtained before laser treatment. The resulting image (*middle*) displayed the heat distribution around the laser fiber as color-encoded pixels within a user-defined window

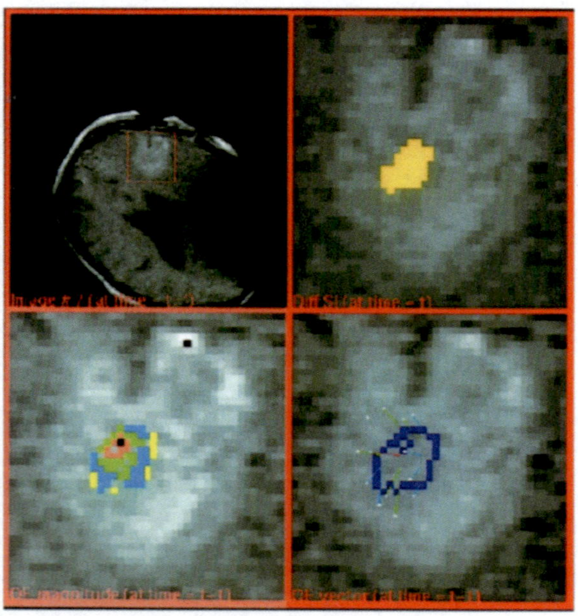

Fig. 31.8. Visualization of thermal distribution with optical flow analysis. On conventional gray-scaled images (*upper left*) a window was selected where the heat distribution could be visualized (*upper right*) after color-encoded pixel subtraction of T1-weighted FSE images. The amount of heat (*lower left*), the speed, and the direction (*lower right*) of the heat distribution during laser therapy were calculated to near real-time

The procedure time has continuously decreased with mounting experience. The time required for a biopsy now averages approximately 45 min once the burr hole is made; tumor resections at present require on average 1.5 h following the craniotomy. The average time of hospitalization of patients undergoing tumor surgery by the conventional method is 6.5 days. Using open intraoperative MRI the length of hospitalization has decreased to 5.3 days.

MR can be used to monitor the therapeutic effect of other non-surgical treatments such as thermotherapy. The potential of this technique is described in Chap. 26. Some preliminary experience is illustrated in Figs. 31.7 and 31.8.

MR image guided therapy combines navigational tools with registration techniques and real-time imaging to achieve image-guided neurosurgery. However, many technical challenges still lie ahead.

Apart from cost and practicability the most important question is how to improve the patient's outcome. There are a few measures to evaluate the usefulness of image-guided surgery, such as length of hospital stay, hospitalization cost, extent of tumor resection, postoperative functional status, symptom-free period, and survival period (Nazzaro and Neuwelt 1990; Curran et al. 1992; Albert et al. 1994; Kowalczuk et al. 1996). While a preliminary review of image-guided surgical cases is encouraging in this regard, a formal study comparing success rates of conventional neurosurgery and image-guided neurosurgery is still outstanding.

Acknowledgement. The authors gratefully acknowledge many of their colleagues for their contribution, and support in this book chapter by the following individuals: Shin Nakajima, MD, PhD, Richard Bradley Schwartz, MD, PhD, Nobuhiko Hata, MS Thomas M. Moriarty, MD, PhD, Eben Alexander III, Phillip Stieg, MD, PhD, and Peter McL. Black, MD, PhD.

References

Albert FK, Forsting M, Sartor K, et al (1994) Early postoperative magnetic resonance imaging after resection of malignant glioma: objective evaluation of residual tumor and its influence on regrowth and prognosis. Neurosurgery 34:45–61

Anzai Y, Desalles AA, Black KL, et al (1993) Interventional MR imaging. Radiographics 13:897–904

Aoki S, Sasaki Y, Machida T, et al (1992) Cerebral aneurysms: detection and delineation using 3-D-CT angiography. AJNR Am J Neuroradiol 13:1115–1120

Barnett GH, Kormos DW, Steiner CP, et al (1993a) Intraoperative localization using an armless, framless stereotactic wand. J Neurosurg 78:510–514

Barnett GH, Kormos DW, Steiner CP, et al (1993b) Use of a frameless, armless stereotactic wand for brain tumor localization with two-dimensional and three-dimensional neuroimaging. Neurosurgery 33:674–678

Castillo M, Wilson JD (1994) CT angiography of the common carotid artery bifurcation: comparison between two techniques and conventional angiography. Neuroradiology 36: 602–604

Curran WJ Jr, Scott CB, Horton J, et al (1992) Does extent of surgery influence outcome for astrocytoma with atypical or anaplastic foci (AAF)? A report from three Radiation Therapy Oncology Group (RTOG) trials. J Neurooncol 12:219–227

Gibson S, Samosky J, Mor A, et al (1997) Simulating arthroscopic knee surgery using volumetric object representations, real-time volume rendering, and haptic feedback. In: Troccaz J, Grimson E, Mösges R (eds) CVRMed-MRCAS'97. Springer, Berlin Heidelberg New York, pp 369–378

Gleason PL, Kikinis R, Altobelli D, et al (1994) Video registration virtual reality for nonlinkage stereotactic surgery. Stereotact Funct Neurosurg 63:139–143

Golfinos JG, Fitzpatrick BC, Smith LR, et al (1995) Clinical use of a frameless stereotactic arm: results of 325 cases. J Neurosurg 83:197–205

Grimson WEL, Ettinger GJ, White SJ, et al (1996) An automatic registration method for frameless stereotaxy, image guided surgery, and enhanced reality visualization. IEEE Trans Med Imaging 15:129–140

Gronemeyer DHW, Kaufman L, Rothschild P, et al (1989) New possibilities and aspects of low-field magnetic resonance tomography. Radiol Diagn 30:519–527

Gronemeyer DHW, Seibel RM, Kaufman L, et al (1991) Low-field design eases MRI-guided biopsies. Diagn Imaging 47:139–143

Gronemeyer DHW, Seibel RM, Schmidt A (1995) Image-guided access techniques. Endosc Surg 3:69–75

Guttmann CRG, Ahn SS, Hsu L, et al (1996) The evolution of multiple sclerosis lesions on serial MR. AJNR Am J Neuroradiol 16:1481–1491

Hata N, Wells WM III, Halle M, et al (1996) Image guided microscopic surgery system using mutual-information based registration. (abstract) Proceedings of 4th international conference on visualization in biomedical computing (VBC '96). Hamburg, Germany, pp 307–316

Hsiang JNK, Liang EY, Lam JMK, et al (1996) The role of computed tomographic angiography in the diagnosis of intracranial aneurysms and emergent aneurysm clipping. Neurosurgery 38:481–448

Hu X, Tan KK, Levin DN, et al (1990) Three-dimensional magnetic resonance images of the brain: application to neurosurgical planning. J Neurosurg 72:433–440

Jolesz FA, Blumenfeld SM (1994) Interventional use of magnetic resonance imaging. Magn Reson Q 10:85–96

Jolesz FA, Lorensen WE, Shinmoto H, et al (1997) Interactive virtual endoscopy. AJR Am J Roentgenol (in press)

Katada K, Kato R, Anno H, et al (1996) Guidance with real-time CT fluoroscopy: early clinical experience. Radiology 200:851–856

Kato A, Yoshimine T, Hayakawa T, et al (1991) A frameless, armless navigational system for computer assisted neurosurgery. Technical note. J Neurosurg 74:845–849

Kaufman L, Arakawa M, Hale J, et al (1989) Accessible magnetic resonance imaging. Magn Reson Q 5:283–297

Kelly PJ (1986) Computer-assisted stereotaxis: new approaches for management of intracranial intra-axial tumors. Neurology 36:535–541

Kelly PJ (1988) Volumetric stereotactic surgical resection of intra-axial brain mass lesions. Mayo Clin Proc 63:1186–1198

Kelly PJ, Kall BA, Goerss S, et al (1986) Computer-assisted stereotactic laser resection of intra-axial brain neoplasms. J Neurosurg 64:427–439

Kelly PJ, Kall BA, Goerss SJ (1988) Results of computed tomography-based computer-assisted stereotactic resection of metastatic intracranial tumors. Neurosurgery 22:7–17

Kettenbach J; Jolesz FA, Kikinis R, (1997) Surgical planning laboratory: a new challenge for radiology? In: Lemke HU, Vannier MV, Inamura K (eds) Proceeding of 11th International Symposium and Exhibition, Computer Assisted Radiology and Surgery, CAR 97. Elsevier, Amsterdam, pp 855-860

Kikinis R, Gleason PL, Moriarty TM, et al (1996) Computer-assisted interactive three-dimensional planning for neurosurgical procedures. Neurosurgery 38:640–651

Kowalczuk A, Macdonald RL, Amidei C, et al (1996) Quantitative postoperative imaging study of the effect of surgical resection of malignant astrocytomas on survival. (abstract) Poster Program of the 64th annual meeting of The American Association of Neurological Surgeons, Park Ridge, pp 304–305

Koyama T, Okudera H, Kobayashi S (1995) Computer-assisted geometric design of cerebral aneurysms for surgical simulation. Neurosurgery 36:541–547

Lu DSK, Lee H, Farahani K, et al (1997) Biopsy of hepatic dome lesions: semi-real-time coronal MR guidance technique. AJR Am J Roentgenol 168:737–739

Matsumae M, Kikinis R, Mórocz IA, et al (1996a) Intracranial compartment volumes in patients with enlarged ventricles assessed by MRI based image processing. J Neurosurg 84:972–981

Matsumae M, Kikinis R, Mórocz IA, et al (1996b) Age-related changes in intracranial compartment volumes in normal adults assessed by magnetic resonance imaging. J Neurosurg 84:982–991

Moriarty TM, Kikinis R, Jolesz FA, et al (1996) Magnetic resonance imaging therapy – intraoperative MR imaging. Neurosurg Clin N A 7:323–331

Nakajima S, Atsumi H, Kikinis R, et al (1997a) Use of cortical surface vessel registration for image-guided neurosurgery. Neurosurgery (in press)

Nakajima S, Atsumi H, Bhalerao AH, et al (1997b) Computer-assisted surgical planning for cerebrovascular neurosurgery. Neurosurgery (in press)

Nazzaro JM, Neuwelt EA (1990) The role of surgery in the management of supratentorial intermediate and high-grade astrocytomas in adults. J Neurosurg 73:331–344

Ortendahl DA, Kaufman L (1995) Real-time interactions in MRI. Comput Biol Med 25:293–300

Pillay PK (1997) Image-guided stereotactic neurosurgery with thermulticoordinate manipulator microscope. Surg Neurol 47:171–177

Reinhardt HF, Horstmann GA, Gratzl O (1993) Sonic stereometry in microsurgical procedures for deep-seated brain tumors and vascular malformations. Neurosurgery 32:51–57

Roberts DW, Strohbehn JW, Hatch J, et al (1986) A frameless stereotaxic integration of computerized tomographic imaging and the operating microscope. J Neurosurg 65: 545–549

Schenck JF, Jolesz FA, Roemer PB, et al (1995) Superconducting open-configuration MR imaging system for image-guided therapy. Radiology 195:805–814

Schwartz RB (1994) Neuroradiological applications of spiral CT. Semin Ultrasound CT MR 145:139–147

Schwartz RB, Jones KM, Chernoff DM, et al (1992) Common carotid artery bifurcation: evaluation with spiral CT - work in progress. Radiology 185:513–519

Shelden CH, McCann G, Jacques S, et al (1980) Development of a computerized microstereotaxic method for localization and removal of minute CNS lesions under direct 3-D vision. Technical report. J Neurosurg 52:21–27

Shenton ME, Kikinis R, Jolesz FA, et al (1992) Abnormalities of the temporal lobe and thought disorders in schizophrenia. A quantitative magnetic resonance imaging study. N Engl J Med 327:604–612

Silverman SG, Collick BD, Figueira MR, et al (1995) Interactive MR-guided biopsy in an open-configuration MR imaging system. Radiology 197:175–181

Tampieri D, Leblanc R, Pleszek J, et al (1995) Three-dimensional computed tomographic angiography of cerebral aneurysms. Neurosurgery 36:749–755

Tan KK, Grzeszczuk R, Levin DN, et al (1993) A frameless stereotactic approach to neurosurgical planning based on retrospective patient-image registration. Technical note. J Neurosurg 79:296–303

Watanabe E, Watanabe T, Manaka S, et al (1987) Three-dimensional digitizer (neuro-navigator): new equipment of CT-guided stereotaxi surgery. Surg Neurol 27:543–547

Watanabe E, Mayanagi Y, Kosugi Y, et al (1991) Open surgery assisted by the neuronavigator, a stereotactic, articulated, sensitive arm. Neurosurgery 28:792–800

Interventional MR Angiography

32 Intravascular Applications of Field Inhomogeneity Catheters: In Vivo Results

G. ADAM

CONTENTS

32.1 Introduction

MR angiography (MRA) is a rapidly evolving technique for noninvasive *vascular imaging* (EDELMAN 1993). Hardware and software improvements in MR imagers and advanced imaging techniques have already made MRA essentially a routine procedure for certain anatomic regions and pathologies such as the extracranial carotid arteries (LEVY and PRINCE 1996), intracerebral aneurysms (RONKANINEN et al. 1995) and cerebral sinus thrombosis (VOGL et al. 1994). In addition, optimized *contrast-enhanced MR angiography* using bolus tracking techniques has improved imaging of the abdominal vessels such as the abdominal aorta and the renal arteries (SNIDOW et al. 1996; PRINCE 1994).

However, since MRA has, until recently, remained a purely noninvasive technique, the logical "next step" of appropriate intravascular intervention such as dilation, occlusion or embolization that frequently accompanies conventional angiography has not yet been possible. Compared with other imaging modalities, MR imaging offers unique advantages such as *multiplanar imaging capabilities*, 3D reformatting, superior soft tissue contrast, and the absence of *ionizing irradiation*. The combination of these imaging advantages with MRA's ability to delineate vessels, and the possibility of intravascular MR-guided instrument manipulation could enhance and facilitate interventional techniques for several procedures. In time-consuming procedures such as transjugular porto-systemic shunt, MRI guidance may reduce the total radiation exposure, and its 3D capabilities may reduce both the time and complication rate by visualization and localization of the portal vein. In embolization procedures it may be possible to display the distribution of the embolized material and the resultant tissue changes immediately.

A prerequisite for intravascular MR angiography is an MR compatible catheter. Several concepts have been evaluated for an appropriate catheter design, and several of them have already undergone in vitro and in vivo testing and are described in this book or previous reports. (ADAM et al. 1997a; BAKKER et al. 1997; GLOWINSKI et al. 1997; WILDERMUTH et al. 1997).

In this chapter we will present our experience with intravascular MR angiography using *field inhomogeneity catheters* in vivo.

32.2 Concept of Field Inhomogeneity Catheters

The concept of field inhomogeneity catheters has been developed by GLOWINSKI et al. (1977) and is described in detail in Chap. 7 of this book. The principle is simple and can be adapted to every catheter configuration and to all instruments for interventional MR. For angiographic purposes, a thin copper wire is wrapped around the catheter shaft and connected to a battery. When the current is switched on, a local field inhomogeneity is induced, leading to intravoxel spin dephasing and therefore to signal loss around the catheter. Increasing the current increases the effect, making the catheter blacker and larger.

G. ADAM, MD, Department of Diagnostic Radiology, University of Technology Aachen, Pauwelsstrasse 30, 52074 Aachen, Germany

32.3 Animal Experiments

32.3.1 Catheter Prototypes

The first experiments were undertaken with 7-F *prototype catheters* of which several were constructed with different configurations. The catheters were manufactured and provided to us by Cordis, Roden, The Netherlands. The *catheter designs* included a 5-F multipurpose catheter, a 5-F pigtail catheter and a variety of 5-F balloon dilation catheters with different sized balloons ranging from 5 to 10 mm in diameter.

All of the catheters have a conventional lumen and can be introduced over a 0.89-mm (0.035-in.) guidewire. After withdrawing the guidewire, the catheter can be flushed with heparinized saline solution or contrast material like any conventional angiographic catheter. In addition, the catheters are radiopaque, allowing good visualization under fluoroscopic control (Fig. 1).

32.3.2 In Vivo Experiments: Experimental Set-up

All of the catheters were evaluated in animals during in vivo experiments that had been approved by the local animal protection committee. For these experiments we used 80–120 kg pigs which were placed under general anesthesia. The studies were carried out on a prototype interventional MR system which consists of a 1.5 T MR imager (Philips ACS NT 1.5 T) coupled via a floating table top to an X-ray fluoroscopy unit equipped with complete vascular imaging capabilities such as DSA and roadmapping (Philips BV 212). Both systems were installed "in line" in one room (Adam et al. 1997b). Details of this set-up for interventional MR imaging have been described in detail in Chapter 3. After securing the animals supine on the floating table top, a variety of *intravascular procedures* were performed.

All of the experiments were performed via *femoral access* which was obtained under fluoroscopic control. In two animals the common femoral vein was punctured, and in eight animals the common femoral artery. After puncture of the vessel using a 16-G venous access needle (Abbocath, Abbot, Ireland), a 5-F or 7-F introducer sheath (Terumo, Germany) was placed over a guidewire into the vessel lumen. The *MR-visible catheters* were introduced through the sheath, and the vessels which were to be

a

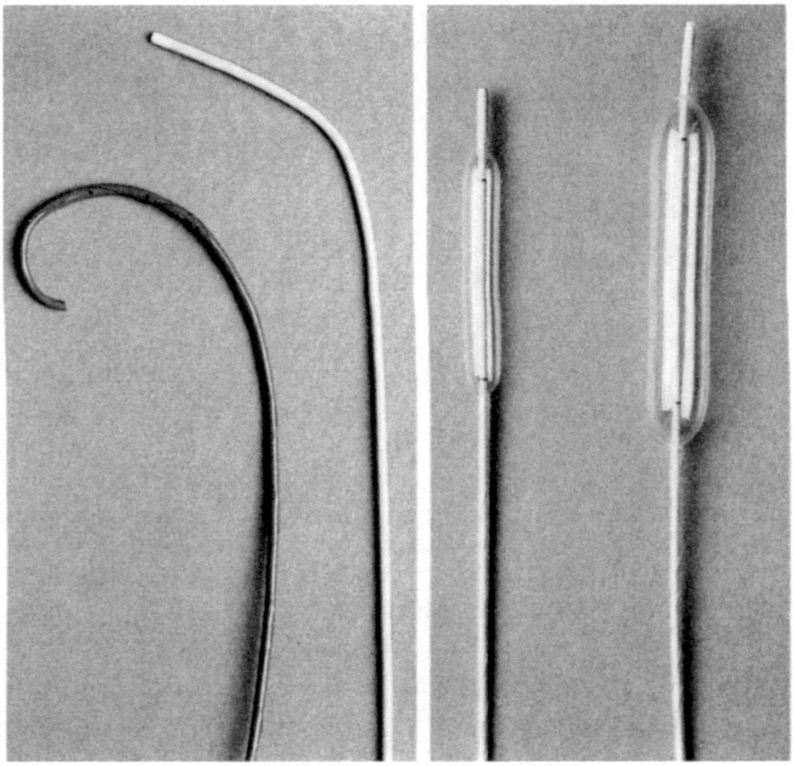

b

Fig. 32.1. a Prototype field inhomogeneity catheters: (*left*) pigtail configuration, (*right*) multipurpose configuraton. **b** Six- and ten-millimeter balloon field inhomogeneity catheters imaged under MR control were first examined with digital subtraction angiography using a conventional iodinated contrast agent (Ultravist, Schering, Germany). We performed angiograms of the inferior *vena cava*, the *abdominal aorta*, the *iliac arteries*, the *renal arteries*, the *superior mesenteric artery*, and the *celiac trunk* using the multipurpose and pigtail catheters.

The balloon catheters were tested in the abdominal aorta where they were inflated using saline solution, room air and a dilute solution of gadopentetate dimeglumine (Magnevist, Schering, Germany).

32.3.3 MR Imaging

MR imaging was performed on a 1.5-T machine using the body coil. For localization of the vessel of interest we applied a fast spin echo localizer in all three orthogonal planes (sagittal, coronal, axial). The optimal slice and plane is selected using a single-slice fast gradient echo sequence (*turbo field echo*) with a contrast preparation pulse in the same plane. This yields a high signal of the inflowing blood and the eventual imaging plane is selected when the vessel is "maximally" displayed. Sequence parameters were TR 17 ms, TE 3.3 ms, flip angle 7 degrees, inversion pulse 940 ms, FOV 370 mm, matrix size 128 × 256, resulting in a pixel size of 1.45 mm. This single-shot sequence was loaded at the main console of the MR imager outside the magnet room, allowing, for example, 50 or more repetitions. Each image sequence was started from a panel at the front of the magnet to interactively visualize the position of the catheter after each movement. The images were displayed immediately after acquisition on LCD screens, which were mounted in front of and beside the magnet.

In one experiment a special fast gradient echo technique, the radial scan mode, was used for catheter visualization, using fast gradient echo techniques. This mode uses *radial k-space sampling* and allows changes of flip angle, slice thickness and scan plane during the study, thus permitting "on-the-fly" adaptation of the scan parameters. Once the sequence is loaded it may be repeated 10 000 times. Due to the great flexibility of this sequence, the scan plane may be adjusted in any desired plane, allowing visualization of tortuous *vascular anatomy* such as the iliac arteries. However, for smaller vessels the spatial resolution is not high enough, a problem which still needs to be overcome.

32.3.4 Results

All of the experiments were completed successfully. No complications relating to the catheters were observed. From the standpoint of steerability and torque control the prototype catheters performed well. Those with the multipurpose configuration were easily manipulated into the branches of the abdominal aorta. Thus it was possible to visualize the catheter within the renal arteries or the iliac vessels (Fig. 2). The repetition of the single shot sequence allowed the operator to visualize the entire catheter, not only the catheter tip, every 2 s. Thus, it was possible to document movement of the entire catheter step by step in arteries and veins using MR imaging (Fig. 3). However, it rapidly became clear that trying to localize smaller and particularly small and tortuous vessels was a major problem. As opposed to conventional angiography, it was impossible to display the vascular anatomy while the catheter was in the vessel lumen of a smaller vessel such as the renal artery. Once the renal artery, for example, was entered, only the catheter artifact was visible, thus making it impossible to use MR imaging to display the normal vascular anatomy.

The performance of the balloon catheters was also good. Once introduced into the vessel lumen, they tracked easily over the wire and could be quickly manipulated into different anatomic regions. The inflation with saline solution and gadopentetate dimeglumine or air resulted in a strong signal loss that allowed excellent delineation of the balloon. The balloons were easy to deflate and could be removed through the introducer sheath without difficulty (Fig. 4).

If the current passing through the wire in the wall of the catheter was switched on while doing MR imaging, no movement of the catheter was observed on MR images. In addition, no clotting of blood around the catheter shaft or the tip of the catheter was noted. As all animals survived the experiments and were not killed thereafter, no pathohistologic examination of the vessel walls was performed. Thus, we have no proof that there is no electrically induced damage to the vessel wall.

32.3.5 Discussion

Our experiments demonstrate that the principle of local field inhomogeneity induction provides a feasi-

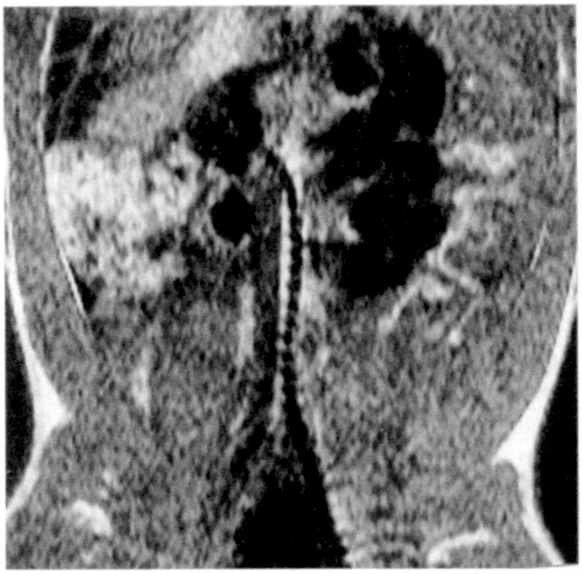
a

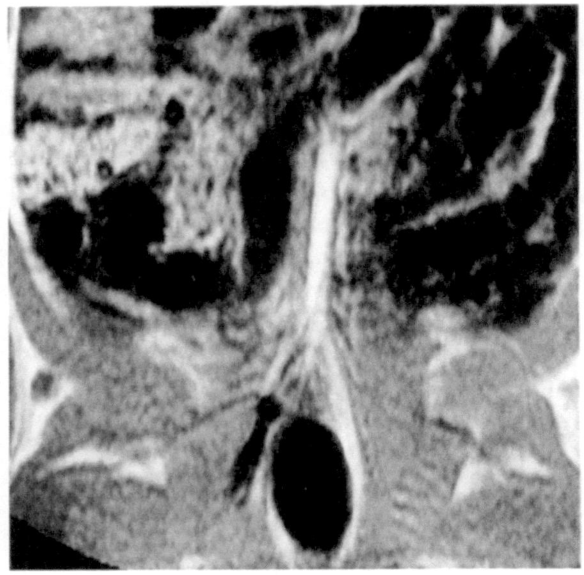
b

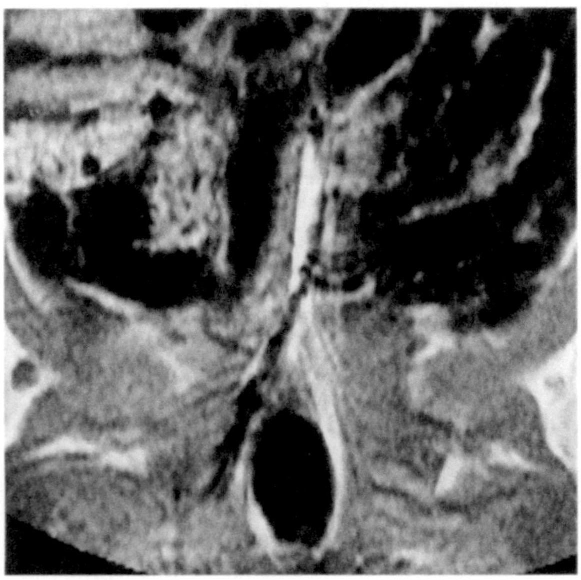
c

Fig. 32.2. **a** Field inhomogeneity catheter in the right renal artery with the current switched on. **b** Field inhomogeneity catheter in the right common iliac artery and distal aorta. **c** Current switched on

a b
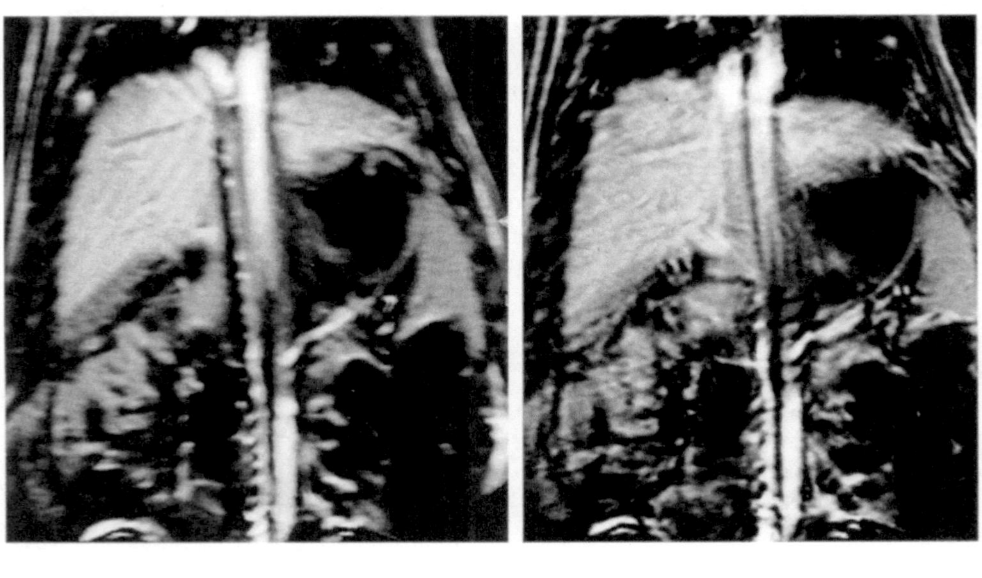

Fig. 32.3. Field inhomogeneity catheter in the inferior vena cava. **a** Without current; **b** with current switched on

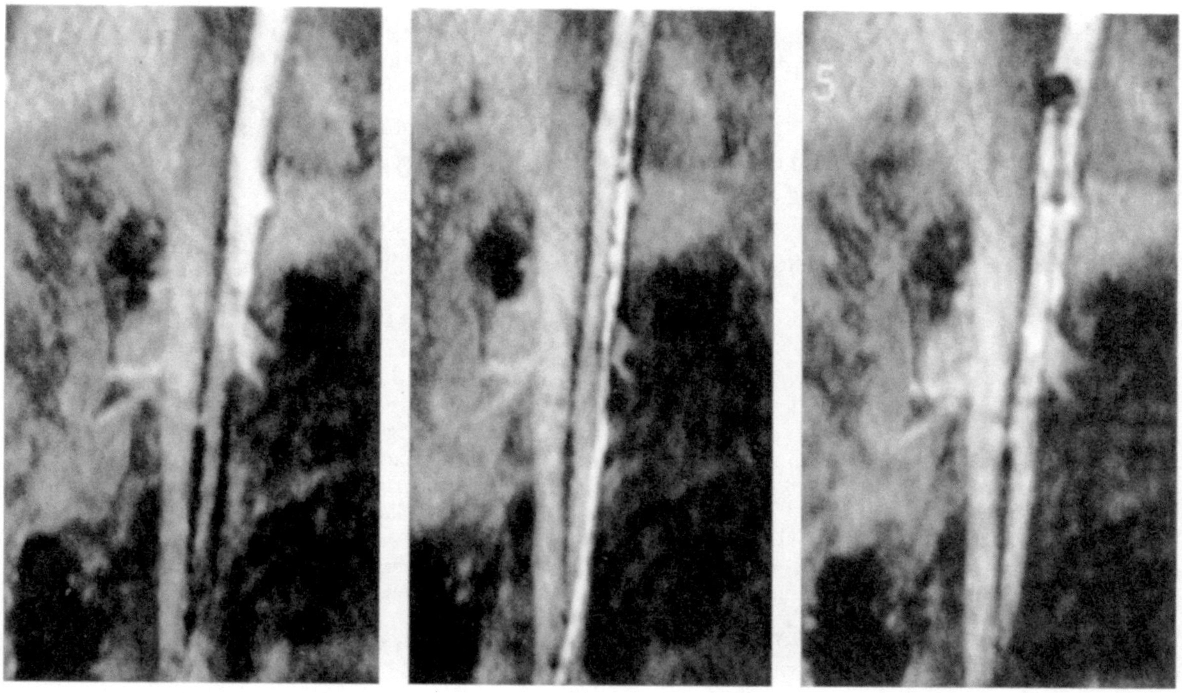

b c

Fig. 32.4. Field inhomogeneity balloon catheter in the aorta. **a** Without current; **b** with current; **c** with the balloon inflated with diluted gadolinium

ble basis for *catheter visualization* under MR guidance using a fast gradient echo technique in animals. This has also been demonstrated in phantom experiments in vitro and the results have been summarized in an earlier chapter of this book. The key to the success of this technique lies in the fact that a fast gradient echo sequence with a contrast preparation prepulse yields a *bright blood effect* also seen with time-of-flight techniques. It therefore displays an excellent contrast between the vessels and signal detoriation caused by the local field inhomogeneity induced by the current flowing through the copper wire around the catheter.

The design of the field inhomogeneity catheter thus allows not only imaging of the catheter tip, but of the whole catheter. It thus differs from other techniques which have also been described in this book, such as the tip-tracking technique (Leung et al. 1994) or the susceptibility-based techniques using dysprosium spheres (Bakker et al. 1997). The advantage of visualization of the whole catheter is obvious, as the images acquired by MR imaging are similar to those from fluoroscopy and digital subtraction angiography. Moreover, the single-slice technique using fast gradient echo scanning is relatively insensitive to respiratory or vessel wall motion, which is not the case for the 3D sequences that are used to provide the roadmaps of the *tip-tracking* techniques.

There is, however, one major shortcoming of the time-of-flight technique. If the vessel runs tortuously through the scan plane, the time of flight effect is diminished, and the vessel is no longer displayed in its entirety on the MR images. Thus, the scan plane has to be adapted to the anatomy. However, this requires multiple sequence reloads in order to secure the appropriate scan plane and increases the imaging time. In vessels such as the aorta or the IVC this is not a problem, because they are almost always parallel throughout their length to a single coronal scan plane. However, as soon as one moves into the iliac region, it becomes more difficult. In tortuous branches of the celiac or the superior mesenteric artery it is currently impossible to display the catheter within the vessel lumen. One method to overcome this disadvantage has been recently attempted in our MR scanner. Fast radial scanning allows adaption of the scan plane "on the fly", as well as changes of the slice thickness which can also be made during scanning without reloading the sequence. Our experience is still limited with this technique and more experimental work needs to be carried out. However, it has already shown promise as a method to overcome the drawbacks of rapidly repeated single-slice, gradient echo images for catheter visualization.

Another very important and as yet unanswered question relating to the field inhomogeneity catheter is its *electrical safety*. Generally, a wire within the body of a patient may behave like an antenna. The more the catheter is tuned to the resonance frequency of the radiofrequency pulses, the greater the chance of energy deposition around the catheter. It is extremely difficult to simulate using computers or in vivo, but prior to any clinical study in humans this question must be answered satisfactorily.

32.4 Conclusions

Our animal studies have demonstrated the feasibility of field inhomogeneity catheters for intravascular visualization of angiography catheters. The principle can be adapted to any catheter configuration, and the technique allows visualization of the whole catheter in a manner that feels comfortably familiar from conventional angiography.

It may be used on any MR scanner on which fast gradient echo techniques are available. However, visualization of the catheter in tortuous vessels remains a major problem. In addition, if the vessel lumen is relatively small compared to the diameter of the field inhomogeneity catheter, the vascular anatomy may be obscured. Thus, it remains unclear whether this technique may be applied to interventional procedures such as angioplasty, where high spatial resolution is required. In addition, the electrical safety of this type of catheter still needs to be elucidated.

The potential clinical applications of intravascular MR angiography have yet to be defined. When one thinks of the temporal and spatial resolution that can be achieved with conventional techniques such as X-ray fluoroscopy and digital subtraction angiography, the MR methods are obviously still in their infancy. However, MR tracking and profiling, the susceptibility-based concepts of catheter visualization at least afford us the unique opportunity to develop meaningful opportunities to use MR as an imaging tool for intravascular procedures.

References

Adam G, Glowinski A, Neuerburg J et al (1997a) Kathetervisualisierung in der MR-Tomographie: erste tierexperimentelle Erfahrungen mit Feldinhomogenitätskathetern. Fortschr Roentgenstr 166:324–328

Adam G, Neuerburg J, Bücker A et al (1997b) Interventional magnetic resonance: initial clinical experience with a 1.5 T magnetic resonance system combined with c-arm fluoroscopy. Invest Radiol 32:191–197

Bakker CJ, Hoogeween RM, Hurtak WF et al (1997) MR-guided endovascular interventions: susceptibility-based catheter and near-real-time imaging technique. Radiology 202:273–276

Edelman RR (1993) MR angiography: present and future. AJR Am J Roentgenol 161–22

Glowinski A, Adam G, Bücker A et al (1997) Catheter visualization using locally induced, actively controlled field inhomogeneities. Magn Reson Med (in press)

Leung DA, Debatin JF, Wildermuth SW et al (1995) Intravascular MR tracking catheter. Preliminary experimental evaluation. AJR Am J Roentgenol 164:1265–1270

Levy RA, Prince MR (1996) Arterial-phase three-dimensional contrast enhanced MR-angiography of the carotid arteries. AJR Am J Roentgenol 167:211–215

Prince MR (1994) Gadolinium-enhanced MR angiography. Radiology 191:155–164

Ronkaninen A, Puranen MI, Hernesmieni JA et al (1995) MR angiographic screening in 400 asymptomatic individuals with increased familial risk. Radiology 195:35–40

Vogl TJ, Bergman C, Villringer A et al (1994) Dural sinus thrombosis: value of venous MR-angiography for diagnosis and follow up. AJR Am J Roentgenol 162:1191–1198

Snidow JJ, Johnson MS, Harris VJ et al (1996) Three-dimensional gadolinium enhanced MR-angiography for aorto iliac inflow assessment plus renal artery screening in a single breathhold. Radiology 198:155–164

Wildermuth S, Debatin JF, Leung DA et al (1997) MR imaging-guided intravascular procedures: initial demonstration in a pig model. Radiology 202:578–583

33 Intravascular Interventions with Active MR Tracking

J. F. Debatin, S. Wildermuth, and G.K. von Schulthess

CONTENTS

33.1 Introduction

Fundamental to the success and safety of intravascular procedures, such as embolization or percutaneous transluminal angioplasty (PTA), is the visualization of the catheter and guidewire relative to the area of treatment. To-date this is achieved with X-ray fluoroscopy. Exposure to ionizing radiation, limited soft tissue contrast, and the inability to image in cross section have motivated the exploration of alternative imaging strategies.

Magnetic resonance imaging (MRI) seems well suited for monitoring vascular interventions. MRI causes no radiation exposure, is capable of combining high temporal and spatial resolution (Edelman 1993), and provides cross-sectional images in any desired plane. The influence of flow on both amplitude and phase of spins provides the basis for "time-of-flight" (TOF) and "phase contrast" MR angiography (MRA). Their dependence on flow effects makes these techniques vulnerable to pulsatility and saturation artifacts. These limitations can be overcome by contrast-enhanced three-dimensional (3D) MRA – a technique based on the use of intravenously administered paramagnetic contrast agents in combination with ultrafast 3D acquisition strategies (Leung et al. 1996).

With contrast-enhanced 3D MRA arterial signal is no longer dependent on flow effects. Rather, in analogy to catheter or CT angiography, signal within the arterial system is based on the presence of paramagnetic contrast material. The intravenously administered paramagnetic contrast agent induces a T1 shortening of blood (Prince et al. 1993) translating into a selective signal intensity increase in the arterial system. This increase is maximal during the first pass of the extracellular contrast agent. While early implementations of 3D MRA were hampered by long acquisition times and motion artifacts, the increasing availability of high-performance gradient systems has reduced imaging times to allow data collection within a single breath-hold of under 30 s (Leung et al. 1996; Holland et al. 1996; Snidow et al 1995, 1996). The breath-hold implementation of 3D MRA has been shown to render high diagnostic accuracy in the detection of vascular disease affecting the aorta and its major branches (Prince et al. 1995), including peripheral vascular segments like the distal renal arteries (Hany et al. 1997). Reflecting its reliability, robustness, and accuracy, the technique has already been implemented in clinical practice in centers around the world. The 3D data sets can be post-processed to provide a comprehensive exoscopic and endoscopic appreciation of the vascular morphology (Davis et al. 1996).

Other features inherent in the MR experiment increase the attractiveness of MRA with regard to guidance and monitoring of vascular interventions. MRI's soft tissue contrast is vastly superior to that of fluoroscopy, permitting the concurrent evaluation of

J.F. Debatin, MD, Institute of Diagnostic Radiology, Zurich University Hospital, Rämistrasse 100, CH-8091 Zurich, Switzerland
S. Wildermuth, MD, Institute of Diagnostic Radiology, Zurich University Hospital, Rämistrasse 100, CH-8091 Zurich, Switzerland
G.K. von Schulthess, MD, PhD, Division of Nuclear Medicine, Zurich University Hospital, Rämistrasse 100, CH-8091 Zurich, Switzerland

tissues surrounding the vessel of interest. Furthermore, quantitative velocity and flow volume characterization can be integrated in the same non-invasive vascular evaluation (PELC et al. 1991a). In addition, the MR experiment is sensitive to temperature changes, thus enabling, in principle, monitoring of intravascular thermosensitive therapies, such as laser or radiofrequency (RF) therapies.

Patient access remains a significant problem for any scenario involving MR guidance and control of intravascular interventions. The "ideal" interventional MRA scanner has yet to be designed. At this time, high field strength and fast gradient systems seem unnegotiable specifications of any such scanner. Recent hardware developments have provided better patient access by shortening the bore while maintaining field strength and gradient performance. For the concept of interventional MRA to evolve from a hypothetical concept to a practical possibility further progress will be needed.

A difficult challenge with regard to MR-guided intravascular interventions pertains to the actual visualization of the catheter or guidewire within the vascular system. There are two fundamental approaches to device localization with MRI: electrically passive techniques based on visualization of the susceptibility-induced signal void caused by the instrument (DUMOULIN et al. 1991; LEUNG et al. 1995a) and electrically active techniques first suggested by Ackerman et al. (1986). Both techniques are described in detail in this book (Chaps. 4–9). This chapter will focus on MR-guided intravascular interventions based on active visualization of catheters and guidewires.

33.2 MR Tracking: The Technique

MR tracking was developed by DUMOULIN et al. (1993) for active monitoring of devices under real-time conditions. As first suggested by ACKERMAN et al. (1986), a small receive-only coil is incorporated into the tip of the device (Fig. 33.1). Following non-selective RF excitation of a volume defined in size by the dimensions of the field of view (FOV), a gradient-recalled echo (GRE) is generated by the miniature receive coil. Following Fourier transformation, a signal peak is obtained, the frequency of which corresponds to the position of the coil on a particular axis. A Hadamard multiplexed pulse sequence is used in which positional information from all three axes is multiplexed and acquired simultaneously (DUMOULIN et al. 1991). Thus, the 3D position of the coil is encoded with only four excitations. With a short TR, the coil's position can be computed up to 16 times per second. The coil position is displayed by graphic overlay as a cursor on any previously acquired MR "roadmap" image (Fig. 33.2). Ultrafast data links and a powerful processor limit the delay between the end of data acquisition and display of the coil position to less than 10 ms, assuring true real-time tracking. The composite image is projected onto a screen visible to the operator in the scan room and video-taped for archiving purposes (Fig. 33.3).

By separating the positional information from the data contained within the image, MR tracking of a device is possible without having to update images. The real-time position of the coil within the catheter or guidewire is simply superimposed on previously acquired MR images (Figs. 33.2, 33.3). This strategy works only as long as the area of interest has re-

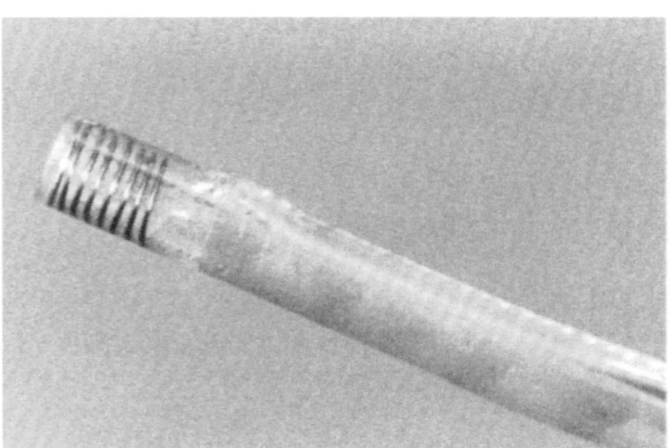

Fig. 33.1. The miniature radiofrequency (RF) coil is incorporated in the tip of a 5-F catheter. The coaxial cable, embedded in the catheter wall, is also seen

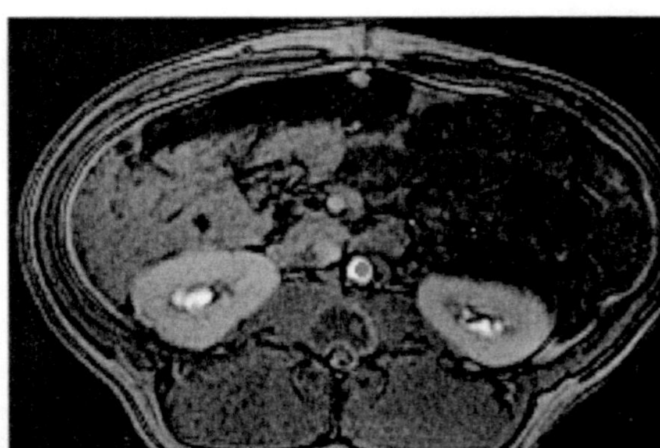

Fig. 33.2. The catheter tip, represented as a red cursor, is seen in the aorta of an axial time-of-flight (TOF) image

mained unchanged in position. As soon as patient motion occurs, updated images need to be obtained to provide a new basis for tracking of the device. Periodic motion processes, such as respiration induced motion in the craniocaudal plane, may be compensated for by incorporation of some sort of gating or "navigator" sequence. The latter provides an adaptive correction system based on specially encoded "navigator" echoes which could be interleaved into the tracking sequence and thus compensate for gross patient motion.

For real-time control, update images can, however, easily be obtained. The actively available positional information of the coil can be used to guide the imaging plane so that new images are acquired in a position always corresponding to the position of the coil integrated into the tip of the catheter or guidewire. For this purpose the acquisition of fast gradient echo images is most useful. The images can be acquired in any plane relative to the tip of the device. The center of the image will always correspond to the position of the tracking coil. In this mode the scanner intermittently switches between image acquisition and tracking. Hence, the position of the coil is updated discontinuously and its movement is not displayed as smoothly as in the continuous tracking mode. In the present implementation, "update" images are acquired using a fast conventional GRE sequence. Data acquisition and subsequent reconstruction take several seconds and are clearly not performed in real time. Improving the temporal resolution of update images would require the implementation of ultrafast echoplanar data acquisition strategies necessitating additional hardware.

33.2.1 Multiplanar MR Tracking

The coil position can be projected onto multiple images simultaneously without loss in temporal resolution. For multiplanar tracking, the coil position is projected onto two or more images covering the same imaging volume in different planes (Leung et al. 1995a) (Fig. 33.4). Biplanar tracking vastly enhances the ability to target any desired area provided the area under consideration is contained within the imaging volume. The simultaneous display of the catheter tip on a coronal and a sagittal roadmap image of the aorta greatly facilitates positional determinations relative to the celiac trunk and the superior mesenteric artery, as well as both renal arteries.

With the biplanar tracking option, updated images can also be displayed in two different planes. The operator is free to choose whether to track the catheter or guidewire on previously acquired images or to have the scanner provide update images on one or both displays corresponding to the position of the RF coil. Any combination of update image and positional display is also possible.

33.2.2 Multicoil MR Tracking

Simultaneous tracking of up to four coils has recently become possible. This is accomplished by attaching each of the four coils to separate receivers. Separate tracking symbols and colors are assigned to the four different receivers, permitting easy separation of the tracking devices. The number of coils that can be tracked simultaneously is dependent on the number of receivers available.

33.3 Material and Methods

33.3.1 In Vivo Experimental Setup

To-date, the in vivo experience with intravascular MR tracking of catheters and guidewires has been limited to experiments performed on fully anesthetized pigs with a body weight ranging between 40 and 55 kg. All experiments were approved by the appropriate governmental regulatory bodies.

As premedication 2.0 ml azaperon and 0.7 ml atropine were administered. The pigs were ventilated at all times with an anesthetic containing halothane and oxygen. The arterial system of the animals was accessed surgically by arteriotomy of the carotid arteries; the venous system by cutdown to the jugular veins. Under fluoroscopic guidance an introducer sheath was passed over a conventional 0.035-in. (0.89 mm) guidewire made out of MR-compatible nitinol into either the carotid artery or the jugular vein. On some occasions both vessels were accessed. The introducer sheath was secured by suture and the guidewire was subsequently removed. Through the indwelling introducer, MR-tracking catheters and guidewires were advanced into the descending aorta or the superior vena cava.

The animals were subsequently transferred to the MRI suite, where they were placed in the bore of the magnet system in the supine position. Experiments were performed on either a 1.5-T MR system (SIGNA, General Electric, Milwaukee, Wis.) or an open configuration 0.5-T system (SIGNA-SP, General Electric, Milwaukee, Wis.), interfaced via high speed data link with a Sparc 20 and Sparc 10 (Sun Microsystems, Palo Alto, Calif.) workstation (Figs. 33.3, 33.4). Various torso surface coils (conventional and phased-array) were used for signal transmission and reception. Two-dimensional time-of-flight angiograms [TR 30/TE 8, 30° flip angle, 36-40 cm FOV, 256×192 matrix, 1 excitation (NEX)] of the abdominal arterial and venous vascular systems were acquired in the coronal and axial plane using 5-mm sections. Maximum intensity projection (MIP) images containing different regions of vascular anatomy were obtained and used as roadmaps for the positional display of the tracked intravascular devices. For biplanar tracking, roadmap images covering the same vascular territory needed to be available in two planes. Depending on the number of 5-mm images required for a particular MIP projection, time for data acquisition in one plane ranged between 1 and 3 min. Acquisition times were broken up into 20 to 30-s packages so that the data could be collected during breath-hold (respirator was stopped) in end-expiration. Based on these images, the MR-tracking catheters and guidewires were manipulated under active MR guidance.

Continuous MR tracking was based on non-selective RF excitation of a volume defined in size by the dimensions of the FOV (36–40 cm) using the following parameters: TR 15–30/TE 8, flip angle 60°. Depending on the TR length, the coil position was sampled every 60–120 ms, or 8–16 times/second. The signal-to-noise ratio (SNR) of the frequency peak based on which the coil position is determined is directly related to the length of the TR used for the RF excitations, as well as the number of spins encompassed by the receive coil. The latter is mainly determined by the coil diameter. To assure robust MR tracking, the TR should thus be chosen in inverse proportion to the diameter of the receive coil used.

To compensate for motion, TOF roadmaps were updated every 15 min. In addition, fast gradient echo "updates" were acquired during the catheter tracking process using the following parameters: TR 20/TE 4, flip angle 20°, 10-mm sections, FOV 36–40 cm, 256×128 matrix, 1 NEX. The tracking information was used to assure that each acquired update image, regardless of the chosen imaging plane, was centered on the most recent coil position. The update images were fed into one of the two displays on a "need-basis", defined by the interventionist.

33.3.2
MR-Tracking Catheter Design

Prototype MR-tracking catheters for all MR-guided intravascular interventions were constructed by Schneider Europe (Bülach, Switzerland). An untuned, receive-only copper RF coil consisting of 8–16 loops with an outer diameter of 1.1 mm is integrated in the catheter tip. The use of 8-16 windings had been found to provide optimal signal in phantom experiments (Leung et al. 1995b). These coils are incorporated into the catheter material itself and connected to a plug at the base of the catheter via a fully insulated coaxial cable with a diameter of

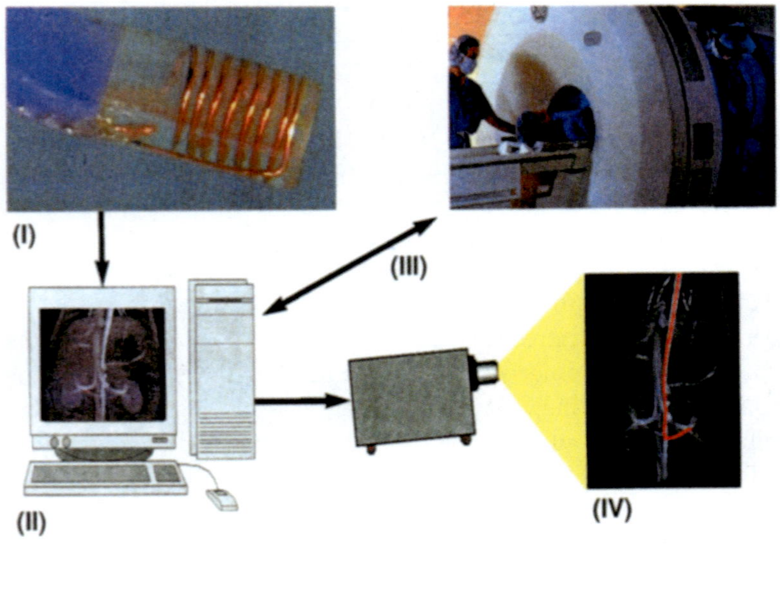

Fig. 33.3. Real-time tracking of catheters is made possible by incorporating a small RF coil in the catheter tip and connecting it to a coaxial cable (*I*). The coaxial cable is interfaced to a workstation (*II*). The tracking software is implemented on the workstation which computes the three-dimensional position of the coil and displays it on a preacquired MR image (*III*) as a moving graphic overlay (*IV*)

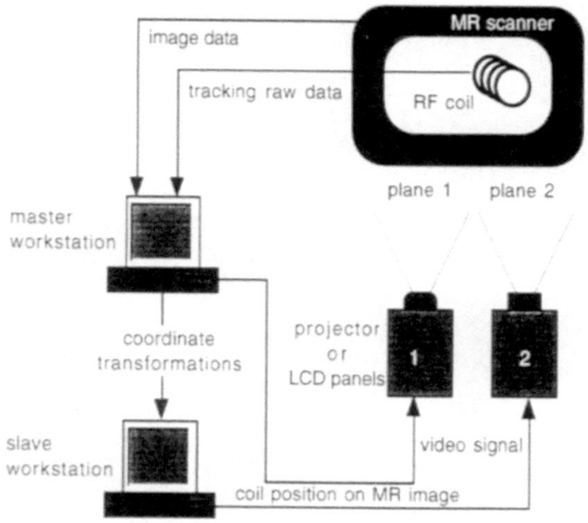

Fig. 33.4. A schematic shows the various components of the multiplanar MR-tracking system (LCD, liquid crystal display)

0.38 mm, embedded in the catheter wall. The need for fully insulated coaxial cables was documented in in vitro experiments. Use of other, less expensive cable designs, such as twisted pair cables, had resulted in corruption of the tracking signal (LEUNG et al. 1995b).

MR-tracking catheters were manufactured at a length of 120 cm out of polyamide (PM 200, Schneider, Bülach, Switzerland), a flexible material providing optimum force transmission and covered with softglide coating. The material is approved for human use and found in commercially available catheters. The catheters contain a standard 0.035-in. (0.89 mm) lumen for placement of a guidewire or application of contrast agent or other materials.

Catheter force transmission (trackability) was assessed for a 5-F coil-tipped catheter in comparison to a standard 5-F catheter (Schneider) in a guidance system (inside diameter of 2.5 mm) with several preformed bends. Force transmission, monitored continuously over distance as the catheters were mechanically advanced 140 mm around a 90° bend with a 12-mm radius, was 18% poorer for the coil-tipped catheter than for the standard catheter (WILDERMUTH et al. 1997b; Fig. 33.5).

33.3.3 MR-Tracking Guidewire Design

An MR-tracking guidewire was constructed with a 0.6-mm diameter solenoid coil integrated in the tip (Schneider). The solenoid coil consisted of 16 windings in two layers. The coil was attached to a coaxial cable. The distal 10 cm portion, including the coil itself, was coated by a sheath of fluoroethylenepropylene (FEP). The remainder of the 1.8-m long wire was sheathed with a polyamide to lend some mechanical stability. FEP, a less rigid polymer, provided a very flexible tip.

The outer diameter of the guidewire was 0.75 mm, small enough to fit into the standard 0.035-in. (0.89 mm) lumen of a 5-F catheter. Small holes were made both proximal and distal to the RF coil (Fig. 33.6). A lumen was left in the interior of the coil so that, during use, fresh blood continually flowed between the holes and through the center of the coil, thus providing a signal source where the coil is most sensitive.

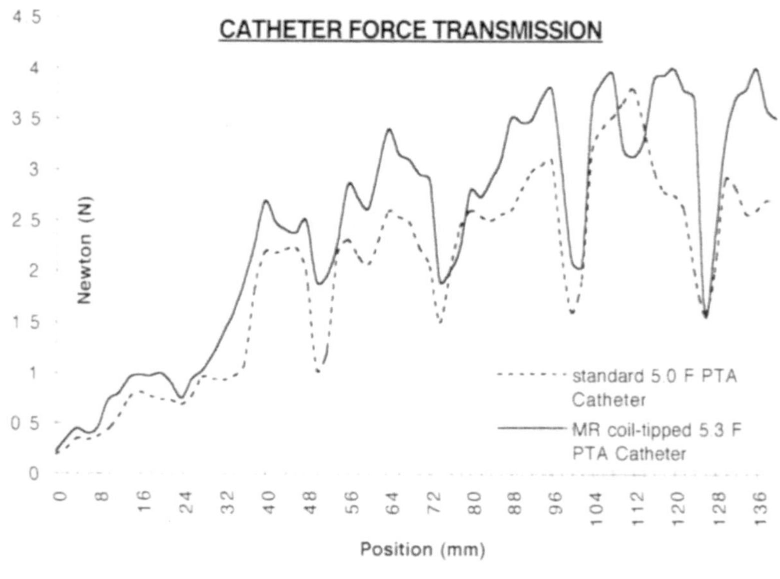

Fig. 33.5. Assessment of catheter force transmission (trackability), expressed in newton (N), of a normal 5.0-F SMASH PTA catheter and a coil-tipped 5.3-F MR catheter over a 140- mm distance, negotiating a preformed 90° turn (radius 12 mm). The area under the MR catheter curve exceeds that of the conventional catheter by 18%

33.4 Positional Accuracy and Robustness of MR Tracking

In vitro phantom experiments demonstrated the MR-tracking technique to be highly accurate with regard to positioning of the tracking coil (LEUNG et al. 1995b). Over an entire 40-cm FOV the coil positions determined with MR tracking agreed well with those determined with X-ray fluoroscopy. A linear regression analysis revealed good correlation (r = 0.99, slope = 1, y-intercept = 0; LEUNG et al. 1995b).

For the in vivo evaluation of the positional accuracy inherent in MR tracking a 5-F MR-tracking catheter was advanced into the descending aorta of a pig via an introducer placed in the carotid artery. Based on TOF MIP projection images, depicting the abdominal aorta with its branch vessels in the coronal projection, the catheter was maneuvered under MR guidance into the splenic artery, as well as both renal arteries (Fig. 33.7). After each placement, a radiograph was obtained to confirm the position of the catheter following the administration of an iodinated contrast material through the catheter. These confirmed the correct positions in the respective vessels as had been indicated by the MR-tracking position on the roadmap MIP images.

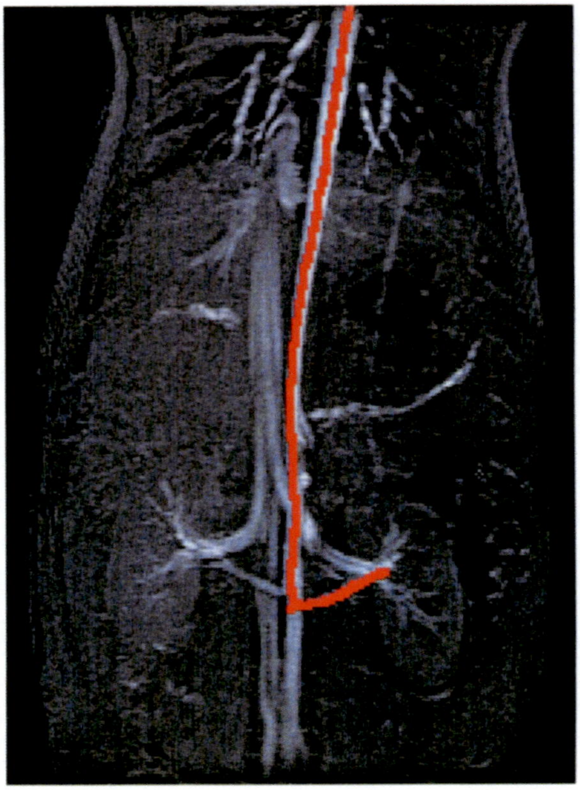

Fig. 33.7. Coronal MR TOF angiographic roadmap images (computer screen shots) of the pig's abdominal arterial system. With the cursor in continuous mode, the path of the catheter tip into the left renal artery is displayed

33.5 MR-Guided Intravascular Procedures

33.5.1 Embolization

A 5-F MR-tracking catheter, 120 cm in length, was inserted through the carotid introducer and tracked into the right renal artery based on previously acquired TOF MIP roadmap images. To enhance maneuverability, the catheter tip had been slightly curved manually over hot steam prior to insertion. Following secure positioning of the catheter tip in the proximal right renal artery (Fig. 33.8), an MR contrast agent (Gd-DTPA, Schering, Berlin, FRG) was injected through the catheter lumen at a concentration of 0.01 mmol/kg. Prior to, as well as at 10-s intervals following contrast agent administration, eight contiguous 10-mm coronal sections were acquired through the kidneys using a fast, multiplanar spoiled gradient echo sequence (FMPSPGR; TR 90/TE 2.1, flip 60°, 1 NEX). These dynamically acquired images revealed isolated early enhancement of the right kidney with subsequent enhancement of the contralateral kidney 30 s after contrast agent administration.

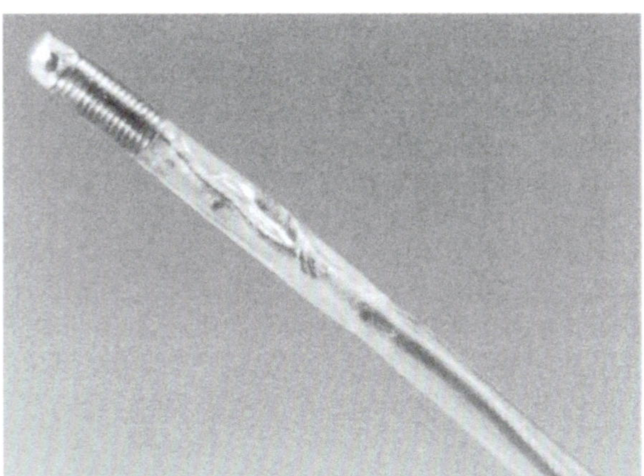

Fig. 33.6. A close-up of the guidewire tip showing the built-in RF coil

Subsequently the right renal artery was embolized by injecting Ethibloc (Ethicon, Germany) embolization material through the lumen of the catheter, the tip of which was lodged in the right renal artery. Dynamic FMPSPGR imaging was repeated. The images now demonstrated isolated enhancement of the contralateral kidney commencing 10 s after contrast agent application due to backflow out of the occluded right renal arterial system. Merely some threadlike areas of signal reduction were seen in the central regions of the affected kidney. These corresponded to T2-shortening effects in the central renal arterial branches induced by the high concentration of paramagnetic contrast agent. Owing to the embolization of the more distally located arteriolar and capillary system, there is no blood flow diluting the contrast agent in the renal arterial branches (Fig. 33.9).

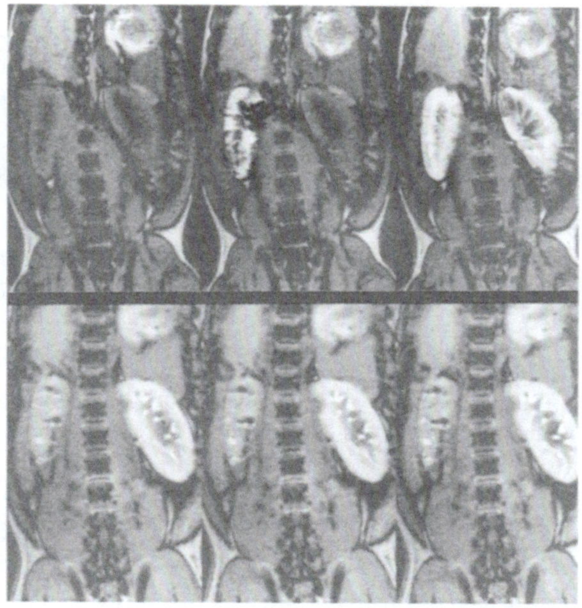

Fig. 33.9. Coronal fast multiplanar spoiled gradient echo images through both kidneys acquired before (*top row*) and following (*bottom row*) embolization. Images were collected prior to (*left*), 10 s after (*middle*) and 30 s after contrast agent application through the MR-tracking catheter, which remained lodged in the right renal artery throughout the procedure. Before embolization, enhancement of the right kidney is seen at 10 s, with enhancement of the contralateral kidney at 30 s. Following embolization, there is enhancement only of the contralateral kidney due to backflow after contrast administration

33.5.2 Balloon Occlusion and Percutaneous Transluminal Angioplasty (PTA)

The design of the PTA MR-tracking catheter (Fig. 33.10), 5.3-F in diameter, was based on the commercially available SMASH model (Schneider, Bülach, Switzerland). The cylindrical balloon portion extends over 40 mm, from 10 to 50 mm proximal of the tracking coil at the catheter's tip. The balloon is made out of a special polyamide (PM 300, Schneider, Switzerland). The inflated balloon is 6 mm in diameter and has a recommended pressure range of 5–10 ATM (burst pressure 14-18 ATM; Fig. 33.11).

The function of the MR-tracking PTA catheter was assessed in vitro using a flow phantom, as well as in vivo in a fully anesthetized, 45-kg pig. For the in vitro experiment, a harvested 12-cm segment of human common femoral artery was connected to 9-mm tygon tubing at both ends and placed in a gel-filled Plexiglas container. The proximal end of the tubing was connected to a roller flow pump, adjusted to deliver 300 ml/min. The distal end of the tubing merged into a vented reservoir from which the pump was supplied. A 2-cm long, high-grade stenosis was created in the center of the harvested vessel segment by placing soft modelling dough around it. The stenosis was depicted on a TOF roadmap MIP image (Fig. 33.12). Subsequently, the PTA catheter was introduced into the phantom through a Luer-Lok proximal to the harvested vessel segment. The stenosis was crossed under MR-tracking guidance. A TR of 15 ms rendered 18 updates/s. Based on the TOF roadmap, the MR-tracking PTA catheter was correctly positioned, assuring complete coverage of the stenosis by the balloon. The balloon was inflated to 4 ATM and the TOF roadmap image acquisition was repeated following withdrawal of the PTA catheter. Tracking remained possible with the ballon inflated. Inflating the balloon reduced the stenosis as documented by the post-dilatation MR angiogram (Fig. 33.12).

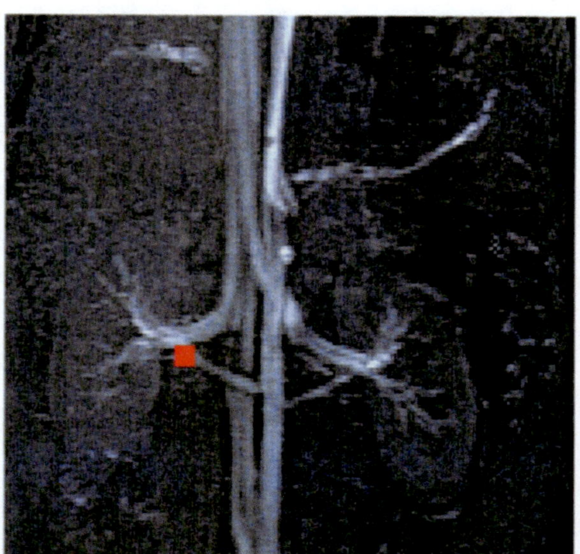

Fig. 33.8. The catheter tip, represented as a red cursor, is seen in the right renal artery on a coronal TOF image, acquired on the interventional 0.5-T system

To assess the in vivo functioning of the MR-tracking PTA catheters, in vivo occlusion of the right sacral artery with the PTA catheter was attempted in two animals. The sacral artery was chosen to minimize stress to the animal. Owing to abundant collateral flow, occlusion of the vessel would not result in any significant tissue ischemia. Coronal TOF images of the abdominal aorta and pelvic arterial system were acquired. Based on these MIP roadmap images, the PTA catheter was tracked into the right sacral artery of the pig (Fig. 33.13). To evaluate the functioning of the PTA balloon, it was inflated with water while the catheter was positioned in the sacral artery. To demonstrate the effect of balloon inflation in the sacral artery, the MRA acquisition of the pelvic arterial system was repeated while the balloon remained inflated (Fig. 33.14).

The effect of balloon inflation was easily demonstrated. Over the entire 40-mm length of the balloon, the vessel was in effect occluded, as shown by the total lack of intravascular signal. Signal distal to the balloon results from abundant collateral flow from the contralateral sacral artery. Tracking remained possible throughout the entire in vivo experiment, even while the balloon was inflated.

In subsequent experiments, the right renal artery was occluded with the PTA MR-tracking catheter. Through the indwelling introducer, the MR-tracking PTA catheter was advanced into the descending aorta of a pig. Based on coronal TOF roadmaps of the abdominal aorta and its branches, the PTA catheter was manipulated under active MR-tracking guidance into the right renal artery. The balloon was inflated with undiluted Gd-DTPA (Magnevist, Schering, Berlin Germany) to 2 ATM. Contrast agent inflation of the balloon, situated within the right renal artery, rendered the outline of the inflated balloon dark. On subsequently acquired TOF roadmap images this dark signal contrasted well with the high signal from surrounding flowing spins. TOF roadmaps confirmed occlusion of the right renal artery when the balloon, situated in the renal artery, was inflated.

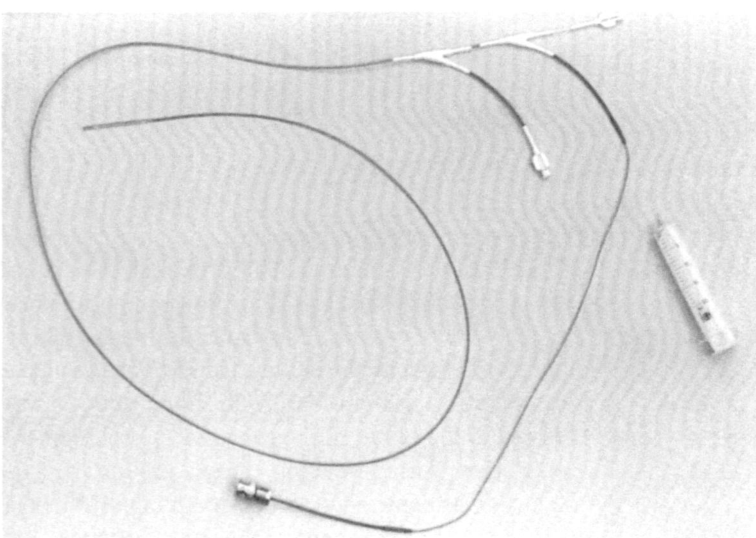

Fig. 33.10. An overview of the PTA MR-tracking catheter with a deflated balloon. Next to two Luer-Loks the coaxial plug is visible from which the signal is fed into the scanner

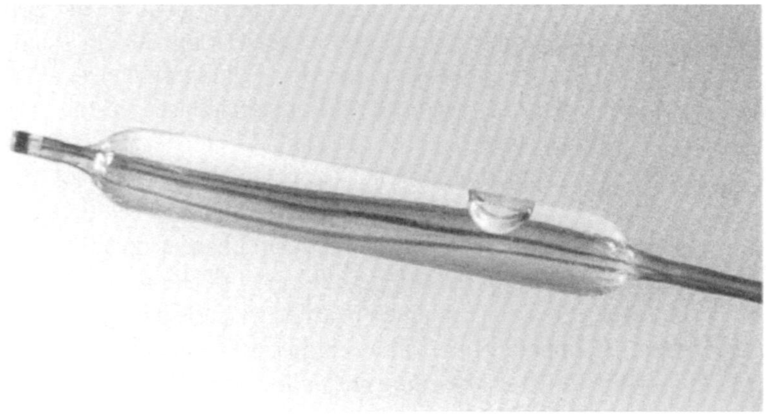

Fig. 33.11. The proximal portion of the 5.3-F PTA MR-tracking catheter contains the cylindrical balloon, which extends over 40 mm and can be inflated to a diameter of 6 mm. The coaxial cable, embedded in the catheter wall, is also seen. The coil is positioned at the catheter's tip, 10 mm distal to the balloon

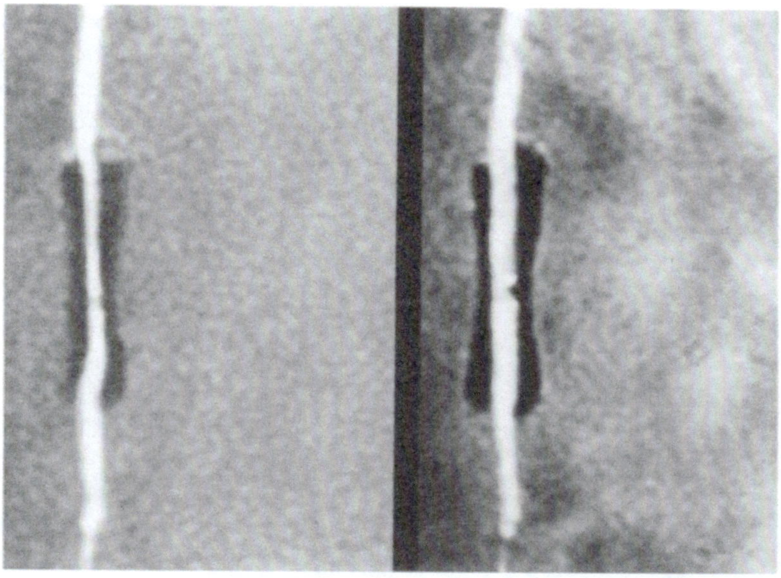

Fig. 33.12. MRA roadmap images of the vascular phantom. A stenosis is seen on the pre-PTA image (*left*). Following PTA with the MR-tracking catheter (*right*), the stenosis is reduced

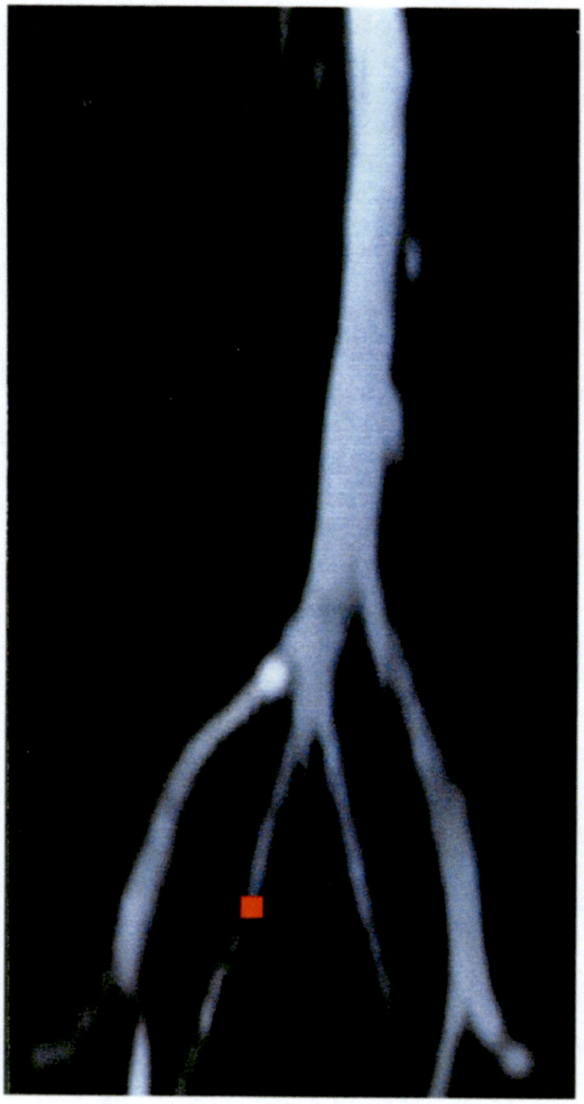

Fig. 33.13. Coronal TOF roadmap of the pelvic arteries of a pig. The tip of a PTA catheter is seen in the right sacral artery

33.5.3 Transjugular Intrahepatic Puncture of the Portal System

For this procedure a modified MReye TIPS (Transjugular intrahepatic porto-systemic shunt) set (William Cook Europe, Bjaeverskov Denmark) was used. It consisted of the following components: a 41-cm long 10-F introducer; a curved 10-F TFE catheter; a 51.5-cm long, 14-Gauge curved MRI-compatible MReye cannula; a 5-F, 59.5-cm long TFE catheter equipped at its tip with a tracking coil (Schneider Europe, Bülach, Switzerland); and a 60-cm long, 20-Gauge flexible MRI-compatible MReye puncture needle. The puncture needle was contained within the 5-F tracking catheter. Since both components are advanced at the same time for the puncture, the needle tip could in effect be tracked by virtue of its position 5 mm distal to the tracking coil incorporated in the tip of the catheter (Figs. 33.15, 33.16).

The procedure was performed with biplanar MR tracking. For this purpose, axial and coronal roadmap images were acquired of the inferior vena cava and the hepatic veins, as well as of the portal venous system. Based on these MIP roadmap images, the coil-tipped tracking catheter, placed within the introducer sheath, was advanced into the middle hepatic vein. Based on the axial and coronal roadmap images, a course for puncturing the right portal vein from the middle hepatic vein was mapped. The actual puncture was performed with the pig in suspended respiration using biplanar tracking of the coil-tipped catheter covering the puncture needle. The intraportal position of the 5-F catheter was subsequently verified fluoroscopically. A stent was not placed.

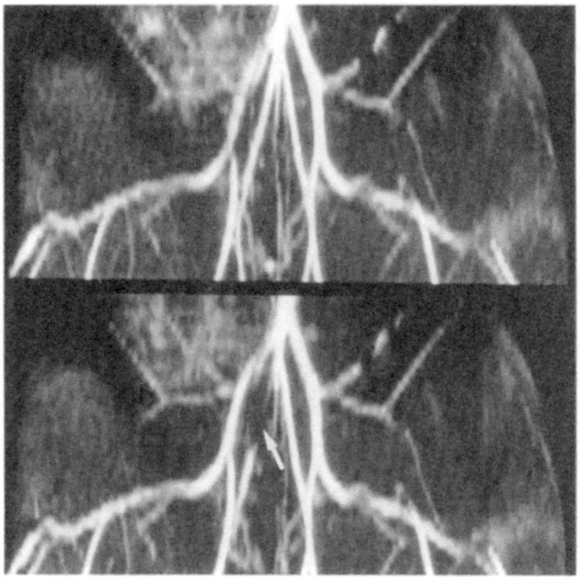

Fig. 33.14. Coronal reprojections of axially acquired MRA TOF images (TR 33/TE 8) of the pelvis of a pig. Based on an MRA roadmap image (Fig. 4c) a PTA catheter was placed into the right sacral artery. MRAs were acquired before (*top*) and during (*bottom*) balloon inflation. The balloon inflation causes a signal void in the right sacral artery (*arrow*)

Transjugular intrahepatic puncture of the portal system was possible in both animals. The entire procedure lasted 90 min. Based on the MIP roadmaps acquired in both the axial and the coronal plane, the parenchymal puncture was in effect guided in real time from the middle hepatic vein into the right portal vein (Fig. 33.17). Five puncture attempts were required in the first experiment, eight in the second. Tracking remained robust as the puncture unit consisting of the needle and tracking catheter was maneuvered from the hepatic vein into the portal vein. Once the introducer sheath was advanced over the catheter into the portal system, it was possible to probe the portal venous system with the 5-F tracking catheter.

33.5.4
MR Tracking of Guidewire-Catheter Composition

In order to perform any vascular intervention, both catheters and guidewires need to be visible to the interventionist. An MR-tracking guidewire with an outer diameter of 0.75 mm, compatible with a standard 5-F catheter was evaluated in a glass phantom with three paired branches of different sizes (2, 4, and 6 mm) and a 60° bifurcation simulating the abdominal aorta, its vessels, and the iliac bifurcation. On one side, the take-off angle of the branch vessels was 90°, on the other side, 129°. The phantom was connected to a pulsatile roller flow pump and contained water doped with 0.003 mol/l Gd-DTPA. Based upon TOF MIP roadmap images depicting the morphology of the phantom, various branches of the phantom were targeted. The guidewire-catheter composition was successfully manipulated into various branches of the phantom. These experiments demonstrate the ability to selectively navigate into branch vessels using the combination of a 5-F MR-tracking catheter and a 0.035-in. (0.89 mm) MR-tracking guidewire. The tracking signal of the guidewire was depicted as a narrow peak in the frequency spectrum. Signal-to-noise ratios ranged between 12 and 20, depending on the orientation of the guidewire within the main magnetic field. These experi-

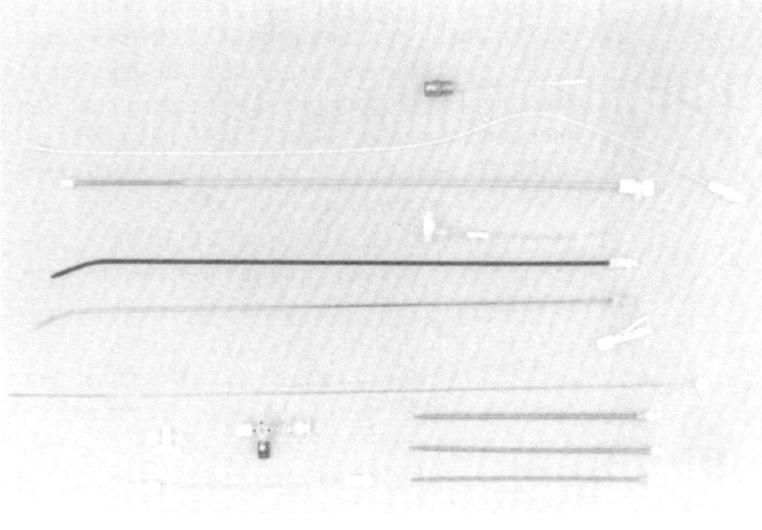

Fig. 33.15. The complete transjugular intrahepatic portosystemic shunt set is shown. To achieve MR compatibility, all metallic components were replaced by hard plastics

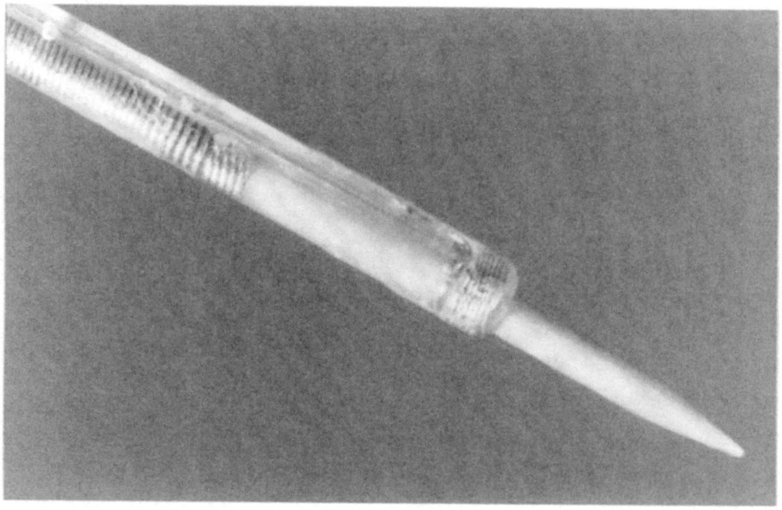

Fig. 33.16. A small RF coil is integrated in the catheter tip enclosing the puncture needle

ments demonstrated the ability to actively track two devices simultaneously, accomplished by attaching the coils within each device to separate receivers.

The guidewire-catheter composition was also assessed in an in vivo experiment, conducted on a fully anesthetized pig in the usual manner. Via a left carotid access both an MR-tracking catheter and an MR-tracking guidewire were inserted into the descending aorta. Based on coronal and sagittal TOF MIP roadmaps, the combined guidewire-catheter composition was maneuvered through the thoracic and abdominal aorta into the superior mesenteric artery as well as both renal arteries, with ease (Fig. 33.18). Tracking of both the catheter tip and the guidewire tip remained robust in the presence of pulsatile flow throughout the in vivo experiment. MR tracking of the guidewire was possible inside and outside the catheter. The relationship of the catheter tip to the guidewire tip was visible at all times. Even superimposition of the two receive coils did not result in any interruption of the tracking process.

33.6 Discussion

The experiments described here demonstrate that robust MR tracking and precise positioning of cathe-

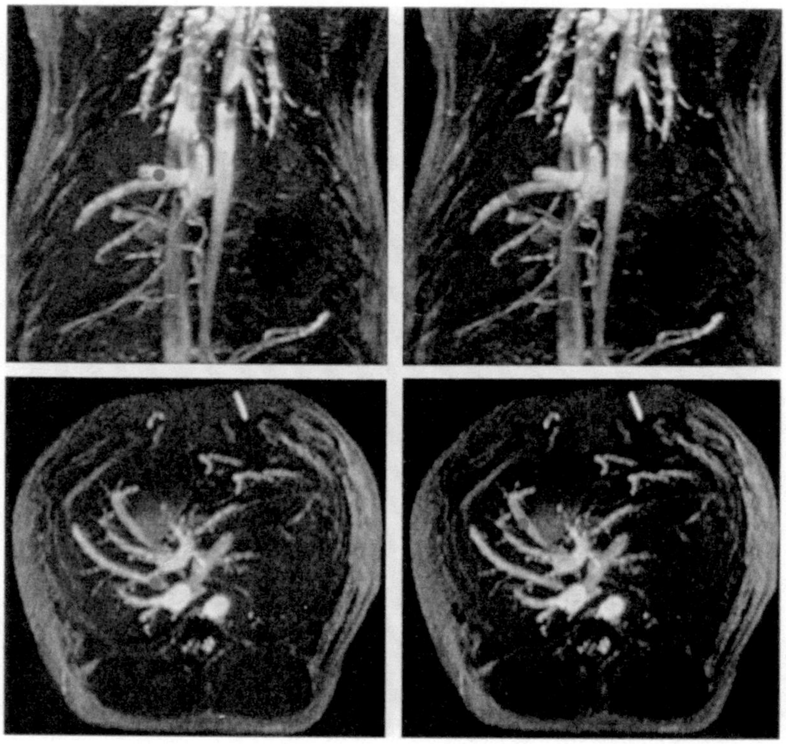

Fig. 33.17. Based on the roadmap MR angiograms acquired in the axial (*top*) and coronal (*bottom*) planes, the parenchymal transhepatic puncture was in effect guided in real time from the middle hepatic vein (*left*) into the right portal vein (*right*)

ters and guidewires equipped with small RF coils at their tip can be achieved under in vivo conditions on standard as well as "open configuration" MR-scanning systems. The high precision of the MR-tracking technique with regard to positional accuracy was documented in phantom experiments (Leung et al. 1995ab). The linear regression analyses of positional data obtained by X-ray fluoroscopy and MR tracking revealed that accurate device placement was possible over a distance of 40 cm. This is an important observation, since, in analogy to conventional fluoroscopy, a large FOV is necessary to monitor interventional procedures with MR imaging.

The accuracy and robustness of MR-tracking positioning is ultimately determined by the signal-to-noise ratio (SNR) of the detected MR signal. Maximizing SNR enhances accuracy and tracking reliability. To eliminate background noise that might impede robust tracking, a fully shielded coaxial cable must be used to transmit the signal from the coil to the catheter base (Leung et al. 1995b). Based on in vitro data, which documented a linear relationship between the height of the MR-tracking signal peak and the number of coil turns (Leung et al. 1995b), the miniaturized receiver coils integrated in the tip of the intravascular devices were constructed with 8 and 16 turns. In addition to the number of turns, signal amplitude is dependent on the diameter of the coil. While coils mounted in the tip of 5-F catheters could be constructed with a diameter of 1.1 mm, coils mounted in the tip of guidewires required significantly smaller diameters in order to fit through the standard 0.035-in. (0.89 mm) lumen of a 5-F catheter. Despite the miniaturized coil design with a diameter of only 0.6 mm, robust MR tracking of guidewires was indeed possible. This success is a reflection of the coil design. It allowed blood to flow through the coil lumen, thereby providing signal-rich spins within the most sensitive region of the coil. For this purpose, the guidewire needed to be open at the tip. Signal could further be augmented by filling the solenoid lumen of the coil with a solution doped with paramagnetic contrast agent. The shorter T1 of such a contrast solution would make even more signal available for tracking. In view of the additional manufacturing complexity, this approach was not implemented in the current set of experiments. It is likely, however, that such an approach would permit the use of even smaller diameter coils, making even smaller vessels accessible with MR-tracking techniques.

There are several unique characteristics of the MR-based active tracking technique. The technique is virtually independent of device orientation and provides maximal flexibility with regard to the characteristics of the underlying MR image on which MR tracking is based. A position update of 18 updates per second with a display delay of under 10 ms ensures real-time tracking of the instrument (Leung et al. 1995a, 1995b). A great advantage, compared with passive visualization, lies in the electronic availability of the position of the interventional device, in this case the catheter or guidewire. It can therefore be used to automatically control image acquisition at a location corresponding to the updated position of the coil. Another characteristic inherent in MR imaging is that the position of the coil can be determined in any desired plane. With biplanar display implementation, it is possible to track any instrument in real time simultaneously in any two planes (Leung et al. 1995a). Thus, the catheter position could be continuously tracked on a coronal or sagittal roadmap image while its progress was monitored on serially updated axial images traversing the tip of the catheter. This feature was found to be particularly helpful in cannulating the renal arteries.

The concept of active tracking has been extended to the guidance of up to four devices. The availability of active multi-device MR tracking must be considered a significant step toward the clinical realization of interventional MRA. Considerable challenges,

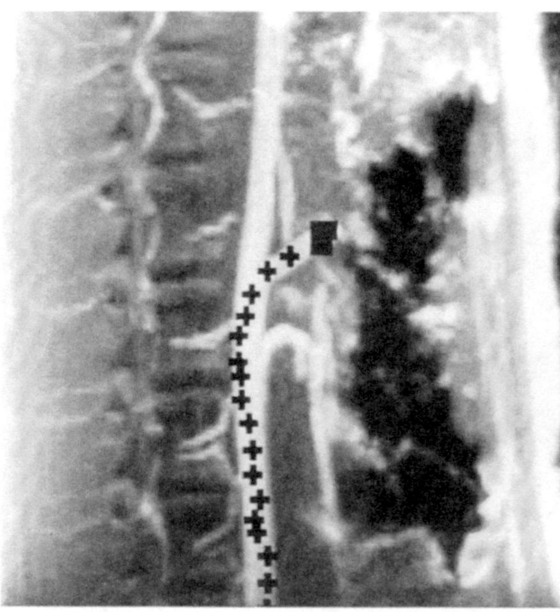

Fig. 33.18. Tracking of both the catheter tip and the guidewire tip (combined guidewire-catheter composition) in the in vivo experiment based on a sagittal TOF maximum intensity projection roadmap. The tip of the catheter has been placed in the superior mesenteric artery. While the catheter was left in position, the guidewire was slowly withdrawn

however, still need to be overcome. Visualization of the guidewire and possibly also the catheter must extend beyond the mere tip. This could be accomplished by implementing multiple coils or integrating other active device visualization techniques, as described elsewhere (LADD et al. 1997), as well as in Chapter 9.

Based on active, biplanar MR tracking, three separate intravascular procedures were successfully performed (WILDERMUTH et al. 1997a). Arterial and venous vessels in abdomen and pelvis were selectively cannulated with specially manufactured MR-tracking catheters. The course of the catheter tips was monitored in real time simultaneously in two planes, permitting active steering into the vessels of interest. Catheters were successfully steered even into small vessels, as illustrated by the balloon occlusion of the right sacral artery. The ability to track catheters was not confined to vessels, as shown by the transhepatic puncture of the portal system. MR tracking permitted active monitoring of the puncture needle, enclosed by the tracking catheter, as it was advanced through the hepatic parenchyma into the portal vein. The availability of both vascular and parenchymal information was shown to be useful in assessing the extent of embolization of the right kidney.

MR-tracking catheters were designed to emulate the characteristics of catheters currently available for fluoroscopically guided interventions. The MR catheters were found to be quite maneuverable, negotiating tight turns as dictated by unusually angled vascular origins, particularly of the renal arteries.

Tracking of the catheters was possible on the MR angiographic TOF roadmap images. Their acquisition remains time consuming. Similar to angiographic roadmap techniques, the tracking process on roadmap images is sensitive to patient motion. Motion should thus be avoided if at all possible. Once motion does occur, the roadmap image needs to be updated or at least modified to avoid localization errors. In the fully anesthetized and relaxed animals used for the presented experiments, motion was less of a problem. The development of ultrafast imaging techniques (MANSFIELD 1977; WETTER et al. 1995) will reduce the time required to update such roadmaps. In addition, cyclical motion, such as breathing, could be compensated for by the use of "navigator sequences" (PELC et al. 1991b; HAUSMANN et al. 1991), obviating the need for the acquisition of a totally new roadmap image. The spatial tracking coordinates of the instrument's tip could be displayed on the roadmap image relative to the concurrent position of the diaphragm. The latter would be continuously updated in real time by means of the navigator sequence. Up to the implementation of these techniques in an interventional MRA environment, however, the motion-related need for time-consuming roadmap updates will remain a significant hurdle.

Despite these limitations, intravascular interventions were possible with MR-tracking catheters. The in vivo embolization of a kidney by means of an MR-guided 5-F embolization catheter is well demonstrated on the dynamic contrast-enhanced FMPSPGR images. Beyond documenting the intervention's feasibility, the experiment also demonstrates the flexibility of MRI with regard to imaging characteristics. While the tracking was guided on roadmap images sensitive to flowing spins, the embolization results were documented on images sensitive to changes in T1 relaxation times induced by the application of paramagnetic contrast agent.

The functionality of balloon inflation was demonstrated by occlusion of a sacral artery. The vessel was occluded over the length of the balloon. Collaterals filled the vessel distal to the occlusion. The experiment demonstrates the ability to place the balloon in a predefined vascular segment.

The transhepatic puncture of the portal system from the hepatic vein represents the most critical step in the placement of a transjugular intrahepatic portosystemic shunt (TIPS; SKEENS et al. 1995; ROIZENTAL et al. 1995). While ultrasound can provide some guidance, the puncture is generally performed with the interventionist more or less blind to the exact position of the portal vein. This can result in suboptimal positioning of the shunt, leaving the shunt subject to early stenosis and even occlusion (SKEENS et al. 1995; ROIZENTAL et al. 1995). With MRA, the perihepatic vascular anatomy is easily displayed in any desired plane. Based on these images, the puncture could be accurately targeted and monitored in real time with MR tracking. By bridging the blind spot between hepatic and portal vein, the procedure is greatly facilitated. The real-time monitoring ability in two planes, allowed for the interactive correction of the needle's course. Still, multiple puncture attempts were necessary. In large part this was due to the restricted maneuverability of the interventionist. This experiment must be considered only a small first step toward MR-guided TIPS placement. The ability to guide the transhepatic puncture in real time in two planes simultaneously does, however, emphasize a potential advantage of MR guidance over conventional techniques: motion of the instrument can be tracked outside the vascular confines on images displaying the vascular anatomy without the need to repeatedly administer contrast agent.

The concept of interventional MRA can be further enhanced by the application of intravascular receiver coils for high-resolution imaging of blood vessels. The ensuing chapter (Chap. 34) will shed some light on the potential of such techniques. Together with conventional MRA and non-invasive flow quantitation, the possibilities of MR tracking of catheters and guidewires outlined in this chapter constitute a fascinating, integrative MR-based approach to intravascular interventions.

References

Ackerman JL, Offut MC, Buxton RB, Brady TJ (1986) Rapid 3D tracking of small RF coils. (abstract) Proceedings of the Society of Magnetic Resonance in Medicine, Berkeley, Calif., p 1131

Davis CP, Ladd M, Romanowski B, Wildermuth S, Knoplioch J, Debatin JF (1996) Human aorta: preliminary results with virtual endoscopy based on three-dimensional MR imaging data sets. Radiology 199:37–40

Dumoulin CL, Souza SP, Darrow RD, Pelc NJ, Adams WJ, Ash SA (1991) Simultaneous acquisition of phase contrast angiograms and stationary tissue images with Hadamard encoding of flow-induced phase shifts. J Magn Reson Imaging 1:399–404

Dumoulin CL, Souza SP, Darrow RD (1993) Real-time position monitoring of invasive devices using magnetic resonance. Magn Reson Med 29:411–415

Edelmann RR (1993) MR angiography: present and future. AJR Am J Roentgenol 161:1–11

Hany TF, Debatin JF, Pfammatter T, Leung DA - 1977: 3D MRA of the Pelvic and Renal Arteries: Comparison with Conventional Angiography. Radiology; 204:357–362

Hausmann R, Lewin JS, Laub G (1991) Phase-contrast MR angiography with reduced acquisition time: new concepts in sequence design. J Magn Reson Imaging 1:415–422

Holland GA, Dougherty L, Carpenter JP, Axel L (1996) Breath-hold ultrafast three-dimensional gadolinium-enhanced MR angiography of the aorta and the renal and other visceral abdominal arteries. AJR Am J Roentgenol 166:971–981

Ladd ME, Erhart P, Debatin JF, Hofmann E, Boesiger P, von Schulthess GK, McKinnon GC (1997) Guide wire antennas for MR fluoroscopy. Magn Reson Med (in press)

Leung DA, Debatin JF, Wildermuth S et al (1995a) Real-time biplanar needle tracking for interventional MR imaging procedures. Radiology 197:485–488

Leung DA, Debatin JF, Wildermuth S et al (1995b) Intravascular MR-tracking catheter: Preliminary experimental evaluation. AJR Am J Roentgenol 164:1265–1270

Leung DA, McKinnon GC, Davis CP, Pfammatter T, Krestin GP, Debatin JF (1996) Breath-hold, contrast-enhanced, three-dimensional MR angiography. Radiology 201:569–571

Lufkin RB, Teresi L, Hanafee WN (1987) New needle for MR-guided aspiration cytology of the head and neck. AJR Am J Roentgenol 149:380–382

Mansfield P (1977) Multiplanar image formation using NMR spin-echoes. J Phys Chem 10:L55–L58

Pelc NJ, Herfkens RJ, Shimakawa A, Enzmann DR (1991a) Phase contrast cine magnetic resonance imaging. Magn Reson Q. 7:229–254

Pelc NJ, Bernstein MA, Shimakawa A, Glover GH (1991b) Encoding strategies for three-direction phase-contrast MR imaging of flow. J Magn Reson Imaging 1:405–413

Prince MR, Yucel EK, Kaufman JA, Harrison DC, Geller SC (1993) Dynamic gadolinium-enhanced three-dimensional abdominal MR angiography. J Magn Reson Imaging 3:877–881

Prince MR, Narasimham DL, Stanley JC, Chenevert TL, Williams DM, Marx MV, Cho KJ (1995) Breath-hold gadolinium-enhanced MR angiography of the abdominal aorta and its major branches. Radiology 197:785–792

Roizental M, Kane RA, Takahashi J, et al (1995) Portal vein: US-guided localization prior to transjugular intrahepatic portosystemic shunt placement. Radiology 196:868–870

Skeens J, Semba C, Dake M (1995) Transjugular intrahepatic portosystemic shunts. Annu Rev Med 46:95–102

Snidow JJ, Aisen AM, Harris VJ, Trerotola SO, Johnson MS, Sawchuk AP, Dalsing MC (1995) Iliac artery MR angiography: comparison of three-dimensional gadolinium-enhanced and two-dimensional time-of-flight techniques. Radiology 196:371–378

Snidow JJ, Johnson MS, Harris VJ, Trerotola SO (1996) Three-dimensional gadolinium-enhanced MR angiography for aortoiliac inflow assessment plus renal artery screening in a single breath hold. Radiology 198:725–732

Wetter DR, McKinnon GC, Debatin JF, von Schulthess GK (1995) Cardiac echo-planar MR imaging: comparison of single- and multiple-shot techniques. Radiology 194: 765–770

Wildermuth S, Debatin JF, Leung DA, Dumoulin CE, Darrow R, Uhlschmidt U, von Schulthess GK (1997a) MR-guided intravascular prodedures: initial demonstration in a pig model. Radiology 202:578–583

Wildermuth S, Dumoulin CL, Pfammatter T et al (1997) MR guided angioplasty: assessment of tracking safety, catheter handling and functionality. Cardiovasc Intervent Radiol (in press)

34 Intravascular MRI

G.G. Zimmermann, H.H. Quick, G K. von Schulthess, and J.F. Debatin

CONTENTS

34.1 Introduction

Although atherosclerotic disease is the leading cause of death in economically developed countries, its evolution, risk manifestations and inconsistent response to therapy remain poorly understood. Atherosclerotic plaque is believed to originate with the incorporation of fatty streaks into the vessel's intima, and later evolves to appear typically as a fibrous cap overlying a central region of necrosis within the vascular wall (Small 1988). The variation in the structure of plaque, which is composed of fat, fibrous tissue and calcification, is wide (Gotlieb and Havenith 1991; Ross 1993). There is mounting evidence that the make-up of an individual plaque represents an important determinant of the clinical risks associated with it, as well as of its response to therapy (Davies and Woolf 1993; Falk 1985; Forrester et al. 1991; Fuster et al. 1992).

To date, conventional X-ray angiography has been the primary means for detecting and characterising atherosclerotic disease. The technique renders a luminogram of the vessel under consideration. It provides no direct data about the vascular wall itself. Plaque structure and even wall thickness remain unexplored. This limitation has motivated the evaluation of other techniques, the most promising of which is high-frequency intravascular ultrasound (Di Mario et al. 1992). The enthusiasm for this technique has been dampened by the high cost of intravascular ultrasound wires and the inability of sound waves to penetrate calcific plaque.

Recently, the potential of CT and MR angiography to evaluate vascular morphology has been investigated (Dumoulin and Hart 1986; Prince et al. 1993; Rubin et al. 1993). Both cross-sectional imaging techniques are less invasive than conventional angiography and can also provide data about vascular walls. While vessel wall thickness can be determined with both cross-sectional imaging techniques, the superior contrast resolution inherent in the MR experiment favours MR imaging for characterisation of plaque structure (Boos et al. 1996). Despite considerable efforts, signal-to-noise (SNR) limitations associated with external surface coils cannot provide the spatial resolution necessary to resolve vascular wall structure. Higher spatial resolution can be achieved with intravascular receiver probes (Hurst et al. 1992; Martin et al. 1992; Ocali and Atalar 1997; Zimmermann et al. 1997a, 1997b). Their clinical application has been limited to date by lack of patient access and the inability to monitor the probes' position in an MR environment.

The availability of "open-configuration" MR systems now permits direct access to the patient while imaging is ongoing. In addition, MR-based instrument guidance systems (MR Tracking) have been developed. These allow real time visualisation of catheter tips (Dumoulin et al. 1993) relative to

G.G. Zimmermann, MD, Institute of Diagnostic Radiology, University Hospital Zurich, Rämistrasse 100, CH-8901 Zurich, Switherland
H.H. Quick, MS, Institute of Diagnostic Radiology, University Hospital Zurich, Rämistrasse 100, CH-8091 Zurich, Switzerland
G.K. von Schulthess, MD, PhD, Division of Nuclear Medicine, Zurich University Hospital, Rämistrasse 100, CH-8091 Zurich, Switzerland
J.F. Debatin, MD, Institute of Diagnostic Radiology, University Hospital Zurich, Rämistrasse 100, CH-8091 Zurich, Switzerland

surrounding structures in two planes simultaneously (LADD et al. 1996; LEUNG et al. 1995). These systems have transformed the concept of clinically relevant in vivo intravascular MR imaging from a hypothetical consideration to a practical possibility.

34.2 Catheter Design

34.2.1 Theoretical Basis

The concept of intravascular MR imaging has been explored for some time now (HURST et al. 1992; MARTIN et al. 1992; KANDARPA et al. 1993; ATALAR et al. 1996). For an intravascular MR-imaging concept to succeed, the design of the imaging coils needs to fulfil various safety and image quality requirements.

High spatial resolution imaging of blood vessels requires coil designs which provide high SNR to compensate for the small voxel dimensions required to resolve the vascular walls. By placing the coil in an internal cavity a high SNR can be achieved in voxels located adjacent to the coil. Since the tissue to be imaged is external to the receiver coil, an "inside-out" variation of a surface or local coil must be considered. The local sensitivity profile of such coils can be considered an advantage, since it facilitates the use of small field of view (FOVs) necessary for high resolution imaging without the drawback of image aliasing.

Other desirable properties of such coils include (MARTIN et al. 1992): (a) minimized radial sensitivity falloff to the coil to improve the penetration depth, (b) homogeneous response to radially equidistant objects, (c) homogeneous response to axially equidistant objects and (d) insensitivity to the orientation of the coil with respect to the main magnetic field B_0. For in vivo use, features like the suppression of flow artefacts, a small diameter of the receiver coil system and a non-rigid, flexible catheter-based design for easy insertion into small vessels have to be considered essential prerequisites.

A large number of inside-out coil designs have been evaluated with varying degrees of success (HURST et al. 1992; MCDONALD et al. 1993). These include loops, "birdcage", "multipole", "center return" and opposed solenoid coils (Fig. 34.1). Recently a new loopless antenna has also been introduced by OCALI and ATALAR (1997).

The center return designs consist of a cylindrical array of coil windings with current flowing in one direction along the central axis of the cylinder. Numerous evenly spaced return lines, running parallel to the axis of the cylinder, lie on the outer surface of the coil. This type of coil geometry is limited by a

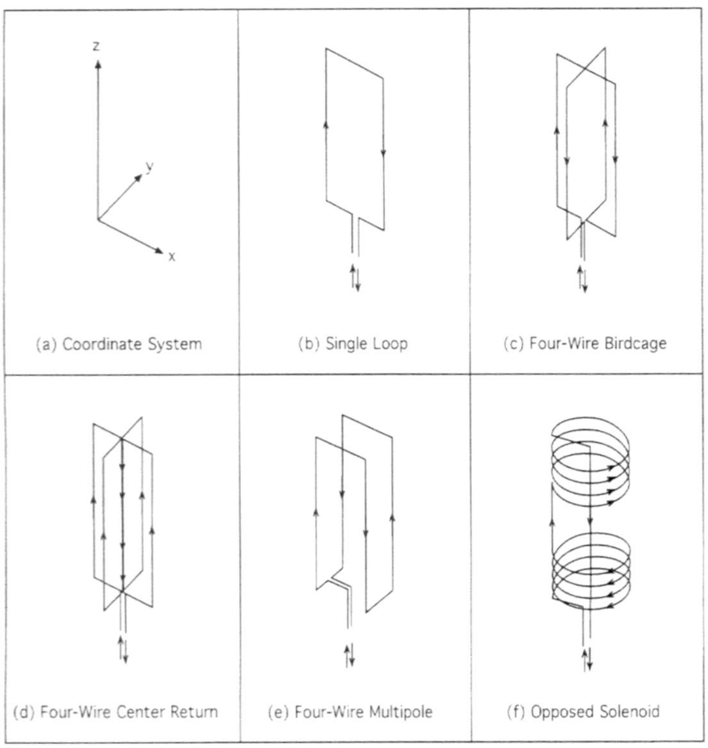

Fig. 34.1a-f. Different "inside-out" coil designs for intravascular imaging. The z axis represents the direction of the main magnetic field B_0. Conductor patterns are shown schematically. Arrows indicate the current direction

rapid radial sensitivity falloff and regions of zero sensitivity external to the coil. The birdcage designs have a geometry similar to that of the center return design. Here, the current winds up and down at evenly spaced intervals on the outer surface of the cylinder. Both coil designs provide a reasonably homogeneous response to axially equidistant objects. This is needed for the acquisition of contiguous slices or for the acquisition of 3D data sets. Their sensitivity to radially equidistant objects, on the other hand, is characterised by great disparity in the vicinity of the coil. While increasing the number of conductors in these configurations enhances angular homogeneity, there is also more rapid radial falloff (Hurst et al. 1992).

The following paragraphs provide a short overview over some of the coil designs that have been developed and tested for in vitro and in vivo intravascular applications up to now.

34.2.2 Opposed Solenoid Coils

Initial assessments favoured opposed solenoid coils reflecting their superior in-plane signal homogeneity and penetration depth (Hurst et al. 1992; Martin et al. 1992). The design of the opposed solenoid coils is based on two solenoids, separated by a gap, whose field lines are in opposition to one another. The region between the two solenoids experiences a large flux extrusion and, therefore, achieves high sensitivity to regions external to the coil. Because of this geometry the coil is physically decoupled during externally applied radiofrequency (RF) pulses. Although the opposed solenoid design provides excellent axial homogeneity, its longitudinal homogeneity is relatively poor. While this is sufficient for the acquisition of a defined single slice, it does not permit the collection of contiguous slices. Another disadvantage is that the high homogeneity region between the solenoids is much lower in absolute sensitivity than regions nearer to the ends of the solenoids.

This coil type was used with some success in phantom and animal experiments (Hurst et al. 1992; Martin et al. 1992; Martin and Henkelmann 1994). Image quality in in vivo experiments was significantly reduced, reflecting trembling motion of the coil in the pulsatile blood stream. As a consequence the opposed solenoid coil was equipped with a "bullet tip" at the distal end to keep the coil stable in the middle of the vessel. Further modifications aimed at stabilising the coil within the vessel of interest resulted in a relatively large and rigid device, virtually impossible to introduce into a patient. Even with these modifications, the opposed solenoid coil design remained highly sensitive to motion and flow effects, compromising image quality.

34.2.3 Loopless Catheter Antenna

To overcome the disadvantages of mechanically rigid designs and the lack of longitudinal coverage of most coil geometries, Atalar et al. (1996) presented an alternative catheter coil design. Their coil was formed by short-circuiting one end of a two-conductor transmission line, which allows for a smaller coil size, enlarged longitudinal coverage, and greater flexibility compared with previous designs. The loopless catheter antenna was tested on various phantoms, animals and isolated human aortas. The signal received by these catheter coils was small compared with conventional coil designs resulting in a poor penetration depth.

Ocali and Atalar (1997) recently modified this catheter probe design. They presented a loopless catheter antenna designed to overcome the limitations in physical dimensions and electromagnetic properties inherent in catheter coils with loops. The catheter antenna is essentially a dipole, which makes a very narrow diameter possible. A piece of conducting wire serves as one of the poles. The second pole is constructed over the outer surface of a thin coaxial cable that carries the MR signal to the matching, tuning and decoupling circuit. The whole dipole antenna and part of the coaxial cable are inserted into the blood vessels. The signal power acquired by this antenna is very high, which allows the tuning and matching circuits to be placed outside the blood vessels.

Both the transmission line concept and the loopless catheter antenna show a comparable axial signal intensity profile. They provide an extremely high SNR in their immediate vicinity which shows a strong falloff in the radial direction. With regard to penetration depth the loopless antenna is superior to the catheter coil (Ocali and Atalar 1997). The homogeneity to radially equidistant objects is enhanced compared with loop coils, birdcages, multipoles, and centre returns, whose conductors have an inherently greater distance to one another.

These catheter probe designs, characterised by good longitudinal coverage, flexibility and a small diameter, do indeed appear suitable for in vivo use. A detailed examination of their suitability for such applications and their sensitivity to flow artefacts, however, remain outstanding at this time.

34.2.4 Balloon-Mounted Single Loop Receiver Coil

As the concept of intravascular MRI is transferred from an in vitro to an in vivo environment, suppression of motion artifacts caused by the presence of pulsatile flow within the vessel under consideration emerges as the central challenge (Hurst et al. 1992). Motion artefacts are caused by surrounding flowing blood, as well as the propagation of pulsatility through the arterial vascular system. Various mechanical concepts have been explored to compensate for these undesired effects, including the introduction of a "bullet-tip" designed to stabilize the coil in the vessel (Martin and Henkelmann 1994). A more promising concept is based on the integration of an intravascular single loop copper wire coil into a balloon catheter (Erhart et al. 1996) (Fig. 34.2). The latter has recently been successfully evaluated both in vitro and in vivo in animal experiments (Zimmermann et al. 1997b).

The design of this intravascular imaging catheter is based on a standard 5-F (1.67 mm) balloon catheter (Schneider, Bülach, Switzerland) with an inflatable balloon of 40-mm length and different diameters (4, 6 or 8 mm). A receive-only coil, consisting of a single loop copper wire 40 mm in length, is mounted longitudinally on the surface of the balloon. To protect the coil and isolate the non-biocompatible copper from the vessel, the wire is covered by a second balloon. A fully insulated coaxial cable was employed to conduct the MR signal from the tip to the base of the catheter (110 cm). Owing to the spatial constraints of the catheter, all coil tuning and matching was performed remotely.

The inflatable balloon allows optimisation (as large as possible) of the coil diameter in different vessel lumen sizes to achieve maximal SNR. The direct contact of the receiver coil to the vessel wall optimises the local SNR. In this manner the highest sensitivity region of the coil is employed for analysis of the vessel wall. The availability of different balloon sizes (4–8 mm) further augments the adaptability of this technique. In the deflated state the flexible coil can be easily manoeuvred through the vascular tree. Owing to the basic design of a 5-F balloon catheter a 0.035-in. (0.89 mm) lumen is available to combine the system with a guidewire (Ladd et al. 1996). In vitro as well as in vivo experiments have demonstrated the concept of a balloon-mounted receiver coil to be capable of overcoming many previously existing limitations related to the presence of motion artefacts.

34.3 In Vitro Intravascular MRI with a Balloon-Mounted Single Loop Receiver Coil

34.3.1 Experimental Set-Up

In an in vitro phantom study, we evaluated the balloon-mounted single loop receive coil design (Fig. 34.2). The evaluation was performed on 12 harvested ex vivo human femoral artery segments excised during autopsy from patients aged between 52 and 84 years. The degree of vascular pathology ranged

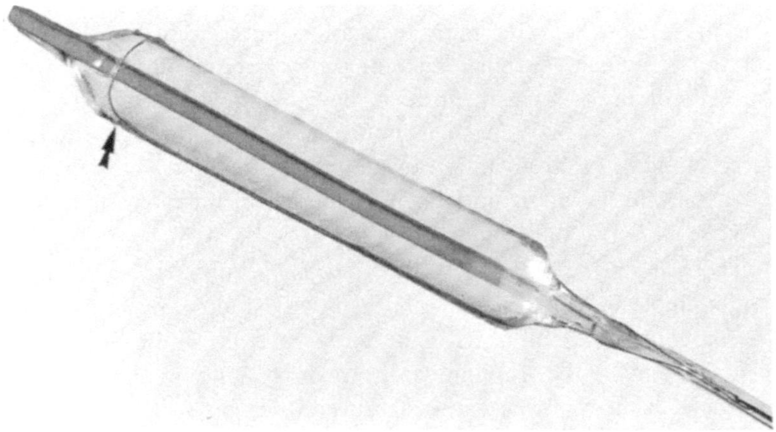

Fig. 34.2. Catheter design of a single loop copper wire (*arrow*) mounted on an inflatable balloon catheter

from mild atherosclerosis with mere intimal thickening to severe atherosclerotic disease with complicated plaques occupying up to 75% of the true luminal diameter. The experimental set-up simulated in vivo flow conditions by integrating the vessel into a closed tubing circuit driven by a pulsatile roller flow pump. For imaging, the balloon was inflated with water to a pressure of 2 atm. At this pressure the balloon filled the vascular lumen, thereby occluding it. Circulation was maintained by activation of a high-pressure bypass contained within the circuit.

For MR imaging, the phantom was placed in the centre of the gantry. To ensure positional identity of MR and subsequent histological sectioning, a thread was attached to the vessel segment positioned at the centre of the MR acquisition volume. Six specimens were imaged in a conventional 1.5-T MR system (Signa EchoSpeed, General Electric Medical Systems, Milwaukee, Wis.) and six other specimens in an open-configuration "interventional" 0.5-T MR system (Signa SP, General Electric Medical Systems, Milwaukee, Wis.). In both systems, identical sequences were used for intravascular imaging:

1. T1-weighted spin-echo (TR 5000/TE 25, bandwidth 5.82 kHz, 6×4 cm FOV, number of excitations (NEX) 4, 4-mm section thickness)
2. T2-weighted fast spin-echo (TR 5000/TE 104, bandwith 5.82 kHz, 6×4 cm FOV, 4 NEX, 4-mm section thickness).

In the 0.5-T system a 256×224 matrix rendered an in-plane resolution of 234×178 mm. Exploiting the higher SNR inherent in a 1.5-T system, a 512×384 matrix was employed, resulting in an in-plane resolution of 117×104 mm. Ten contiguous sections were acquired with each sequence. Only the most central three sections were analysed.

Wall thickness and plaque area were measured in each of the three central 4-mm MR sections. In each image the thickness was measured at two sites. The relation of the measurement sites to the fatty marker along the side of the vessel was marked to assure correlation with histological analysis. Plaque area was measured by tracing its contours and quantitating the surrounded area. The inner demarcation of the plaque was defined by the lumen of the vessel; the outer lineation by the signal-intense media.

The plaque structure was analysed by plotting the signal intensities along a straight line traversing the plaque. For comparison with histological sectioning, the line plot was placed in a sagittal plane through the plaque, originating in a pre-defined position relative to the fatty marker. The signal intensities along the plaque were recorded for every other pixel. Based upon pixel size, the different pixel values were directly correlated with findings at histological sectioning. Separate analysis was performed for the six specimens imaged at 1.5-T and 0.5-T. Mean values and standard deviation of signal intensities for various plaque components were determined. Student's t-test was employed to assess for a statistical difference of pixel values associated with different plaque components.

Following MR imaging, the specimens were immediately fixed in 10% buffered formalin for at least 24 h. In cases of severe calcification the arterial segments were decalcified with acid before sectioning. Three sections, 4 mm in thickness, corresponding to the centre of the three analysed MRI sections were cut from the specimens, mounted on slides and embedded in paraffin. For subsequent histopathological evaluation the slides were stained with haematoxylin-eosin and elastic van Gieson stain.

Morphometric measurements of wall thickness and plaque area were performed on a planimeter (MOP-OM3, Kontron, Eiching, Germany). The plaque area was defined as the area between the lumen of the vessel and the internal elastic membrane seen best on the elastic van Gieson stain. Plaque structure analysis was provided by an experienced pathologist viewing the histological cross-sections independently along the pre-defined line traversing the plaque. Each analysed pixel location was characterised as corresponding to one of three plaque components: calcification, fibrous material and fat.

34.3.2 Results

Intravascular images were obtained from all 12 specimens. Despite the presence of pulsatile flow within the phantom, motion artefacts were not apparent. Figure 34.3 shows a representative cross-section of the femoral artery with the inflated balloon adjacent to the inner wall of the vessel in correlation with histological findings. Image resolution ranged from 117×104 mm at 1.5-T to 234×178 mm at 0.5-T. Resolution was sufficient to discriminate the vessel wall layers.

On T2-weighted FSE images the three different vessel wall layers – adventitia, media and thickened intima – could be discriminated. The intima was only visualised if it was thickened. T1-weighted

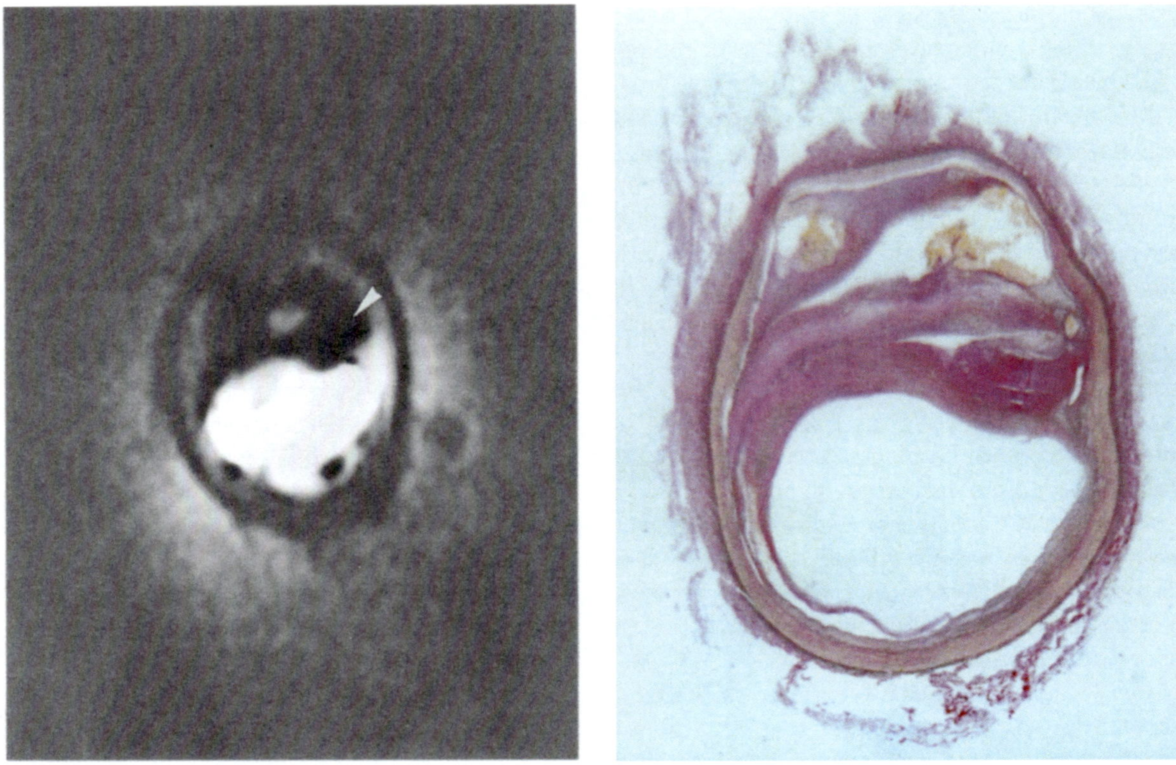

Fig. 34.3 In vitro image of an atherosclerotic femoral artery in comparison with **b** the histological appearance. Plaque structure including collagen, fat and calcification (*arrowhead*) can be identified on the MR image

images did not permit differentiation between the wall layers. Only calcified plaque was readily identified as an area of reduced signal. Wall thickness and plaque characterisation analysis was thus based on the T2-weighted images.

There was a good correlation of MR measurements and histological analysis of wall thickness with a correlation coefficient of 0.97 (Fig. 34.4a). There was some systematic overestimation of wall thickness with MRI, as evidenced by the mean thickness of 3.5 mm measured on MR images versus 2.8 mm at histology.

Demarcation of plaque from the vascular lumen filled by the balloon was possible in all cases. The media, demarcating the plaque against the vessel wall, was identified in all but one specimen. In that specific case, histology confirmed a severely diminished media and, therefore, the adventitia was used for plaque demarcation. Plaque area was systematically overestimated with MRI (mean 9.6 mm^2) compared with histological analysis (mean 7.2 mm^2). Here, too, there was an excellent correlation between the two measurements with $r = 0.98$ (Fig. 34.4b).

Plaque characterisation was possible based on T2-weighted images. There was less overlap on 0.5-T images than on 1.5-T images, reflecting the higher signal intensity of fibrous tissue at 1.5 T. The adventitia was seen as an outer ring of reduced signal intensity (385±112 at 0.5 T vs 134±78 at 1.5 T). The media was significantly brighter (2178±678 at 0.5 T vs 692±371 at 1.5 T). Calcified plaque was identified as areas of low signal intensity (134±98 at 0.5 T vs 38±27 at 1.5 T). The fibrous structures containing collagen showed much higher signal intensities with a mean of 1968±680 at 0.5 T compared to 783±542 at 1.5 T. Fat components were seen with a signal mean 762±394 at 0.5 T vs 321±214 at 1.5 T (Table 34.1).

Table 34.1. Differentiation of wall layers and pathological intima with calcification, collagen and fat on 0.5 and 1.5 Tesla numbers represent means ± standard devitation

Tesla	Adventitia	Media	Calcium	Collagen	Fat
0.5	385±112	2178±678	134±98	1968±680	762±394
1.5	134±78	692±371	38±27	783±542	321±214

34.4 In Vivo Intravascular MRI with a Balloon-Mounted Single Loop Receiver Coil

34.4.1 Experimental Set-Up

To prove the concept of intravascular imaging with a balloon-mounted receiver coil, in vivo experiments were performed in a pig model ($n = 4$) in full accordance with governmental regulations. With the animals under full anaesthesia, a 12-F introducer sheath was inserted over the left carotid artery into the descending aorta. Prior to insertion of the MR-imaging catheter conventional angiography was performed of the iliac arteries (Multiskop Siemens, Erlangen, Germany) by administering a 10-ml bolus of contrast material for each series through the indwelling aortic sheath. To assure correct placement of the MR-imaging catheter in the right common iliac artery a 0.035-in. (0.89 mm) MR-tracking guidewire system was used. Once the imaging catheter was positioned in the common iliac artery, the balloon was inflated with water spiked with paramagnetic contrast medium (Gd-DTPA, 2 mmol/l). The presence of the contrast medium in the balloon allowed confirmation of the correct placement.

Experiments were performed in a 0.5-T open-configuration interventional MR system (Signa SP, General Electric Medical Systems, Milwaukee, Wis.). T1-weighted images were acquired with a spin-echo sequence (TR 400/TE 12, FOV 6×4 cm, matrix 256×128, 6 NEX) over 5 min 12 s. T2-weighted images were collected with an FSE sequence employing a TR of 3000 and a TE of 108 ms (FOV 6×4 cm, matrix 256×128, 8 NEX). The imaging time amounted to 6 min 24 s. Images of the iliac arteries were acquired.

34.4.1.1 Model of atherosclerosis

To prove the sensitivity of the imaging coil regarding plaque structure analysis, in vivo experiments were performed using an animal model of atherosclerosis. Four Watanabe hereditary hyperlipidemic rabbits (WHHL) suffering from a low-density lipoprotein receptor defect and developing atherosclerotic lesions similar to humans, as well as two healthy New Zealand rabbits were fully anaesthetized after tracheotomy. A 4-F introducer sheath was placed via the left carotid artery into the aortic arch. Conventional angiography of the abdominal aorta and its branches was performed with bolus administration of 3 ml of iodinated contrast material for each series via the aortic sheath. Imaging results obtained with the WHHL rabbits were compared with those from the healthy New Zealand rabbits.

The animals were then transferred to the MRI suite where high resolution T1-weighted and T2-weighted images of the suprarenal aorta were acquired with an externally applied surface coil: T1 spin echo: TR 500/TE 12, FOV 12×12cm, matrix

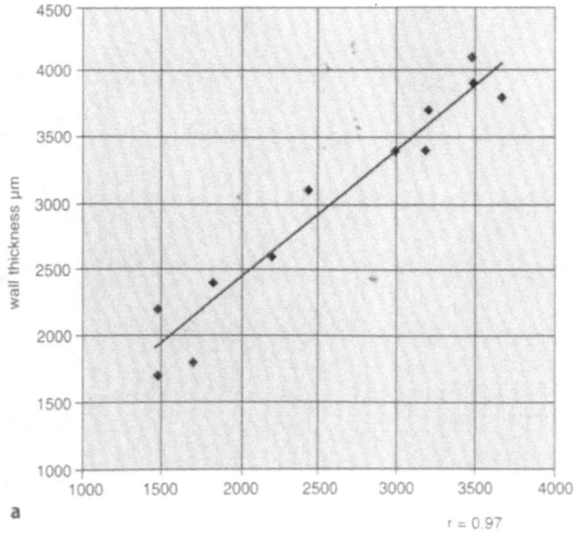

Fig. 34.4. Linear regression analysis correlating **a** wall thickness and **b** plaque area measurements based on histopathological analysis and MR images

512×256, 4 NEX, resulting in an imaging time of 8 min 36 s; T2 FSE TR 2000/TE 80, FOV 12×12 cm, matrix 512×256, 8 NEX, resulting in an imaging time of 8 min 36 s.

Subsequently, the intravascular MR-imaging catheter was surgically inserted via the right iliac artery into the suprarenal aorta. For signal transmission the body coil was used. T1-weighted SE images (TR 400/TE 20, FOV 2×1 cm, matrix 256×64, 8 NEX) were collected over 3 min 45 s followed by a 3 min 16 s acquisition of T2-weighted FSE images (TR 2000/TE 80, FOV 2×1 cm, matrix 256×64, 8 NEX).

Following sacrifice of the animals, the aorta including the iliac arteries was excised, fixed in 10% buffered formalin for at least 24 h and sectioned corresponding to the centre of the MRI sections in 4-mm thickness. Specimens were mounted on slides and embedded in paraffin. For subsequent histopathological evaluation the slides were stained with haematoxylin-eosin and elastic van Gieson stain. Wall thickness was measured using morphometry (MOP-OM3, Kontron, Eiching, Germany).

34.4.2 Results

Placement of the catheter in the right iliac artery through a trackable guidewire was expeditiously accomplished with MR tracking. The intravascular high resolution MR images of the common iliac artery vascular wall obtained under in vivo conditions were of high quality and free of motion artefacts. In one of the animals, conventional angiography revealed wall-adherent thrombus in the right iliac artery with concomitant occlusion of the contralateral iliac artery (Fig. 34.5a). The thrombus was visible on the high resolution images acquired with the intravascular catheter as an inhomogeneous ring of increased signal intensity (Fig. 34.5b). Macropathology confirmed it as representing mural thrombus (Fig. 34.5c).

34.4.2.1 *Model of Atherosclerosis*

In the atherosclerotic rabbit both conventional angiography and high resolution MR imaging with external and intravascular surface coils could be performed. The small diameter of the balloon in the collapsed state allowed easy insertion of the catheter into the fine iliac arteries of the rabbits.

Conventional angiography of atherosclerotic rabbits did not reveal any wall irregularities in the abdominal aorta (Fig. 34.6a). In fact, the appearance of the angiograms was indistinguishable from those obtained in the healthy rabbits. High resolution imaging with external surface coils, on the other hand, depicted excentric wall thickening in the aorta

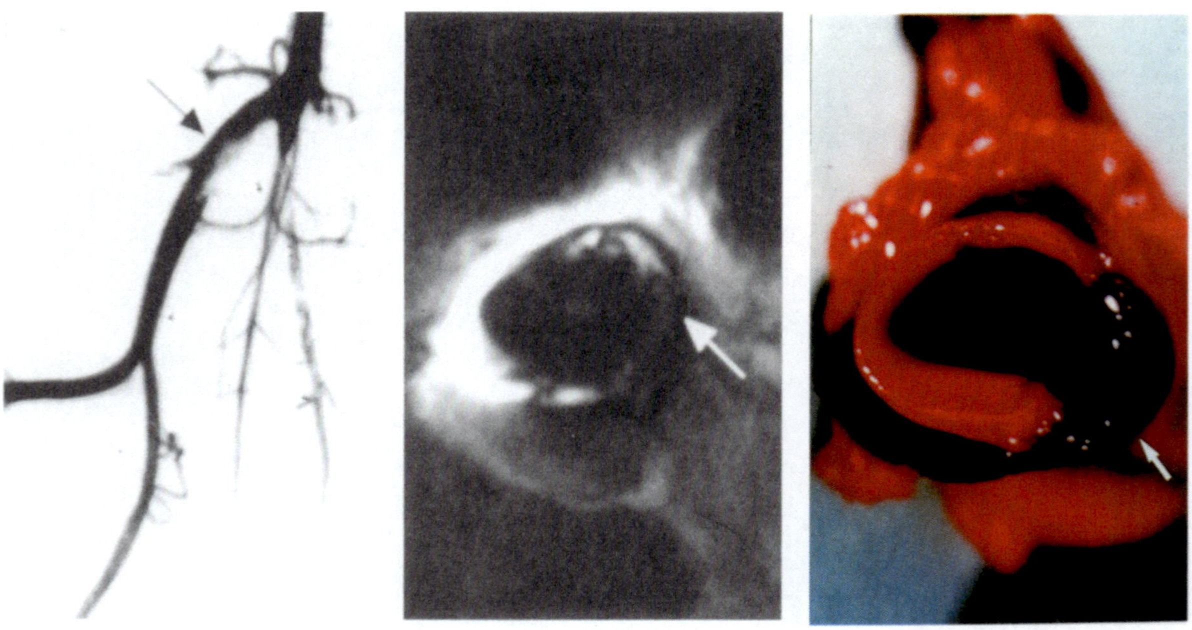

a, b c

Fig. 34.5a-c. MR guidance with the MR tracking technique permitted exact placement of the imaging catheter in the right common iliac artery of a pig. Wall-adherent thrombus (*arrow*), seen on **a** conventional angiography, is identifed as an inhomogeneous ring of increased signal intensity (*arrow*) on **b** the intravascular scan **c** Macropathology confirmed the presence of mural thrombus (*arrow*) of the atherosclerotic rabbits. Discrimination of plaque components or wall layers, however, was not possible (Fig. 34.6b). Based on a data acquisition time of 8-min 36 s a spatial resolution of 234×468 mm was achieved.

Atherosclerotic changes were well visualised on MR images acquired with the intravascular imaging catheter. Inflation of the balloon suppressed flow and pulsatility artefacts. Due to the reduced FOV, image resolution could be increased to 78×156 mm. Imaging and thus vessel occlusion times did not exceed 3 min 45 s. Intimal thickening and a calcified lesion in the case of a 4-year-old WHHL rabbit were depicted on the intravascular MR images (Fig. 34.6c). Intravascular MRI correlated well with histology (Fig. 34.6d). The calcified plaque, characterised by signal intensities of 123±83 was easily distinguished from areas of proliferated muscle and collagen fibres with signal intensities of 812±330.

34.5 Assessment of Intravascular MRI

Although percutaneous transluminal angioplasty (PTA) and stenting procedures have been in clinical use for many years, their effectiveness remains contested in at least some vascular territories. Restenosis rates of up to 30% (Bonelli et al. 1995) underscore the need for a more detailed analysis of the underlying pathomorphology and pathophysiology of atherosclerotic plaque formations. Although the

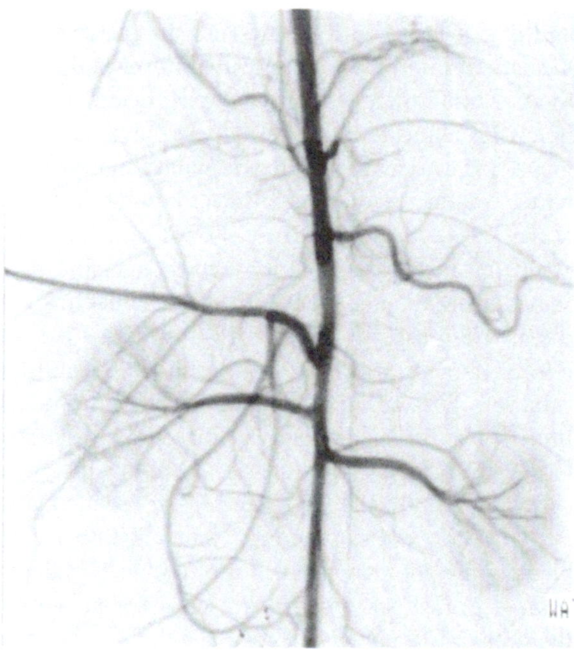

a

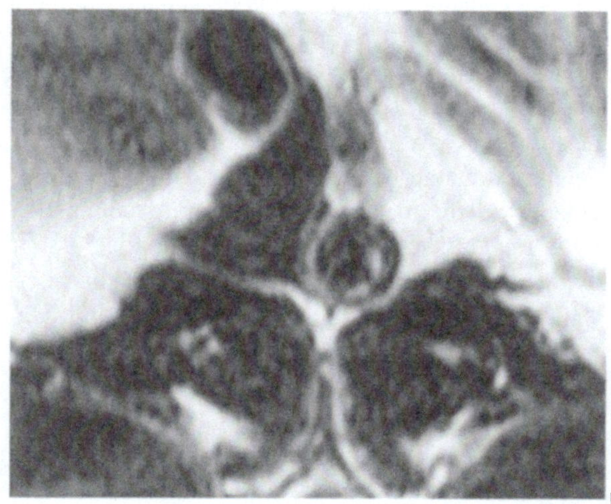

b

Fig. 34.6a Conventional angiography does not reveal any wall irregularities in the abdominal aorta of a 4-year-old atherosclerotic Watanabe hereditary hyperlipidemic rabbit. **b** While high resolution imaging with an external surface coil depicts excentric wall thickening, an analysis of plaque strucure is not possible. **c,d** On the intravascular images, the calcified plaque (*arrow*) is identified as an area of reduced signal intensity **c** correlating well with histological findings **d**

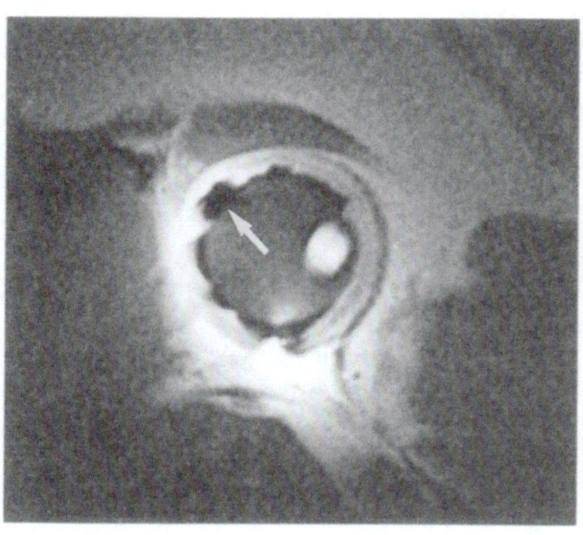

c

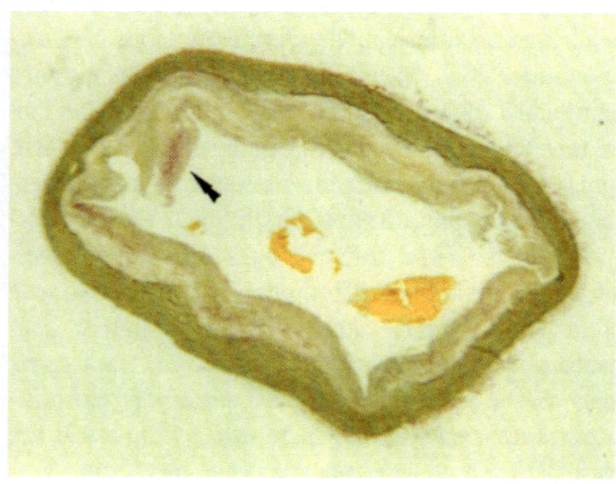

d

mechanisms of restenosis have not yet been fully identified, platelet aggregation, intimal proliferation and wound contraction do appear to be contributing factors (Willensky et al. 1995).

The presented in vitro and in vivo experiments in animal models suggest that intravascular MRI is indeed capable of providing the required plaque analysis with differentiation of calcification, collagen and fat. It is conceivable that these "prognostic" morphological data could be used to guide treatment decisions with regard to PTA and/or stenting. In addition, availability of these data may aid in the development, treatment monitoring and application of new therapeutic agents such as peptides (Tcheng 1996). In contrast to the mechanical approach inherent in PTA and stenting, these substances treat plaque locally on a molecular basis (Matsuno et al. 1995). In such a setting, the inflatable balloon might not only be used to assure an optimal coil position adjacent to the vascular wall, but may also be used for application of therapeutic agents through small perforations in a second balloon layer.

The evaluated balloon-mounted coil design provided excellent image quality. The improved sensitivity in imaging vessel wall structure is made possible by the direct contact of the receiver coil to the vessel wall. The design assures maximal spatial and contrast resolution with a minimum of flow-related motion artefacts. By positioning the coil next to the vascular wall, the latter lies within the maximal sensitivity area of the single loop imaging coil. Hence, the vascular walls could be displayed in great detail to a penetration depth of up to 10 mm. Individual wall layers were delineated even on 0.5-T images.

The concept of a balloon-mounted intravascular imaging coil also overcame the greatest challenge of intravascular MRI: suppression of motion artefacts due to flow within the vessel under consideration (Hurst et al. 1992; Martin and Henkelmann 1994). The inflatable balloon immobilises the coil against the vessel wall, thereby transiently occluding the vessel (Zimmermann et al. 1997a, 1997b). Flow artefacts are thus eliminated while, simultaneously, motion of the coil relative to the vessel wall is minimised. The excellent image quality achieved in the presented in vitro experiments under pulsatile flow conditions, as well as the in vivo results in two different animal models demonstrate the feasibility of this approach. The vascular wall is displayed in great detail without corrupting artefacts. Although the depth of signal reception is dependent on the coil, i.e. balloon diameter, under most circumstances penetration will be sufficient to assess the vascular walls without incurring shading effects.

This study confirms T2 contrast to be better suited for plaque analysis than T1 contrast. The contrast resolution inherent in both the 1.5-T and the 0.5-T images was sufficient to discriminate the components of plaque structure, including calcification, fibrous tissue and fat. Indeed, the in vitro results seem to suggest that signal differences between collagen and fat are more pronounced on 0.5-T images than on those collected at 1.5-T. At 0.5-T the various plaque components could be distinguished without overlap. The better contrast properties at 0.5-T likely reflect the specifics of the FSE sequence. With systematic variation of parameters, contrast resolution at 1.5-T could be similarly optimised, whilst exploiting the significantly better spatial resolution for even easier plaque characterisation.

Recently, Boos et al. (1996) reported on the acquisition of high resolution images of the femoral and iliac arteries with an external surface coil. The in-plane resolution of about 250 mm was sufficient to assess wall thickness but appeared insufficient to precisely delineate the different vessel wall components. Intravascular imaging provides significantly better spatial resolution (Martin and Henkelmann 1994; Zimmermann et al. 1997a, 1997b). At 1.5-T, the in-plane resolution achieved in the presented experiments was 117×104 mm. Reflecting the direct relationship between SNR and field strength (Hoult and Richards 1976), the spatial resolution achieved at 0.5-T was somewhat lower (234×178 mm). It was sufficient, however, to accurately quantitate wall thickness and atherosclerotic plaque area, as evidenced by the high correlation coefficients. Systematic overestimation of wall thickness and plaque area compared with histology likely reflects some degree of specimen shrinkage associated with the preparation for histological analysis (Di Mario et al. 1992).

To optimise SNR, four excitations were averaged, resulting in a considerable lengthening of imaging times of up to 5 and 8 min for T1- and T2-weighted images, respectively. The proposed imaging concept stipulates occlusion of the vessel during this time. While ischaemic times of similar lengths associated with PTA treatments appear to be of very limited consequence in the lower extremities, they seem unacceptably long when imaging of the renal or coronary arteries is considered (Eltchaninoff et al. 1996). Possible solutions include the use of fast and ultrafast gradient-echo based sequences, which could reduce imaging times to below 60 s (Rubin et al. 1994), particularly if the number of acquired images were reduced.

There are several impediments to the widespread use of intravascular MRI at this time. Accurate placement of the imaging catheter in conjunction with the possibility of interactive repositioning must be assured, and has been shown in animal experiments. Furthermore, the invasiveness of the procedure demands the ability to provide treatment in the same sitting. Basic to the fulfilment of both requirements in an MR environment is patient access.

In combination with other recent hardware and software developments, intravascular MRI promises to become an integral element in the overall concept of interventional MR angiography.

References

Atalar E, Bottomley PA, Ocali O, Correia LCL, Kelemen MD, Lima JAC, Zerhouni EA (1996) High resolution intravascular MRI and MRS by using a catheter receiver coil. Magn Reson Med 36:596–605

Bonelli U, Cerruti R, Baglietto F, Arnuzzo L, et al (1995) Iliac PTA: long-term results and current prospects. Minerva Chir 50:105–108

Boos M, Böttcher U, Laub G, Jakob AL (1996) Clinical value of high resolution MRI of vessel wall lesions in peripheral atherosclerosis disease. First in vivo experience before and after PTA. MAGMA 127:94

Davies MJ, Woolf N (1993) Atherosclerosis: what is it and why does it occur? Br Heart J 69:3–11

Di Mario C, The SHK, Madretsma S, et al (1992) Detection and characterization of vascular lesions by intravascular ultrasound: an in vitro study correlated with histology. J Am Soc Echocardiogr 5:135–146

Dumoulin CL, Hart HR (1986) Magnetic resonance angiography. Radiology 161:717–720

Dumoulin CL, Souza SP, Darrow RD (1993) Real-time position monitoring of invasive devices using magnetic resonance. Magn Reson Med 299:411–415

Eltchaninoff H, Cribier A, Koning R, Chan C, et al (1996) Effects of prolonged sequential balloon inflations on results of coronary angioplasty. AJR Am J Roentgenol 77: 1062–1066

Erhart P, Ladd ME, Zimmermann GG, Hoffmann E, von Schulthess GK, Debatin J (1996) Balloon-mounted intravascular coils for MR imaging of vessel walls. MAGMA 94:129

Falk E (1985) Unstable angina with fatal outcome: dynamic coronary thrombosis leading to infarction and/or sudden death. Autopsy evidence of recurrent mural thrombosis with peripheral embolization culminating in total vascular occlusion. Circulation 71:699–708

Forrester JS, Litvack F, Grundfest W (1991) Initiating events of acute coronary arterial occlusion. Annu Rev Med 42:35–45

Fuster V, Badimon L, Badimon JJ, Chesebro JH. (1992) The pathogenesis of coronary artery disease and the acute coronary syndromes. N Engl J Med 326:242–250

Gotlieb AI, Havenith MG (1991) Atherosclerosis: lesions and pathogenesis. In: Silver MD (ed) Cardiovascular pathology. Churchill Livingstone, New York, pp. 225–266

Hoult DI, Richards RE (1976) The signal-to-noise ratio of the nuclear magnetic resonance experiment. J Magn Reson Imaging 24:71–85

Hurst GC, Hua J, Duerk JL, Cohen AM (1992) Intravascular (catheter) NMR receiver probe: preliminary design analysis and application to canine iliofemoral imaging. Magn Reson Med 24:343–357

Kandarpa K, Jakob P, Patz S, Schoen FJ, Jolesz FA (1993) Prototype miniature endoluminal MR imaging catheter. J Vasc Interv Radiol 4:419–427

Ladd ME, Erhart P, Zimmermann GG, Debatin JF et al (1996) MR trackable vascular guide wires. MAGMA 144 [Suppl 2]: 264

Leung DA, Debatin JF, Wildermuth S, McKinnon GC, et al (1995) Active visualization of intravascular catheters with MRI: in vitro and in vivo evaluation. AJR Am J Roentgenol 164:1265–1270

Martin AJ, Plewes DB, Henkelmann RM (1992) MR imaging of blood vessels with an intravascular coil. J Magn Reson Imaging 2:421–429

Martin AJ, Henkelmann RM (1994) Intravascular MR imaging in a porcine animal model. Magn Reson Med 32:224–229

Matsuno H, Hoylaerts MF, Vermylen J, Deckmyn H (1995) Inhibition of integrin function prevents restenosis following vascular injury. (in Japanese) Nippon Yakurigaku Zasshi 106:143–155

McDonald GG, Chwialkowski M, Peshock RM (1993) Performance comparison of several coil geometries for use in catheters. Radiology 189:319

Ocali O, Atalar E (1997) Intravascular magnetic resonance imaging using a loopless catheter antenna. Magn Reson Med 37:112–118

Prince MR, Yucel EK, Kaufmann JA, Harrison DC, et al (1993) Dynamic gadolinium-enhanced three dimensional abdominal MR arteriography. J Magn Reson Imaging 3:877–881

Ross R (1993) The pathogenesis of atherosclerosis: a perspective for the 1990s. Nature 362:801–809

Rubin GD, Dake MD, Napel SA, McDonnell CH, Jeffrey RB Jr (1993) Three-dimensional spiral CT angiography of the abdomen: initial clinical experience. Radiology 186:147–152

Rubin GD, Herfkens RJ, Pelc NJ, et al (1994) Single breath-hold pulmonary magnetic resonance angiography: optimization and comparison of three imaging techniques. Invest Radiol 29:766–792

Small DM (1988) Progression and regression of atherosclerotic lesions. Arteriosclerosis 8:103–129

Tcheng JE (1996) Glycoprotein IIb/IIIa receptor inhibitors: putting the EPIC, IMPACT II, RESTORE, and EPILOG trials into perspective. Am J Cardiol 78:35–40

Willensky RL, March KL, Gradus-Pizlo I, Sandusky G, et al (1995) Vascular injury, repair and restenosis after percutaneous transluminal angioplasty in the atherosclerotic rabbit. Circulation 92:2995–3005

Zimmermann GG, Erhart P, Schneider J, von Schulthess GK, Schmidt M, Debatin J (1997a) Intravascular MR imaging of atherosclerotic plaque: 'ex vivo' analysis of human femoral arteries with histologic correlation. Radiology (in press)

Zimmermann GG, Quick HH, Hilfiker P, Giovanoli P, von Schulthess GK, Debatin J (1997b) Intravascular MR imaging in vivo: Preliminary results in an atherosclerotic animal model. RoFo Fortschr Geb Roentgenstr Neuen Bildgeb Verfahr 167(2):74-80

A Critical Perspective

35 Interventional Radiology and Interventional MRI

D. Vorwerk and R.W. Günther

CONTENTS

35.1 State of the Art in Interventional Radiology

Fifty years of interventional radiology make this subspeciality a major field in radiology. Each decade has been highlighted by a new, important therapy development having a major impact on interventional radiology. While, in the 1950s, biliary drainage and nephrostomies were introduced, the 1960s were marked by vascular recanalization using the Dotter technique, the 1970s, by the introduction of balloon angioplasty and the 1980s, by stent technologies. Moreover, the process of development has not yet come to an end: there is a trend toward more complex interventions, such as transjugular intrahepatic shunt (TIPS) or endoluminal graft techniques for the treatment of fistulas and aortic aneurysms. Development of new materials, metal alloys and coverings enable production of highly specialized instruments needed for complex inventions. Image guidance is essential to successful intervention: fluoroscopy and digital subtraction angiography are the most important guiding tools, computer tomography (CT) and ultrasound playing a more limited role, especially in vascular interventions. These are mainly focussed on nonvascular applications, such as biopsies and drainages.

D. Vorwerk, MD, Department of Diagnostic Radiology, University of Technology Aachen, Pauwelsstrasse 30, D-52074 Aachen, Germany
R.W. Günther, MD, Department of Diagnostic Radiology, University of Technology Aachen, Pauwelsstrasse 30, D-52074 Aachen, Germany

35.2 MR-Guided Interventions

MRI has revolutionized diagnostic imaging with its numerous possibilities, offering multiplanar imaging, tissue information, and vascular and functional imaging. Since MRI is a cross-sectional imaging modality, the idea to apply it as a guiding tool in "classical" CT-guided interventions, such as organ biopsy and drainage, seemed very attractive. The various possibilities MRI offers, however, make it useful as a tool for vascular interventions as well (Jolesz and Blumenfeld 1994).

Four major potential benefits recommend application of MRI:

1. Guidance with freedom to choose nearly any imaging plane, thus allowing nonaxial planning of access routes that are not feasible by other modalities such as fluoroscopy and CT.
2. In vivo monitoring of tissue alterations induced percutaneously or transluminally.
3. Simultaneous imaging of the vascular lumen and the surrounding tissue in order to guide intervention instruments safely to the target area.
4. Avoidance of X-ray exposure.

These benefits make MRI guidance potentially attractive for both vascular and nonvascular applications. Limitations, however, are related to current unit configuration, sensitivity to artefacts and inherent limitations of spatial and temporal resolution.

35.3 MR-Guided Biopsy

Presently, the most important clinical application is MR-guided percutaneous biopsy. MRI is well suited in this case since free angulation allows safe routes via nonaxial pathways, which gains special interest in examinations of the subphrenic space or in the head and neck area. Moreover, MRI enhances lesions in the breast, in bone and in brain that would remain otherwise invisible (FISCHER et al. 1995; SCHENCK et al. 1995) and renders them amenable to biopsy.

The requirement of continuous or rapid monitoring of the procedure makes availability of open or partially open magnetic systems desirable. Conventional full magnets may also be used when a technique is applied such as CT-guided biopsy: repeat control scans allow the operator to check the needle's pathway through the body while the needle is advanced blindly. Imaging of needles and instruments still remains a problem even when MR-compatible instruments are used, since artefacts are dependent on the angle of the needle to the static magnetic field B_0 and may alter according to the sequences used. This is especially important when small lesions are targeted. Furthermore, the lack of dedicated nonferromagnetic instruments is still compromising the use of MRI for more complex nonvascular interventions, such as purely MR-guided abscess drainage.

Although MRI offers attractive alternatives to CT, one should keep in mind that, even under CT guidance, nonaxial access routes are feasible if simple geometric rules are applied in planning biangulated accesses. Moreover, B-scan ultrasound is an easy and low-cost means to perform biopsies with free choice of angulation. Furthermore, CT fluoroscopy is being developed to allow real-time monitoring of needle movement, thus offering an attractive alternative to MR-guided biopsies.

35.4 In Vivo Monitoring by MRI and Functional Imaging

MR-guided percutaneous biopsy is certainly of interest in cases where a lesion cannot be visualized by other means or a nonaxial access route is mandatory, but its impact on interventional radiology is much too small to justify the development of dedicated systems for this sole purpose. However, additional abilities of MRI are even more fascinating, particularly in the field of visualization and monitoring of physical changes of stationary tissue, such as functional imaging of the brain.

These mainly include laser coagulation, focussed ultrasound, cryotherapy and ethanol ablation, as well as localized hyperthermia (GEWIESE et al. 1994; HONG et al. 1994; HYNYNEN et al. 1995; VOGL et al. 1995). In vitro experiments were able to visualize the damage related to temperature or the amount of contrast agent that was applied. This offers several potentials for clinical application. To carry out tumor ablation by these methods, however, several access routes are frequently required in one patient. Moreover, with many procedures ultrasound also offers possibilities to monitor tissue changes, e.g., with ethanol ablation or cryotherapy. A direct comparison of ultrasound guidance and MR guidance is, however, still pending. The future role of MR monitoring in local tumor therapy will depend on how accurately MR changes can predict the acute and late effect on tumors in relation to temperature and size. Moreover, MRI will only play a major role in clinical therapy if these methods can show a significant effect on the morbidity rate and survival time in patients with metastatic tumor disease.

35.5 Combined Imaging of Extravascular and Intravascular Spaces

Simultaneous imaging of the endoluminal spaces and surrounding tissue and organs offers intriguing new perspectives for interventional radiology. These include MR monitoring of catheter-guided drug delivery regimes, such as embolization (Fig. 35.1), chemoembolization and thrombolysis, which may make it possible to directly visualize the efficacy of the chosen therapy, especially within organs. Additionally, the combined information might be used to establish a spatial orientation which cannot be depicted from a selective endoluminal image alone. Potential advantages could be gained for secure transversal or arterial or venous occlusions, aortic fenestration or TIPS procedures (Fig. 35.2). However, none of these possible applications have been sufficiently tested so far and, in some cases, alternative guiding tools are already available, such as endoluminal ultrasound (e.g., for aortic fenestration) and transcutaneous ultrasound (for TIPS).

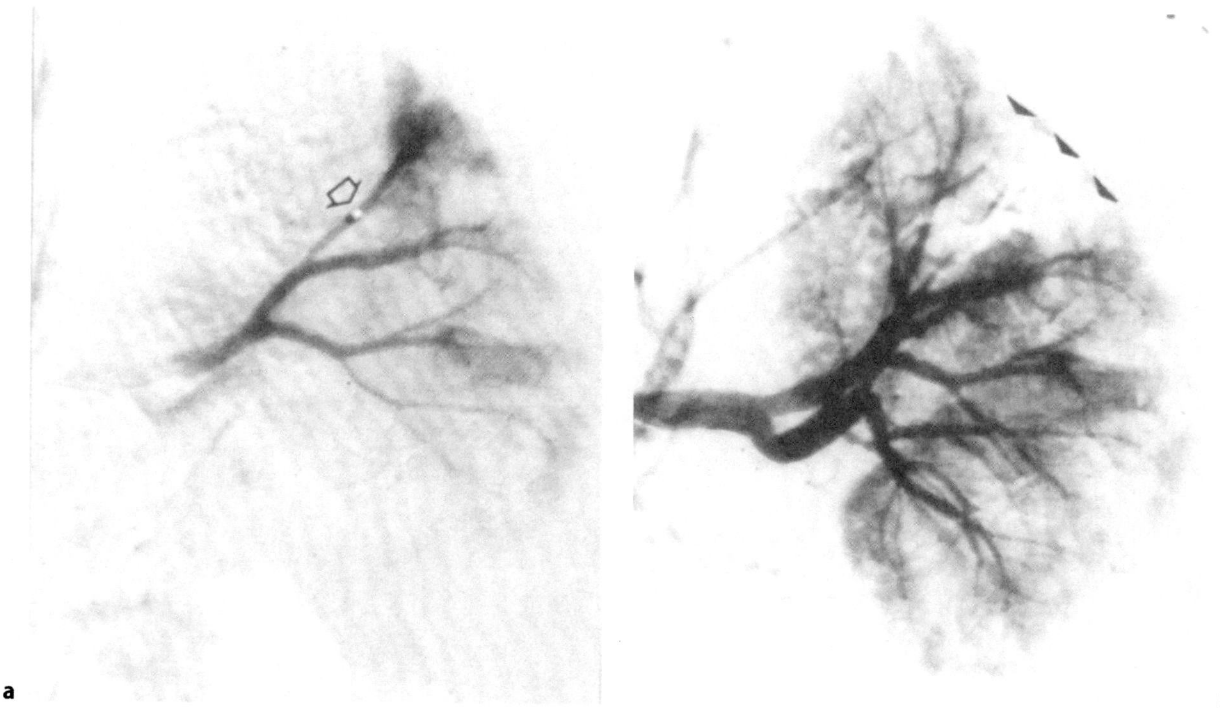

Fig. 35.1a,b. Selective embolization: **a** Exact placement of a coaxial catheter (*arrow*) within a segmental artery before embolization. **b** After glue embolization a triangular filling defect (*arrowheads*) indirectly indicates the extension of the embolized area.

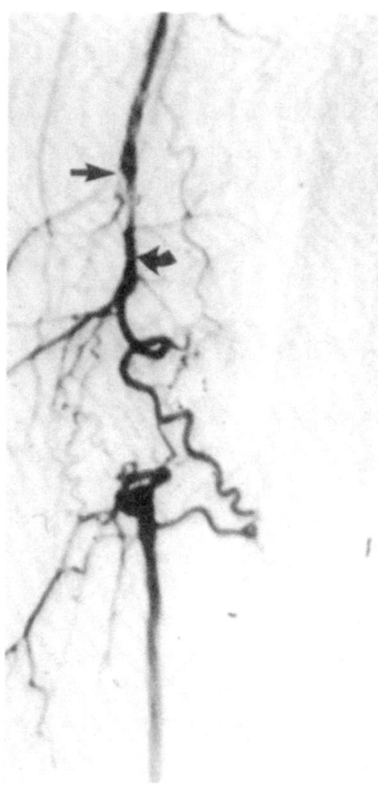

Fig. 35.2. Extraluminal and intraluminal information: Short occlusion of a superficial femoral artery (*arrow*). Under fluoroscopy guidance it is difficult to enter the occluded lumen instead of a straight collateral (*curved arrow*). Visualization of the occluded channel would facilitate the procedure

35.6 Vascular interventions using MRI

The most challenging interventions under MR guidance are certainly endovascular procedures, such as balloon dilation, implantation of stents and filters, superselective embolization, and TIPS. In order to perform such interventions safely and adequately, several requirements have to be met: a fluoroscopy-type sequence technology that allows near real-time demonstration of all manipulations performed and a high spatial resolution in order to reduce the risks of the intervention (Fig. 35.3). The sequences used should be flexible enough to change image plane or modalities rapidly, and free access to the patient is preferable. While these requirements are sufficiently fulfilled for X-ray techniques, MR guidance is still suffering from incomplete solutions in most fields.

35.6.1 Hardware

While excellent angiographic units have been developed over the years, reaching a high standard of technology, optimized dedicated MR systems are not available for vascular interventions. Although there are open and semi-open magnets available from dif-

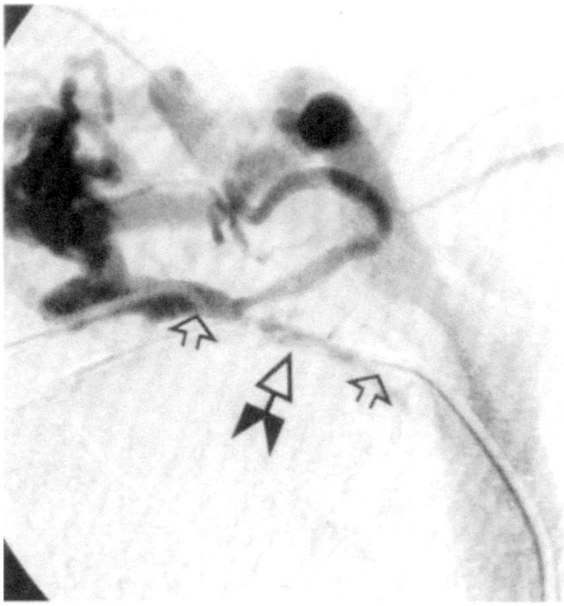

a

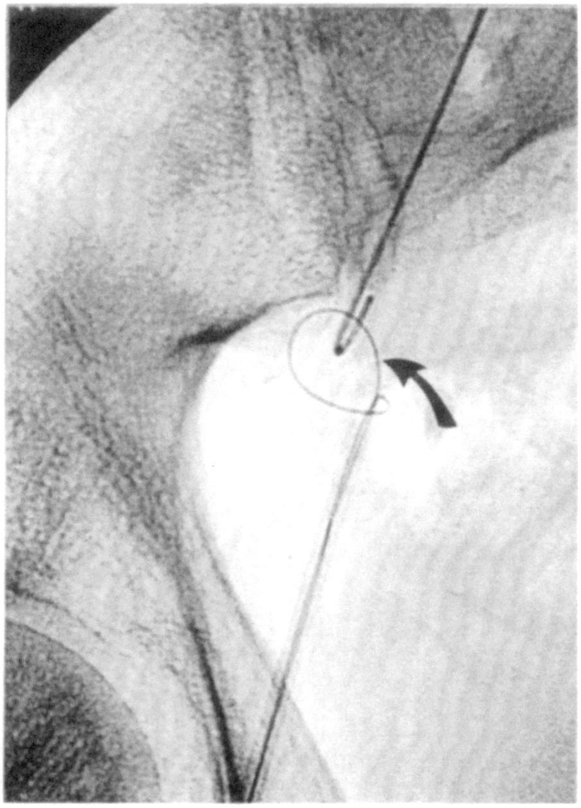

b

Fig. 35.3a,b. Complex vascular interventions: **a** Difficult occlusion of a subclavian vein (*large arrow*) that required recanalization from both sides (*open arrows*). **b** Capturing a guidewire with a snare to perform a pull-through maneuver for recanalization of an occluded iliac artery (*arrow*). For success, high spatial and temporal resolution is mandatory

ferent suppliers, these represent a compromise with regard to field strength. Field strength is a limiting factor in ultrafast imaging which in turn is a major requirement for high-quality MR angiography. High field strength units, on the other hand, restrict free access to the patient, while allowing adequate vascular imaging (Adam et al. 1996; Schenck et al. 1995).

35.6.2 MRI

A true real-time MRI system which could be compared with X-ray fluoroscopy has not yet been developed. Once such a system does become reality, it would be decisive for the role of vascular interventions under MR guidance. For the time being, there are different sequences available that offer active catheter visualization. Topographic information is delivered via a "roadmapping" technique (Leung et al. 1995). Roadmapping, however, is highly prone to artefacts due to breathing or movement, thus limiting its application to only some parts of the body, e.g. the head, extremities, and pelvis. Safe and reliable imaging of catheters and instruments requires continuous visualization, preferably along the whole length independent of the imaging plane used as it is achieved by projection imaging during X-ray fluoroscopy.

Much research will be necessary to develop optimized, tailored sequences that allow simultaneous imaging of vessel, instrument, and target lesion with equal quality.

35.6.3 MR-Compatible Instruments

The development of MR-compatible instruments is another important step in establishing endovascular MR procedures and is still only in the first stages. The material used for the instruments should not only be MR compatible without creating major artefacts but should also be easily detectable within the body with respect to position and true size.

Two concepts in a first attempt to meet these requirements are based on active visualization by coil technology and passive visualization by incorporation of gadolinium or dysprosium. These techniques have been applied using simple catheters or balloon catheters and first guidewires and caval filters have been developed. There are, however, no new developments in highly specialized instruments such as atherectomy catheters, stents, grafts, superselective catheters, and embolization coils.

Due to these complex problems, which remain unsolved in many details, intravascular MR interventions represent the greatest challenge in this field, and it seems certain that the significance of the role played by MRI will depend on satisfying solutions being found in all three fields outlined above.

35.7 Radiation Protection and Safety Issues

Avoidance of radiation exposure has been frequently used as an argument in favor of MR-guided interventions, and it is well known that, especially in interventional procedures, exposure can be high under X-ray guidance. This consideration is of less importance for the older patient in that the majority suffer from malignant or chronic disease that limits the general prognosis. Thus, it is more of interest for the younger patient but, more particularly, for the staff, who is exposed to high radiation doses during their professional lives. Significant reduction of this exposure would be more than desirable, and MRI would be one tool helpful to this aim. On the other hand, it is not yet known whether long-term exposure to high magnetic fields, which both patient and operator would experience if major interventions were able to be performed under MR guidance, is without any significant impact on human health. Furthermore, avoidance of X-ray exposure is not a strong enough argument for performing MR interventions unless other major prerequisites, such as MR fluoroscopy, are met that might help to increase the safety of the patient. The intervention procedure itself, as well as the fragility of diseased vessels and the general health of most patients require rapid and adequate action in case of complications (Fig. 35.4). From this point of view, risks of radiation exposure become of limited relevance for the patient.

35.8 Conclusions

Interventional MRI is a new, attractive and challenging field in radiology that offers broad opening for research and development. The potentials of this technology seem to be at least as numerous as the technical problems facing us in clinical practice.

The rapid progress that is still being made in X-ray-guided interventional radiology does not help to speed up the establishment of interventional MRI, since this new modality has not only still to prove it-

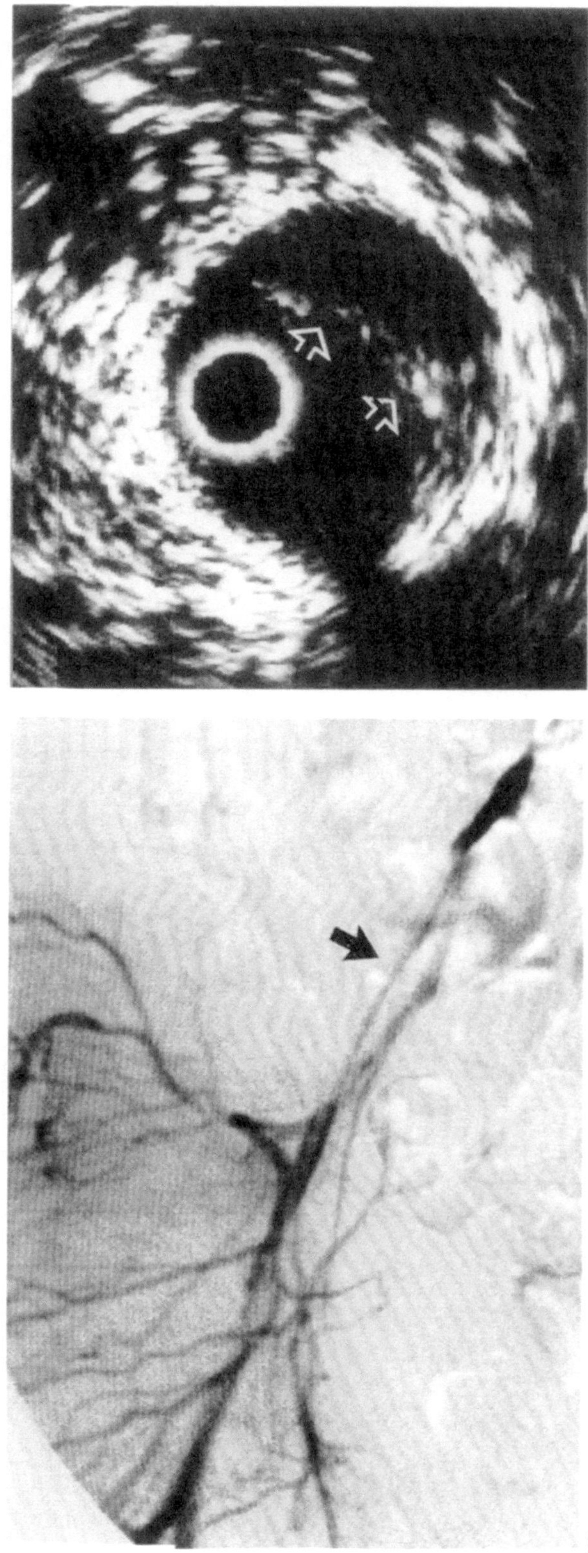

Fig. 35.4a,b. Complications of interventions: **a** Membrane-like dissection material floating within the vascular lumen (*arrows*) seen by intravascular ultrasound. These thin structures are sometimes only faintly visible, even on fluoroscopy. **b** Near complete occlusion of the right external iliac artery (*arrow*) after balloon angioplasty requiring immediate stenting to prevent thrombotic occlusion. Excellent fluoroscopy conditions are mandatory for success

self equal to modern X-ray methods in interventions but must also keep up with new developments and procedures. This is of major importance since it would make no sense to perform only simple and basic interventions under MRI guidance, while difficult and lengthy interventions still remained under X-ray guidance.

Thus, it is realistic that interventional MRI with all its fascinating potentials will more and more become a part of this subspeciality. Whether MRI will completely replace X-ray fluoroscopy as the leading guiding tool, however, seems unlikely from the current point of view.

References

Adam G, Neuerburg J, Glowinski A, Stargardt A, van Vaals J, Günther RW (1996) Erste Erfahrungen mit einem neuen Hybridsystem zur interventionellen MR-Tomographie bei 1,5 T. Rofo Fortschr Geb Roentgenstr Neuen Bildgeb Verfahr 164:110

Fischer U, Vosshenrich R, Doler W, Hamadeh A, Oestmann J, Grabbe E (1995) MR-guided breast intervention: experience with two systems. Radiology 195:533–538

Gewiese B, Beuthan J, Fobbe F, Stiller D, Müller G, Bose-Landgraf J, Wolf KJ, Deimling M (1994) Magnetic resonance imaging-controlled laser-induced interstitial thermotherapy. Invest Radiol 29:345–351

Hong J, Wong S, Pease G, Rubinsky B (1994) MR imaging assisted temperature calculations during cryosurgery. Magn Reson Imaging 12:1021–1031

Hynynen K, Damianou C, Colucci V, Unger E, Cline H, Jolesz F (1995) MR monitoring of focused ultrasonic surgery of the renal cortex: experimental and simulation studies. J Magn Reson Imaging 5:259–266

Jolesz FA, Blumenfeld S (1994) Interventional use of magnetic resonance imaging. Magn Reson Q 10:85–96

Leung D, Debatin J, Wildermuth S, et al (1995) Intravascular MR tracking catheters. AJR Am J Roentgenol 164:1265–1270

Schenck J, Jolesz F, Roemer P, et al (1995) Superconducting open-configuration MR imaging system for image guided therapy. Radiology 195:805–814

Vogl TJ, Mack M, Muller P, et al (1995) Recurrent nasopharyngeal tumors: preliminary clinical results with interventional MR imaging-controlled laser-induced thermotherapy. Radiology 196:725–733

Instrumentation Vendors

36 MR-Compatible Instrumentation

B.J. Romanowski

CONTENTS

36.1 Introduction

Various instruments and devices are required for diagnostic imaging, as well as for all kinds of interventions. As indicated by its name, magnetic resonance imaging is based on the use of a magnetic field. Various scanner designs with different field strengths and shielding techniques have been introduced over recent years. The inherent magnetism of the imaging system itself has remained common to all of these innovations. Hence, the earliest and most fundamental definition of "MR compatibility" is synonymous with non-ferromagnetic. For safety reasons, only non-ferromagnetic devices and instruments should be allowed in the MRI suite (Fig. 36.1). All personnel must receive safety training in order to prevent the accidental introduction of ferromagnetic devices into the MR suite, as these can cause serious injury to both the patient and the medical team.

With the availability of open-configuration magnet designs allowing for MR monitoring of interventional procedures, the definition of MR compatibility has evolved beyond lack of attraction to the magnet and now focuses on the issue of instrument- or device-induced susceptibility effects (Fig. 36.2). The magnitude of these effects is dependent on the underlying material, as well as on the field strength of the magnet, the sequence parameters and even the orientation of the device within the magnetic field. All materials, including titanium and nickel alloys, ceramics, plastics and polymer composites have some degree of susceptibility effect. Different materials cause effects of different magnitude, ranging from minor distortions limited to a millimeter or less in distance from the instrument to total obliteration of the imaging field.

Minor susceptibility-induced signal voids can be taken advantage of to help guide instruments to target lesions (Fig. 36.3) in the case of rapid imaging. They can also be used in conjunction with stereotactic referencing devices for target guidance (Fig. 36.4). Instruments which must remain within the imaging field should generate the least amount of artifact possible, while instruments that are only temporarily within the field can be made from a material with higher susceptibility effects. Testing all instruments and devices is therefore crucial before any intervention can take place in patients.

36.2 Testing

The first and simplest method of instrument testing for ferromagnetism is the use of a hand-held magnet. It should be sufficiently strong as to exert some force on even mildly ferromagnetic objects. If there is a strong attraction to this type of magnet, the user can be assured that the instrument would be impossible to control near a strong magnetic field and it should, therefore, be removed from the interventional procedure inventory. Objects which show only slight attraction in this type of precursory testing should also be replaced because the attraction will increase within a stronger field, rendering it potentially dangerous and difficult to control. Any remaining instruments showing no attraction to the hand-held magnet can go on to the next compatibility test.

The next step is to see how the instrument will react within the scanner itself. Only a single object should be taken in at one time. The magnetic field should be approached slowly. *Under no circumstances should this be done while there is someone in the magnet.* Only the instruments which show no

B.J. Romanowski, Research Coordinator, MRI Center, Institute of Diagnostic Radiology, University Hospital Zurich, Rämistrasse 100, CH-8091 Zurich, Switzerland

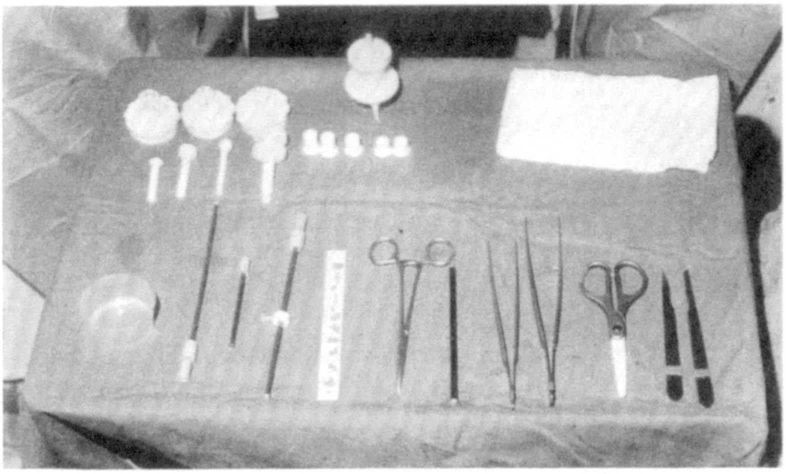

Fig. 36.1. MR-compatible interventional biopsy instruments: a polymer composite "Snapper" fixation device and biopsy needles, titanium alloy clamps and forceps, and ceramic scissors and scalpels. All instruments are specially color coded for identification as MR safe

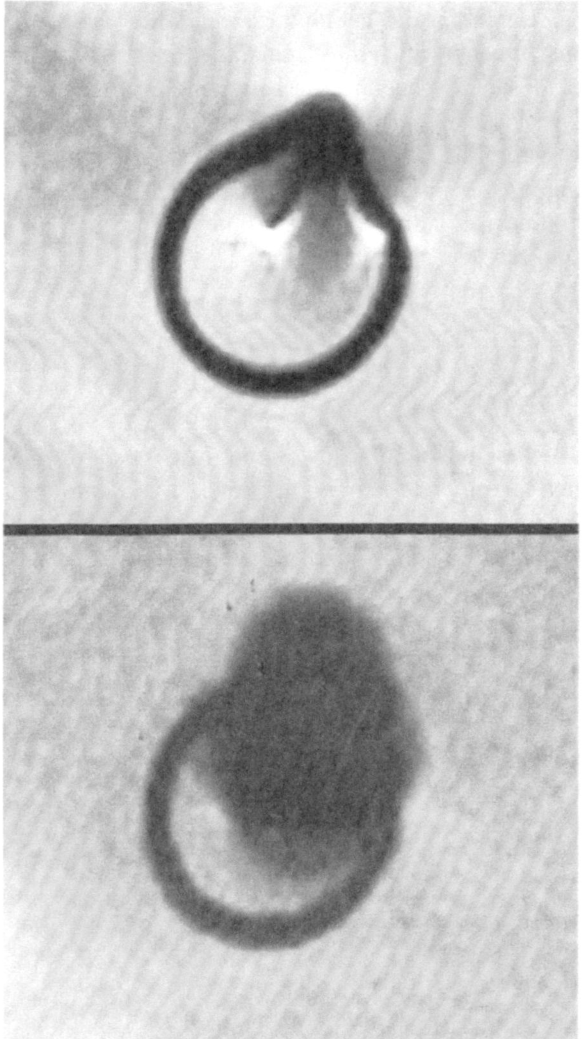

Fig. 36.2. The artifact given off by two "MR-compatible" metallic needles. Samples were scanned inside a plastic tube (*circular* signal void) to exhibit distortion effects. The tube was suspended in agar gel. Neither sample is considered acceptable

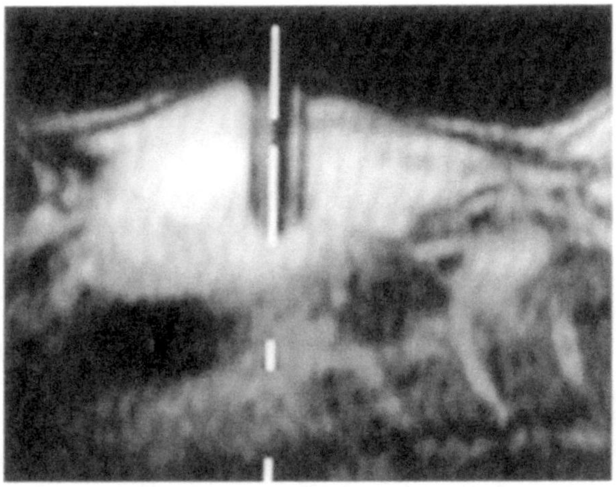

Fig. 36.3. Susceptibility artifact from an MR-compatible needle during a thyroid biopsy. The *dotted line* shows good correlation between the needle position and the stereotactic referencing system

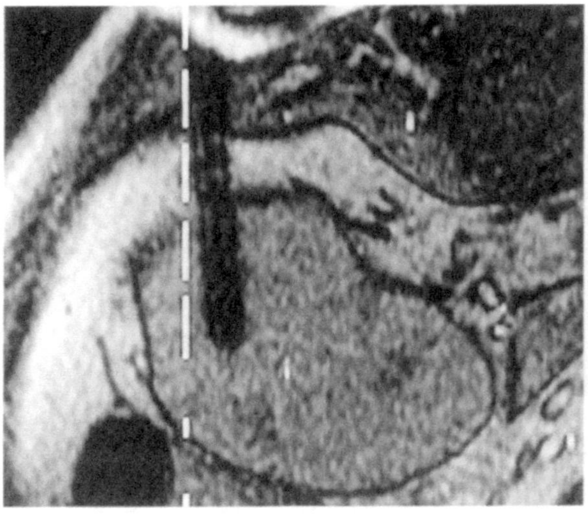

Fig. 36.4. A susceptibility artifact from an MR-compatible needle shows deflection from the stereoscopically projected trajectory (*dotted line*) during a pelvic biopsy. Artifacts can be used to check for correct instrument position, as well as for guidance system accuracy

attraction within the field should be considered acceptable.

Once the issue of safety has been satisfied, the instruments must be tested for the amount of associated susceptibility artifact. Since interventional imaging requires rapid updates, gradient-echo sequences are often employed during patient procedures. These sequences are also highly sensitive to fluctuations in field homogeneity and, therefore, susceptibility artifacts will be enhanced, ultimately effecting image quality. A standardized screening protocol for instrumentation utilizing a gradient-echo sequence is recommended. This will ensure reproducible results under a common "worst case" imaging sequence. Possible imaging parameters could be as follows: gradient echo, TR 25/TE 8, 30° flip angle, 10-mm section thickness, 256×256 matrix, 1 excitation, approximately a 30-s scan. Objects should be scanned in either a water bath or in agar gel, the gel holding instruments in place better. Depending upon their size, objects should be positioned far enough apart that susceptibility artifacts can be distinguished from individual instruments. A marker placed at one side of the container can help identify orientation if multiple objects are being scanned.

Instruments with little or no susceptibility artifact are acceptable for use even close to the area of interest. Instruments or devices with high susceptibility artifact should be kept outside the imaging field.

36.3 List of Vendors Offering Various MR-Compatible Instruments

The following list contains the names of companies, both in the United States and throughout Europe, who presently offer alternative instrumentation for use in an interventional MR environment. By no means is this list exhaustive. It is intended to provide a point at which to start the often tedious search for adequate instrumentation and accessories. Vendors may add to or discontinue specific product lines in the future. An effort has been made to provide an updated list. The author would like to acknowledge the support of Susan Koran of General Electric Medical Systems, Milwaukee, Wis. In compiling this list. *(Note: phone and fax numbers in the United States and Canada are listed with their respective area codes. European numbers are listed with their respective country codes in parentheses.)*

Aesculap, 1000 Gateway Boulevard, South San Francisco, CA 94080
Products: general surgical instruments, MR-compatible scissors
USA: Tony Messer, Manager, research and development (R&D)
Phone: 800-282-9000
415-876-7000
Fax: 415-876-7027
International: Theodore Lutze, Manager, R&D, Applications Research Aesculap AG, AM Amesculap-Platz, P.O. Box 40, D-78501 Tuttlingen, Germany
Phone: (49) 7461-95-2354
Fax: (49) 7461-146-14

Baxter Custom Sterile, 1500 Waukegan Road, McGaw Park, IL 60085
Products: sterile drapes
USA: Jan McDonnell
Phone: 708-473-1500

BIP, Am Brand 1, P.C. 0, D-82299 Tuerkenfeld, Germany
Products: core biopsy gun
International: Norbert Heske
Phone: (49) 8193-60-26
(49) 8193-65-48

Bruker Odam, 34, rue de l'industrie, F-67160 Wissembourg, France
Products: patient monitoring devices
International: Laurent Sigrist, Secretaire General
Phone: (33) 88-63-36-06
Fax: (33) 88-54-36-32
Sales Department:
Phone: (33) 88-63-36-00
Fax: (33) 88-94-12-82

Cogent Light, 26145 Technology Drive, Santa Clarita, CA 91355-1137
Products: Surgical headlamp/light source
USA/International: Richard B. Davies
Phone: 805-294-2989
Fax: 805-294-2904

Contour Fabricators Inc., PO Box 56, Grand Blanc, MI 48439
Products: custom magnet drapes
James D. Miller, Sales and Marketing
Phone: 810-695-2910
Fax: 810-695-5336

Cook Medical, PO Box 489, Bloomington, IN 47402
Products: needles, biopsy guns, catheters
USA/International: John DeFord, PhD, Product Development Manager (MRI-compatible biopsy needles)
Phone: 800-346-2686
812-339-2235
Fax: 812-339-5369
Customer Service: 800-457-4500

Cryomedical Sciences, 1300 Piccard Drive Suite 102, Rockville, MD 20850
Products: cryotherapy equipment
USA: J.J. Finkelstein, President
Phone: 301-417-7070
Fax: 301-417-7077

Cuda Products, 600 Powers Avenue, Jacksonville, FL 32217
Products: light source adaptors (for endoscope)
Phone: 904-737-7611
Fax: 904-733-4832

Daum Medical Devices GmbH, Hangenower Strasse 73, D-19061 Schwerin, Germany
Products: MR-compatible needles
International: Martin Tscherkow, Sales and Marketing
Phone: (49) 385-6344-109
Fax: (49) 385-6344-152

Elekta Instrument AB, Birger Jarlsgatan 53, PO Box 7593, S-103 93 Stockholm, Sweden
Products: neurosurgical instruments
International: Raymond Rau, Product Manager
Phone: (46) 8-402-5429
Fax: (46) 8-402-5500

E-Z-EM Inc., 717 Main Street, Westbury, NY 11590
Products: needles/catheters/biopsy guns/MR-compatible devices (interested in development of prototype devices for investigational use only)
USA/
International: Ben Gonzalez, Product Manager for Interventional Devices (contact Product Manager for name and address of distributor in a specific country)
Phone: 516-333-8230, ext. 304
Fax: 516-333-8278

Hess, Im Schossacher 15, CH-8600 Dubendorf, Switzerland
Products: MR-compatible trolleys with wheels
International: Matthias Angst
Phone: (41) 1-821-6435
Fax: (41) 1-821-6433

Intermetro Industries, North Washington Street, Wilkes-Barre, PA 17805
Products: drug/storage systems
USA:
Phone: 717-825-2741

In-Vivo GE Medical Diagnostic Imaging Accessories, PO Box 414, W-462, Milwaukee, WI 53201
Products: general MR imaging accessories
USA/
International: Phone: 800-472-3666
Fax: 414-827-3347

ITI Medical Technologies, 7000 East Avenue, PO Box 808, L-433, Livermore, CA 94550
Products: "prototype" Weitlander instrumentation, Bookwalter table post, Bookwalter endoscope holder
USA/
International: Roger W. Werne, PhD
Phone: 510-371-8305
Fax: 510-422-1680

Johnson & Johnson Professional Inc., (Codman Division), 41 Pacella Park Drive, Randolph, MA 02368
Products: will manufacture custom device once only. No duplication of custom devices
USA: Direct sales through representatives; Paula Papineau, Product Manager
Phone: 800-451-2006
508-828-3065
International: Blair Fraser, Manager, new business development for European operation
Phone: (44) 344-86-40-30

J&J Ethicon Inc., Route 22, Somerville, NJ 08876
Products: needles with sutures
USA: Bill McJames
Phone: 908-218-2297
Fax: 908-218-2531

Kerwin Surgical Products, 83 East Water Street, PO Box 545, Rockland, MA 02370
Products: bi-polar cable #10-6000s
USA: James A. Hannan
Phone: 617-878-2706

Life Instruments, 14 Wood Road, Suite 002, Braintree, MA 02184
Products: Penfields, curets, mini-Cobbs
USA: Larry Foley
Phone: 800-925-2995
617-849-0209
Fax: 617-849-0128

Lone Peak Engineering, 12660 South Fort Street, Draper, UT 84020
Products: ceramic sissors
USA: Vickey Coombes
Phone: 801-553-1732
Fax: 801-553-1734

Magnetic Resonance Equipment Corporation, PO Box 5489, 5 Grant Avenue, Bay Shore, NY 11706
Products: patient monitors, communication and music systems
USA/
International: John V. Plump (contact for name and address of the distributor in a specific country)
Phone: 516-243-3500
Fax: 516-243-3516

Magnetic Vision GmbH, Lochacher 6, CH-8630 Rüti, Switzerland
Products: MR-compatible skull fixation device (Snapper) and custom biopsy needles
International: Dr. Adriano Vigano
Phone: (41) 55-260-18-55
Fax: (41) 55-260-18-56

Medilas AG, Grindlenstrasse 3, CH-8954 Geroldswil, Switzerland
Products: surgical drapes
International: Mark Kleger
Phone: (41) 1-748-4000
Fax: (41) 1-748-0105

Medilink S.A., Via al Fiume 3a, CH-6962 Viganello-Lugano, Switzerland

Products: EZ-Em/Somatex needles
International: Christopher Jackson, General Manager
Phone: (41) 91-972-84-17
Fax: (41) 91-972-85-68

Medrad, 240 Alpha Drive, Pittsburgh, PA 15238-2870

Products: MR injector (contrast media only)
USA:
Phone: 800-633-7237
412-967-9700
Fax: 412-963-1964
International: Medrad Europe, Postbus 3084, 6202 N.B. Maastricht, The Netherlands
Phone: (31) 43-364-08-08
Fax: (31) 43-365-00-20

Microsurgical Techniques Inc., Seven Lakes Industrial Park, 2290 East Prospect, Suite 3, Fort Collins, CO 80525

Products: ceramic scalpels
USA/
International: Richard Rosenthal CEO
Phone: 970-221-4988
Fax: 970-221-9493

Midas Rex, 3001 Race Street, Ft. Worth, TX 76111

Products: MRI-compatible pneumatic drill
USA: Ray Umber, PhD
Phone: 800-433-7639
817-831-2604
Fax: 817-834-4835

Möller Microsurgical, 7 Industrial Park, Waldwick, NJ 07463

Products: MRI-compatible microscope
USA: Dick Montgomery, Vice President, Marketing and Sales
Phone: 201-251-9592
Fax: 201-251-9516
International: Martin Schmidt, PhD, President; J.D. Möller, Optische Werke GmbH, Rosengarten 10, D-22880 Wedel, Germany
Phone: (04) 103-70-93-33
Fax: (04) 103-70-93-50

MR Resources Inc., 158R Main Street, PO Box 880, Gardner, MA 01440

Products: MR parts and accessories, stethoscopes
USA/
International: Ann Cochran, Catalog Manager
Phone: 800-443-5486
508-632-7000

Ohmeda Inc., Ohmeda Drive, PO Box 7550, Madison, WI 53707-7550

Products: anesthesia machines, vaporizers, breathing circuit
USA: Deb Schmaling, Product Manager
Phone: 800-345-2700, ext. 3357
Fax: 608-223-2476
International: Canada: Gary Williamson, Ohmeda, 5865 McLaughlin Road, Suite 101, Mississauga, Ontario L5R 1BR
France: Pascal Robert, Ohmeda, Parc de Pissaloup, 8 Avenue Jean d'Alembert, F-78109 Trappes
Phone: (33) 1-30-686-000
Sweden/Norway: Hans Danielson, Ohmeda, PO Box 6331, Helsingborg, S-251 06
United Kingdom: Rob McCue, Ohmeda House, 71 Grant North Road, Hatfield, Herts., AL9 SEN
Phone: (44) 1707-263570
Malaysia (Distributor): Malaysian Oxygen Berhad, PO Box 10633, Kuala Lumpur, Kuala Lumpur 50720
Germany (Distributor): Anders Herdevall, HP GmbH, Schickardstrasse 4, D-71034 Böblingen
Switzerland (Distributor): Willem Jan Hofmans, HP Switzerland, In der Luberzen 29, CH-8902 Urdort
Phone: (41) 1-735-7228

Olympus America, 4 Nevada Drive, Lake Success, NY 11042-1179

Products: endoscopes/light sources/video systems
USA: Toshiyuki Takara, Senior Design Engineer, R&D, Medical Instruments Division
Phone: 516-488-0525
Fax: 516-326-9085

OMI Surgical Products, 3924 Virginia Avenue, Cincinnati, OH 45227

Products: Mayfield skull clamp
USA/
International: James McCafferty, Marketing; Chuck Dinkler, R&D
Phone: 800-755-6381
513-561-2705
Fax: 513-561-0195

Omnivent, Topeka, Kansas

Products: patient ventilators and ventilator monitors
USA/
International: Bill Gates, President
Phone: 800-933-7902
913-273-8924

Pacific Surgical Innovations, Inc. (aka S.E.C.), 871 Industrial Road, Unit A, San Carlos, CA 94070

Products: surgical instruments
USA: Terry Johnston
Phone: 800-810-6610
415-802-6988
Fax: 415-802-0120

PINA-Vertriebs AG, Langrietstrasse 17A, Neuhausen, CH-8212 Switzerland
Products: surgical instruments, development of MR-compatible custom devices
International: Axel Hoehn, Director of Sales and Marketing
Phone: (41) 52-672-40-42
Fax: (41) 52-672-40-48

Research, 4420 Metric Drive, Suite A, Winter Park, FL 32792
Products: vital sign monitoring equipment (ECG, respiratory, invasive and NIBP, CO^2, $SP0^2$ and temperature)
USA: (Direct sales representatives with some distributors)
Christopher Dedyo, Director of Marketing
Phone: 407-275-3220
Fax: 407-249-2022

Schneider Europe (Pfizer), PO Box, Ackerstrasse 6, CH-8180 Bülach, Switzerland
Products: diagnostic catheters
International: Eugen Hofmann, Manager, R&D
Phone: (41) 1-872-1111
Fax: (41) 1-862-0504

Smith and Nephew Spine, 1450 Brooks Road, Memphis, TN 38116
Products: Arthroscopic Microdiscectomy (AMD) instrumentation, ear, nose, throat (ENT) instrumentation, spinal instrumentation
USA/
International: Robert Brosnahan, Thomas McGahan
Phone: 901-396-2121
Fax: 901-348-6140

Snowden-Pencer, 5175 South Royal Atlanta Drive, Tucker, GA 30084
Products: titanium surgical instruments
USA/
International: Customer Service Department
Phone: 800-367-7874
Fax: 404-934-4922

Somatex, Postfach 42 06 20, D-12066 Berlin, Germany
Products: needles
International: Frank Kniep
Phone: (49) 30-625-30-46
Fax: (49) 30-625-30-47

Stortz Instrument Co., 3365 Tree Court Ind. Boulevard, St. Louis, MO 63122-6694
Products: endoscopes, ENT instrumentation
USA: John Meyer, ENT Product Manager
Phone: 800-325-9929, ext. 5433

Studer Medical Engineering AG, Rundbuckstrasse 2, CH-8212 Neuhausen am Rheinfall, Switzerland
Products: MR-compatible microscope and stand
International: Karl Weissbach, Vice Preisdent
Phone: (41) 52-674-08-78
Fax: (41) 52-674-08-79

Tri-anim Health Services, 13170 Telfair Avenue, Sylmar, CA 15697
Products: copper stylette
USA: John McLane
Phone: 800-874-2646
412-925-1091
Fax: 800-309-6436

United Metal Fabricators, 409 Eisenhauer Boulevard, Johnstown, PA 15904
Products: instrument tables, basin stands, operating-room (OR) furniture
USA: Peter Terry
Phone: 800-359-1335

US Surgical Auto Suture, 150 Glover Avenue, Norwalk, CT 06856
Products: 10-mm Surgiview Scope #176608
USA/
International: Phone: 617-533-1017

Valley Forge Scientific Corp., 136 Green Tree Road, Suite 100, Oaks, PA 19456
Products: VFS-200 bi-polar electrocoagulation unit
USA: Jerry Malis, PhD; Bonnie Ritchie
Phone: 610-666-7500
Fax: 610-666-7565

Valleylab, 5920 Longbow Drive, Boulder, CO 80301
USA: Claude Mott, Director, R&D
Phone: 303-581-6701
International:
Europe/Africa/Middle East:
Nieuwegein, The Netherlands
Phone: (31) 3402-50171
Fax: (31) 3402-39064
Canada: Toronto
Phone: 416-764-6800
Latin America: Boulder, Colorado
Phone: 303-530-6210
Fax: 303-530-6285
Australia/ASEAN/Far East: Sydney, Australia
Phone: (61) 2-688-4888
(61) 2-688-4575

Veenstra Instruments, Madame Curieweg 1, PO Box 115, 8500 AC Joure, The Netherlands
Products: MR-compatible OR furniture
International:
Phone: (31) 513-41-69-64
Fax: (31) 513-41-69-19

Wilson Great Batch, 10,000 Wehrle Drive, Clarence, NY 14031
Products: lithium batteries
USA/
International: Charles L. Mozeko, Market Manager (contact for name and address of a distributor in a specific country)
Phone: 716-759-5426
Fax: 716-759-2562

Subject Index

List of Contributors

Gerhard Adam, MD
Department of Diagnostic Radiology
University of Technology Aachen
Pauwelsstrasse 30
D-52057 Aachen
Germany

Chris J.G. Bakker, PhD
Department of Radiology
University Hospital Utrecht
Huispostnr E.01.1.32
Heidelberglaan 100
3584 CX Utrecht
The Netherlands

René Bernays, MD
Department of Neurosurgery
University Hospital Zurich
CH-8091 Zurich
Switzerland

Travis L. Boaz, MD
Department of Radiology
Case Western Reserve University
University Hospitals of Cleveland
11100 Euclid Avenue
Cleveland, OH 44106
USA

Chris Boesch, MD, PhD
MR Center 1
University and Inselspital
CH-3010 Bern
Switzerland

René Botnar, PhD
MRI Center
Department of Medical Radiology
Zurich University Hospital
Rämistrasse 100
CH-8091 Zurich
Switzerland

A. Bücker, MD
Department of Diagnostic Radiology
University of Technology Aachen
Pauwelsstraße 30
D-52057 Aachen
Germany

Jörg F. Debatin, MD
Institute of Diagnostic Radiology
Zurich University Hospital
Rämistrasse 100
CH-8091 Zurich
Switzerland

Matthias Drobnitzky, PhD
Siemens AG
Medical Engineering
MR Applications
P.O. Box 3260
D-91050 Erlangen
Germany

Charles L. Dumoulin
General Electric
Research and Development Center
P.O. Box 8
Schenectady, NY 12301
USA

Jaques Felblinger, PhD
MR Center 1
University and Inselspital
CH-3010 Bern
Switzerland

Christian Frahm, MD
Institute of Radiology
Lübeck Medical University
Ratzeburger Allee 160
D-23538 Lübeck
Germany

Hans-Björn Gehl, MD
Institute of Radiology
Lübeck Medical University
Ratzeburger Allee 160
D-23538 Lübeck
Germany

Arndt Glowinski, MS
Department of Diagnostic Radiology
University of Technology Aachen
Pauwelsstraße 30
D-52057 Aachen
Germany

Susanne Göhde, MD
Institute of Diagnostic Radiology
Zurich University Hospital
Rämistrasse 100
CH-8091 Zurich
Switzerland

R.W. Günther, MD
Department of Diagnostic Radiology
University of Technology Aachen
Pauwelsstraße 30
D-52057 Aachen
Germany

Margaret A. Hall-Craggs, MD
MR Unit
The Middlesex Hospital
University College London Hospitals
Mortimer Street
London W1N 8AA
United Kingdom

Andreas F. Heuck, MD
Institute of Diagnostic Radiology
Ludwig Maximilians-Universität München
Klinikum Großhadern
Marchioninistraße 15
D-81377 Munich
Germany

Kullervo Hynynen, PhD
Department of Radiology
Harvard Medical School and
Brigham and Women's Hospital
75 Francis Street
Boston, MA 02115
USA

Ferenc A. Jolesz, MD
MR Division
Image Guided Therapy Program
Department of Radiology
Harvard Medical School and
Brigham and Women's Hospital
75 Francis Street
Boston, MA 02115
USA

Georg M. Kacl, MD
Department of Medical Radiology
Zurich University Hospital
Rämistrasse 100
CH-8091 Zurich
Switzerland

Thomas Kahn, MD
Institute for Diagnostic Radiology
Heinrich-Heine-University
Moorenstrasse 5
D-40225 Düsseldorf
Germany

Joachim Kettenbach, MD
Department of Radiology
Image Guided Therapy Program and
Surgical Planning Laboratory
Harvard Medical School and
Brigham and Women's Hospital
75 Francis Street
Boston, MA 02115
USA

Ron Kikinis, MD
Surgical Planning Laboratory
Department of Radiology
Harvard Medical School and
Brigham and Women's Hospital
75 Francis Street
Boston, MA 02115
USA

Spiros Kollias, MD
Institute of Neuroradiology
Zurich University Hospital
Rämistrasse 100
CH-8091 Zurich
Switzerland

Christiane Katharina Kuhl, MD
Department of Radiology,
University of Bonn,
Sigmund-Freud-Strasse 25
D-53105 Bonn
Germany

Mark E. Ladd, MSEE
MRI Center
Department of Medical Radiology
University Hospital Zurich
Rämistrasse 100
CH-8091 Zurich
Switzerland

Gerald Lenz, PhD
Siemens AG
Medical Engineering
MR Applications
P.O. Box 3260
D-91050 Erlangen
Germany

Jonathan S. Lewin, MD
Department of Radiology
Case Western Reserve University
University Hospitals of Cleveland
11100 Euclid Avenue
Cleveland, OH 44106
USA

Martin G. Mack
Department of Radiology
Virchow Hospital
Humboldt University
Augustenburger Platz 1
D-13353 Berlin
Germany

Gerd Ullrich Müller-Lisse, MD
Institute of Diagnostic Radiology
Ludwig Maximilians-Universität München
Klinikum Großhadern
Marchioninistraße 15
D-81377 Munich
Germany

Jörg-Michael Neuerburg, MD
Department of Diagnostic Radiology
University of Technology Aachen
Pauwelsstraße 30
D-52057 Aachen
Germany

Robert Newman, MS
General Electric Company
P.O.B. 414
Milwaukee, WI 53201-0414
USA

Erik A. Penner, PhD
GE Medical Systems Germany
Praunheimer Landstrasse 50
D-60488 Frankfurt am Main
Germany

Harald H. Quick, MS
Institute of Diagnostic Radiology
Zurich University Hospital
Rämistrasse 100
CH-8091 Zurich
Switzerland

Benjamin J. Romanowski, RT
MRI Center
Institute of Diagnostic Radiology
Zurich University Hospital
Rämistrasse 100
CH-8091 Zurich
Switzerland

John F. Schenck, MD, PhD
General Electric Company
Corporate Research and Development Center
Research Circle
Schenectady, NY 12309
USA

Hans-Joachim Schwarzmaier, MD
Institute of Laser Medicine
Heinrich-Heine-University
Moorenstrasse 5
D-40225 Düsseldorf
Germany

Henk F.M. Smits, MD
Department of Radiology
University Hospital Utrecht
Huispostnr E.01.1.32
Heidelberglaan 100
3584 CX Utrecht
The Netherlands

Ralf Speetzen, BEng
Helmholtz Institute for Biomedical Engineering
University of Technology Aachen
Pauwelsstraße 20
D-52057 Aachen
Germany

Uwe Spetzger, MD
Department of Neurosurgery
University of Technology Aachen
Pauwelsstraße 30
D-52057 Aachen
Germany

Paul Steiner, MD
MR Center
Department of Medical Radiology
Zurich University Hospital
Rämistrasse 100
CH-8091 Zurich
Switzerland

Josef Tacke, MD
Department of Diagnostic Radiology
University of Technology Aachen
Pauwelsstraße 30
D-52057 Aachen
Germany

Frank Ulrich, MD
Department of Neurosurgery
Krefeld Municipal Hospital
Lutherplatz 40,
D-47805 Krefeld,
Germany

Joop J. van Vaals, PhD
Philips Medical Systems
Clinical Science MR
P.O. Box 10.000
5680 DA Best
The Netherlands

Thomas J. Vogl, MD
Department of Radiology
Virchow Hospital
Humboldt University
Augustenburger Platz 1
D-13353 Berlin
Germany

Gustav K. von Schulthess, MD, PhD
Division of Nuclear Medicine
Zurich University Hospital
Rämistraße 100
CH-8091 Zurich
Switzerland

Dierk Vorwerk, MD
Department of Diagnostic Radiology
University of Technology Aachen
Pauwelsstraße 30
D-52057 Aachen
Germany

Simon Wildermuth, MD
Institute of Diagnostic Radiology
Zurich University Hospital
Rämistrasse 100
CH-8091 Zurich
Switzerland

Gesine G. Zimmermann, MD
Institute of Diagnostic Radiology
Zurich University Hospital
Rämistrasse 100
CH-8091 Zurich
Switzerland

MEDICAL RADIOLOGY
Diagnostic Imaging and Radiation Oncology

Titles in the series already published

DIAGNOSTIC IMAGING

Innovations in Diagnostic Imaging
Edited by J.H. Anderson

Radiology of the Upper Urinary Tract
Edited by E.K. Lang

The Thymus - Diagnostic Imaging, Functions, and Pathologic Anatomy
Edited by E. Walter, E. Willich, and W.R. Webb

Interventional Neuroradiology
Edited by A. Valavanis

Radiology of the Pancreas
Edited by A.L. Baert, co-edited by G. Delorme

Radiology of the Lower Urinary Tract
Edited by E.K. Lang

Magnetic Resonance Angiography
Edited by I.P. Arlart, G.M. Bongartz, and G. Marchal

Contrast-Enhanced MRI of the Breast
S. Heywang-Köbrunner and R. Beck

Spiral CT of the Chest
Edited by M. Rémy-Jardin and J. Rémy

Radiological Diagnosis of Breast Diseases
Edited by M. Friedrich and E.A. Sickles

Radiology of the Trauma
Edited by M. Heller and A. Fink

Biliary Tract Radiology
Edited by P. Rossi

Radiological Imaging of Sports Injuries
Edited by C. Masciocchi

Modern Imaging of the Alimentary Tube
Edited by A. R. Margulis

Diagnosis and Therapy of Spinal Tumors
Edited by P. R. Algra, J. Valk, and J. J. Heimans

Interventional Magnetic Resonance Imaging
Edited by J. F. Debatin and G. Adam

RADIATION ONCOLOGY

Lung Cancer
Edited by C.W. Scarantino

Innovations in Radiation Oncology
Edited by H.R. Withers and L.J. Peters

Radiation Therapy of Head and Neck Cancer
Edited by G.E. Laramore

Gastrointestinal Cancer – Radiation Therapy
Edited by R.R. Dobelbower, Jr.

Radiation Exposure and Occupational Risks
Edited by E. Scherer, C. Streffer, and K.-R. Trott

Radiation Therapy of Benign Diseases - A Clinical Guide
S.E. Order and S.S. Donaldson

Medical Radiology
Diagnostic Imaging and Radiation Oncology

Titles in the series already published

Radiation Oncology

Interventional Radiation Therapy Techniques - Brachytherapy
Edited by R. Sauer

Radiopathology of Organs and Tissues
Edited by E. Scherer, C. Streffer, and K.-R. Trott

Concomitant Continuous Infusion Chemotherapy and Radiation
Edited by M. Rotman and C.J. Rosenthal

Intraoperative Radiotherapy – Clinical Experiences and Results
Edited by F.A. Calvo, M. Santos, and L.W. Brady

Radiotherapy of Intraocular and Orbital Tumors
Edited by W.E. Alberti and R.H. Sagerman

Interstitial and Intracavitary Thermoradiotherapy
Edited by M.H. Seegenschmiedt and R. Sauer

Non-Disseminated Breast Cancer
Controversial Issues in Management
Edited by G.H. Fletcher and S.H. Levitt

Current Topics in Clinical Radiobiology of Tumors
Edited by H.-P. Beck-Bornholdt

Practical Approaches to Cancer Invasion and Metastases
A Compendium of Radiation Oncologists' Responses to 40 Histories
Edited by A.R. Kagan with the Assistance of R.J. Steckel

Radiation Therapy in Pediatric Oncology
Edited by J.R. Cassady

Radiation Therapy Physics
Edited by A.R. Smith

Late Sequelae in Oncology
Edited by J. Dunst and R. Sauer

Mediastinal Tumors. Update 1995
Edited by D.E. Wood and C.R. Thomas, Jr.

Thermoradiotherapy and Thermochemotherapy
Volume 1: Biology, Physiology, and Physics
Volume 2: Clinical Applications
Edited by M.H. Seegenschmiedt, P. Fessenden, and C.C. Vernon

Carcinoma of the Prostate
Innovations in Management
Edited by Z. Petrovich, L. Baert, and L.W. Brady

Radiation Oncology of Gynecological Cancers
Edited by H.W. Vahrson

Carcinoma of the Bladder
Innovations in Management
Edited by Z. Petrovich, L. Baert, and L.W. Brady

Blood Perfusion and Microenvironment of Human Tumors
Implications for Clinical Radiooncology
Edited by M. Molls and P. Vaupel

Radiation Therapy of Benign Diseases. A Clinical Guide
2nd revised edition
S.E. Order and S.S. Donaldson

SPRINGER NATURE

GPSR Compliance

The European Union's (EU) General Product Safety Regulation (GPSR) is a set of rules that requires consumer products to be safe and our obligations to ensure this.

If you have any concerns about our products, you can contact us on ProductSafety@springernature.com

In case Publisher is established outside the EU, the EU authorized representative is:

Springer Nature Customer Service Center GmbH
Europaplatz 3
69115 Heidelberg, Germany

Kolibri 360 GmbH
Ferdinand-Jühlke-Straße 7
99095 Erfurt, Deutschland
produktsicherheit@kolibri360.de